Saffron

The Age-Old Panacea in a
New Light

Saffron

The Age-Old Panacea in a New Light

Edited by

MARYAM SARWAT
Amity Institute of Pharmacy
Amity University
Noida, Uttar Pradesh, India

SAJIDA SUMAIYA
Amity Institute of Pharmacy
Amity University
Noida, Uttar Pradesh, India

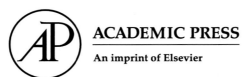

Saffron   ISBN: 978-0-12-818462-2

Notices

Practitioners and researchers must always rely on their own experience and knowledge in evaluating and using any information, methods, compounds or experiments described herein. Because of rapid advances in the medical sciences, in particular, independent verification of diagnoses and drug dosages should be made. To the fullest extent of the law, no responsibility is assumed by Elsevier, authors, editors or contributors for any injury and/or damage to persons or property as a matter of products liability, negligence or otherwise, or from any use or operation of any methods, products, instructions, or ideas contained in the material herein.

Publisher: Andre Gerhard Wolff
Acquisition Editor: Erin Hill-Parks
Editorial Project Manager: Anna Dubnow
Production Project Manager: Kiruthika Govindaraju
Cover Designer: Alan Studholme

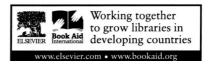

List of Contributors

Mir Ajaz Akram
Government
NMV Hoshangabad (Barkatullah University)
Bhopal, Madhya Pradesh, India

Rajendra Awasthi
Amity Institute of Pharmacy
Amity University, Uttar Pradesh
Noida, Uttar Pradesh, India

Hamid A. Bakshi
Department of Pharmacy
School of Applied Sciences
University of Huddersfield
Queensgate, Huddersfield, HD13DH, United Kingdom
SAAD Centre for Pharmacy and Diabetes
School of Pharmacy and Pharmaceutical Science
Ulster University
Coleraine, County Londonderry, BT52 1SA,
    Northern Ireland, United Kingdom
School of Biomedical Sciences
University of Ulster
Coleraine, BT52 1SA, Northern Ireland,
    United Kingdom

K. Hüsnü Can Başer
Near East University
Faculty of Pharmacy
Nicosia, North Cyprus, Turkey

Sabeeha Bashir
Department of Botany
University of Kashmir
Srinagar, Jammu and Kashmir, India

Silvia Bisti
Department of Biotechnology and Applied
    Clinical Sciences (DISCAB)
Università degli Studi dell'Aquila
L'Aquila, AQ, Italy
IIT Istituto Italiano di Tecnologia
Genova, GE, Italy
Istituto Nazionale Biosistemi e Biostrutture
Roma, Italy

Mohammad Hossein Boskabady
Department of Physiology
School of Medicine
Mashhad University of Medical Sciences
Mashhad, Iran
Neurogenic Inflammation Research Center
Mashhad University of Medical Sciences
Mashhad, Iran

Nathalie Chahine
Faculty of Public Health
La Sagesse University
Beirut, Lebanon
Faculty of Sciences and Faculty of Agronomy
Lebanese University
Beirut, Lebanon

Ramez Chahine
Faculty of Public Health
La Sagesse University
Beirut, Lebanon

Neerupma Dhiman
Amity Institute of Pharmacy
Amity University
Noida, Uttar Pradesh, India

Benedetto Falsini
Facolta' di Medicina e Chirurgia
Fondazione Policlinico A. Gemelli
Universita' Cattolica del S. Cuore
Roma, Italy

Tahereh Farkhondeh
Cardiovascular Diseases Research Center
Birjand University of Medical Sciences
Birjand, Iran

Hakkim L. Faruck
Department of Mathematics and Sciences
College of Arts and Applied Sciences
Research Center
Dhofar University
Salalah, Oman

Research center
Dhofar University
Salalah, Oman

Homa Fatma
Molecular Cancer Genetics & Translational
    Research Laboratory
Section of Genetics
Department of Zoology
Aligarh Muslim University
Aligarh, Uttar Pradesh, India

Zahra Gholamnezhad
Department of Physiology
Faculty of Medicine
Mashhad University of Medical Sciences
Mashhad, Iran

Neurogenic Inflammation Research Center
Mashhad University of Medical Sciences
Mashhad, Iran

Vahideh Ghorani
Department of Physiology
School of Medicine
Mashhad University of Medical Sciences
Mashhad, Iran

Pharmaceutical Research Center
Mashhad University of Medical Sciences
Mashhad, Iran

Gamze Guclu
Department of Food Engineering
Faculty of Agriculture
Cukurova University
Adana, Turkey

Mortaza Hajyzadeh
Central Laboratory of Technology and Research
    (SUTAM)
Sirnak, Turkey

Ruqaya Jabeen
University College
Addarb
Jazan University
Jazan, Kingdom of Saudi Arabia

Riffat John
Department of Botany
University of Kashmir
Srinagar, Jammu and Kashmir, India

Parisa Pourali Kahriz
Ardahan University
Ardahan Technical Sciences Vocational School
Ardahan, Turkey

Prachi Kaushik
Amity Institute of Pharmacy
Amity University Uttar Pradesh
Noida, Uttar Pradesh, India

Hasim Kelebek
Department of Food Engineering
Adana Science and Technology University
Adana, Turkey

Mohammad Afsar Khan
Molecular Cancer Genetics & Translational Research
    Laboratory
Section of Genetics
Department of Zoology,
Aligarh Muslim University
Aligarh, Uttar Pradesh, India

Harsha Kharkwal
Amity Institute of Phytomedicine and
    Phytochemistry
Amity University
Noida, Uttar Pradesh, India

Khalid Mahmood Khawar
Department of Field Crop
Faculty of Agriculture
Ankara University
Ankara, Turkey

Mohammad Reza Khazdair
Torbat Jam Faculty of Medical Sciences
Torbat Jam, Iran

Müberra Koşar
Eastern Mediterranean University
Faculty of Pharmacy
Famagusta, North Cyprus, via Mersin-10, Turkey

G.T. Kulkarni
Amity Institute of Pharmacy
Amity University Uttar Pradesh
Noida, Uttar Pradesh, India

Hariom Kumar
Amity Institute of Pharmacy
Amity University Uttar Pradesh
Noida, Uttar Pradesh, India

Maria Anna Maggi
Hortus Novus srl
Canistro, AQ, Italy

Department of Physical and Chemical Sciences (DSFC)
Università degli Studi dell'Aquila
L'Aquila, AQ, Italy

Stefano Di Marco
Department of Biotechnology and Applied Clinical
    Sciences (DISCAB)
Università degli Studi dell'Aquila
L'Aquila, AQ, Italy

Istituto Nazionale Biosistemi e Biostrutture
Roma, Italy

Arghavan Memarzia
Department of Physiology
Faculty of Medicine
Mashhad University of Medical Sciences
Mashhad, Iran

Roohi Mirza
Amity Institute of Pharmacy
Amity University Uttar Pradesh
Noida, Uttar Pradesh, India

Amin Mokhtari-Zaer
Department of Physiology
Faculty of Medicine
Mashhad University of Medical Sciences
Mashhad, Iran

Dhondup Namgyal
Amity Institute of Neuropsychology & Neuroscience
Amity University
Noida, Uttar Pradesh, India

Tanveer Naved
Amity Institute of Pharmacy
Amity University
Noida, Uttar Pradesh, India

Fatih Olmez
Department of Plant Protection
Faculty of Agriculture
Sirnak University
Sirnak, Turkey

Mattia Di Paolo
Department of Biotechnology and Applied Clinical
    Sciences (DISCAB)
Università degli Studi dell'Aquila
L'Aquila, AQ, Italy

Marco Piccardi
Facoltà di Medicina e Chirurgia
Fondazione Policlinico A. Gemelli
Universita' Cattolica del S. Cuore
Roma, Italy

Nikolaos Pitsikas
Department of Pharmacology
School of Medicine, Faculty of Health Sciences
University of Thessaly
Larissa, Greece

Shaista Qadir
Department of Botany
Government Degree College for Women
Cluster University
Srinagar, Jammu and Kashmir, India

Saeideh Saadat
Department of Physiology
School of Medicine,
Mashhad University of Medical Sciences
Mashhad, Iran

Saeed Samarghandian
Department of Basic Medical Sciences
Neyshabur University of Medical Sciences
Neyshabur, Iran

Ercument Osman Sarihan
Department of Field Crops
Agriculture and Natural Science Faculty
Usak University
Usak, Turkey

Maryam Sarwat
Amity Institute of Pharmacy
Amity University
Noida, Uttar Pradesh, India

Serkan Selli
Department of Food Engineering
Faculty of Agriculture
Cukurova University
Adana, Turkey

Archana Sharma
Amity Institute of Pharmacy
Amity University
Noida, Uttar Pradesh, India

Bhupesh Sharma
Amity Institute of Pharmacy
Amity University Uttar Pradesh
Noida, Uttar Pradesh, India

Muzafar Ahmad Sheikh
Department of Zoology
Government Degree College, Ganderbal
Ganderbal, Jammu and Kashmir, India

Hifzur R. Siddique
Molecular Cancer Genetics & Translational Research
  Laboratory
Section of Genetics
Department of Zoology
Aligarh Muslim University
Aligarh, Uttar Pradesh, India

Sajida Sumaiya
Amity Institute of Pharmacy
Amity University
Noida, Uttar Pradesh, India

Murtaza M. Tambuwala
SAAD Centre for Pharmacy and Diabetes
School of Pharmacy and Pharmaceutical Science
Ulster University
Coleraine, County Londonderry, BT52 1SA,
  Northern Ireland, United Kingdom
School of Biomedical Sciences
University of Ulster
Coleraine, BT52 1SA, Northern Ireland,
  United Kingdom

Sangilimuthu Alagar Yadav
Department of Biotechnology
Karpagam Academy of Higher Education
Coimbatore, Tamil Nadu, India

Mehmet Ugur Yildirim
Department of Field Crops
Agriculture and Natural Science Faculty
Usak University
Usak, Turkey

Foreword

In the context of human health, a large number of natural products have been collected, collated, characterized, and made available to mankind. Some of these products target the diseases, whereas others simply work for the rejuvenation of the body by their immunomodulatory actions. Yet another ones work beyond the human body and perhaps reach to the soul. Of all the plant-derived herbs, saffron has always attracted a great deal of attention of common man and elites alike. The actual saffron is the dried stigma of *Crocus sativus* L., family Iridaceae. A sizable part of the literature is devoted to describe its health potentials and beneficial effects on the human body. Although mind and body are connected, they still maintained functional compartmentalization. Saffron has very positive effects on a large number of vital systems of the human body encompassing central nervous, cardiovascular, digestive, locomotor, urogenital, ophthalmic, integumentary, and immune systems. Saffron's safranal is an aromatic aldehyde, a vital component of plant volatile oil. In addition, saffron has more than 150 different types of components. The present book on saffron truly reflects deep and wide understanding of the authors accumulating crucial fact about this much sought-after and wonderful gift of nature. I found the book unputdownable and sincerely hope that it would evoke a great deal of interest among people who respect nature and believe in naturopathy. I envisage that this book would prove to be an eye-opener to students, teachers, and researcher. I found that this book reflects deep scientific understanding and academic prowess of the editors, Maryam Sarwat and Sajida Sumaiya, who have complemented each other to bring about their very best on saffron.

Professor Dr. Sher Ali, PhD, FNA, FASc, FNASc, FSASc,
J C Bose National Fellow, DST, New Delhi
Av-Humboldt Fellow, Germany
Professor, Center for Interdisciplinary
Research in Basic Sciences
Ramanujan Block, Room 108
Jamia Millia Islamia,
Jamia Nagar, New Delhi — 110025
Alumni: USA, UK, Germany, and Australia
Email: alis@jmi.ac.in
Former Senior Staff Scientist and Head
Molecular Genetics Division
National Institute of Immunology
New Delhi — 110067

Preface

With advancements in the field of science over the years, the section of medicine and pharmacology has greatly benefited the society. Remarkable contributions have been made both in understanding drugs at the molecular level as well as in developing more selective drugs. The search for newer therapeutic agents has created a new ray of hope for physicians, pharmacists, researchers, medicine experts, and most importantly the patients consuming such drugs. Herbs and spices cover a major aspect of these alternative therapeutic agents. Sustained research is being carried out worldwide to study their efficiency and mechanism of action among many other aspects. This research is constantly promoted as it has negligible side effects (if any) on patients even after long-term use.

Books that are available in the market describing the benefits and pharmacological activities of herbs and spices especially saffron (a stigma of *Crocus sativus* L.) have limited sections, perhaps insufficient information devoted to its medicinal aspect. To overcome this inadequacy, we planned to write this comprehensive book. This book will expand and also bring together scattered information on saffron. It will cater to the needs of pharmacologists, molecular biologists, medicine experts, researchers, and students.

In our book, we have extensively highlighted various phytochemical studies as well as medicinal and pharmacological aspects of saffron. This book is divided into four sections, with the fourth section covering major chunk of this book. Section one provides the introduction, while sections two and three describe cultivation, biosynthesis, and phytochemistry, respectively. The fourth section is further divided into six parts. It covers various medicinal benefits of saffron in treating diseases of nervous system, cardiovascular system, ocular diseases, and cancers and saffron's immunomodulatory effect.

Each chapter has been meticulously elaborated with its unique style of presentation. The chapters have been arranged in such a way that foundation laid in the initial chapters will be helpful for understanding the subsequent chapters. Furthermore, detailed studies have been explained with the help of figures, images, and tables to make it even more interesting and descriptive. Even after our best efforts, we do feel that there may still be scope for improvement and addition in this work especially given the rapidly evolving and ever-advancing nature of this field. Helpful criticism and suggestions from the readers are dearly welcome.

We are thankful to Elsevier for their keen interest and attention in bringing out this book in its present form.

Maryam Sarwat
Sajida Sumaiya

Acknowledgment

We wish to express our deepest appreciation to our institute and all faculty members from Amity Institute of Pharmacy, Amity University, Noida, India, for their expert insights, discussions, and communications throughout the process of book writing and editing that greatly assisted and enhanced the final outlook of our book.

The authors are sincerely indebted to **Prof. Ashok Chauhan**, Founder President of Amity University, **Prof. W. Selwamurthy**, President of Amity Science, Technology and Innovation Foundation, and **Prof. B. C. Das**, Dean of Amity Health and Allied Sciences, Amity University, Noida, for the all-time help and encouragement during the process of writing of this book.

We owe special thanks to the Joint Heads of Amity Institute of Pharmacy; Dr. Tanveer Naved and Prof. G.T. Kulkarni and the research scholars Dhondup Namgyal, Ms. Meenakshi Gupta, and Ms. Kumari Chandan for assistance with comments and innovative ideas that greatly improved the manuscript.

We are immensely thankful to our funding agency "Central Council for Research in Unani Medicine (CCRUM)," Ministry of AYUSH, Government of India for their continuous support, encouragement, and faith in us.

This book would not have any essence of thoughts, concerns, and feel without having Ms. Faria Zafar (Daughter of MS) on board. She is our inspiration, encouragement, and vision in deciding the topic of the book and selecting which contents must be included, simply because she is among the various kids which belong to our future generation. Both the authors want to express their gratitude to their friends and families, especially Dr. Fakhre Alam (Father of SS), for providing moral support, valuable comments, and suggestions while writing the book. Our thankfulness and appreciation are beyond measure.

Finally, we would like to acknowledge with gratitude all the authors, reviewers, publishers, and their team members for sharing their pearls of wisdom with us during the course of writing and compilation of this book.

Contents

CHAPTER 1

Amelioration of Liver Ailments by Saffron (*Crocus sativus*) and Its Secondary Metabolites

SAJIDA SUMAIYA • TANVEER NAVED • ARCHANA SHARMA • MARYAM SARWAT

INTRODUCTION

The use of spices has been recorded from past many decades across the world as condiments as they exhibit flavor, aroma, and pigment (Zheng et al., 2016). Apart from being used as condiments, they have been used for medicinal purposes in traditional prescriptions including Chinese, Ayurveda, and Unani medicine (Rahmani et al., 2017). One such reputed condiment is saffron (Chermahini et al., 2010). Saffron is the dried stigma of *Crocus sativus* L., of the family Iridaceae. It is a perpetual bulb cultivated mainly in Iran, India, and the Mediterranean countries (Bathaie et al., 2010; Christodouloua et al., 2015). It is estimated that around 75,000 crocus blossom or around 2,00,000 dried stigmas produce just around 1 kg of saffron and cost somewhere around $500, making it the costliest spice in the world (Melnyk et al., 2010). It is hand plucked and handpicked to preserve its volatile compounds and stored in air-tight containers for best results (Jan et al., 2014).

Saffron's major active constituents include crocin ($C_{44}H_{64}O_{24}$), crocetin ($C_{20}H_{24}O_4$), picrocrocin ($C_{16}H_{26}O_7$), and safranal ($C_{10}H_{14}O$) (Rezaee Khorasany and Hosseinzadeh., 2016) (Fig. 1.1).

Crocin is a water-soluble carotenoid, which is accountable for most of saffron's color and also represents the major component of saffron's extract. Crocetin is the dicarboxylic carotenoid, and when it gets glycosylated, it is converted into crocin. Saffron's bitter taste is attributed to picrocrocin, which is a monoterpene glycoside precursor of safranal and also a degradation product of zeaxanthin carotenoid. Safranal is an aromatic aldehyde that is the main component of plant volatile oil

(Tavakkol-Afshari et al., 2008; D'Alessandro et al., 2013; Festuccia et al., 2014).

Since the past 3600 years, saffron is being used as a medicine (Ferrence et al., 2004; Al-Sanafi, 2016), as an emmenagogue, an antispasmodic, and a carminative agent; as a thymoleptic and cognition enhancer; and an aphrodisiac in the Middle East. In Chinese medicine, its use was considered in deliveries of high risk and also in postpartum lochiostasis, in menorrhagia, and also in amenorrhea. In India, it was used for headache and vomiting, sore throat, bronchitis, and also for fever (Al-snafi, 2016).

Various studies have reported the beneficial effects of saffron on liver diseases. Damage to the liver may be a result of autoimmune diseases; alpha toxins; contaminated food; and parasitic, viral, or fungal infection. This damage is directly related to increased levels of biochemical markers such as serum glutamate pyruvate transaminase and serum glutamate oxaloacetate transaminase, malondialdehyde (MDA) and triglycerides, nonprotein sulfhydryls (NP-SH), bilirubin and alkaline phosphatase, and sometimes hepatocytes necrosis (Sharma et al., 2015).

Although science and technology are advancing at a fast pace, treatment of diseases related to the liver still demands search for newer therapeutics. The present chapter highlights various beneficial and medicinal aspects of saffron in liver diseases.

Cellular Structure of the Liver

The liver is a major organ of the human body and is composed of a variety of cells comprising hepatocytes,

Saffron. https://doi.org/10.1016/B978-0-12-818462-2.00001-2

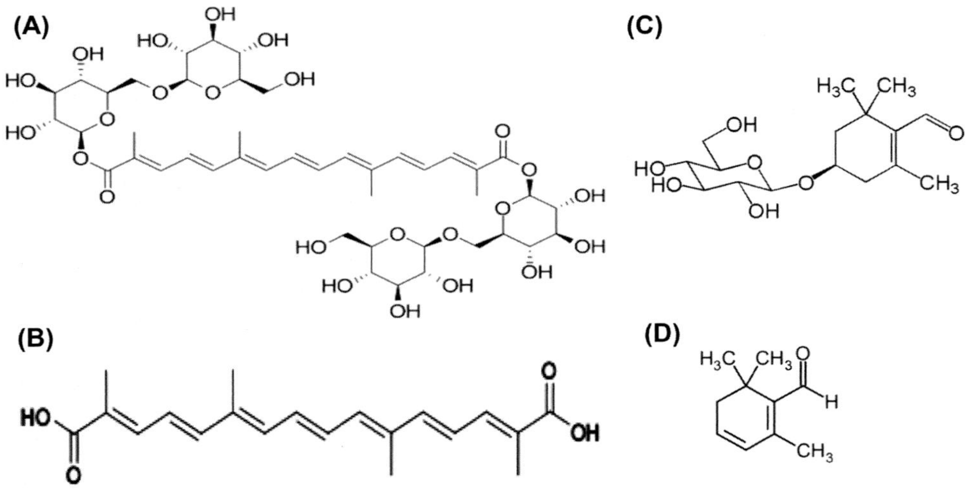

FIG. 1.1 Structure of saffron's metabolites. **(A)** Crocin, **(B)** Crocetin, **(C)** Picrocrocin, **(D)** Safranal.

cholangiocytes (biliary epithelial cells), ito cells (stellate cells), liver sinusoidal endothelial cells, and Kupffer cells. Every cell has its own special function and collectively work at various levels to govern the functions of the liver (Trefts et al., 2017; Malarkey et al., 2005).

1. Hepatocytes:
   - primary epithelial cells
   - comprise major population of liver cells
2. Cholangiocytes:
   - second most abundant epithelial cells of the liver
   - line the lumen of bile ducts
3. Stellate cells:
   - dynamic cell population
   - exist in two forms: quiescent or activated
   - quiescent state stores vitamin A in the form of lipid droplets
   - damage to liver cells activate these cells and cell loses stores of vitamin A
   - responsible for deposition of collagen in injured liver
   - major contributors in scarring the liver
4. Kupffer cells:
   - native macrophages of the liver
   - recognize foreign particles in portal circulation
5. Liver sinusoidal epithelial cells:
   - specialized endothelial population
   - form fenestrated sieve plates at the lumen of sinusoid
   - form a space of disse for exchange of blood and proteins

(Braet and Wisse, 2002; Vekemans and Braet, 2005; Malarkey et al., 2005; Si-Tayeb et al., 2010; Trefts et al., 2017; Ma et al., 2017)

The functional structural unit of the liver around which these liver cells are arranged is called lobule (Mac Sween et al., 2002) (Fig. 1.2). It consists of hexagon-shaped chords of hepatocytes. The vertices of this hexagon are surrounded by branches of hepatic artery, portal vein, and bile duct (portal triad) (Kalra and Tuma, 2018).

The units of circulation inside the hepatocyte chord do not form tight junctions that produce networks of sinusoids in between and lower the barrier between blood flowing through the sinusoid and the hepatocytes. The composition of blood changes in these sinusoids, as hepatic artery blood that is rich in oxygen mixes with portal circulation blood rich in nutrient before going toward the lobule cells and drains into the central vein. The cells of lobule use this blood and produce metabolites and wastes that make the blood deoxygenated. At different lobular locations, gradients of nutrients, oxygen, and wastes are created across sinusoids of lobule, which result in partitioning of functions. This partitioning is termed as "metabolic zonation," and it divides the lobules into three separate zones. Each of these zones constitutes hepatocytes with a distinct function and metabolic gene expression. The metabolic zones are discrete regions, but hepatic zonation works flexibly. In case of any damage or loss of function to any specific zone, another zone takes over and helps the liver to maintain its functions properly (Saxena et al., 1999; Trefts et al., 2017).

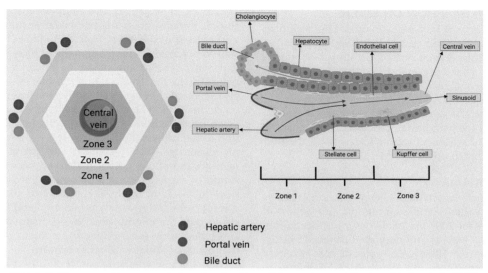

FIG. 1.2 Diagrammatic representation showing the cellular anatomy of the liver (Trefts et al., 2017).

Physiology of the Liver

The liver constitutes various physiological processes. Some of them are metabolism of macronutrients, regulation of blood volume, support to immune system, endocrine control of growth-signaling pathways, homeostasis of cholesterol and lipid, and disintegration of xenobiotic compounds, comprising of a lot of present drugs. It stores glucose as glycogen with feeding and accumulates glucose via gluconeogenesis in the fasting state. It oxidizes lipids and can also pack excess lipid for other tissues such as adipose. Also, the liver handles the metabolism of protein and amino acids (Tortora and Derrickson, 2012; Guyton and Hall, 2006).

- Carbohydrate metabolism: The liver plays an important role in maintenance of normal level of blood glucose. As this level goes down, glycogen is broken down into glucose and released into the blood stream. It can also convert amino acids and lactic acid to glucose via gluconeogenesis and other forms of sugars such as fructose and galactose into glucose.
- Lipid metabolism: Triglycerides are stored in hepatocytes; fatty acids are broken down to produce adenosine triphosphate (ATP), and lipoproteins are synthesized here, which are helpful to transport cholesterol, fatty acids, and triglycerides to and from body cells.
- Protein metabolism.: Deamination of amino acids (removal of NH_2 from the amino group) is carried out by hepatocytes, so that it can be used for the production of ATP or converted to fats or carbohydrates. The byproduct in the form of toxic ammonia (NH_3) is further transformed into quite less toxic urea and excreted in urine. Synthesis of plasma protein is also carried out by hepatocytes such as albumin, globulin, prothrombin, fibrinogen, and alpha and beta globulins.
- Processing of drugs and hormones: The liver carries out detoxification of alcohol and excretion of drugs such as erythromycin, penicillin, and sulfonamides into the bile along with chemical alteration and excretion of thyroid and steroid hormones.
- Excretion of bilirubin and synthesis of bile salts: Bilirubin derived from the heme part of hemoglobin is taken from the blood and secreted into bile. Liver synthesizes bile salt that is used for emulsification and absorption of lipids in the intestine.
- Storage: The liver stores vitamin A, D, E, K, and B12 and minerals such as iron and copper that are released as per requirement of the body.
- Phagocytosis: Kupffer cells of the liver phagocytize some bacteria, white blood cell, and aged red blood cell.
- Activation of vitamin D: Synthesis of the active form of vitamin D is carried out by the involvement of skin, the kidneys, and the liver (Tortora and Derrickson, 2012).

EFFECT OF SAFFRON ON LIVER

A number of researches have been carried out regarding the activities of saffron on the liver (Fig. 1.3). Studies have proved that saffron possesses antioxidant, antiinflammatory, chemopreventive, antitumor and anticancer, antigenotoxic, and antidiabetic activities. It is also reported that saffron prevents from hepatic ischemia-reperfusion, reduces liver enlargement, and reduces morphine-withdrawal syndrome. The possible mechanism of actions of saffron's activity on the liver has been summed up in Table 1.1.

Antioxidant Activity

Oxygen participates in high-energy electron transfers because of reactivity and supports the production of high amount of ATP via oxidative phosphorylation. As a result, our body is continuously threatened by reactive oxygen species (ROS). A complex defense system of antioxidants balances this attack, but on many instances, this balance gets disturbed which leads to oxidative stress. Thus, oxidative stress in broad terms can be defined as variation in balance of prooxidants and antioxidants. This oxidative stress is now known to be a critical part in pathophysiology of numerous disorders (Burton and Jauniaux, 2011; Halliwell and Gutteridge, 2015), such as neurodegenerative disease, inflammation of the liver (Djordjevic et al., 2010), cirrhosis of the liver, conditions of the liver due to acute and chronic consumption of alcohol, increased cholesterol in blood, chronic disease of the kidney, etc (Dalle-Donne et al., 2006; Bandegi et al., 2014).

Bandegi et al. (2014), in a study on rats, stated that chronic restraint stress induced oxidative stress damage in the tissue of the brain, liver, and kidney when they were kept restrained for 6 h/day for 21 days. Treatment with saffron extract and crocin indicated a noteworthy reduction in the level of ROS. Ochiai et al. (2004) also reported that neuronally differentiated pheochromocytoma (PC-12) cells deprived of serum/glucose when treated with 10 mM crocin inhibited the formation of peroxidized lipids, partly restored the Superoxide dismutase (SOD) activity, and maintained the neuron's morphology. Crocin also suppressed the activation of caspase-8 caused by serum/glucose deprivation. In the same study, they examined the effect of α-tocopherol at the same concentration and found crocin to be more effective then α-tocopherol and hence concluded crocin to be unique and a potent antioxidant that combats oxidative stress in neurons.

Aqueous and ethanolic extract of saffron attenuated the oxidative stress, inflammation, and apoptosis in rats after subjecting them to chronic constriction injury (CCI). The possible mechanism behind this was augmented level of GSH and MDA and reduction in proinflammatory cytokines such as TNF-α, IL-6, and IL-1β (Amin et al., 2014).

In 2017, Hassani et al. aimed their study to investigate the hepatoprotective effect of crocin against Bisphenol- A (BPA)-induced liver toxicity; increased levels of AST, glucose, and lactate dehydrogenase; triglyceride. Reduction in GSH level and periportal inflammation was also seen in animals subjected to BPA. Treatment

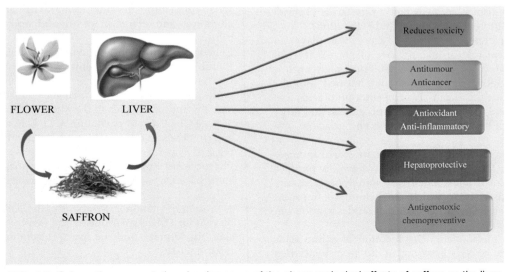

FIG. 1.3 Schematic representation showing some of the pharmacological effects of saffron on the liver.

TABLE 1.1

Pharmacological Activities of Saffron and its Active Metabolites on Liver.

Biological Activity	Saffron Constituent Tested	Aim of Study	*IN VITRO*		*IN VIVO*			Reference
			Types of Cells	Doses Used	Models Used	DOSES USED	Result of Study	
Antioxidant	Ethanolic extract of saffron	Effect of saffron on aged liver	—	—	Male Wistar rats	5, 10, 20 mg/kg	Saffron ameliorated increased serum nitric oxide and MDA levels and reduced GST activity in the liver, protects susceptible aged liver.	Samarghandian et al. (2016)
	Ethanolic and aqueous extract of saffron	Antioxidant activity of saffron	—	—	Adult male Wistar rats	200 mg/kg, 200 mg/kg	Saffron alleviates neuropathic pain, through attenuation of antioxidant activity	Amin et al. (2014)
	Saffron extract, crocin	Effect of saffron against chronic stress	—	—	Adult male Wistar rats	30 mg/kg, 30 mg/kg	Saffron extract reduced MDA levels, GPx, GR, and SOD levels increased total antioxidant reactivity (TAR) in the stressed animals.	Bandegi et al. (2014)
	Ethanolic extract of saffron, Crocin	Activity of saffron against STZ-induced diabetes	—	—	Male Wistar rats — Mohammad et al. (2011); female wistar rats — Altinoz et al. (2014); male Wistar rats— Yaribeygi et al., 2018	40 mg/kg— Mohammad et al., 2011; 20 mg/kg — Altinoz et al. (2014); 40 mg/kg- Yaribeygi et al., 2018	Crocin deduced glucose level of blood in STZ-induced diabetic rats and shielded their liver by reducing the oxidative stress.	Mohammad et al. (2011); Altinoz et al. (2014); Yaribeygi et al., 2018
	Crocin	Effect of crocin on liver of BPA treated rats.	—	—	Male Wistar albino rats	5, 10, or 20 mg/kg	Crocin reduced liver damage and improved elevated levels of TG and liver enzymes of BPA-treated rats.	Vahdati Hassani et al., 2017

Continued

TABLE 1.1
Pharmacological Activities of Saffron and its Active Metabolites on Liver.—cont'd

| Biological Activity | Saffron Constituent Tested | Aim of Study | *IN VITRO* | | | *IN VIVO* | | | |
			Types of Cells	Doses Used		Models Used	DOSES USED	Result of Study	Reference
	Crocin	Crocin's effect on hemorrhagic shock–induced organ damage.	—	—		Male Wistar rats	60 mg/kg	Crocin reduced myeloperoxidase levels in the liver and protected organs from hemorrhagic shock–induced damages due to its antioxidative role.	Yang and Dong, 2017
Anticancer	Ethanolic and aqueous extract of saffron	Saffron's effect on liver cancer	HepG2- Amin et al. (2011); HepG2 cells- Amin et al., 2016	Various concentrations of saffron (0.1–6 mg/mL)- Amin et al. (2011); 0.01, 0.03, 0.1, 0.31 mM- Amin et al. (2016)		Adult male albino Wistar rats – Amin et al. (2011); Adult male albino Wistar rats- Amin et al. (2016)	75, 150, and 300 mg/kg in Rats – Amin et al. (2011); 100, 200mg/kg- Amin et al. (2016)	Saffron inhibited cell proliferation and induced apoptosis in liver cancer cell line and experimental animal models.	Amin et al. (2011); Amin et al. (2016)
	Free crocin, crocin-coated magnetic nano particles	Assessment of crocin-coated MNPs on liver cell.	HepG2 cells	(0.025,0.05, 0.5, 3, 5, 8, 10, 15 or 20 mg/mL)—Free crocin (0.05, 0.07, 0.09 or 0.1 mg Fe/mL)- MNPs HepG2 cells		—	—	Crocin-coated magnetite nano particles showed regression of precancerous lesions when compared to free crocin treatment.	El-Kharrag et al. (2017)
	Crocin	Crocin's role on telomerase activity of HepG2 cells.	Various concentrations			—	—	Crocin reduced telomerase activity of HepG2 cells by downregulating the expression of catalytic subunit of the enzyme.	Noureini and Wink (2012)
Anticancer (cont.)	Aqueous extract of saffron	Role of saffron on HepG2 and Hep2 cells	HepG2, Hep2 cells	0, 200, 400, 800 µg/mL.		—	—	Saffron reduced nitric oxide production in HepG2 and Hep2 cells lines.	Parizadeh et al. (2011)

	Compound	Study focus	Cell line	Concentration	Animal model	Dose	Results	References
	Crocin	Crocin's effect against STAT3 in HepG2	Hep3B, HepG2, HCT116, MDA-MB-231	0, 5, 10, 20 µM	—	—	Crocin inhibited STAT3 activation induced by IL-6 in HepG2 cell line	Kim and Park (2018)
Hepato-protective	Crocin	Role of crocin on liver enzymes	—	—	Male Wistar rats	200 mg/kg	Crocin decreased levels of antioxidants activity, improved level of liver enzymes. The expression of miR-122, miR-34a, and P53 decreased, while Nrf2 increased in male wistar rats.	Akbari et al. (2017)
	Crocin	Probable mechanisms of hepatoprotective activity of crocin	—	—	Male Sprague–Dawley rats	5, 10, 25, 50 and 100 µg/mL	Crocin prevented liver injury by preventing subcellular organelle damage, proteolysis and apoptosis in isolated hepatocytes of male Sprague–Dawley rats.	Yousefsani et al. (2018)
Reduced toxicity Reduces toxicity	Ethanolic extract of saffron	Role of saffron on acetaminophen- and rifampicin-induced toxicity	—	—	Adult male Wistar rats	40 and 80 mg/kg	Saffron decreased liver enzyme levels and ameliorated oxidative stress against hepatotoxicity induced by acute acetaminophen and rifampicin in male Wistar rats.	Moossavi et al., 2017
	Aqueous extract of saffron	Saffron against aluminum chloride–induced toxicity	—	—	Mice strain BALB/c and C57BL/6	200 mg/kg of saffron extract	Saffron and honey improved liver biochemical markers and alleviated the increase of lipid peroxidation against aluminum chloride–induced toxicity in mice strains.	Shati et al., 2010

Continued

TABLE 1.1

Pharmacological Activities of Saffron and its Active Metabolites on Liver.—cont'd

Biological Activity	Saffron Constituent Tested	IN VITRO			IN VIVO			Reference
		Aim of Study	Types of Cells	Doses Used	Models Used	DOSES USED	Result of Study	
	Aqueous and ethanolic extract of saffron, crocin, safran, safranal.	Saffron's metabolites against CCl4-induced toxicity of the liver	–	–	Male white Razi mice-Iranshahi et al., (2011); male Sprague Dawley rats-Bahashwan et al., 2014; Wistar albino male rats-Arihan et al. (2016)	0.56 and 0.8 g/kg of aqueous extract, 1.4 and 2 g/kg of ethanolic extract -Iranshahi et al., (2011); 100 mg/kg/day of crocin -Bahashwan et al., 2014; Safran (100 mg/kg), Safranal (100 mg/kg), Crocin (100 mg/kg) -Arihan et al. (2016)	Saffron ameliorated condition of liver against carbon tetrachloride induced hepatotoxicity due to its active ingredients.	Iranshahi et al., (2011); Bahashwan et al., 2015; Arihan et al. (2016)
	Crocin	Crocin against nicotine-induced liver toxicity	–	–	Balb/c male mice	12.5, 25, and 50 mg/kg	Crocin partly protected liver against nicotine-induced toxicity in male mice.	Jalili et al. (2015)
	Crocin	Effect of crocin on diazinon induced hepatotoxicity	–	–	Male Wistar rats	12.5, 25, and 50 mg/kg	Crocin reduced diazinon induced hepatotoxicity in rats.	Lari et al., 2015
	Crocin	Crocin against morphine-induced liver damage	–	–	Balb/c male mice	12.5, 25, and 50 mg/kg	Crocin ameliorated condition of liver and protected the liver from the damage induced by morphine.	Salahshoor et al. (2016)
	Crocin	Activity of crocin against acrylamide liver toxicity	–	–	Male Wistar albino rats	50 mg/kg	Crocin protected liver from acrylamide induced liver toxicity due to its antioxidant property.	Gedik et al. (2017)

Category	Compound	Study		Species	Dose	Findings	Reference
	Crocin	Role of crocin on cisplatin—induced liver damage	—	Kunming mice	6.25 and 12.5 mg/kg	Crocin protected liver against cisplatin induced toxicity	Sun et al. (2014)
	Crocin	Crocin against 5-FU—induced liver injury	—	Male Wistar rats	40 mg/kg	Crocin supplementation ameliorated 5-Fluorouracil-induced oxidative stress and liver injury in rat	Afolabi et al. (2016)
	Crocin	Effect of crocin against iron overload on the liver.	—	Male Wistar albino rats	200 mg/kg	Crocin ameliorated biochemical changes induced by iron overload in rat liver	EL–Maraghy et al. (2009)
Anti-genotoxic	Extract of saffron; crocin; safranal.	Activity of saffron and it's constituent against DNA damage	—	Adult male NMRI mice - Hosseinzadeh et al., 2007; Adult male NMRI mice- Hosseinzadeh et al. (2008)	72.75 & 363.75 mg/kg, ip Hosseinzadeh et al., 2007; 50, 200, and 400 mg/kg, ip- Hosseinzadeh et al. (2008)	Saffron and its constituent protected liver from DNA damage induced by methyl methanesulfonate.	Hosseinzadeh et al., 2007; (2008)
Fatty liver disease	Extract of saffron; crocin	Effect of saffron on nonalcoholic fatty liver disease	—	Male Sprague Dawley rats	40 and 80 mg/kg	Saffron extract and crocin protected liver against nonalcoholic fatty liver disease and high fat diet induce liver damages.	Mashmoul et al. (2016)
	Saffron	Evaluation of saffron's activity against nonalcoholic fatty liver disease diabetic rats.	—	Sprague—Dawley male rats	100 mg/kg/day	Saffron exhibited hypoglycemic and hepatoprotective activity on nonalcoholic fatty liver disease of diabetic rats.	Konstantopoulos et al. (2017)

with crocin improved the damage of the liver probably by antioxidant activity, downregulation of miR-122 expression, and lowering of the phosphorylation of ERK 1/2, JNK, and MAPKAPK (Hassani et al., 2017).

Saffron extract and crocin reduce MDA and glutathione S-transferase in STZ-induced diabetic rats

Oxidative stress plays a leading role in developing complications that arise from diabetes mellitus (DM). Saffron has been found to show protective effect in rodents suffering from DM. In a study conducted by Mohammad et al. (2011) on streptozotocin-induced diabetic Wistar rats, a significant increase in the level of Reduced Glutathione (GSH), Superoxide dismutase (SOD), Catalase (CAT), and GSH-Px was observed in rats treated with ethanolic extract of saffron as compared with untreated diabetic rats. Treatment with saffron extract significantly decreased the level of MDA in rats, which concluded that the antioxidant property of saffron lessens oxidative stress of liver tissue in artificially induced diabetic rats (Mohammad et al., 2011). In another study by Yaribeygi et al., 2018, it was reported that hyperglycemia mitigated the elements of antioxidant defense system by decreasing the activity of SOD and CAT and further instigated damage because of increase in reactive nitrogen species (RNS) and generating MDA in liver tissues of male Wistar rats. Treatment with crocin attenuated the levels of nitrate and MDA and substantiated the impact of oxidative stress (Yaribeygi et al., 2018).

Hepatoprotective Activity of Saffron

Avicenna, in his book "Canon", has mentioned many herbs having hepatoprotective activity. One among them is *Crocus sativus* L. which is considered to have its temperament as "hot and dry" in first grade (Shamsi-Baghbanan et al., 2014).

Saffron protects susceptible aged liver

The liver is an important organ that helps the body in detoxification. Its function declines gradually with age due to structural atrophy. Increase in age also impairs functions of mitochondria, which may be a chief reason underlying upsurge in the production rate of ROS. An antioxidant nutrient may be a good diet strategy for prevention of age-related liver disease. Samarghandian et al. (2016) demonstrated that aging causes a noteworthy enhancement in the serum NO (nitric oxide) and MDA and decrease in the activities of SOD, glutathione S transferase (GST), and CAT in the liver of a 20-month-old rat. Treatment was found to be effective in protecting susceptible aged liver by modulation of liver peroxidation, antioxidants, and detoxification systems. This study is another confirmation for the use of antioxidants as a health beneficial food component during aging (Samarghandian et al., 2016).

Crocin alleviates hemorrhagic shock—induced organ damages

Hemorrhage is considered to be the key reason of death globally under the age of 44 years and comprises about 40% of the death among trauma patients (Curry et al., 2011). It produces adverse injuries in various organs as there is a swift loss of volume intravascularly and tissue reperfusion. This results in hypotension and hypoxemia along with ischemia-reperfusion injuries during recovery (Alam and Rhee, 2007). Studies have revealed the potential effect of saffron extract and crocin in alleviating the organ damage caused by hemorrhagic shock. Yang and Dong (2017) assessed the antioxidant activity of crocin in relieving hemorrhagic shock—induced damage of organs. They noticed betterment in the levels of wet-to-dry ratio, quantitative assessment ration, creatinine, blood urea nitrogen (BUN), AST, and ALT. Elevation in the level of glutathione in serum and deduction in the level of MDA and myeloperoxidase were observed in the animals treated with crocin. The possible mechanism behind recovery is via the antioxidant activity of crocin (Yang and Dong, 2017). In another study carried out by Yang et al. (2011), it was reported that administration of Crocetin during resuscitation resulted in reduced activation of hepatic apoptosis and therefore an increase in survival rate (Yang et al., 2011).

Crocin protects the liver from ischemia-reperfusion (IR) injury

Although various pharmacological, genetic, and surgical protocols are available for alleviating the side effects of hepatic IR injury, the treatment still remains unsatisfactory (Khowailed et al., 2011). Damages associated such as hypovolemic shock, trauma, liver transplantation, and resection interventions demand the development of a newer candidate to curb the disease (Teoh et al., 2003).

Akbari et al. (2017) assessed the effect of crocin being an hepatoprotective agent on IR injury and microRNA (miR-122 and miR-34a) expression on rat models. Molecular, biochemical, and histopathological examinations showed that crocin improved histopathological changes and protected the liver against IR injury by improving serum levels of liver enzymes through increasing the activity of antioxidant enzymes and downregulating miR-122, miR-34a, and P53 and through upregulating Nrf2 expression (Akbari et al., 2017).

Crocin protects the liver by preventing proteolysis and subcellular organelle damage and apoptosis

It is clear that compounds that show antioxidant property, inhibit lipid peroxidation, and scavenge free radicals are found to possess hepatoprotective action. Previous studies have reported the protective effect of crocin in liver diseases. Yousefsani et al. (2018) examined the effect of crocin on cumene hydroperoxide (CHP)-induced toxicity on isolated rat hepatic cell preparation. It was noted that crocin attenuated the cell lysis, lipid peroxidation, level of ROS generation, and cellular proteolysis. Reduction in lysosomal membrane damage and mitochondrial membrane potential was observed in cells treated with crocin along with an increase in the levels of GSH/GSSG in rats fed with crocin (Yousefsani et al., 2018).

Saffron reduces toxicity in the liver

Several studies have been conducted on saffron which shows that saffron reduces the toxicity induced artificially in the liver of mice and rats. A study was conducted by Moossavi et al., 2017 to evaluate the hepatoprotective activity of three medicinal plants *Crocus sativus* (petal and stigma), *Ziziphus jujube*, and *Berberis vulgaris* in acetaminophen- and rifampicin-induced hepatotoxicity in Wistar rats. It was noted that treatment with the medicinal plants decreased levels of liver enzymes such as ALT, AST, ALP, and LD (lactate dehydrogenase) and ameliorated the status of oxidative stress in hepatotoxic rats. This impact was noted in a considerable amount in *C. sativus* and *Z. jujube*. More importantly, the experimental plants effectively treated the group of acetaminophen when compared with rifampicin group (Moossavi et al., 2017).

Crocin ameliorates biochemical alterations due to iron overload in the liver

Iron is a vital nutrient found in trace amount and is required for the growth, development, and sustenance of most of the organisms. Meanwhile, no active process is found in human beings to maintain and control excretion of iron. Excess iron, irrespective of the course of entry, gets stored in parenchymal organs and in turn jeopardizes the viability of cell (Yajun et al., 2005). Syndromes of iron overload are categorized as genetic (hereditary hemochromatosis) or secondary (for long-term blood transfusions, like in patients of severe anemia and thalassemia). Additionally, a lot of diseases such as chronic hepatitis-C, alcoholic liver disease, and nonalcoholic steatohepatitis display mild deposition of iron or imbalance in distribution of body iron (Britton et al., 1994; Kohgo et al., 2008). The cell damage arises due to oxidative stress in the liver when iron-buffering ability in the liver is overwhelmed as the liver is the main site of storage of iron in body (Yajun et al., 2005; Kohgo et al., 2008). Study undertaken by El-Maragy et al. (2009) to assess the possible enhancing effect of crocin and curcumin on iron overload–induced hepatic damage in rats revealed alterations in the indices of liver function, decreased level of serum urea and hyperammonemia, changes in liver energy metabolism along with reduced ureagenesis, and a decrease in dimethylarginine dimethylaminohydrolase activity. Treatment with either curcumin or crocin resolved most of the biochemical changes induced by overload of iron in the liver of rat, an outcome which can be helpful for people experiencing iron overload (El-Maraghy et al., 2009).

Crocin reduces 5-fluorouracil–induced liver toxicity and injury

5-Fluorouracil, antagonist/antimetabolite, is chiefly used as an antineoplastic drug because of its efficiency in various malignancies (Grem et al., 2000; Longley et al., 2003), but its beneficial effect is limited by its hepatotoxicity. Aflobi et al. (2016) investigated the effect of crocin against 5-Fluorouracil–induced liver injury. In their study, some of the rats were treated with crocin prior to administration of 5-FU, some treated along with 5-FU administration, and some were treated with crocin after administration of 5-FU, while some were not treated at all with crocin after administration of 5-FU. Treatment of crocin given prior, concurrent, and after administration of 5-FU significantly reduced MDA, advanced oxidized protein products (AOPP), and lipid hydroperoxides (LOOH) levels and elevated total antioxidant capacity when compared with the 5-FU–alone group, with enhancement in the actions of the antioxidant enzymes, SOD, CAT, and PONase. Liver injury was distinctly reversed when AST, ALT, and ALP activities were estimated in the three treatment groups when pitched against the 5-FU group, but the repair was incomplete, when compared to the control. Histopathological examinations supported the aforementioned biochemical changes, which indicated that crocin treatment can be beneficial in reducing 5-FU–induced oxidative stress and liver injury in rats (Afolabi et al., 2016).

Crocin protects the liver from CCl₄-induced liver injury

Carbon tetrachloride (CCl_4) is a nonflammable, transparent lethal chemical which may swiftly evaporate from its liquid form (Kus et al., 2005). Pharmacologically, it is a cytotoxic xenobiotic which causes cellular damage by augmenting lipid peroxidation. Experimental or unintended contact to CCL_4 causes severe problems to an organism. Hepatotoxicity is the main aftereffect caused by CCL_4 exposure. Various herbs including saffron are found to possess protective effect against CCL_4-induced hepatotoxicity. In a study conducted on CCL_4-exposed experimental rats, it was noted that CCl_4 significantly increased the weight of the liver as compared to the weight of body, active caspase-3, IL-6, and TNF-α plasma levels, and liver MDA content. In addition to this, CCl_4 also distressed histology of the liver, metabolizing enzymes (CYP2E1 and GST), and LFT (liver function tests). It considerably decreased the activities of SOD, CAT, GSH-Px, and GSH content. After administering crocin with CCl_4, it was noted that it modified all the parameters that were disturbed by CCl_4 and conserved via modulation of liver metabolizing enzymes, inhibition of inflammatory cytokines, caspase 3, and oxidative stress along with favoring elimination of CCl_4 toxic metabolites (Bahashwan et al., 2015). Iranshahi et al. focused on precautionary effects of ethanolic and aqueous extracts of saffron's petal and stigma against liver toxicity produced by CCl_4 in rats. CCl_4-induced fatty degeneration and vacuole formation significantly increased the levels of ALT and AST in plasma. Treatment with ethanolic and aqueous extracts of *C. sativus* L. petals and stigmas considerably reduced AST and ALT levels in plasma. The histopathological results displayed that it reduced the occurrence of lesions in the liver, which was previously produced by CCl_4. The influence shown by ethanolic and aqueous extracts of saffron can be attributed to

- reduction of CCl_4 metabolic activation by cytochrome P450 inhibition
- antioxidant effects and radical scavenging activity
- fixation of hepatic cell membrane

The outcome proposed that the aqueous and ethanolic extracts of saffron safeguard the liver from damages induced by CCl_4 in mice (Iranshahi et al., 2011).

Crocin removes acrylamide-induced liver damages

Acrylamide (AA) is used in industrial wastewater treatment as a preservative chemical, in industry of textile, and also in printing and production of cosmetics. Studies have reported that high levels of acrylamide can have neurotoxic, genotoxic, and carcinogenic consequence on living beings. Gedik et al. (2017) noticed that administration of acrylamide considerably reduced the level of hepatic GSH and TAS in rats in comparison to the control group while it increased AST, ALT, ALP, SOD, and CAT activities and TOS and MDA levels. Their histopathological examinations showed that cells had inflammatory infiltration, hepatocellular necrosis, and hemorrhagic parts in liver segments. Moreover, hepatocytes showed intracytoplasmic vacuolization. Upon treatment with crocin, levels of GSH and TAS were elevated, whereas activities of ALT, ALP, AST, SOD, and CAT and TOS and MDA levels were reduced. A considerable amount of decrease was noted after the treatment of crocin in inflammatory cell infiltration and vascular congestion in parts of the liver, and intracytoplasmic vacuolization in hepatocytes and no degree of hemorrhages and hepatocellular necrosis were seen. The hepaprotective effect of crocin here might be due to its antioxidant activity, and as a result, it protected the liver from the damage caused by acrylamide (Gedik et al., 2017).

Crocin provides partial protection from nicotine-induced toxicity

Cigarette contains nicotine which is a major pharmacologically active substance responsible for addiction and negative health consequence worldwide (Prah-Ruger et al., 2014). Its metabolism largely takes place in the liver, and it causes distressing impacts. A study was designed by Jalili et al. to examine the protective effect of crocin against toxicity induced by nicotine on the mice liver for which they treated mice with crocin, which were initially administered with nicotine. Histology and weight of the liver and levels of AST, ALT, ALP, and S. nitric oxide were examined. The outcome specified that the administration of nicotine considerably reduced the total weight of the liver while it increased the mean diameter of hepatocyte, central hepatic vein, liver enzymes level (ALP, AST, ALT), and blood serum nitric oxide level when compared with the mice who were not administered with nicotine. Conversely, when crocin and crocin plus nicotine was given, it considerably enhanced the weight of the liver and deduced the mean diameter of hepatocyte and also that of central hepatic vein, hepatic enzymes levels (ALP, AST, ALT), and S. nitric oxide (NO) levels in each group when matched to the group which was not treated with nicotine (Jalili et al., 2015).

Pesticides are widely used in agriculture which causes environmental pollution and is a main concern as its outreach is enormous. Lari et al. (2015) studied the consequences of exposure of subacute DZN and crocin's enriching influence on peroxidation of lipid and alterations that occurred pathologically in the liver of male Wistar rats.

Crocin, which has shown antioxidant activity in previous studies, was used by Lari et al. (2015) to evaluate its hepatoprotective effect against DZN-induced hepatoxicity. They studied the consequences of exposure of subacute DZN and crocin's enriching influence on peroxidation of lipid and alterations that occurred pathologically in the liver of male Wistar rats. Also, levels of protein of activated and total caspases −3 and −9 and Bax/Bcl-2 ratio were assessed. The rats were exposed to diazinon, and some of them were later on treated with crocin after DZN exposure. The MDA level got elevated considerably in the DZN group when compared with that in the group not exposed to diazinon. Also, the MDA level reduced notably in the DZN plus crocin–treated group. DZN generated the process of apoptosis by activation of caspases −9 and −3 and increased Bax/Bcl-2 ratio. Crocin lessened the activation of caspases and reduced the ratio of Bax/Bcl-2, which brought the study of Lari et al. (2015) to a conclusion that apoptosis occurs when there is an exposure of subacute type due to DZN which is mediated by oxidative stress, while the treatment of crocin can diminish the DZN-generated liver toxicity (Lari et al., 2015).

Crocin reduces morphine-induced liver damage

Morphine is an opioid analgesic drug which is the main psychoactive chemical in opium. Morphine has a high potential for addiction, tolerance, and psychological dependence (Stoops et al., 2010). Its metabolism largely takes place in the liver, and that causes some disturbing impacts such as enhancing the production of free radicals. A study was planned by Salahshoor et al. (2016) to assess the crocin's shielding effect against toxicity produced by morphine on mouse liver. Multiple dosages of crocin and crocin plus morphine were given intraperitoneally on daily basis. The histology and liver weight and ALP, AST, ALT, and S. nitric oxide levels were examined. The outcome showed that when morphine was given, it considerably reduced the weight of the liver and enlarged the mean diameters of hepatocyte and central hepatic vein, liver enzymes levels, and S. nitric oxide level in blood when compared with the group which was treated with saline. However, administration of crocin enhanced considerably the weight of the liver and deduced the mean diameter of hepatocyte and central hepatic vein, nitric oxide levels, and liver enzymes in each group in comparison to the morphine treated group (Salahshoor et al., 2016). The outcome

seems quite helpful, but it needs to be studied on humans as toxicity caused by morphine is on a high these days and crocin can be used as a protective agent against morphine-induced toxicity of the liver.

Saffron and honey provide protection to the liver from aluminum chloride–induced injury

Aluminum (Al) is an integral part of utensils used for cooking, medications, sprays, and deodorants, as well as of food preservatives, as a result, it easily enters human body (Yokel et al., 2000), and when human body is exposed to it for a longer period of time, it can cause toxicity. The hepatotoxicity induced by aluminum chloride (AlCl3), its biochemical and molecular aspect, and also the shielding impact of saffron along with honey in contradiction to such type of toxicity were studied by Shati et al. in 2010.

BALB/c and C57BL/6 mice strains were used and treated in groups with AlCl3 and saffron and honey. Modification in levels of Gamma-glutamyl transferase (GGT), ALT, AST, ALP, total bilirubin, and lipid peroxidation was tested. They examined the suppressed and induced mRNA in the homogenate of the liver and carried out isolation of upregulated and downregulated genes, and later on, it was cloned and then sequenced. It was seen that AlCl3 induced considerable rise in the levels of triglyceride and cholesterol, GGT, AST, ALT, ALP, and lipid peroxidation, and there was occurrence of hyperglycemia when compared with the control group. However, when these rats were treated with saffron and honey, improvement was seen in all the disrupted biochemical markers along with reduction in lipid peroxidation. Five upregulated genes (2 BALB/c and three C57BL/6) and seven downregulated genes (3 BALB/c and four C57BL/6) were viewed. The *Aa2-245* gene was detected as being upregulated (Shati et al., 2010) concluding that the toxic effect caused due to exposure of AlCl3 could be minimized by treatment of saffron and honey; however, it needs to be studied and experimented further to bring it into use in day-to-day life.

Crocin relieved cisplatin-induced hepatic damage

Cisplatin (CDDP) is a chief antitumor agent, but owing to its hepatotoxicity, its use is getting restricted. Sun et al. (2014) conducted a study to investigate the effect of crocin on cisplatin-induced hepatotoxicity in mice liver. It was noted that crocin treatment considerably improved CDDP-induced liver damage which was assessed by measurement of serum AST and ALT levels. Crocin also alleviated oxidative stress which was induced by CDDP by lowering the level of MDA and recuperating glutathione and antioxidant enzymes levels. Also, hepatic histopathology showed improvement in CDDP-induced focal necrosis due to crocin. Western blot analysis and immunohistochemical staining revealed that crocin notably reduced the levels of P53 (tumor protein 53) and MAPK (phospho-p38 mitogen-activated protein kinase) and cleaved caspase-3. The activity of crocin against CDDP-induced hepatotoxicity may be attributed to its antioxidant activity and inhibition of activation of P38 MAPK, P53, and caspase-3 (Sun et al., 2014).

Anticancer Activity of Saffron on the Liver

Cancer is one of the major burdens on health globally, although a lot of efforts are being concerted to treat and detect it at early stages. Among cancers of different organs of the body, hepatic cancer turns out to be the fifth commonest cancer in males and the ninth in females. Still, it happens to be the second leading cause of deaths due to cancer (Torre et al., 2015). Hepatocellular carcinoma (HCC) accounts for over 70% of the primary liver cancer cases (Cancer Incidence and Mortality Worldwide, 2015). Median survival span counts up to 8 months without treatment, and the period can be extended only by 3 months when the chemotherapy is given. Hepatitis (B and C) and viral infections of the liver often progress to form HCC. Likewise, HBV and HCV count up to 70%—90% of the cases of patients with HCC (Sherman et al., 2010). Other factors that contribute to the formation of HCC include fatty liver disease, iron overload (Nahon et al., 2010), alcoholism, and exposure to environmental carcinogens (Starley et al., 2010) such as diethylnitrosamine (DEN) (Park et al., 2009; Amin et al., 2016). The side effects encountered by most of the chemotherapeutic agents happen to be their nonspecificity and subsequently cytotoxicity. Hence, the invention of novel anticancer therapies and utilization of an advance system of drug delivery would enhance the specificity to cancer cells and lessen the adverse effects of chemotherapy (Tietze et al., 2015; El-Kharrag et al., 2017).

Crocin averts early lesions in liver cancer

Study carried out by Amin et al., in 2011, demonstrated that crocin exhibited antiproliferative and proapoptotic properties when administered in DEN-induced HCC model. For their study, saffron was administered in the DEN-treated rats, which reduced the quantity and incidence of dyschromatic nodules along with reduction in the development of neoplastic foci of altered hepatocytes. It was related by considerable reduction in

the number of positive foci of GST-P and the level of plasma alpha fetoprotein that are distinct indicators of preneoplasia and neoplasia.

The physiological changes that are seen in cancerous cells during their continuous growth are the rise in proliferation of cell and loss of apoptotic mechanisms (Reuter et al., 2010). It was marked that saffron demonstrated significant antiproliferative activity by significantly arresting cell cycle in vitro and decreasing the number of proliferative cells (Ki-67-positive cells 18) in DEN-administered rats. Saffron's antiproliferative activity was also related to the initiation of apoptosis as demonstrated in vitro by caspase-3 cleavage and the pre-G predominant fraction in Propidium Iodide- Fluorescence Activated Cell Sorting (PI-FACS) analysis. The initiation of apoptosis must have occurred due to the damage to DNA as revealed by the upregulation of the double-stranded DNA breakage marker, p-H2XA, which suggested saffron's additional function in transforming the cells of cancer through the impacts of different chemotherapeutic agents. Treatment of saffron consistently elevated the TUNEL- and M30 Cyto Death-positive cell's numbers in vivo. Saffron's administration in DEN-treated rats reduced the oxidative stress which was induced earlier by DEN, and it was marked by refurbishment of the levels of antioxidants SOD, CAT, and GST in the liver and minimizing of important indicators of oxidative stress, such as oxidized lipids (MDA) and proteins (P.Carbonyl). Along with saffron's antioxidant activity, it shielded the liver from damage by reducing serum ALT and GGT. It also displayed ABTS and DPPH radical scavenging activities and showed considerable reducing power as exhibited by the FRAP assay. The credit to Saffron's antioxidant activity could be given to the phenolic content it has and to the ingredients actively found in it such as crocetin, crocin, safranal, and carotene (Karimi et al., 2010).

Saffron shielded the liver against inflammation induced by DEN by diminishing numbers of Kupffer cells and liver MPO level (indicator of neutrophil infiltration). It seemed to be linked to NF-κB signaling pathway's early inactivation as shown in the initial in vitro inhibition of p-IκB and IL-8, and also, the inhibition of the in vivo protein expressions of iNOS and COX-2 was seen. The administration of saffron downregulated the activation of TNFα receptor in vivo along with its expression in vitro. Collectively, the results suggested that saffron's shielding effect against carcinogenesis can be credited to its anti-inflammatory property via downregulation of COX-2 and iNOS expressions and by reducing the numbers of tumor cell's active TNFα receptors (Fig. 1.4). Also, the DEN induced inflammation

(A) Cancerous state

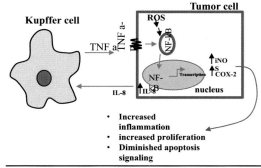

(B) Saffron treatment

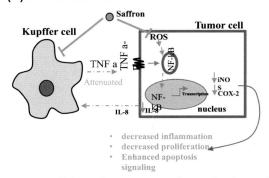

FIG.   1.4 Schematic   representation   showing   the antiinflammatory and antiproliferatory effects of saffron on tumor cell signaling. **(A)** In cancerous state, Kupffer cells increase TNFα signaling to the tumor cells, resulting in increased reactive oxygen species (ROS), localization of NF-kB to the nucleus for increased transcription, ultimately increasing the levels of iNOS and COX-2. These two components further feed forward the inflammation and proliferation signals, and apoptosis signaling is diminished. **(B)** Saffron reduces Kupffer cell proliferation and attenuates TNF-αR signaling of the tumor cell. Saffron also directly reduces the ROS. Together, these mechanisms bring down the levels of inflammatory and proliferatory signaling components and enhance apoptosis signaling, providing a check on cancer cell proliferation.

by an oxidative-dependent mode which involved ROS. Saffron's administration to DEN-treated rats swapped DEN-induced upregulation of NF-kB-p65 subunit. Parallel result was reported in *in vitro* studies, where saffron treatment caused an early decrease in the phosphorylation state of IkB (Amin et al., 2011, 2016).

Crocin inhibits STAT3 activation induced by IL-6

It is well known that signal transducer and activator of transcription 3 (STAT3) takes part in the proliferation, angiogenesis, endurance, annexation, and metastasis of the tumor cells. Also, reports have suggested interleukin-6 (IL-6) to be intimately linked to the activity of STAT3. A research conducted by Kim and Park in 2018 investigated that crocin, which is saffron's major glycosylated carotenoid, can modify the pathway IL-6/STAT3 to instigate sensitivity and growth restraint to apoptosis of cancer cells. Also, it was assessed that crocin suppressed the activation of STAT3 which was produced by IL-6 in HepG2 and Hep3B cells in HCC. STAT3 clampdown was directed via the inactivation of Src kinase and Janus kinase 1/2(JAK1, JAK2) in the aforementioned cancer cell lines of the liver. Moreover, crocin was noted to induce the protein tyrosine phosphatase (PTP) SHP-1 expression, leading to dephosphorylation of STAT3. Also when *SHP-1* gene was deleted by siRNA, crocin's inhibitory effects were recovered, which suggested the vital role of SHP-1. Crocin also helped in downregulating of the expression of STAT3-regulated antiapoptotic (Bcl-2, survivin), proliferative (cyclin D1), invasive (CXCR4), and angiogenic (VEGF) proteins. Contrarily, crocin amplified the proapoptotic (BAX) protein that was associated with the inhibition of proliferation and induction of apoptosis. These outcomes presented affirmation that crocin had the prospective capability to inhibit the IL-6/STAT3 signaling pathway specifically in hepatic cancer (Kim and Park, 2018).

Crocin inhibits telomerase activity and downregulates Human telomerase reverse transcriptase (hTERT)

Telomerase is a reverse transcriptase enzyme. It plays a vital role in immortality of cell by maintaining the repeats of telomere at the ends of chromosomes in cells that proliferate. Ninety percent of the cancer cells have many fold telomerase overexpression when matched with normal cells. As a result, telomerase inhibitors are recommended as significant targets for the anticancer agents as apoptosis and proliferative senescence are induced by short telomeres (Patel et al., 2017). The study of Noureini and Wink in 2012 provided an understanding of crocin, a carotenoid of saffron with the telomeric quadruplex sequences, which is a catalytic subunit of telomerase enzyme along with *hTERT* gene transcription's downregulation. They used FRET analysis and quantitative real-time PCR. Their study proved that crocin inhibited the telomerase activity in liver cancer cell line HepG2.

The test was carried out to check the possible interaction between crocin and telomeric sequences by calculating the melting points of a synthetically synthesized telomere with the help of FRET analysis. The analysis showed that there was roughly no increment of T1/2 in the existence of crocin. The measurements done using quantitative real time amplification protocol (qTRAP) of protein extracts in equivalent amount indicated a significant decrease in activity of telomerase of nontreated control cells, 48 hours after the treatment of crocin. The result exhibited that a decrease happened in the telomerase activity in a concentration-dependent mode (Patel et al., 2017).

Aqueous extract of saffron reduces nitric oxide production and has antitumour effect on HepG2 and Hep2 cell lines

Various researches have verified the possible antitumor effect of saffron and its constituents on numerous malignant cells. A study carried by Parizadeh et al. (2011) investigated the effect of aqueous extract of saffron on production of nitric oxide by HepG-2 and Hep2 cell lines. They treated the cell lines with different concentration of saffron and observed and recorded the morphological changes after varying hours of incubation. The cell viability was assessed by MTT assay, and NO production was evaluated by Griess test. The morphological images showed an upsurge in cytotoxic effect by increasing the concentrations of extract, and there was a considerable decrease in NO production when the time of incubation was increased. The IC_{50} for HepG2 cells was obtained to be 400 µg/mL, while no response to any concentration of extract was seen in L929 cells and Hep2 (Parizadeh et al., 2011). A lot of researches have revealed that elevated and constant production of nitric oxide (NO) play an important part in the regulation of oncogenic processes (Ying and Hofseth, 2007). As seen in the study, extract of saffron reduced the production of NO at different concentrations in cancer cell lines, which probably might be the reason behind its antitumour effect.

Magnetite nanoparticles coated with crocin enhances liver cancer treatment

In 2017, El-Kharrag et al. suggested in their study that since saffron was noticed to hamper liver cancer in rat models, some new and effective techniques can be proposed and implemented to enhance the effects of saffron by using magnetite nanoparticles (MNPs). It can be prepared by coating the MNPs with crocin, which is an active constituent of saffron. MNPs were coated at the beginning with a cross-linker to augment the coalition of crocin and dextran by using a revised method of coprecipitation. Hepatic cancer cells (HepG2) which were cultured and DEN-administered mice were tended with crocin-layered MNPs and examined using cell proliferation assay and immune-histochemical test, respectively. It was noted that HepG2 cells when tended with crocin-coated MNPs culminated to a notable hampering of their development when matched to those which were treated with uncoated MNPs or free crocin or the control group. Histological assessment of DEN-administered mice livers displayed many precancerous modifications: hyperplastic or dysplastic changes of bile ductules/ducts, numerous proliferative hepatic foci, and nuclear atypia related with polyploidy, vacuolation, and karyomegaly. Immunohistochemistry involving antibodies meant for apoptosis and cell propagation exhibited their upregulation all through the expansion of precancerous lesions. The inflammation antibody cyclooxygenase-2 and antibodies meant for oxidative stress (glutathione) and angiogenesis were used, which revealed the participation of several signaling pathways in the generation and growth of precancerous lesions. Treatment by crocin-coated MNPs displayed lapse of precancerous lesions, marked apoptotic cell's upregulation along with downregulation of Bcl-2 labeling and the indicators of inflammation, cell proliferation, angiogenesis, and oxidative stress.

It concluded that crocin-coated MNPs were found to be more effective than free crocin for cure of precancerous lesions of the liver in mice models, and these findings may further help in initial recognition and cure of precancerous lesions of liver (El-Kharrag et al., 2017).

Genoprotective Property of Saffron in the Liver

A toxin that has the capability to damage DNA or chromosome is considered as a genotoxin. When this type of damage occurs in a germ cell it can cause a germline mutation, while in a somatic cell, it may result in a somatic mutation, which may further transform into malignancy (Phillips et al., 2009). In a study carried by Hosseinzadeh et al., in 2008, it was displayed that extracts of saffron and crocin have shielding activity against damage to DNA. They used methyl methanesulfonate on mice which is a chemical that can induce DNA damage. These mice were further treated with extract of saffron and crocin which suggested that damage to DNA was lessened in the lung, kidney, spleen, and liver, concluding that saffron has a genoprotective property (Hosseinzadeh et al., 2008). In a similar study, it was established by Hosseinzadeh et al., in 2007, that safranal has a protecting activity against DNA damage similar to crocin. Going by the results shown here, metabolites of saffron have proved to be genoprotective in nature when used in animal models, but some clinical trials on humans and in-depth studies may be helpful in introducing saffron as a potent antigenotoxic agent against genomic abnormalities originating from various reasons.

Saffron's Activity on Fatty Liver

Nonalcoholic fatty liver disease (NAFLD) is associated with type 2 diabetes mellitus and is the result of the buildup of adipose tissue deposits in the liver. Saffron is recognized for its possible hypoglycemic activity and potential antioxidant effects. As a result, a study was conducted by Konstantopoulos et al. (2017) to investigate the role of saffron on NAFLD in diabetic rats. Streptozotocin was used to induce diabetes in these rats, followed by treatment of saffron. Histopathological investigation and metabolic profile of the liver showed high levels of glucose and a higher percentage of steatosis in the STZ-induced group; on the contrary, the rats that were treated with saffron showed no such levels of glucose and steatosis. It further implied that saffron exhibits both hypoglycemic and hepatoprotective actions. Yet, further studies enlightening the exact mechanisms of saffron's mode of actions are required (Konstantopoulos et al., 2017).

In a separate study, protective activity of saffron extract and crocin on fatty hepatic tissues were evaluated on obese male Sprague Dawley rats. Some of the rats were give normal diet, while others received high-fat diet. Blood sample was collected to determine levels of hepatic marker enzymes, including AST, ALT, ALP, and albumin, along with the histopathological examination of the liver. It was seen that saffron extract and crocin, in a dose-dependent manner, improved hepatic enzyme levels and histopathological variations in obese rat model which suggested that saffron extract and crocin supplements helped in contrary to the fatty liver. This activity may occur as a result of modification of hepatic enzymes as well as stabilization of hepatic structure and size along with a marked decrease in infiltration of fat in hepatocytes of high-fat diet administered to obese rats (Mashmoul et al., 2016).

CONCLUSION AND FUTURE PERSPECTIVE

Saffron, similar to other herbs, has a long history to be used as condiment and for therapeutic purposes. Several researches have been going on to assess its beneficial properties on the liver especially liver cancer. HCC is a widespread disease globally and is highly associated to the increase in mortality. The development of HCC has multiple intermediate steps such as molecular and transcriptional proceedings that transform the normal functioning of hepatocytes into malignant one. A lot of factors participate in these steps including oxidative stress, NAFLD, HCV (hepatitis C virus), HBV (hepatitis B virus), chronic inflammation, some genetic metabolic errors, atmospheric toxins, some drugs, etc.

The literature and research articles reviewed here indicate that saffron could be used to protect the liver as an antioxidant from free radicals, as anticancer agent to prevent adverse effects of chemotherapeutics. Various studies show that saffron and its constituents can be used as antitoxic agent against overdose of various chemicals such as CCL_4, STZ, acrylamide, cisplatin, morphine, etc. Saffron is also effective in treating the fatty liver of nonalcoholic-type diabetic obese rats. Although these studies show promising results on rats, mice, and some cell lines, clinical trials are required to be carried on humans to verify all the aforementioned activities of saffron on the liver. Also, their comprehensive and in-depth studies need to be conducted to define therapeutic mechanisms involved.

The use of saffron for the purpose of research work is limited because of its high cost; it is further suggested that in-door cultivation of saffron can help in achieving the highest of quality of saffron which can be made available at relatively low-price compared to its availability in market.

CONFLICT OF INTEREST

All authors listed report no conflict of interest.

ACKNOWLEDGMENTS

This work was funded by Central Council for Research in Unani Medicine (F.No. 3−31/2014-CCRUM/Tech) Ministry of AYUSH, Government of India.

REFERENCES

Afolabi, O.K., Adeleke, G.E., Ugbaja, R.N., 2016. Crocin alleviates 5-fluorouracil-induced hepatotoxicity through the abrogation of oxidative stress in male wistar rats. Asian Pac. J. Health Sci. 3 (2), 58−68.

Akbari, G., Mard, S.A., Dianat, M., Mansouri, E., 2017. The hepatoprotective and microRNAs downregulatory effects of crocin following hepatic ischemia-reperfusion injury in rats. Oxid. Med. Cell Longev. 2017.

Al-Snafi, A.E., 2016. The pharmacology of *Crocus sativus*-A review. IOSR J. Pharm. 6 (6), 8−38.

Alam, H.B., Rhee, P., 2007. New developments in fluid resuscitation. Surg. Clin. 87 (1), 55−72.

Altinoz, E., Oner, Z., Elbe, H., Turkoz, Y., Cigremis, Y., 2014. Protective effect of saffron (its active constituent, crocin) on oxidative stress and hepatic injury in streptozotocin induced diabetic rats. Gene Ther. Mol. Biol. 16, 160−171.

Amin, A., Hamza, A.A., Bajbouj, K., Ashraf, S.S., Daoud, S., 2011. Saffron: a potential candidate for a novel anticancer drug against hepatocellular carcinoma. Hepatology 54 (3), 857–867.

Amin, A., A Hamza, A., Daoud, S., Khazanehdari, K., Al Hrout, A., Baig, B., Salehi-Ashtiani, K., 2016. Saffron-based crocin prevents early lesions of liver cancer: in vivo, in vitro and network analyses. Recent Pat. Anti-cancer Drug Discov. 11 (1), 121–133.

Amin, B., Abnous, K., Motamedshariaty, V., Hosseinzadeh, H., 2014. Attenuation of oxidative stress, inflammation and apoptosis by ethanolic and aqueous extracts of Crocus sativus L. stigma after chronic constriction injury of rats. An Acad. Bras Ciências 86 (4), 1821–1832.

Arihan, O., Oto, G., Bayram, I., Aras, I., 2016. Effect of safran, safranal and crocin which are active ingredients of Saffron (Crocus) on erythrocyte fragility and hematological parameters in carbon tetrachloride intoxicated rats. East. J. Med. 21 (4), 173–177.

Bahashwan, S., Hassan, M.H., Aly, H., Ghobara, M.M., El-Beshbishy, H.A., Busati, I., 2015. Crocin mitigates carbon tetrachloride-induced liver toxicity in rats. J. Taibah Univ. Med. Sci. 10 (2), 140–149.

Bandegi, A.R., Rashidy-Pour, A., Vafaei, A.A., Ghadrdoost, B., 2014. Protective effects of Crocus sativus L. extract and crocin against chronic-stress induced oxidative damage of brain, liver and kidneys in rats. Adv. Pharmaceut. Bull. 4 (Suppl. 2), 493–499.

Bathaie, S.Z., Mousavi, S.Z., 2010. New applications and mechanisms of action of saffron and its important ingredients. Crit. Rev. Food Sci. Nutr. 50 (8), 761–786.

Braet, F., Wisse, E., 2002. Structural and functional aspects of liver sinusoidal endothelial cell fenestrae: a review. Comp. Hepatol. 1 (1), 1.

Britton, R.S., Ramm, G.A., Olynyk, J., Singh, R., O'Neill, R., Bacon, B.R., 1994. Pathophysiology of iron toxicity. In: Progress in Iron Research. Springer, Boston, MA, pp. 239–253.

Burton, G.J., Jauniaux, E., 2011. Oxidative stress. Best Pract. Res. Clin. Obstet. Gynaecol. 25 (3), 287–299.

Cancer Incidence and Mortality Worldwide: IARC Cancer Base. No.11, January 4, 2015. Retrieved January 4, 2015, from. http://globocan.iarc.fr.

Chermahini, S.H., Majid, F.A.A., Sarmidi, M.R., Taghizadeh, E., Salehnezhad, S., 2010. Impact of saffron as an anti-cancer and anti-tumor herb. Afr. J. Pharm. Pharmacol. 4 (11), 834–840.

Christodoulou, E., Kadoglou, N.P., Kostomitsopoulos, N., Valsami, G., 2015. Saffron: a natural product with potential pharmaceutical applications. J. Pharm. Pharmacol. 67 (12), 1634–1649.

Curry, N., Hopewell, S., Dorée, C., Hyde, C., Brohi, K., Stanworth, S., 2011. The acute management of trauma hemorrhage: a systematic review of randomized controlled trials. Crit. Care 15 (2), R92.

Dalle-Donne, I., Rossi, R., Colombo, R., Giustarini, D., Milzani, A., 2006. Biomarkers of oxidative damage in human disease. Clin. Chem. 52 (4), 601–623.

D'Alessandro, A.M., Mancini, A., Lizzi, A.R., De Simone, A., Marroccella, C.E., Gravina, G.L., Festuccia, C., 2013. Crocus sativus stigma extract and its major constituent crocin possess significant antiproliferative properties against human prostate cancer. Nutr. Cancer 65 (6), 930–942.

Djordjevic, J., Djordjevic, A., Adzic, M., Niciforovic, A., Radojcic, M.B., 2010. Chronic stress differentially affects antioxidant enzymes and modifies the acute stress response in liver of Wistar rats. Physiol Res 59 (5), 729–736.

El-Kharrag, R., Amin, A., Hisaindee, S., Greish, Y., Karam, S.M., 2017. Development of a therapeutic model of precancerous liver using crocin-coated magnetite nanoparticles. Int. J. Oncol. 50 (1), 212–222.

EL-Maraghy, S.A., Rizk, S.M., El-Sawalhi, M.M., 2009. Hepatoprotective potential of crocin and curcumin against iron overload-induced biochemical alterations in rat. Afr. J. Biochem. Res. 3 (5), 215–221.

Ferrence, S.C., Bendersky, G., 2004. Therapy with saffron and the goddess at Thera. Perspect. Biol. Med. 47 (2), 199–226.

Festuccia, C., Mancini, A., Gravina, G.L., Scarsella, L., Llorens, S., Alonso, G.L., D'Alessandro, A.M., 2014. Antitumor effects of saffron-derived carotenoids in prostate cancer cell models. Biomed. Res. Int. 2014.

Gedik, S., Erdemli, M.E., Gul, M., Yigitcan, B., Bag, H.G., Aksungur, Z., Altinoz, E., 2017. Hepatoprotective effects of crocin on biochemical and histopathological alterations following acrylamide-induced liver injury in Wistar rats. Biomed. Pharmacother. 95 (11), 764–770.

Grem, J.L., 2000. 5-fluorouracil: forty-plus and still ticking. A review of its preclinical and clinical development. Investig. New Drugs 18 (4), 299–313.

Guyton, A.C., Hall, J.E., 2006. Textbook of Medical Physiology, eleventh ed. WB Sounders Company, Philadelphia.

Halliwell, B., Gutteridge, J.M., 2015. Free Radicals in Biology and Medicine. Oxford University Press, USA.

Hassani, F.V., Mehri, S., Abnous, K., Birner-Gruenberger, R., Hosseinzadeh, H., 2017. Protective effect of crocin on BPA-induced liver toxicity in rats through inhibition of oxidative stress and downregulation of MAPK and MAP-KAP signaling pathway and miRNA-122 expression. Food Chem. Toxicol. 107 (Pt A), 395–405.

Hosseinzadeh, H., Abootorabi, A., Sadeghnia, H.R., 2008. Protective effect of Crocus sativus stigma extract and crocin (trans-crocin 4) on methyl methanesulfonate–induced DNA damage in mice organs. DNA Cell Biol. 27 (12), 657–664.

Hosseinzadeh, H., Sadeghnia, H.R., 2007. Effect of safranal, a constituent of Crocus sativus (Saffron), on methyl methanesulfonate (MMS)–induced DNA damage in mouse organs: an alkaline single-cell gel electrophoresis (Comet) assay. DNA and cell biology 26 (12), 841–846.

Iranshahi, M., Khoshangosht, M., Mohammadkhani, Z., Karimi, G., 2011. Protective effects of aqueous and ethanolic extracts of saffron stigma and petal on liver toxicity induced by carbon tetrachloride in mice. Pharmacologyonline 1, 203–212.

Jalili, C., Tabatabaei, H., Kakaberiei, S., Roshankhah, S., Salahshoor, M.R., 2015. Protective role of Crocin against nicotine-induced damages on male mice liver. Int. J. Prev. Med. 6.

Jan, S., Wani, A.A., Kamili, A.N., Kashtwari, M., 2014. Distribution, chemical composition and medicinal importance of saffron (*Crocus sativus* L.). Afr. J. Plant Sci. 8 (12), 537−545.

Kalra, A., Tuma, F., 2018. Physiology, liver. In: StatPearls. StatPearls Publishing.

Karimi, E., Oskoueian, E., Hendra, R., Jaafar, H.Z., 2010. Evaluation of *Crocus sativus* L. stigma phenolic and flavonoid compounds and its antioxidant activity. Molecules 15 (9), 6244−6256.

Khorasany, A.R., Hosseinzadeh, H., 2016. Therapeutic effects of saffron (*Crocus sativus*L.) in digestive disorders: a review. Iran. J. Basic Med. Sci. 19 (5), 455−469.

Khowailed, E.A., Mubarak, H.A., Seddeek, H.A., 2011. Protective xanthine oxidase inhibition on ischemia/reperfusion injury in rat liver. Med. J. Cairo Univ. 79 (2), 667−677.

Kim, B., Park, B., 2018. Saffron carotenoids inhibit STAT3 activation and promote apoptotic progression in IL-6 stimulated liver cancer cells. Oncol. Rep. 39 (4), 1883−1891.

Kohgo, Y., Ikuta, K., Ohtake, T., Torimoto, Y., Kato, J., 2008. Body iron metabolism and pathophysiology of iron overload. Int. J. Hematol. 88 (1), 7−15.

Konstantopoulos, P., Doulamis, I.P., Tzani, A., Korou, M.L., Agapitos, E., Vlachos, I.S., Perrea, D.N., 2017. Metabolic effects of *Crocus sativus* and protective action against non-alcoholic fatty liver disease in diabetic rats. Biomed. Rep. 6 (5), 513−518.

Kus, I., Ogeturk, M., Oner, H., Sahin, S., Yekeler, H., Sarsilmaz, M., 2005. Protective effects of melatonin against carbon tetrachloride-induced hepatotoxicity in rats: a light microscopic and biochemical study. Cell Biochem. Funct. 23 (3), 169−174.

Lari, P., Abnous, K., Imenshahidi, M., Rashedinia, M., Razavi, M., Hosseinzadeh, H., 2015. Evaluation of diazinon-induced hepatotoxicity and protective effects of crocin. Toxicol. Ind. Health 31 (4), 367−376.

Longley, D.B., Harkin, D.P., Johnston, P.G., 2003. 5- fluorouracil: mechanisms of action and clinical strategies. Nat. Rev. Cancer 3 (5), 330−338.

Ma, Y.Y., Yang, M.Q., He, Z.G., Wei, Q., Li, J.Y., 2017. The biological function of kupffer cells in liver disease. Biol. Myelomonocytic Cells 53−84.

MacSween, R.N.M., Desmet, V.J., Roskams, T., Scothorne, R.J., 2002. Developmental anatomy and normal structure. In: MacSween, R.N.M., Burt, A.D., Portmann, B.C., Ishak, K.G., Scheuer, P.J., Anthony, P.P. (Eds.), Pathology of the Liver. Churchill Livingstone, New York, pp. 1−66.

Malarkey, D.E., Johnson, K., Ryan, L., Boorman, G., Maronpot, R.R., 2005. New insights into functional aspects of liver morphology. Toxicol. Pathol. 33 (1), 27−34.

Mashmoul, M., Azlan, A., Mohtarrudin, N., Yusof, B.N.M., Khaza'ai, H., Khoo, H.E., Boroushaki, M.T., 2016. Protective effects of saffron extract and crocin supplementation on fatty liver tissue of high-fat diet-induced obese rats. BMC Complement. Altern. Med. 16 (1), 401.

Melnyk, J.P., Wang, S., Macrone, M.F., 2010. Chemical and biological properties of the world's most expensive spice: saffron. Food Res. 43 (8), 1981−1989.

Mohammad, R., Daryoush, M., Ali, R., Yousef, D., Mehrdad, N., 2011. Attenuation of oxidative stress of hepatic tissue by ethanolic extract of saffron (dried stigmas of *Crocus sativus* L.) in streptozotocin (STZ)-induced diabetic rats. Afr. J. Pharm. Pharmacol. 5 (19), 2166−2173.

Moossavi, M., Hoshyar, R., Hemmati, M., Farahi, A., Javdani, H., 2017. An invivo study on the hepato-protective effects of *Crocus sativus*, *Ziziphus jujuba* and *Berberis vulgaris* against acute acetaminophen and rifampicin-induced hepatotoxicity. Clin. Phytosci. 2 (1), 16.

Nahon, P., Ganne-Carrié, N., Trinchet, J.C., Beaugrand, M., 2010. Hepatic iron overload and risk of hepatocellular carcinoma in cirrhosis. Gastroenterol. Clin. Biol. 34 (1), 1−7.

Noureini, S.K., Wink, M., 2012. Antiproliferative effects of crocin in HepG2 cells by telomerase inhibition and hTERT down-regulation. Asian Pac. J. Cancer Prev. 13 (5), 2305−2309.

Ochiai, T., Ohno, S., Soeda, S., Tanaka, H., Shoyama, Y., Shimeno, H., 2004. Crocin prevents the death of rat pheochromyctoma (PC-12) cells by its antioxidant effects stronger than those of α-tocopherol. Neurosci. Lett. 362 (1), 61−64.

Parizadeh, M.R., Ghafoori Gharib, F., Abbaspour, A.R., Tavakol Afshar, J., Ghayour-Mobarhan, M., 2011. Effects of aqueous saffron extract on nitric oxide production by two human carcinoma cell lines: hepatocellular carcinoma (HepG2) and laryngeal carcinoma (Hep2). Avicenna J. Phytomed. 1 (1), 43−50.

Park, D.H., Shin, J.W., Park, S.K., Seo, J.N., Li, L., Jang, J.J., Lee, M.J., 2009. Diethylnitrosamine (DEN) induces irreversible hepatocellular carcinogenesis through overexpression of G1/S-phase regulatory proteins in rat. Toxicol. Lett. 191 (2−3), 321−326.

Patel, S., Sarwat, M., Khan, T.H., 2017. Mechanism behind the anti-tumour potential of saffron (*Crocus sativus* L.): the molecular perspective. Crit. Rev. Oncol. Hematol. 115 (7), 27−35.

Phillips, D.H., Arlt, V.M., 2009. Genotoxicity: damage to DNA and its consequences. In: Molecular, Clinical and Environmental Toxicology. Birkhäuser Basel, pp. 87−110.

Prah Ruger, J., Ng, N.Y., 2014. Ethics and social value judgments in public health. Ng NY, and Ruger JP ethics and social value judgments in public health. In: Culyer, A.J. (Ed.), Encyclopedia of Health Economics, vol. 1, pp. 287−291.

Rahmani, A.H., Khan, A.A., Aldebasi, Y.H., 2017. Saffron (*Crocus sativus*) and its active ingredients: role in the prevention and treatment of disease. Pharmacogn. J. 9 (6), 873−879.

Reuter, S., Gupta, S.C., Chaturvedi, M.M., Aggarwal, B.B., 2010. Oxidative stress, inflammation, and cancer: how are they linked? Free Radic. Biol. Med. 49 (11), 1603−1616.

Salahshoor, M.R., Khashiadeh, M., Roshankhah, S., Kakabaraei, S., Jalili, C., 2016. Protective effect of crocin on liver toxicity induced by morphine. Res. Pharmaceut. Sci. 11 (2), 120−129.

Samarghandian, S., Asadi-Samani, M., Farkhondeh, T., Bahmani, M., 2016. Assessment the effect of saffron ethanolic extract (*Crocus sativus* L.) on oxidative damages in aged male rat liver. Der Pharm. Lett. 8 (3), 283–290.

Saxena, R., Theise, N.D., Crawford, J.M., 1999. Microanatomy of the human liver—exploring the hidden interfaces. Hepatology 30 (6), 1339–1346.

Shamsi-Baghbanan, H., Sharifian, A., Esmaeili, S., Minaei, B., 2014. Hepatoprotective herbs, avicenna viewpoint. Iran. Red Crescent Med. J. 16 (1).

Sharma, M.K., Sharma, G.N., Vishal, V., Ranjan, B., 2015. Hepatotoxicity: a major complication with critical treatment. MOJ Toxicol. 1 (3), 00016.

Shati, A.A., Alamri, S.A., 2010. Role of saffron (*Crocus sativus* L.) and honey syrup on aluminum-induced hepatotoxicity. Saudi Med. J. 31 (10), 1106–1113.

Sherman, M., 2010. Hepatocellular carcinoma: epidemiology, surveillance, and diagnosis. Semin. Liver Dis. 30 (1), 3–16.

Si-Tayeb, K., Lemaigre, F.P., Duncan, S.A., 2010. Organogenesis and development of the liver. Dev. Cell 18 (2), 175–189.

Starley, B.Q., Calcagno, C.J., Harrison, S.A., 2010. Non-alcoholic fatty liver disease and hepatocellular carcinoma: A weighty connection. Hepatology 51 (5), 1820–1832.

Stoops, W.W., Hatton, K.W., Lofwall, M.R., Nuzzo, P.A., Walsh, S.L., 2010. Intravenous oxycodone, hydrocodone, and morphine in recreational opioid users: abuse potential and relative potencies. Psychopharmacology 212 (2), 193–203.

Sun, Y., Yang, J., Wang, L., Sun, L., Dong, Q., 2014. Crocin attenuates cisplatin-induced liver injury in the mice. Hum. Exp. Toxicol. 33 (8), 855–862.

Tavakkol-Afshari, J., Brook, A., Mousavi, S.H., 2008. Study of cytotoxic and apoptogenic properties of saffron extract in human cancer cell lines. Food Chem. Toxicol. 46 (11), 3443–3447.

Teoh, N.C., Farrell, G.C., 2003. Hepatic ischemia reperfusion injury: pathogenic mechanisms and basis for hepatoprotection. J. Gastroenterol. Hepatol. 18 (8), 891–902.

Tietze, R., Zaloga, J., Unterweger, H., Lyer, S., Friedrich, R.P., Janko, C., Alexiou, C., 2015. Magnetic nanoparticle-based drug delivery for cancer therapy. Biochem. Biophys. Res. Commun. 468 (3), 463–470.

Torre, L.A., Bray, F., Siegel, R.L., Ferlay, J., Lortet-Tieulent, J., Jemal, A., 2015. Global cancer statistics, 2012. Cancer J. Clin. 65 (2), 87–108.

Tortora, G.J., Derrickson, B., 2012. Principles of Anatomy & Physiology. John Wiley & Sons, Inc., pp. 994–995

Trefts, E., Gannon, M., Wasserman, D.H., 2017. The liver. Curr. Biol. 27 (21), R1147–R1151.

Vekemans, K., Braet, F., 2005. Structural and functional aspects of the liver and liver sinusoidal cells in relation to colon carcinoma metastasis. World J. Gastroenterol. 11 (33), 5095.

Yajun, Z., Hongshan, C., Baoxi, S., Dengbing, Y., Jianhua, S., Xinshun, G., Yi, C., 2005. Translocation of Bax in rat hepatocytes cultured with ferric nitrilotriacetate. Life Sci. 76 (24), 2763–2772.

Yang, L., Dong, X., 2017. Crocin attenuates hemorrhagic shock-induced oxidative stress and organ injuries in rats. Environ. Toxicol. Pharmacol. 52 (6), 177–182.

Yang, R., Vernon, K., Thomas, A., Morrison, D., Qureshi, N., Van Way III, C.W., 2011. Crocetin reduces activation of hepatic apoptotic pathways and improves survival in experimental hemorrhagic shock. J. Parenter. Enteral Nutr. 35 (1), 107–113.

Yaribeygi, H., Taghi, M., Sahebkar, A., 2018. Crocin potentiates antioxidant defense system and improves oxidative damage in liver tissue in diabetic rats. Biomed. Pharmacol. 98 (2), 333–337.

Ying, L., Hofseth, L.J., 2007. An emerging role for endothelial nitric oxide synthase in chronic inflammation and cancer. Cancer Res. 67 (4), 1407–1410.

Yokel, R.A., 2000. The toxicology of aluminum in the brain: a review. Neurotoxicology 21 (5), 813–828.

Yousefsani, B.S., Mehri, S., Pourahmad, J., Hosseinzadeh, H., 2018. Crocin prevents sub-cellular organelle damage, proteolysis and apoptosis in rat hepatocytes: a justification for its hepatoprotection. Iran. J. Pharm. Res. 17 (2), 553–562.

Zheng, J., Zhou, Y., Li, Y., Xu, D.P., Li, S., Li, H.B., 2016. Spices for prevention and treatment of cancers. Nutrients 8 (8), 495.

CHAPTER 2

Ethnomedicinal and Traditional Usage of Saffron (*Crocus sativus* L.) in Turkey

MEHMET UGUR YILDIRIM • ERCUMENT OSMAN SARIHAN • KHALID MAHMOOD KHAWAR

INTRODUCTION

Saffron is an old crop plant of a region that lie across present day Turkey and Greece. Some researchers believe it that it is an autotriploid of *Crocus cartiwrightianus (Brighton, 1977, Ghaffari, 1986, Grilli Caiola 2004)*, whereas, others believe that it originated by an one-time natural cross between *Crocus cartwrightianus herb* and *Crocus thomasii Ten (Tsaftaris et al., 2011, Harpke et al., 2013)*. Therefore, this is not a new plant to this land (Turkey/Anatolia). There is another view that Kashmir and Iran were homeland of saffron (Winterhalter and Straubinger 2000) (Fig. 2.1)

Ancient Greeks named saffron as "Hercules' Blood", and they used it as incense and protective amulets in religious rituals (Kafi et al., 2018). Yellow color in the ancient world had been accepted as the goddess of fertility and the color of women (Barber, 1994). Saffron was named "A-Zupiru" which means queen of herbal drugs in Anatolia during Hittites period (Koç, 2012). The name of saffron (*Crocus sativus* L.) plant, which is almost the same in many languages of the world, derives from the Arabic word "Z'aferan" meaning yellow (Winterhalter and Straubinger, 2000; Ceylan, 2005). The plant is called as "koricos" in ancient Greek "crocum" in Roman period, "kurkum" in some parts of the Middle East, "kesar" in India, "koung" in Kashmir (Fernandez, 2004; Jan et al., 2014), "safran" in Turkish; "Gewurzsafran" in German; hay saffron, "korcom", in Hebrew (Ceylan, 2005), "krokos" in Greek (Kafi et al., 2018), "saffron" in French, "saffron" in English, "shafran" in Russian, "zafferano" in Italian, and "hong hua", "fan hong hua", or "zang hong hua" in China (Mousavi and Bathaie, 2011).

Saffron was cultivated in Izmir by the Byzantines. It was also known that it was grown in Safranbolu, Göynuk, Istanbul, Bolu, Izmir, Adana, Tokat, Sanliurfa, and Mardin during the Ottoman periods (Aktas Yasa, 2013). Saffron cultivation was carried out in Viransehir county of Sanliurfa about 100 years ago (Kafi et al., 2018). The fact that only 9705 kg of saffron was sold to England in 1858 during the Ottoman period is sufficient to explain the importance of saffron production in that period (Arslan, 2016).

The usage of plants for medicinal purposes is as old as the existence of humanity. Almost all archeological records from Turkey give an evidence to the ethnomedicinal uses of medicinal plants including saffron by the local people in their daily life since ancient times. Remains of saffron, yarrow (Achillea), groundsel (Senecio), rose marshmallow (Althaea), cornflower (Centaurea), hibiscus (Malva), and sea grape (Ephedra) have been discovered in an excavation of a 60,000-year-

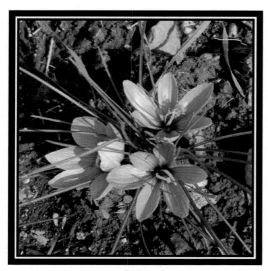

FIG. 2.1 Saffron flowers.

old tomb in caves of Sanidar locality (of Hakkâri province in the South-Eastern Turkey). It is accepted that these remains are the oldest data showing human relationship with plants (Arslan et al., 2015). It is well established that the Sumerians (4000 B.C.) and the Chinese (3750 B.C.) were the first to report medicinal uses of medicinal plants. The land that comprise present day Turkey has hosted many ancient civilizations. The oldest transcriptions in Central Anatolian land of Turkey have been found from the remains belonging to the Hittite dynasty. There are reports of use of 250 plants including saffron, mandrake, henbane, hellebore, poppy (opium poppy), mustard, thyme, tragacanth musilage, mint, pomegranate, fennel, and so forth in writings on tablets in various civilization that lived in Mesopotamian region.

About 600 AD, the people living on lands comprising present day Turkey used approximately 4000 medicinal plants (Keykubat, 2016). Similarly, people who lived during all civilizations (Hatti, Hittite, Urartu, Phrygian, Lydian, İonian, Caria, Lycian, Hellenic civilizations, Roman, Byzantine, Seljuk, and Ottoman Empire) on the present Turkey used saffron and other medicinal plants. Therefore, the use of medicinal plants in Turkish healing industry is not new (Baytop, 1999; Baser, 2009; Özturk, 2011; Altundag and Özturk, 2011).

The Materia Medica written by Dioscorides is considered the first pharmacopoeia in the world and renders great amount of such information (Keykubat, 2016). It is known that 50,000−70,000 plant species including saffron are used traditionally and in the modern medicinal systems (Polat and Satil, 2012). Number of identified and known species and taxa in Flora of Turkey has reached 12,054 in recent years with added new records and identifications. The number of endemic taxon has increased to 4207, and the rates of endemism have been determined as 35%−36% (Özhatay and Kultur, 2006; Özhatay et al., 2009, 2011; Davis et al.,1988; Guner et al., 2000; Paksoy et al., 2016).

Knowledge of the traditional uses of these herbal drugs has and will contribute to the development of the new drugs. Therefore, the number of scientific studies related to traditional and modern medicinal practices and usage of herbal drugs has increased dramatically (Dogan et.l., 2004; Kultur, 2007; Kargioglu et al., 2008; Ugulu et al., 2009; Ugulu and Baslar, 2010; Cakilcioglu and Turkoglu, 2010; Dogan et al., 2011; Polat and Satil, 2012; Heitmar et al., 2019).

The intrusion of saffron into the Turkish culture is seen everywhere, including food, medicine, literature, rituals, construction, cosmetic products, household appliances, musical instruments, firewood, pharmaceuticals, clothing, shelter, and other uses, either verbally or in writings and has been transferred from generation to generation. It has now become a part of ethnobotany in folk cultures of different regions (Balick and Cox, 1996; Ertug, 2004b; Kargioglu et al., 2010; Ugulu, 2011; Polat et al., 2012) among the young and elderly. Therefore, documenting the traditional ethnobotanical knowledge through ethnobotanical studies is important for conservation (Muthu et al., 2006).

The usage of saffron from past to present is summarized briefly in this chapter, starting from history to the usage of saffron in food as spices, cosmetics, perfumery, dyeing, handcrafts, and literature in Turkey. Second, some methodologies used for medical purposes in traditional folk medicine are described in nutshell.

SAFFRON IN TURKISH HISTORY

There is a controversy about origin of saffron, and many records suggest the origin of saffron in the mountainous regions of Anatolia, Greece, West Asia/Asia minor, Egypt, or Kashmir (Vavilov, 1951; Delgado et al., 2006; Salwee and Nehvi, 2013; Kafi et al., 2006). Saffron was previously cultivated in Babylon and Hulwan and has been used in Anatolia since the Hittites period (Ceylan, 2005). The details of archeological and historical records about the distribution of saffron and Crocus species and their emergence have been given by Grilli Caiola (2004).

Today saffron is cultivated in both hemispheres extending from Australia to Kashmir through Mediterranean region, Europe, and North America along tropical, subtropical, and temperate regions (Mathew, 1984; Davis et al., 1988; Koç, 2012; Kafi et al., 2018; Salwee and Nehvi, 2013). Saffron can be grown at a high altitude up to 2000 m above sea level as well as in favorable climatic conditions between 600 and 1700 m altitude (Delgado et. Al. 2006; Salwee and Nehvi, 2013).

The oldest work about pharmacy in Turkey is the Turkish translation of the book named "Mufredat-Ibni Baytar". However, "Edviye-i Mufrede" is the oldest book written in Turkish by Geredeli İshak bin Murad in 1389 (Ozbilgen, 2011). In terms of pharmacy, Turkish physicians benefited from the "el Kanun" of Ibn-i Sina (Avicenna) for many years. They also benefitted from the pharmacopoeias written by Anatolian physicians. They used drugs having herbal (including saffron), animal, mineral, or compound sources to prepare drugs (Ozbilgen, 2011). Saffron is included among medicinal plants in European Pharmacopoeia from the

many values and elements belonging to the Turkish Culture and has become a memory of written culture of Turkish people (Kaya, 2015). In classical Turkish poetry, the poets mostly mention flowers such as saffron (za-feran), rose, tulip, daffodil, jasmine, iris, and water lily. In classical Turkish poetry, saffron is mostly associated with the face of the beloved (Bayram, 2007; Incidagi, 2015), especially by Bolulu Muhammad Hanif who is one of the poets of the 18th century. The poet writes in one of his poems describing his beloved face resembling saffron color. Additionally, poets have mentioned about joyful moment effects and features of saffron in their poems. The word saffron has been mentioned five times in Mesnevi by Maulana Jalâluddin Rumi who is a world-famous thinker and Sufi. The word saffron has been used in Mesnevi with meanings of "on the way to Allah", convergence to Allah (beloved), and union with beloved (Allah), away from worldly desires (Incidagi, 2015).

Similar to classical Turkish poetry, saffron has also made its ways into Turkish folk riddles and rhymes.

Ethnomedicinal Usage of Saffron in Turkey

The traditional medicine practices have a great role in the emergence of modern medicine that uses intensive technological advances. The local and traditional uses of medicinal and aromatic plants are documented by means of the ethnobotanical studies (Muthu et al., 2006). Turkish people have used herbal remedies to treat diseases since a very long time. During the Ottoman Empire, 139 medicinal plants in raw form were exported for herbal use (Yesilada and Sezik, 2002). Ethnomedicinal studies in Turkey have been increasing since 1945 (Baytop, 1999; Altundag Çakir, 2017). Many studies have been carried out on ethnobotanic and medicinal plants used in traditional folk medicinal systems (Sezik et al., 1991, 1997; Ertug 2000, 2004a; Tuzlaci and Tolon, 2000; Ozgokçe and OzCelik, 2004; Simsek et al., 2004; Ozkan and Koyuncu, 2005; Akgul, 2008; Koyuncu et al., 2009; Cansaran and Kaya, 2010; Polat and Satil, 2010, 2012; Bulut, 2011; Çakilcioglu et al., 2011; Gunes and Ozhatay, 2011).

For example, during the Ottoman period, lady Hafsa Sultan, the mother of the Magnificent Suleyman, was ill. Royal physician Merkez Efendi prepared "Mesir" paste using saffron, anise, black cumin, mustard seeds, coconut, cardamom, black pepper, carnation, cumin, coriander, cinnamon, vanilla, ginger, cassia, and fennel for her treatment, and she recovered after using it. The king was very happy and ordered to distribute it among public as charity. This event is remembered every year in the name of Manisa Mesir Festival since 1539. This festival is protected since 2012 under UNESCO's list of intangible cultural heritage.

Saffron is mentioned in literary works such as Edviye-i Mufrede (in 14th century), Tabiatnâme (in 14th century) (Karasoy, 2009), Ebvâb-i Sifâ (in 14th century), Yâdigar (in 15th century), and Kemaliyye (in 16th century).

Saffron has been used to treat insomnia, head and eye aches, impotence, etc. (Pasayeva and Tekiner, 2014). The potential of saffron in reprieving the heart, strengthening the stomach, and relieving spleen and kidney pains was written in the Edviye-i Mufrede by İshak bin Murad in 16th century. At the same time, it has been mentioned that it relieves backache caused by cold, increases sexual power, provides brightness to the eye, and opens urinary tract (Canpolat and Onler, 2007; Pasayeva and Tekiner, 2014). Saffron, with anti-depressive properties, was also added to the pharmaceutical preparations for the treatment of melancholy patients in hospitals (called Darusshifa or bimaristan) during the Ottoman period.

Traditionally, offering zerde and rice with saffron in weddings and a meal with saffron twice a week in the boarding houses of the old İstanbul Schools was a custom (Onay, 1992; Ceylan, 2005; Kaya, 2015).

According to another medicine manuscript Ebvâb-i Sifâ, saffron and puhteç (it is prepared from grape juice and lamb meat boiled together and filtered) soups were taken together to treat eye infections and improve memory (Yaylagul, 2010; Pasayeva and Tekiner, 2014). It is also mentioned in the book "Kitabu'l-Muhimmat" written in the 15th century that if a mixture of milk and saffron extract is dripped in the eyes, it will prevent eye infections (Ozcelik, 2001; Pasayeva and Tekiner, 2014). Physician Ibn al-Sharif in 15th century has mentioned in his book "Yadigâr" that the tablets made up with saffron extracts could be used to prevented headaches. He also mentioned that the sherbet prepared with saffron could cure toothache, stomach coldness, backache, and other aches (Pasayeva and Tekiner, 2014). In the book named Kemâliyye, written in 16th century, the paste that was prepared with saffron, black cumin, ginger, carnation, and walnut could cure urinary incontinence. Saffron was also used in the paste known as chickpea paste used for increased sexual potency. In the book named Cerrahnâme written by Bursali Ali Munsi in the 18th century, saffron was effective in removing bumps and bruises that occur with impact or fall (Aciduman et al., 2008). It was also stated that saffron gives body vitality and refreshment, stimulates the nervous system that regulates sleep, resolves the heart palpitations, and cheers up the person. Saffron also helps regulating digestion, cures asthma and cough, and remedies ear aches. When chewed, it is useful for gums and also eyes. Nowadays, saffron is reported to be effective in the treatment of some types of cancer. Saffron is also an important appetite suppressant (Baytop, 1994; Onay, 1992; Ceylan, 2005; Kaya, 2015). Ethnobotanical studies performed today report that the saffron is among the herbal drugs sold for the purpose of attenuation in the Kirikhan county of Hatay (Altay et al., 2015).

In the province of Nevsehir, saffron flowers have been used as infusion for the purpose of suppressing appetite, for resolving stomach pain, as skin protection, and as a diuretic (Akgul et al., 2016). Saffron tea is prepared and used for its stimulant effect and for healing cough, bronchitis, and asthma in the Erzincan province (Korkmaz et al., 2016). In addition, it is stated that saffron beautifies the skin color and gives vitality. It cures splenic swelling and provides breech and uterine pain relief; it is also stated that saffron helps to remove fungi in the skin (Cicek, 2018).

Daruhifa (hospitals) served as important institutions for the protection and treatment of both human and animals. Tercume-i Baytarnâme and Haza Kitâbu Baytârname are books about veterinary practices in the Ottoman period. In particular, there is information about a number of diseases and treatments in horses which could be treated using saffron (Yigit et al., 2013).

It is mentioned that if saffron is overused, it causes headache. It is also stated that if added into wine, it gives feelings of rapid drunkenness (Canpolat and Önler, 2007; Bayat, 2007; Pasayeva and Tekiner, 2014). Saffron has a toxic effect when used in high doses. The use of 10–20 g can lead to death in adults. The daily dose should not exceed 1.5 g. It causes severe bleeding and miscarriage of pregnant women in high doses. In particular, kidney damage is frequently reported. Excessive vomiting and sweating can be observed. Disorderly behavior and thinking can be observed (Arslan, 2016).

REFERENCES

Aciduman, A., Er, U., Belen, D., 2008. Neurosurgery related sections included in the surgical treatise by Ali Munsi of bursa: a work from the late Ottoman era. Turk Nörosirurji Dergisi cilt 18 (1), 5–15.

Akiniz, S., 2017. Ortaçag Akdeniz'inde Kirmizinin İzinden (In the way of red in the medieval mediterranean). In: 2nd. International Mediterranean Art Symposium 10–12 May, pp. 231–239.

Aktas Yasa, A., 2013. Kulturel Zenginlikleri ile Göynuk. (Göynuk with cultural Wealth), Göynuk El Sanatlari Paneli ve Çalistayi Bildirileri (2), pp. 17–46 (Aktas Yasa A., Göynuk with its cultural richness. (Göynuk with cultural Wealth) Göynuk Handicrafts Panel and Workshop Proceedings) In Turkish.

Altundag, E., Özturk, M., 2011. Ethnomedicinal studies on the plant resources of east Anatolia Turkey. Procedia Soc. Behav. Sci. 19, 756–777.

Altundag Çakir, E., 2017. A comprehensive review on ethnomedicinal utilization of gymnospermae in Turkey. Eurasian J. For. Sci. 5 (1), 35–47.

Arslan, N., Baydar, H., Kizil, S., Karik, U., Sekeroglu, N., Gumusçu, A., 2015. Tibbi Bitkiler Uretiminde Degismeler Ve Yeni Arayislar; Vİİİ. Turkiye Ziraat Muhendisligi Teknik Kongresi, Ankara.

Arslan, N., Özer, A.S., Akdemir, R., 2007. Cultivation of saffron (Crocus sativus L.) and effects of organic fertilizers to the flower yield. In: International Medicinal and Aromatic Plants Conference on Culinary Herbs, vol. 826, pp. 237–240.

Arslan, N., 2016. Penceremden Tibbi Bitkiler: safran uzerine Dusunceler. Turkiye Tohumcular Birligi Dergsi. Turktob dergisi 20, 66–69.

Altay, V., Karahan, F., Sarcan, Y.B., İlçim, A., 2015. An ethnobotanical research on wild plants sold in Kirikhan county (Hatay/Turkey) herbalists and local markets. Biol. Divers. Conserv. 8/2, 81–91.

Atasoy, F. (Ed.), 2016. Yukselen İpek Yolu 3. Cilt; İpek Yolu'nda Kultur Sanat. Turk Yurdu Yayinlari, Ankara. Ss: 480.

Ayverdi, İ., 2006. Misalli Buyuk Turkçe Sözluk, Kubbealti Lugati, İ-İİİ, İkinci Baski, İstanbul: Kubbealti Nesriyati.

Akgul, A., 1993. Baharat Bilimi ve Teknolojisi. Damla Matbaacilik ve Tic, Konya, Turkiye, p. 541.

Akgul, G., 2008. Local names and ethnobotanical features of some wild plants of Çildir (Ardahan) and its vicinity. Herb J. Syst. Bot. 14, 75–88.

Akgul, G., Yilmaz, N., Celep, A., Celep, F., Çakilcioglu, U., 2016. Ethnobotanical purposes of plants sold by herbalists and folk bazaars in the center of Cappadocia (Nevsehir, Turkey). Indian J. Tradit. Knowl. 15 (1), 103–108.

Balick, M.J., Cox, P.A., 1996. Plants, People, and Culture: The Science of Ethnobotany. Scientific American Library, New York, pp. 1–24.

Bakir, A., 2005. Ortacag İslam Dunyasinda Tekstil Sanayi Giyim Kusam ve Moda. Bizim Buro Basimevi, Ankara.

Baser, K.H.C., 2009. Most widely traded plant drugs of Turkey (Chapter 46). In: De Silva, T., et al. (Eds.), Traditional and Alternative Medicine-Research & Policy Perspectives. NAM-Daya Publ. House, Delhi-India, pp. 443–454.

Barber, E.W., 1994. Women's Work –The First 20.000 Years Women, Cloth and Society in Early Times. WW Norton&Company Inc., New York, pp. 101–126.

Batur, M., Binboga, G., Binboga, H., Kucukahmetler, O., Yardimci, E.K., Çolak, A., Kocabas, A., 2013. İzmir Ekoturizm Rehberi, Ege Ormancilik Arastirma Enstitusu Mudurlugu. İzmir Ecotourism Guide, Ege Forestry Research Institute 69 (6), 284. InTurkish.

Bayat, A.H., 2007. Kemaliyye - Erken Anadolu Turkçesi ile Yazilmis Bir Tip Risalesi. Merkez Efendi Geleneksel Tip Dernegi, İstanbul, pp. 14—30.

Bayram, Y., 2007. Klâsik Turk Sirinde Duygularin Dili: Cicekler, Turkish studies international periodical for the languages. Lit. Hist. Turk. 2/4, 209—219. Fall.

Baytop, T., 1994. Turkçe Bitki Adlari Sözlugu. Turk Dil Kurumu Yay, Ankara.

Baytop, T., 1999. Turkiye'de Bitkiler ile Tedavi. Nobel Tip Kitabevleri; Bitkibilim, Sifali Bitkiler,.İİ. baski., Nobel Tip Kitapevleri Ltd. Sti. Tayf Ofset Baski, 480 pp. İstanbul.

Bilgin, A., 2002. In: Koz, S. (Ed.), Seçkin mekânda seçkin damaklar: Osmanli sarayinda beslenme aliskanliklari. (15.-17. Yuzyil). Yemek kitabi tarih halk bilimi edebiyat, İstanbul: Kitabevi.

Brighton, C.A., 1977. Cytology of *Crocus sativus* and its allies (Iridaceae). Plant Syst. Evol. 128, 137—157.

Bulut, G., 2011. Folk medicinal plants of Silivri (İstanbul Turkey). Marmara Pharm. J. 15, 25—29.

Çakilcioglu, U., Khatun, S., Turkoglu, İ., Hayta, S., 2011. Ethnopharmacological survey of medicinal plants in Maden (Elazig-Turkey). J. Ethnopharmacol. 137, 469—486.

Cakilcioglu, U., Turkoglu, I., 2010. An ethnobotanical survey of medicinal plants in Sivrice (Elazığ-Turkey). J Ethnopharmacol 132 (1), 165—175. https://doi.org/10.1016/j.jep.2010.08.017.

Cansaran, A., Kaya, Ö.F., 2010. Contributions of the ethnobotanical investigation carried out in Amasya county of Turkey (Amasya center, baglarustu, bogakoy and Vermis villages; yassiçal and ziyaret towns). Biol. Divers. Conserv. 3, 97—116.

Canpolat, M., Önler, Z., 2007. İshak bin Murad - Edviye-i Mufrede. Turk Dil Kurumu Yayinlari, Ankara, p. 32.

Ceylan, Ö., 2005. Tasranin Altin Çiçegi Safran, Osmanli Tarihi Arastirmalari XXVİ, Prof. Dr Mehmet Çavusoglu'na armagan İİ. İstanbul Kultur Universitesi Fen-Edebiyat Fakultesi, İstanbul, pp. 147—162.

Celik, M.F., 2015. Klasik sirde badem (almond in the classical poetry). Divan Edebiyati Arastirmalari Dergisi 14, 47—66.

Celik, S., Cankurt, H., Dogan, C., 2010. Safran ilavesinin sade dondurmanin bazi özelliklerine etkisi (The effect of Saffron Addition on some properties of plane ice-cream). Gida 35 (1), 1—7.

Cicek, H., 2018. Celaluddin es- Suyuti'nin el- Makamatu'l-Miskiyye ve el-Makamatu'l-Verdiyye'de Konusturdugu Guzel Kokular ve Cicekler, SDU Ilahiyat Fak. Dergisi 40, 147—172.

Davis, P.H., Mill, R., Tan, K., 1988. Flora of Turkey and the East Aegean İslands, vol. 10. Edinburgh University Press, Edinburgh, 278 pp.

Delgado, M.C., Aramburu, A.Z., Diaz-Marta, G.L.A., 2006. The Chemical Composition of Saffron: Color Taste and Aroma İmprenta Junquera S.L. Albacete, pp. 1—213.

Demirgul, F., 2018. Çadirdan saraya Turk Mutfagi (Turkish cuisine from tent to place) uluslararasi Turk Dunyasi Turizm Arastirmalari Dergisi. Int. J. Turk. World Tour. Stud. 3 (1), 105—125.

Dogan, Y., Baslar, S., Mert, H.H., Ay, G., 2004. The use of wild edible plants in western and central Anatolia (Turkey). Econ. Bot. 58 (4), 684—690.

Dogan, Y., Ugulu, İ., Durkan, N., Unver, M.C., Mert, H.H., 2011. Determination of some ecological characteristics and economical importance of *Vitex agnus-castus*. EurAsian J. BioSci. 5, 10—18.

Dolen, E., 1992. Tekstil Tarihi. Marmara Universitesi Teknik Egitim Fakultesi Yayinlari, İstanbul.

Ertug, F., 2000. An ethnobotanical study in Central Anatolia (Turkey). J. Econ. Bot. 54, 155—182.

Ertug, F., 2004a. Wild edible plants of the Bodrum area (Mugla, Turkey). Turk. J. Bot. 28, 161—174.

Ertug, F., 2004b. Etnobotanik çalismalari ve Turkiye'de yeni açilimlar. Kebikeç 18, 181—187.

Faroqhi, S., Neumann, C.K., 2006. Soframiz Nur, Hanemiz Mamur. Osmanlı maddi kültüründe yemek ve barınak (Çeviren: Zeynep Yelçe). İstanbul kitap Yayinevi, İstanbul, p. 38.

Fernandez, J.A., 2004. Biology, biotechnology and biomedicine of Saffron. Recent Res. Dev. Plant. Sci. 2, 127—159.

Finlay, V., 2007. "Renkler —Boya Kutusunda Yolculuklar"(Cev. K.Emiroglu). Dost Yayinevi, Ankara, 190- 223, 210-212.

Ghaffari, S.M., 1986. Cytogenetic studies of cultivated *Crocus sativus* (Iridaceae). Plant Syst. Evol . 53, 199—204.

Grilli Caiola, M., 2004. Saffron reproductive biology. Acta Hortic. 650, 25—37.

Guler, S., 2010. Turkish kitchen culture; eating and drinking habits, Dumlupinar Univ. Sos. Bil. Dergisi 26, 24—30.

Gunes, F., Özhatay, N., 2011. An ethnobotanical study from Kars (Eastern) Turkey. Biol. Divers. Conserv. 4, 30—41.

Guner, A., Özhatay, N., Ekim, T., Baser, K.H.C., 2000. Flora of Turkey and the East Aegean İslands, vol. 11. Edinburgh University Press, Edinburgh, UK.

Harpke, D., Meng, S., Kerndorff, H., Rutten, T., Blattner, F.R., 2013. Phylogeny of Crocus (Iridaceae) based on one chloroplast and two nuclear loci: ancient hybridization and chromosome number evolution. Mol. Phylogenet. Evol. 66, 617—627.

Hazar, M., 2006. Mardin "Kiziltepe-Bozhöyuk"yöresinde Beden İsaretleri (Tattoos in Mardin "Kiziltepe-Bozhöyuk"). SBArD 8, 293—305.

Heitmar, R., Brown, J., Kyrou, I., 2019. Review saffron (*Crocus sativus* L.) in Ocular diseases: a narrative review of the existing evidence from clinical studies. Nutrients 11, 649. https://doi.org/10.3390/nu11030649.

Isin, P.M., 2010. Osmanli Mutfak Sözlugu. Kitap Yayinevi, İstanbul.

Incidagi, A.S., 2015. Mevlana'nin Mesnevi'sinde yer alan itki e meyvelerin tasavvuf dunyasindaki embolik anlamlari. Yuksek Lisas tezi: Selçuk niversitesi, Mevlana Arastirmalari enstitusu Mevlana ve Mevlevilik Arastirmalari Anabilim Dali, p. 403.

Ingram, J.S., 1969. Saffron *Crocus sativus* L. Trop. Sci. 11, 177—184.

Irgin, S., 2017. Boya ve Dogal Boya Anlatisi (Dyes and Natural Dyes). In: International Mediterranean Art Symposium 10-12 May, 2nd, pp. 301—305.

Jan, S., Wani, A.A., Kamili, A.N., Kashtwari, M., 2014. Distribution, chemical composition and medicinal immportance of Saffron (*Crocus sativus* L.). Afr. J. Plant Sci. 8 (12), 537−545.

José Bagur, M., Alonso Salinas, G.L., Jiménez-Monreal, A.M., Chaouqi, S., Llorens, S., Martínez-Tomé, M., Alonso, G.L., 2017. Saffron: an old medicinal plant and a potential novel functional food. Molecules 23 (1), 30.

Kafi, M., Kamili, A.N., Husaini, A.M., Özturk, M., Altay, V., 2018. An expensive spice saffron (Crocus sativus L.): In: Özturk, M., Hakem, K.R., Ashraf, M., Ahmad, M.S.A. (Eds.), A Case Study from Kashmir, İran and Turkey. Global Perspectives on Underutilized Crops. Springer, Switzerland, ISBN 978-3-319-77776-4.

Kafi, M., Koocheki, A., Rashed, M.H., Nassiri, M., 2006. Saffron (*Crocus sativus*) Production and Processing. Science Publishers, United States of America, pp. 1−221.

Karadag, R., 2007. Doğal Boyamacılık, Geleneksel El Sanatları ve Mağazalar İşletme Müdürlüğü 65 Kimyasal Maddelerle Emprenye Edilebilme Özellikleri". Pamukkale Üniversitesi Mühendislik Bilimleri Dergisi 2 (2), 147−156.

Karademir, F., 2007. Halk bilmecelerinde renklerin kullanim sikligi ve islevselligi, (The usage and role of colors in folk riddles), Elektron. Sos. Bil. Dergisi 6 (21), 192−211.

Karasoy, Y., 2009. Eski Oguz Türkcesiyle Yazılmıs Bir Tip Kitabı Tabiatname (A Medical Book Written in Old Oghuz Turkish). Palet Yayınları. In Turkish.

Kargioglu, M., Cenkci, S., Serteser, A., Evliyaoglu, N., Konuk, M., Kok, M.S., Bagci, Y., 2008. An ethnobotanical survey of inner-west Anatolia, Turkey. Hum. Ecol. 36, 763−777.

Kargioglu, M., Cenkci, S., Serteser, A., Konuk, M., Vural, G., 2010. Taraditional uses of wild plants in the Middle aegean region of Turkey. Hum. Ecol. 38, 429−450.

Kaya, B.A., 2015. Klasik turk Sirinde Sifali Bitkiler Uzerine Bir Deneme Divan Edebiyati Arastirmalari Dergisi, vol. 15, pp. 263−314.

Kiliç, Y., 2018. Antik Çag'da Boya ve Boyamacilik. Selçuk Universitesi, Sosyal Bilimler Enstitusu, Arkeoloji Anabilimdali, Konya, p. 245. Yuksek lisans tezi.

Koç, H., 2012. Safran Yetistiriciligi. Bilge Kultur Sanat Yayin Dagitim San. ve Ltd., İstanbul, p. 504. Sti. No.

Koyuncu, O., Yaylaci, O.K., Tokur, S., 2009. A study on Geyve (Sakarya) and its environs in terms of ethnobotanical aspects. Herb J. Syst. Bot. 16, 123−142.

Korkmaz, M., Karakus, S., Özcelik, H., Selvi, S., 2016. An enthnobotanical study on medicinal plants in Erzincan, Turkey. Indian J. Tradit. Knowl. 15 (2), 192−202.

Keykubat, B., 2016. Tibbi Aromatik Bitkiler ve İyi Yasam, İzmir Ticaret Borsasi. Ar-Ge Mudurlugu yayini, İzmir.

Kuban, D., 2009. Turkiye'de Kentsel Koruma. Tarih Vakfi Yurt Yayinlari, İstanbul.

Kultur, S., 2007. Medicinal plants used in kirklareli province (Turkey). J. Ethnopharmacol. 111, 341−364.

Leung, A.Y., 1980. Encyclopedia of Common Natural Ingredients in Food, Drugs and Cosmetics. Wiley, New York, USA.

Mathew, B., 1984. Crocus. In: Davis, P.H. (Ed.), Flora of Turkey and the East Aegean İslands, vol. 8. Edinburgh University Press, Edinburgh, pp. 413−438.

Mousavi, S.Z., Bathaie, S.Z., 2011. Historical uses of saffron: İdentifying potential new avenues for modern research. Nat. Prod. Indian J. 7 (4), 174−180.

Muthu, C., Ayyanar, M., Raja, N., İgnacimuthu, S., 2006. Medicinal plants used by traditional healers in Kancheepuram county of Tamil Nadu, India. J. Ethnobiol. Ethnomed. 2, 43.

Onay, A.T., 1992. Eski Turk Edebiyatinda Mazmunlar Ve İzahi, Hazirlayan: Cemal Kurnaz. Turkiye Diyanet Vakfi Yay, Ankara.

Oral, M.Z., 2008. In: Sabri Koz, M. (Ed.), Selçuk Devri Yemekleri ve Ekmekleri,. Yemek Kitabi İ, Cilt İ. Kitabevi Yayinlari, İstanbul, pp. 18−34.

Oguz, B., 2002. Turkiye Halkinin Kultur Kökenleri 1, vol. 2. Anadolu Aydinlanma Vakfi Yayinlari, Baski, İstanbul, pp. 723−777.

Özbilgen, E., 2011. Butun Yönleriyle Osmanli Adab'i Osmaniyeye. İz yayimcilik, İstanbul, p. 488.

ÖzCelik, S., 2001. Kitab'ul Muhimmat. Ataturk Kultur Merkezi Baskanligi Yayinlari, Ankara, pp. 46−47.

Özdogan, Y., Isik, N., 2007. Geleneksel Turk mutfaginda serbet, 38. In: International Congress of Asian and North African Studies, Ataturk Kultur. Dil ve Tarih Yuksek Kurumu, Ankara, pp. 1059−1077.

Özgökçe, F., Ozcelik, H., 2004. Ethnobotanical aspects of some taxa in East Anatolia (Turkey). Econ. Bot. 58, 697−704.

Özhatay, N., Kultur, S., 2006. Check-list of additional taxa to the supplement Flora of Turkey 3. Turk. J. Bot. 30, 281−316.

Özhatay, N., Kultur, S., Aslan, S., 2009. Check-list of additional taxa to the supplement Flora of Turkey 4. Turk. J. Bot. 33, 191−226.

Özhatay, N., Kultur, S., Gurdal, M.B., 2011. Check-list of additional taxa to the supplement Flora of Turkey 5. Turk. J. Bot. 35, 589−624.

Özkan, A.M.G., Koyuncu, M., 2005. Traditional medicinal plants used in pinarbasi area (Kayseri − Turkey). Turk. J. Pharm. Sci. 2, 63−82.

Özturk, M., 2011. Ethnobotany-time for a new relationship-case study from Turkey. In: 11th National Meeting of Plant Scientists (NMPS) and 2nd İntern. Conf. of Plant Scientists (İCPS-2011), 22−24 Feb. GC University Lahore-Pakistan.

Pakalin, M.Z., 1993. *Osmanli Tarih Deyimleri ve Sözlugu*, 3c. MEB Yayinlari, İstanbul.

Paksoy, M.Y., Selvi, S., Savran, A., 2016. Ethnopharmacological survey of medicinal plants in Ulukisla (Nigde-Turkey). J. Herb. Med. 1−7.

Pasayeva, L., Tekiner, H., 2014. Turk-İslâm tibbinda safranin yeri. Lokman Hekim J. 4 (3), 11−15.

Perez, A., 1995. Analisis biometrico de los cormos de azafran de distintas poblaciones de la provincial de Albacete. Trabajo fin de carrera Ingenieria Tecnica Agricola. Universidad Castilla −La Mancha, Albacete, Espana.

Polat, R., Çakiloglu, U., Ertug, F., Satil, F., 2012. An evaluation of ethnobotanical studies in eastern Anatolia. Biol. Divers. Conserv. 5/2, 23—40.

Polat, R., Satil, F., 2010. Havran ve Burhaniye (Balikesir) Yörelerinde Etnobotanik Arastirmalari, TUBA Kultur Envant. Dergisi 8, 65—100.

Polat, R., Satil, F., 2012. An ethnobotanical survey of medicinal plants in Edremit Gulf (Balikesir —Turkey). J. Ethnopharmacol. 139, 626—641.

Razavi, B.M., Hosseinzadeh, H., Abnous, K., İmenshahidi, M., 2014. Protective effect of crocin on diazinon induced vascular toxicity in subchronic exposure in rat aorta exvivo. Drug Chem. Toxicol. 37 (4), 378—383.

Salwee, Y., Nehvi, F.A., 2013. Saffron as a valuable spice: a comprehensive review. Afr. J. Agric. Res. 8 (3), 234—242.

Samanci, Ö., 2006. 19. Yuzyilda Osmanli Saray Mutfagi" Yemek ve Kultur, Sayi 4. Çiya Yayinlari, İstanbul.

Sevuktekin, A.M., Onat, G.F., Ozturk, E.F., 1997. Ottoman Women's Clothing. Is Bank Publications (ın Turkish), Ankara.

Sezik, E., Tabata, M., Yesilada, E., Honda, G., Goto, K., İkeshiro, Y., 1991. Traditional medicine in Turkey ifolk medicine in North-east Anatolia. J. Ethnopharmacol. 35, 191—196.

Sezik, E., Yesilada, E., Tabata, M., Honda, G., Takaishi, Y., Fujita, T., Tanaka, T., Takeda, Y., 1997. Traditional medicine in Turkey Vİİİ. Folk medicine in east Anatolia; erzurum, erzincan, agri, igdir provinces. J. Econ. Bot. 51, 195—211.

Surucuoglu, M.S., Celik, L., 2003. Pekmez. Turk Mutfak Kulturu Uzerine Arastirmalar. Turk Halk Kulturunu Arastirma ve Tanitma Vakfi Yayinlari Yayin No: 31. Ankara, pp. 22—23.

Simsek, İ., Aytekin, F., Yesilada, E., Yildirimli, S., 2004. An ethnobotanical survey of the Beypazari, Ayas, and Gudul county towns of Ankara province (Turkey). Econ. Bot. 58, 705—720.

Tsaftaris, A., Pasentsis, K., Makris, A., Darzentas, N., Polidoros, A., Kalivas, A., Argiriou, A., 2011. The study of the E-class SEPALLATA3-like MADS-box genes in wild-type and mutant flowers of cultivated saffron crocus (*Crocus sativus* L.) and its putative progenitors. Plant Phys 168, 1675—1684.

Tuzlaci, E., Tolon, E., 2000. Turkish folk medicinal plants, part İİİ: sile (İstanbul). Fitoterapia 71, 673—685.

Ugulu, İ., 2011. Traditional ehnobotanical knowledge abaut medicinal plants used for external therapies in Alasehir, Turkey. Int. J. Med. Aromatic Plants. ISSN: 2249-4340 vol (2), 101—106.

Ugulu, İ., Baslar, S., 2010. The determination and fidelity level of medicinal plants used to make traditional Turkish salves. J. Altern. Complement. Med. 16 (3), 313—322.

Ugulu, I., Baslar, S., Yorek, N., Dogan, Y., 2009. The investigation and quantitative ethnobotanical evaluation of medicinal plants used around İzmir province, Turkey. J. Med. Plants Res. 3 (5), 345—367.

Vavilov, N.I., 1951. The Origin, Variation, Immunity and Breeding of Cultivated Palnts. The Cronica Botanica, Co., Waltham, Mass.

Winterhalter, P., Straubinger, M., 2000. Saffron: renewed interest in an ancient spice. Food Rev. Int. 16, 39—59.

Witcombe, C., 2017. Women in the Aegean Minoan Snake Goddess. arthistoryresources.net.

Yaylagul, Ö., 2010. Ebvâb-i Sifâ - Metin Dilbilimsel Bir İnceleme. Köksav, Ankara, pp. 119—141, 2010.

Yazir, M.B., 1989. Kalem Guzeli (Ceviren: Ugur Derman). Gaye Maatbacilik, Ankara.

Yesilada, E., Sezik, E., 2002. A Survey on the Traditional Medicine in Turkey: Semi-quantitative Evaluation of the Results. In: Ethnomedicine, Pharmacognosy, Singh, V.K., Govil, J.N. (Eds.), Recent Progress in Medicinal Plants, Vol.VII. Gurdip Singh, Research Periodicals - Book Publishing House, New Delhi.

Yildirim, C., 2017. Bereketlilik kultu, safran ve Ekofeminist Dusunce (fertility Cult, saffron and Eco-Feminism). In: 2nd.International Mediterranean Art Symposium 10-12 May, pp. 66—72.

Yigit, A., Izmirli, S., Yasar, A., 2013. An evaluation on joint applications in the field of human medicine and veterinary medicine in *"Haza Kitâbu Baytarnâme"* and *"Tercume-i Baytarnâme"*. Lokman Hekim J. 3 (1), 7—14.

Zor, Z., 2017. Kitap Sanatlarinda Kullanilan Dogal Boya ve Murekkep (natural dyes ink used in book arts). In: 2nd. International Mediterranean Art Symposium 10—12 May, pp. 272—276.

flooding. Generally, saffron is not involved in planting rotation as a field is used for three to five consecutive years. At the end of the third to fifth year in June, the corms are removed from the soil and are kept until next planting time in new fields after the second half of June to October or November (Anonymous, 2019a, b, Pers. Obs 2019).

The farmers also avoid selection of soil previously used for cultivation of other crops to avoid risks of relatively diverse pests, including rodents, insects, plant mites, diseases such as corm rot, and weeds as phytosanitary measures. The farmers prefer to plant saffron corms in fields that have been left fallow at least for one to 2 years. The soil is plowed a number of times until the time of planting. It is important that the soil is thoroughly cleaned from seeds because once the corms germinate, weed control is very difficult. After germination of corms, the farmers clean weeds from the saffron fields using manual hand-held small tractor plows or manually. Weeding a field is necessary to improve yield by protecting the corms by going into negative competition with weeds and destroy plants that act as hiding and breeding place of fungus and insect pests. The farmers avoid to mechanically remove weeds when the crop is in the field to avoid damage to the germinating saffrons and prefer manual weeding. Weeding operation continues throughout year very carefully to avoid growth of perennial woody bushes. Last weeding operation is carried out 15–30 days before corm planting (Pers Observations).

As saffron corms are planted every 3–4 years and can be extended for a few more years depending on the health and frequency of the plants, extreme care is given to the fields before planting. There is no chance to replant corms every year. The planted corms face number of biotic and abiotic stresses underground (Anonymous, 2019b).

Multiple approaches are applied to prepare the soil. Some farmers use mini tractors with rakes and a vibrating cylinder to loosen up soil. Generally, the farmers add 25–35 kg/ha of organic manure with multiple plowing. The farmers do not use chemical fertilizers. However, some farmers may also use these fertilizers.

The next year, saffron cultivation should be carried out in August at the earliest or in early September.

PLANTING DEPTH AND SPACING

Saffron is multiplied by corms, which are modified body structures with buds on them in the form of rings. It is well established that corm planting depth has important significant impacts on the saffron yield,

therefore, most of the farmers prefer to plant saffron at depth of 10–15 cm or more in fields having 15% –20% slanting slopes, to avoid water accumulation in the root zones. The fields are cleaned of weeds and remanured in the summer after cleaning fields of weeds. The fields are then harrowed and given manure once again before planting the corms. The fields are protected from fast blowing winds in the area by planting and erecting wind barriers. Saffron corms are resistant to summer droughts and are frost resistant. Corms prefer dry and sunny weather, especially during the flowering period. Precipitation in this period is not desired as it significantly reduces the quality of the product. Saffron flowers are very sensitive to frost. Cool and humid weather in the vegetation period adversely affects the development of the plant.

The saffron corms are dug up from the fields in summer months, from late June to August. The corms are stored in heaps or split layers. This practice protects the corms from getting infected and makes it easy for cleaning and discarding diseased corms.

Insufficiently decayed and fermented manure is avoided as this can burn and damage corms. To have a high saffron yield in the first year, the diameter of saffron corms should be at least 15–20 mm as was determined in the studies carried out at Eskişehir Transit Zone Agricultural Research Institute. As the corm diameter increases, saffron stigma yield also increases because of the increased number of flower induction per plant. Depending on corm size, they are planted at the rate of 150–600 kg da. The yield of saffron stigma varies from year to year. In a field that has been used for 3 years, yield is 1 kg per decare, or, on average, 80,000–120,000 flowers yield 5 kg of fresh weight and 1 kg of dry product (Anonymous a,b,c).

The farmers plow the land so many times and break the soil surface or any crust formation. Saffron corms are planted in rows with a plant-to-plant distance of 10–20 cm and row-to-row distance of 8–10 cm. This can vary depending on the farmer. These corms grow well under dry summers with mild temperature. The plant can survive the cold winters and can withstand snow under −10°C for a short period of time. However, it requires irrigation if it is not grown in humid climates with an annual precipitation of 1000–1500 mm. There is a need to irrigate fields through sprinklers, drip irrigation system, or other appropriate irrigation systems if the precipitation is less than 1000 mm per annum.

Thereafter, the corms develop roots, and the mother corm induce new daughter corms. Depending on the diameter of corms, they induce 1–12 flowers on each corm. There are large number of components in secondary metabolites of saffron plants such as carotenoids (like α- and β-carotene, lycopene, and zeaxanthin, along with water-soluble C_2O apocarotenoid and its ester derivatives and the trans crocetin [β-D-digentibiosyl] ester), monoterpenoids, flavonoids, and anthocyanins (Lozano et al., 1999; Carmona et al., 2006a,b,c; Rychener et al., 1984). The female organ of the flower consists of an ovary, which is a long pale yellow—colored tube-like structure. The male part of the plant or stigma is made up of three red-colored 2.5- to 3-cm-long filamentous structures. Sometimes, stigmas could get an elongation of upto 5 cm. The stigmas contain coloring pigments (crocin), odorant (safranal), and bitter taste—giving compounds (picrocrocin) (Fernandez, 2004; Grilli Caiola, 2004).

As the corms germinate, they give rise to 6 -7 grass-type leaves from each corm which reach a length of 20—55 cm and remain on the plant from October to June. The farmers take care of watering the crop in the absence of natural precipitation during fall before the flowering season. Rain at the time of flowering affects and mars the quality of flowers and hence the stigmas negatively. To avoid risk of rain or snow fall, the farmers prefer to harvest flowers in the first week after the start of flowering. It is preferable to hand harvest saffron to avoid any damaging due to mechanized farming. Saffron usually begin to bloom in mid-October and lasts for 15—25 days, and under exceptional conditions, it may continue for ~30 days. The farmers hire family members or temporary laborers to carefully pluck flowers in baskets. The farmers prefer to harvest each morning by selecting unopened flowers and cutting them below corolla using a forceps or pair of sharp scissors. A female worker can isolate 50—60 g of stigma per hour from the flower. Considering all these points, it is easily understood that the cultivation of saffron is very laborious. The low yield of saffron and the demand for intensive labor are among the main reasons why saffron stigmas make the most expensive spice in the world (Tammaro, 1990, 1999 Pers. com. With Prof. Dr. K.M. Khawar 2019).

These are dried gently in shade without damaging them during the process. Saffron has a short flowering season; therefore, the farmers are very cautious toward this end to avoid any untoward incident such as prolonged rain or snowfall. Precipitation during flowering results in reducing the quality of saffron. Plucking saffron flowers for harvest is a time-consuming, laborious, and tiring job (Anonymous a, b, c). Depending on the expertise, an average laborer harvests 7—17 kg of saffron flowers per day. Generally, the field labors

prefer to harvest in a sitting position on foot or using a small stool. Mechanical harvest of flowers is not preferred as it catches dirt that affects and influences saffron quality. Catching dirt harms harvested flowers and could damage stigmas. A female worker can pluck 50—60 gr of flowers per hour with a flower yield of 80—90 kg/da (Pers. observations 2019).

It has been observed that the stigma yield is directly related to the corm size. Moreover, the maximum yield is generally obtained at lower altitudes, away from fast moving winds in the area.

Many experiments have been carried out in different parts of Turkey (Koc, 2012a,b) such as Ankara, Eskisehir, Hatay, Istanbul, Izmir, Igdir, Tekirdag, Tokat, Siirt, Sanliurfa Igdir, Sanliurfa, and Tekirdag to understand the adaptation problem of saffron.

After corm harvest in June, saffron enters a long period of sleep in the summer under Turkish conditions. Turkish saffron flowers in late autumn in October to early winter in November and is influenced by temperature and atmospheric humidity and precipitation during flower induction. The harvesting time of the saffron flowers usually coincides with the climatic conditions of year and may sometimes shift to the first half of November. The harvest time of flowers in Safranbolu is between 20—25 October and 10—15 November, in general. Harvest takes 15—20 days. The harvest of saffron is very tiring and is usually done in two stages. The farmer has to take quick decisions to collect unopened flowers in the early morning on nonrainy days. Saffron flowers are carefully collected in baskets by cutting with pair of scissors. Collection of opened flowers reduces the quality of saffron. These unopened flowers or buds are brought back to a clean, ventilated, and dry place to obtain stigma and ovaries by cutting near the place where the crest pieces are separated using a small pair of scissors. The quality of saffron is determined by the length of stigma. The smaller stigmas are priced more than longer stigmas. Drying of stigmas is carried out at 50—80°C for 30—35 min. There is a risk of burning stigmas if the care is not taken. Sometimes, the stigmas are dried at a cool dry shady place away from the breeze (Pers. Observation). At other times, the farmers encapsulate stigmas with bee wax to increase their shelf life. However, the practice is counted as adulteration and reduces the quality and price of saffron in international market. In this way, the yield increases slightly, but the quality is very low. This traditional but poor drying technique has become the most effective factor in the loss of Turkish saffron in world trade, as the buyers consider this as adulteration and cut the imports by turning to other countries. All saffron produced in Turkey are sold without any brand name that quality assurance. Instead of collecting the dried stigmas in dark-colored bottles and keeping them at cool and dark places free of moisture, the saffron are collected and marketed in transparent glass bottles and resold in grams. There is a need to give importance to packing material for retail and wholesale markets. Some local traders contaminate saffron stigmas with safflower stigmas or sell them singly as local saffron, Aspir (local name for safflower) saffron. Some traders also trade turmeric powder as saffron pollen (Pers. Observation).

Soon after flowering, the mother corm enters into generative phase by producing new daughter corms or cormlets under Turkish conditions throughout winter. These daughter corms grow up gradually by consuming nutrients from the mother corm until its total consumption at the end of season (Arslan, 1986; Gumussuyu, 2002; Bakhtavari et al., 2011; Bakhtaveri, 2010, pers. communication with Prof. Dr. K.M. Khawar 2019).

SAFFRON CULTIVATION IN OTHER AREAS OF TURKEY

Since almost same agricultural practices are performed in saffron cultivation at other places in Turkey, no details about those locations are given in this chapter except for their climatic conditions.

WEATHER AND CLIMATE

Turkey lies on the transition or meeting point of three continents, Asia, Africa, and Europe. The land of Turkey is structurally very complex and could be divided into seven regions. All these share a general mountainous terrain with many natural or man-made lakes, rivers, and streams. Successful experiments about saffron cultivation have been performed in all seven regions (Fig. 3.5).

Saffron cultivation has been reported on an experimental scale in the provinces of Istanbul and Tekirdağ that lie in the Marmara region toward the northwest direction.

Experimental saffron production has also been reported in the province of Tokat (Ipek et al., 2009; Koc, 2012a) that lies in the Black Sea region toward north; the climate of the Black Sea region is humid and wet with summer temperatures of 23°C and winter temperatures of 7°C.

There are reports of experimental saffron production from the province of Izmir (Ipek et al., 2009) that lies in

the Aegean region toward the far west with hot dry summers and cool wet winters.

The province of Adana (Ipek et al., 2009) lies in the Mediterranean region toward south with cool wet winters and hot dry summers.

The province of Karabük with Safranbolu county is the main hub of saffron commercial production in Turkey (Ipek et al., 2009, Anonymous, 2019 a,b,c, Unaldi, 2007) Besides this, Prof. Dr. Neset Arslan has also successfully carried out saffron production experiments at Ankara in the Central Anatolian Plateau (Ipek et al., 2009) are places where successful experimental production by Prof. Neşet Arslan has affirmed the potential of production. The Central Anatolia has a steppe climate with large temperature variation during day and night and poor rainfall dominated by snow. The western Anatolia has a moderate Mediterranean climate with temperatures of 9°C−29°C. Similar climate prevail in southern Anatolia. There is a sharp day and night temperature difference. There is low precipitation, and most of it occurs in the form of snow. The mean temperature is around 23°C in summer and about −2°C in winter.

Saffron cultivation has also been reported from the province of SanliUrfa. In the southeast Anatolian region (Ipek et al., 2009), the summer months are very hot and dry, having temperatures above 30°C. The spring and autumn seasons are more or less mild, with sudden change to frequent hot and cold spells.

The province of Igdir in the eastern Anatolian region has a prolonged winter with snow, and the area remains covered with snow from November to the end of April (the mean winter and summer temperatures are around −13°C and 17°C in the same order) in this region.

The black sea region enjoys continental climate.

FUTURE PROSPECTS

Saffron is cultivated in Turkey since very old times as a highly valued food additive for use in traditional medicines (based on their antitumor/anticarcinogenic cytotoxic properties) and for textile dyeing.

There is significant reduction in saffron production in Turkey. The following reasons could be counted as the main ones to decrease saffron production:

a. There is shortage of knowledge about proper cultural practices in saffron production. Practically, the saffron production technology has not changed since centuries, and there is no change in the cultural

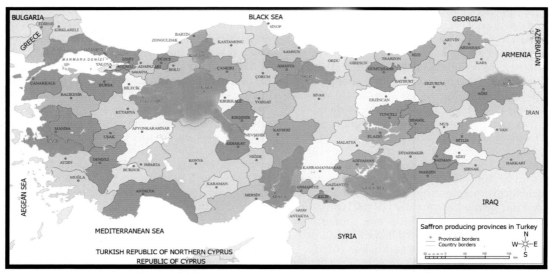

FIG. 3.5 Saffron-producing provinces in Turkey on commercial or experimental scale.

techniques. The farmers culture the plants based on age-old techniques without caring age of fields and the plant density.

b. All production to postharvest processing are very expensive, unprofitable, and done by following old outdated laborious techniques by hand. Although high-quality saffron is produced, Turkish saffron is rarely recognized as the marketing is done without any brand name or practice without International Organization for Standardization (ISO) compliance (ISO 3632, that has a range from I, the finest, to IV, the poorest), which provides no surety to guarantee quality. This results in poor attraction for international buyers. Better packing and sticking to ISO standards could fetch higher price for Turkish saffron.

c. Increasing labor costs, poor postharvest processing and marketing techniques, and no change in saffron production technology and cultural practices since ancient times could be the main reasons.

Possible Solutions

a. There is a need to increase saffron production by exploring new areas for its cultivation in the light of the experiments carried out in various universities and research centers of Turkey. Most appropriate field-management techniques to plant to obtain optimum yield in terms of qualitative and quantitative traits need to be defined and taught to the farmers. Turkey has appropriate climatic conditions for saffron production in all parts. Commercial saffron production is done in Safranbolu only. Saffron production in all other areas is in experimental or transition stage. There is a need to have a change in the status quo in this respect.

b. The farmers should be encouraged to uproot, replace, and replant their fields every 3—4 years.

c. There is a need to introduce new cost-effective cheaper cultivation techniques.

d. The farmers should be encouraged for saffron farming on state level by giving subsidies and incentives.

e. Mechanization should be introduced in saffron cultivation. Introduction of mechanized farming tools could help in significant savings in terms of labor costs and production quality.

f. Greenhouse farming should be encouraged after optimization of techniques. Experiments could be carried out for tunnel, glasshouse, and plastic house farming to optimize the best conditions.

g. There is a need to develop techniques for saffron cultivation on marginal lands as an alternative crop.

h. All practices that involve waxing and lowering of saffron quality should be discouraged.

i. Marketing of saffron is an important practice; the people dealing in marketing should be trained in pricing structure and marketing dynamics approaches for attraction of international buyers.

j. Contamination of saffron stigmas or selling of safflower stigmas as Turkish or local saffron should be discouraged.

REFERENCES

Abdullaev, F., 2007. Biological properties and medicinal use of saffron (Crocus sativus L.). Acta Hortic. 739, 339–345. https://doi.org/10.17660/ActaHortic.2007.739.44.

Abdullaev, F.I., Frankel, G.D., 1999. Saffron in biological and medical research. In: Negbi, M. (Ed.), Saffron: *Crocus Sativus* L. Harwood Academic Publishers, Amsterdam The Netherlands, pp. 103–113.

Abe, T., 1933. Studies on a new dry rot disease of the bulb of *Crocus sativus* L. caused by *Fusarium bulbigenum* Cke. et. Mass var. blasticola (Rostr.) Wr. Trans. Tottori Soc. Agric. Sci. 4 (3), 212–228.

Acikgoz, O.A., 2010. Safran Bitkisinin (*Crocus sativus* L.) yetiştirilmesi, kalitesi ve ticari önemi. (Saffron (*Crocus sativus* L.) Growing, Quality And Commercial Importance). Bartın Üniversitesi Fen Bilimleri Enstitüsü (Institute of natural and applied Sciences, Bartin University. Yüksek Lisans Tezi (M.Sc. thesis), 111s (111 pages) (In Turkish).

Ahmad, M., Zaffar, G., Habib, M., Arshid, A., Dar, N.A., Dar, Z.A., 2014. Saffron (*Crocus sativus* L.) in the light of biotechnological approaches: a review. Sci. Res. Essays 9, 2348–2353.

Alarcon, J., Sanchez, Y.A., 1968. Elazafran heja divulgadora. In: The Saffron Disclosing Sheet Ministeria de Agriculture (Ministry of Agriculture)Madrid, p. 68 (In Spanish).

Allahverdiev, S., Vurdu, N., Kirdar, E., 1998. Perspectives for use of phytohormones for rapid propagation of *Crocus sativus* L.. In: Conference on Introduction of Nonconventional and Unusual Agricultural Plants. Penza, Russia. 24-28 June, 1998, pp. 57–59.

Anonymous 2019a. https://arastirma.tarimorman.gov.tr/gktaem/Belgeler/safran_yetistiriciligi.pdf.

Anonymous 2019b. http://www.tarimkutuphanesi.com/SAFRAN_YETISTIRICILIGI_00003.html.

Anonymous 2019c. https://weather-and-climate.com/average-monthly-Rainfall-Temperature-Sunshine,safranbolu,Turkey.

Arslan, N., 1984. Safran Anbau in der Türkei. (Saffron cultivation in Turkey). HGK releases HGK Mitteilungen 27 (9), 103–107 (In German).

Arslan, N., 1986. Kaybolmaya Yüz Tutan bir kültür safran Tarımı (A disappearing agriculture of saffron cultivation:). Ziraat Mühendisligi (Agric. Eng.) 180, 21–24.

Arslan, N., Gürbüz, B., Gpek, A., Özcan, S., Sarihan, E., 2007. The effect of corm size and different harvesting times on saffron regeneration. Acta Hortic. 749, 113–117.

Asil, H., 2015. Farklı hormon Uygulamalarının ve Soğan Kesme Yöntemlerinin safran (*Crocus sativus* L.) Bitkisinde verim ve verim Öğeleri Üzerine Etkisi (effects of different hormone applications and corm cutting methods on yield and yield components of saffron (*Crocus sativus* L.). Mustafa Kemal Üniversitesi. In: Fen Bilimleri Enstitüsü, Tarla Bitkileri Anabilim Dalı Doktora Tezi, 80 s. Hatay (Mustafa Kemal University Hatay, Turkey. Institute Of Natural And Applied Sciences, Field Crops Department, Ph.D. thesis, 80 pp. (In Turkish).

Azizbekova, N.S., Milyaeva, E.L., 1999. Saffron cultivation in Azerbaijan. In: Negbi, M. (Ed.), Saffron: *Crocus Sativus* L. Harwood Academic Publishers, Amsterdam, The Netherlands, pp. 63–71.

Babaei, T.M., Bahar, M., Zeinali, H., 2014. Analysis of genetic diversity among saffron (*Crocus sativus* L.) accessionsfrom different regions of Iran as revealed by SRAP markers. Sci. Hortic. 171, 27–31.

Bakhtavari, A.S., Khawar, K.M., Neset, A., 2011. Ex vitro shoot regeneration and lateral buds of freshly harvested saffron corms. Afr. J. Agric. Res. 6 (15), 3583–3587.

Bakhtaveri, A.S., 2010. Farklı Soğan (korm) Boylarının ve Bitki Sıklığının Safran (Crocus sativus L.)'nın Verim ve Diğer Bazı Özelikleri Üzerine Etkisi. (Effect of different saffron (Crocus sativus L.) bulb (corm) sızes and plant densıty on the yıeld and factors affectıng yıeld). Ankara Üniversitesi, Fen Bilimleri Enstitüsü, Tarla Bitkileri Anabilim Dalı Doktora Tezi, 79 s. Ankara (Ankara University, Institute of Natural and Applied Sciences, Department of Field Crops, Ph.D. thesis, 79 pp. Ankara). (In Turkish).

Basker, D., Negib, M., 1983. Uses of saffron Crocus sativus. Econ. Bot. 37, 228–236.

Bathaie, S.Z., 2011. Historical uses of saffron: identifying potential new avenues for modern research. Avicenna J. Phytomed. 1, 57–66.

Behnia, M.R., 1996. Saffron: Botany, Cultivation and Production. University of Tehran Press, Iran, p. 285.

Beiki, A.H., Keifi, F., Mozafari, J., 2010. Genetic differentiation of Crocus species by random amplified polymorphic DNA. J. Genet. Eng. Biotech. 18, 1–10.

Cappelli, C., 1994. Occurrence of Fusarium oxysporum f. sp. gladioli on saffron in Italy. Phytopathol. Meditarr. 33 (1), 93–94, 40 (1): 148-149.

Cappelli, C., Buonaurio, R., Polverari, A., 1991. Occurrence of Penicillium corymbiferum on saffron in Italy. Plant Pathol. 40 (1), 148–149.

Carmona, M., Martínez, J., Zalacain, A., Rodríguez-Méndez, M.L., De Saja, J.A., Alonso, G.L., 2006a. Analysis of saffron volatile fraction by TD-GC-MS and e-nose. Eur. Food Res. Technol. 223, 96–101.

Carmona, M., Zalacain, A., Salinas, M.R., Alonso, G.L., 2006b. Generation of saffron volatiles by thermal carotenoid degradation. J. Agric. Food Chem. 54, 6825–6834.

Carmona, M., Zalacain, A., Sanchez, A.M., Novella, J.L., Alonso, G.L., 2006c. Crocetin esters, picrocrocin and its related compounds present in *Crocus sativus* stigmas and Gardenia jasminoides fruits. Tentative identification of seven new compounds by LC-ESI-MS. J. Agric. Food Chem. 54, 973–979.

Carta, C., Flori, M., Franceschini, A., 1982. Charcoal Rot of Saffron (Crocus Sativus L.) Bulbs, vol. 29. Instituto di Patologia Vegetale dell University di Sassari Italy, pp. 193–197.

Castellar, M.R., Montijano, H., Manjon, A., lborra, J.L., 1993. Preparative high-performance liquid chromatographic purification of saffron secondary metabolites. J. Chromatogr. 648, 187–190.

Cavusoglu, A., 2010. The effects of cold storage of saffron (*Crocus sativus* L.) corms on morphology, stigma and corm yield. Afr. J. Agric. Res. 5, 1812–1820.

Chichiricco, G., 1984. Karyotype and meiotic behaviour of the triploid Crocus sativus L. Cayologia 37, 233–239.

Chichiricco, G., 1996. Intra-and interspecific reproductive barriers in *Crocus* (Iridaceae). Plant Syst. Evol. 201 (1), 83–92.

Davis, P.H., Mill, R.R., Kit, T., 1988. Flora of Turkey and the East Aegean Islands Volüme 10. University of Edinburgh, Edinburgh.

Drayton, F.L., 1934. The Gladiolus dry rot caused by Sclerotinia gladioli (Massey) n. Comb. Phytopathology 14 (4), 397–404.

Fernandez, J.A., 2004. Biology, biotechnology and biomedicine of saffron. Recent Res. Dev. Plant Sci. 2, 127–159.

Fluch, S., Hohl, K., Stierschneider, M., Kopecky, D., Kaar, B., 2010. Crocus sativus L. Molecular evidence on its clonal origin. Acta Hortic.) 850, 41–46.

Ghorbani, M., 2007. The economics of saffron in iran. Acta Hortic. 739, 321–331. https://doi.org/10.17660/Acta-Hortic 2007.739.42.

Goliaris, A.H., 1999. Saffron cultivation in Greece. In: Negbi, M. (Ed.), Saffron: Crocus Sativus L. Harwood Academic Publishers, Australia, pp. 73–85.

Greenberg- Kaslasi, D., 1991. Vegetative and Reproductive Development in the Saffron Crocus (*Crocus sativus* L.). M.Sc. thesis. the Hebrew University of Jerusalem, Israel.

Grilli-Caiola, M., Di-Somma, D., Lauretti, P., 2001. Comparative study of pollen and pistil in Crocus sativus L. (Iridaceae) and allied species. Annali Di Botanica 1, 93–103.

Grilli Caiola, M., 2004. Saffron reproductive biology. Acta Hortic. 650, 25–37.

Grilli Caiola, M., Canini, A., 2010. Looking for saffron's (*Crocus sativus* L.) parents. In: Husaini, A.M. (Ed.), Saffron. Global Science Books, UK, pp. 1–14.

Gumussuyu, I., 2002. Dünyanın en pahalı baharatı. Safran. Kültür Bakanlığı'nın yayını, 48 sayfa. (The world's most expensive spice, Saffron. Publication of the Ministry of Culture, 48 pages.) (In Turkish).

Guner, A., Ozhatay, N., Ekim, T., Bafler, K.H.C., 2000. Flora of Turkey and the East Aegean Islands, Second Supplement, vol. 11. University Press, Edinburgh, p. 656.

Hosseinzadeh, H., Younesi, H.M., 2002. Antinociceptive and anti-inflammatory effects of *Crocus sativus* L. stigma and petal extracts in mice. BMC Pharmacol. 15 (2), 7.

Husaini, A.M., 2014. Challenges of climate change. Omics-based biology of saffron plants and organic agricultural biotechnology for sustainable saffron production. GM Crops Food 5 (2), 97–105.

ICARDA. (2007). Caravan (24) June 2007 available at:(hPp://www.icarda.org/Publica;ons/Caravan/Caravan24/Focus_4.htm.

Ipek, A., Arslan, N., Sarihan, E.O., 2009. Effects of different planting depth and bulb sizes on yield and yield components of saffron (*Crocus sativus* L.). Tarım Bilimleri Dergisi 15, 38–46.

Koc, H., 2012a. Farklı ekolojik şartların safranın safranın (*Crocus sativus* l.) bazı özelleiklerine etkileri (Effects of different ecological conditions on some characteristics of saffron (*Crocus sativus* L.).). In: Tıbbi Ve Aromatik Bitkiler Sempasyumu (Symposium on Medicinal and Aromatic Plants) 13–15 September, Tokat.), 13-15 eylül Tokat, Türkiye (13-15 September, Tokat, Turkey).

Koc, H., 2012b. Safran Yetiştiriciliği (Saffron Cultivation). Bilge Kültür Sanat Yayınları, Istanbul, p. 176 (Bilge Culture and Art Publications. Istanbul. pp. 176) (In Turkish).

Koul, K.K., Farooq, S., 1984. Growth and differentiation in the shoot apical meristem of the saffron plant (*Crocus sativus* L.). J. Indian Bot. Soc. 63, 153–160.

Larsen, B., Orabi, J., Pedersen, C., Qrgaard, M., 2015. Large intraspecific genetic variation within the SaffronCrocus group (crocus L., series crocus; Iridaceae). Plant Systamatic Evol. 301 (1), 425–437.

Lozano, P., Castellar, M.R., Simancas, M.J., Ibora, J.L., 1999. A quantitative high-performance liquid chromatographic method to analyze commercial saffron (*Crocus sativus* L.) products. J. Chromatogr. A 830, 477–483.

Madan, C.L., Kapoor, B.M., Gupta, U.S., 1967. Saffron. Econ. Bot 20, 377–385.

Mathew, B., 1977. Crocus turcicus. Plant Systematic Evol. Austria 129, 98.

Mathew, B., 1982. The *Crocus*. A Revision of the Genus *Crocus* (Iridaceae). B.T. Batsford, London.

Mathew, B., Petersen, G., Seberg, O., 2009. A reassessment of *Crocus* based on molecular analysis. Plantsman 8 (1), 50–57.

Milyaeva, E.L., Azizbekova, N.S., 1978. Cytophysiological changes in the course of development of stem apices of saffron crocus. Sov. Plant Physiol. 25, 227–233.

Mizusawa, Y., 1923. A bacterial rot disease of saffrons. Ann. Phytopathol. Soc. Jpn. 1 (5), 1–12.

Molina, R.V., Valero, M., Navarro, Y., Guardiola, J.L., Garcia-Luis, A., 2005. Temperature effects on flower formation in saffron (*Crocus sativus* L.). Sci. Hortic. 103, 361–379.

Moraga, A.R., Trapero-Mozos, A., Gomez-Gomez, L., Ahrazem, O., 2010. Intersimplesequence repeat markers for molecular characterization of Crocus cartwright-ianus cv. albus. Ind. Crops Prod. 32, 147–151.

Nadkarni, K.M., 2000. Indian Materia Medica, vol. 1. Popular Prakashan, Bombay, pp. 390–391.

Negbi, M., 1999. Saffron cultivation: past, present and future prospects. In: Negbi, M. (Ed.), Saffron: Crocus Sativus L. Harwood Academic Publishers, Australia, pp. 1–19.

Nehvi, F.A., Wani, S.A., Dar, S.A., Makhdoomi, M.I., Allie, B.A., Mir, Z.A., 2007. New emerging trends on production technology of saffron. In: Koocheki, A., et al. (Eds.), Proc. II Nd IS on Saffron Bio. And Techno, Acta Horticulturae (ISHS), vol. 739, pp. 375–381.

Nemati, Z., Harpke, D., Gemicioglu, A., Kerndorff, H., Blattner, F.R., 2019. Saffron (Crocus sativus) is an autotriploid that evolved in Attica (Greece) from wild Crocus cartwrightianus. Mol. Phylogenet Evol 136, 14–20.

Ozel, A. ve, Erden, K., 2005. Harran Ovası koşullarında yerli ve Iran safranı (*Crocus sativus* L.)'nın verim ve bazı bitkisel özelliklerinin belirlenmesi. In: . (Determination of Yield and Some Plant Characteristics of Native and Iranian

Saffron (Crocus Sativus L.) under Harran Plain conditions.) GAP IV. Tarım Kongresi (Agricultural Congress), pp. 793−798, 21−23 Eylül (September), Sanlıurfa, Turkey (In Turkish).

Rychener, M., Bigler, P., Pfander, H., 1984. Isolation and structure Elucidation of neapolitanose (O-β-D-Glucopyranosyl-(1→2)-O-[β-D-glucopyranosyl-(1→6)]-D-glucose), new trisaccharide from the stigmas of garden crocusses (crocus neapolitanus var.). Helv. Chim. Acta 67, 386−391.

Schmidt, M., Betti, G., Hensel, A., 2007. Saffron in phytotherapy: pharmacology and clinical uses. Wien. Med. Wochenschr.

Shah, A., Srivastava, K.K., 1984. Control of corm rot of saffron. Progress. Hortic. 16, 141−143.

Skrubis, B., 1990. The cultivation in Greece of *Crocus sativus* L.. In: Proceedings of the International Conference on Saffron (Crocus Sativus L.); L'Àquilla Italy. 27−29 October 1989, pp. 171−182.

Sud, A.K., Paul, Y.S., Thakur, B.R., 1999. Corm rot of saffron and its management. Indian J. Mycol. Plant Pathol. 29 (3), 380−382.

Tammaro, F., 1990. *Crocus sativus* L. − cv. Piano di Navelli (L'Aquila saffron): environment, cultivation, morphometric characteristics, active principles, uses. In: Tammaro, F., Marra, L. (Eds.), Proceedings of the International Conference on Saffron (*Crocus sativus* L.), L'Aquila, pp. 47−57.

Tammaro, F., 1999. Saffron (*Crocus sativus* L.) in Italy. In: Negbi, M. (Ed.), Saffron: *Crocus Sativus* L. Harwood Academic Publishers, Australia, pp. 53−62.

Thakur, R.N., 1997. Corm rot in saffron and its control. In: Handa, S.S., Kaul, M.K. (Eds.), Supplement to Cultivation and Utilization of Aromatic Plants. Regional Research Laboratory, Jammu Tawi, pp. 447−458.

Tomilinson, J.A., 1952. Root rot of Crocus caused by Pythium ultimum. Plant Pathol. 1 (2), 50−51.

Unaldi, E.U., 2007. Tehdit ve tehlike altında bir kültür bitkisi: safran (*Crocus sativus* L.). (An endangered and threatened plant species (*Crocus sativus* L.).). Fırat Üniversitesi Sosyal Bilimler Dergisi (Fırat Univ. J.Soc. Sci.) 4, 53−67 (In Turkish).

Vurdu, H., Şaltu, Z., Ayan, S., 2002. Safran (Crocus sativus L.)'un Yetiştirme Tekniği. Gazi Üniversitesi. Kastamonu Orman Fakültesi Dergisi. 2: 2. (Saffron (Crocus sativus L.) Growing Techniques. Gazi University Journal of Faculty of Forestry, Kastamonu. 2: 2) (In Turkish).

Warburg, L.L., 1957. Crocus. Endeavor. 16, 209−216.

Winterhalter, P., Straubinger, M., 2000. Saffron: renewed interest in an ancient spice. Food Rev. Int. 16, 39−59.

Xu, C.X., Ge, Q.X., 1990. A preliminary study on corm rot in *Crocus sativus* L. Acta Agric. Univ. Zhejangensi 16, 241−246.

Yamamoto, W., Maeda, M., Oyasu, N., 1956. Studies on the Penicillium diseases occurring on cultivated plants. Scientific 137 Reports of the Hyogo University of Agriculture 2, 23−28.

Zadoks, J.C., 1981. Treatise on the violet root of saffron Crocus. Mededelingen Landbouwhoge School Wageningen Nederland is Landbouwhogeschool Wageningen. 81 (7), 1−8.

Zeybek, E., Önde, S., Kaya, Z., 2012. Improved *in vitro* micropropagation method with adventitious corms and roots for endangered saffron. Cent. Eur. J. Biol. 7 (1), 138−145.

Zouahri, A., El Madani, N., Lage, M., Douaik, A., Alilou, H., 2017. Characterization of soils used for saffron production in the main saffron producing zone in Morocco. Acta Hortic. 1184, 131−136.

CHAPTER 4

Ex Vitro Macropropagation of Saffron (*Crocus sativus* L.) Corms

KHALID MAHMOOD KHAWAR • MEHMET UGUR YILDIRIM • ERCUMENT OSMAN SARIHAN

INTRODUCTION

Saffron (*Crocus sativus* L. of family Iridaceae) is a perennial herb that grows widely in Iran and many other countries. Commercial saffron consists of dry red stigma and a small yellowish style (Zargari, 1990). The first reference to its cultivation dates back to 2300 B.C. by King Sargon (Acadian empire), who was born at Azupirano close to the Euphrates (Gadd, 1971). A clear identification of the plant goes back to about 1700−1600 B.C., as a fresco painting at the palace of Knossos (Greek island of Crete) in a palace at Minos. Negbi (1989) has described that saffron corms are produced and reproduced vegetatively since centuries and has been documented as early as 300 B.C. by Theophrastus in *Historia Plantarum* and 1 A.C. by Pliny in *Natural History*.

It is believed that first documentation of saffron was done in 7th century B.C. by Ashurbanipal an Assyrian. Thereafter, saffron is being cultivated and documented, presently is mentioned in treatment of about 90 diseases (Grisolia, 1974; Verma and Bordia, 1998). The perfumes made by the Lydians from saffron have been collected from Bozdag (Tmolos) which were among the luxury goods in antiquity and were exported. Strabon (60−24 B.C. born at present day Anatolian city of Amasya) reports high-quality saffron production in Cilicia. A famous physician Dioscorides (40−90 B.C.), who lived in the Kozan (Anavarza/Anazarbos/Anazarba/Anazarbus/Aynızarba-Ancient City) district of Adana, also report the highest quality of saffron production from Cilicia, Korikos, lying in the vicinity of present day Kizkalesi (close to Mersin and Silifke) and foothills of Mount Olympus (Tahtali), in the Aegean region (Arslan et al., 1984).

Saffron plants have an average height of 25−30 cm that rarely goes to 40−60 cm under natural and cultivated conditions (Husaini et al., 2010, Pers. Observations 2019). Triploid Saffron—C. sativus (2n = 3x = 24 chromosomes)—can be reproduced vegetatively only and are sterile. Saffron—(C. sativus) is commercially used in industries related to spice, dye, and processing and manufacturing of drugs (Arslan, 1984; Husaini et al., 2010; Schnittler et al., 2009). Bulbils contra seeds: reproductive investment in two species of Gagea (Liliaceae). Commercially produced saffron is a 3-lobed 2.5- to 3.2-cm-long stigma with dark red or orange color. The active ingredients of the stigma are compounds such as essential oils, carotenes, and picrocrocin. Carotenes (10%, especially crosin 2%) give the staining properties of saffron; bitterness and aroma are due to picrocrocin and safranal (4%). The proportion of essential oil of saffron ranges 0.4%−1.5%; cineol and the essential oil are also effective in the smell of saffron. The saffron also contains fat (7%), pentosans (5%), pectin (6%), and B vitamins (Mathew, 1982, 1999; Mathew et al., 1979; Frello et al., 2004, Arslan, 1984).

Anonymous (2019a) has described a Crocus list that includes 320 species in the genus Crocus, and of these, 94 are accepted and are listed below (Table 4.1).

According to the Red List and Tubives 2019b, 35 crocus species are included in the list of the endangered species in the world (Davis, 1984,1988; Anonymous, 2019b,c). Of these, 3 are species that are endangered (EN), 3 are vulnerable (VU), 3 are near threatened (NT), 2 are data deficient (DD), and 24 of them are in the least concern (LC) level. There are 62 species, subspecies, and taxon of saffron found in Turkey (Anonymous, 2019b - Table 4.2). This list shows 28 taxons that are included in the red book of endangered species. Nine (9) of these taxons are VU, 7 are NT, 5 are LC 3 of them are EN, 2 are CD (LC), 1 is critically endangered (CR), and another one is found at the DD level of

Saffron. https://doi.org/10.1016/B978-0-12-818462-2.00004-8

TABLE 4.1
Some Important Saffron Species, Their Status, and Their Confidence Level.

No.	Name	Confidence Level	Source
1	*Crocus abantensis* T.Baytop & B.Mathew	a	iPlants
2	*C. aerius* Herb.	a	iPlants
3	*C. adanensis* T.Baytop & B.Mathew	a	iPlants
4	*C. alatavicus* Regel & Semen.	a	iPlants
5	*C. aleppicus* Baker	a	iPlants
6	*C. almehensis* C.D.Brickell & B.Mathew	a	iPlants
7	*C. ancyrensis* (Herb.) Maw	a	iPlants
8	*C. angustifolia* Weston	b	TRO
9	*C. angustifolius* Weston	a	iPlants
10	*C. antalyensis* B.Mathew	a	iPlants
11	*C. asumaniae* B.Mathew & T.Baytop	a	iPlants
12	*C. autranii* Albov	a	iPlants
13	*C. banaticus* J.Gay	a	iPlants
14	*C. baytopiorum* B.Mathew	a	iPlants
15	*C. biflorus* Mill.	a	iPlants
16	*C. boissieri* Maw	a	iPlants
17	*C. boryi* J.Gay	a	iPlants
18	*C. boulosii* Greuter	a	iPlants
19	*C. cambessedesii* J.Gay	a	iPlants
20	*C. cancellatus* Herb.	a	iPlants
21	*C. candidus* E.D.Clarke	a	iPlants
22	*C. carpetanus* Boiss. & Reut.	a	iPlants
23	*C. cartwrightianus* Herb.	a	iPlants
24	*C. caspius* Fisch. & C.A.Mey. ex Hohen.	a	iPlants
25	*C. chrysanthus* (Herb.) Herb.	a	iPlants

TABLE 4.1
Some Important Saffron Species, Their Status, and Their Confidence Level.—cont'd

No.	Name	Confidence Level	Source
26	*C. corsicus* Vanucchi	a	iPlants
27	*C. cvijicii* Kosanin	a	iPlants
28	*C. cyprius* Boiss. & Kotschy	a	iPlants
29	*C. dalmaticus* Vis.	a	iPlants
30	*C. danfordiae* Maw	a	iPlants
31	*C. etruscus* Parl.	a	iPlants
32	*C. fleischeri* J.Gay	a	iPlants
33	*C. flavus*[b] Weston	a	iPlants
34	*C. gilanicus* B.Mathew	a	iPlants
35	*C. gargaricus* Herb.	a	iPlants
36	*C. goulimyi* Turrill	a	iPlants
37	*C. graveolens* Boiss. & Reut.	a	iPlants
38	*C. hadriaticus* Herb.	a	iPlants
39	*C. hartmannianus* Holmboe	a	iPlants
40	*C. herbertii* (B.Mathew) B.Mathew	a	iPlants
41	*C. hermoneus* Kotschy ex Maw	a	iPlants
42	*C.* × *hybridus* Petrovic	a	iPlants
43	*C. hyemalis* Boiss. & Blanche	a	iPlants
44	*C. imperati* Ten.	a	iPlants
45	*C. kerndorffiorum* Pasche	a	iPlants
46	*C. karduchorum* Kotschy ex Maw	a	iPlants
47	*C. korolkowii* Maw & Regel	a	iPlants
48	*C. kosaninii* Pulevic	a	iPlants
49	*C. kotschyanus* K.Koch	a	iPlants
50	*C. laevigatus* Bory & Chaub.	a	iPlants
51	*C. leichtlinii* (Dewer) Bowles	a	iPlants
52	*C. ligusticus* Mariotti	a	iPlants
53	*C. longiflorus* Raf.	a	iPlants

(continued)

TABLE 4.1
Some Important Saffron Species, Their Status, and Their Confidence Level.—cont'd

No.	Name	Confidence Level	Source
54	*C. malyi* Vis.	a	iPlants
55	*C. mathewii* Kerndorff & Pasche	a	iPlants
56	*C. michelsonii* B.Fedtsch.	a	iPlants
57	*C. minimus* DC.	a	iPlants
58	*C. moabiticus* Bornm.	a	iPlants
59	*C. naqabensis* Al-Eisawi & Kiswani	a	iPlants
60	*C. nerimaniae* Yüzb.	a	iPlants
61	*C. nevadensis* Amo & Campo	a	iPlants
62	*C. niveus* Bowles	a	iPlants
63	*C. nudiflorus* Sm.	a	iPlants
64	*C. ochroleucus* Boiss. & Gaill.	a	iPlants
65	*C. olivieri* J.Gay	a	iPlants
66	*C. oreocreticus* B.L.Burtt	a	iPlants
67	*C. paschei* Kerndorff	a	iPlants
68	*C. pulchellus* Herb.	a	iPlants
69	*C. × paulineae* Pasche & Kerndorff	a	iPlants
70	*C. pestalozzae* Boiss.	a	iPlants
71	*C. pelistericus* Pulevic	a	iPlants
72	*C. robertianus* C.D.Brickell	a	iPlants
73	*C. reticulatus* Steven ex Adam	a	iPlants
74	*C. pallasii* Goldb.	a	iPlants
75	*C. rujanensis* Randjel. & D.A.Hill	a	iPlants
76	*C. sativus* L.	a	iPlants
77	*C. scardicus* Kosanin	a	iPlants
78	*C. scharojanii* Rupr.	a	iPlants
79	*C. serotinus* Salisb.	a	iPlants
80	*C. speciosus* M.Bieb.	a	iPlants
81	*C. sieheanus* Barr ex B.L.Burtt	a	iPlants
82	*C. sieberi* J.Gay	a	iPlants

TABLE 4.1
Some Important Saffron Species, Their Status, and Their Confidence Level.—cont'd

No.	Name	Confidence Level	Source
83	*C. suaveolens* Bertol.	a	iPlants
84	*C. suwarowianus* K.Koch	a	iPlants
85	*C. thomasii* Ten.	a	iPlants
86	*C. tommasinianus* Herb.	a	iPlants
87	*C. tournefortii* J.Gay	a	iPlants
88	*C. vallicola* Herb.	a	iPlants
89	*C. veluchensis* Herb.	a	iPlants
90	*C. wattiorum* (B.Mathew) B.Mathew	a	iPlants
91	*C. vitellinus* Wahlenb.	a	iPlants
92	*C. versicolor* Ker Gawl.	a	iPlants
93	*C. vernus* (L.) Hill	a	iPlants
94	*C. veneris* Tapp. ex Poech	a	iPlants

[a] High confidence.
[b] Medium confidence.
Source: Anonymous, 2019a. http://www.theplantlist.org/browse/A/Iridaceae/Crocus/ All details related to the Status of each name and High Confidence level could be found at (Anonymous, 2019a).

classification in the red list of endangered plants (Anonymous, 2019b,c).

Considering the present distribution of crocus species in the world and in Turkey, most of the crocus species are under threat of genetic erosion because of loss of land to fast urbanization, greenhouse effect, and global warming—based climate changes (Frello et al., 2004; Walia et al., 2016; Khorramdel et al., 2017). It seems inevitable to protect these plant species for the future of our generations. Therefore, there is a need to protect and conserve these species, locally and at international levels, by establishing Crocus gene banks under the authority of mutually agreed local or international consortiums. All these grow under natural conditions, and there is no clear information about the multiplication pattern of these species, except for —ffron—Crocus sativus L. (Piqueras et al., 1999; Khorramdel et al., 2017).

Culturing of these species along with establishment of gene bank/s and the development of rapid propagation protocols for them is one of the most important needs to conserve them and to reduce loss of genetic

TABLE 4.2
List of 62 Crocus Taxa Found in Turkey (Anonymous, 2019b).

No.	Name of Taxon	Status According to the Red Book of Endangered Species	Endemizm
1	*Crocus baytopiorum*	VU	Endemic
2	*C. fleischeri*	LC	Endemic
3	*C. reticulatus* sub sp. reticulatus	—	Not endemic
4	*C. reticulatus* sub sp. hittiticus	VU	Endemic
5	*C. abantensis*	NT	Endemic
6	*C. gargaricus* sub sp. gargaricus	NT	Endemic
7	*C. gargaricus* sub sp. herbertii	EN	Endemic
8	*C. ancyrensis*	LC	Endemic
9	*C. sieheanus*	VU	Endemic
10	*C. chrysanthus*	—	Not endemic
11	*C. danfordiae*	LC	Endemic
12	*C. pestalozzae*	VU	Endemic
13	*C. biflorus* sub sp. biflorus	—	Not eendemic
14	*C. biflorus* sub sp. crewei	VU	Not eendemic
15	*C. biflorus* sub sp. nubigena	LC	Endemic
16	*C. biflorus* sub sp. isauricus	LC	Endemic
17	*C. biflorus* sub sp. punctatus	NT	Endemic
18	*C. biflorus* sub sp. pseudonubigena	—	Endemic
19	*C. biflorus* sub sp. adamii	—	Not eendemic
20	*C. biflorus* sub sp. artvinensis	—	Endemic
21	*C. biflorus* sub sp. pulchricolor	—	Endemic
22	*C. biflorus* sub sp. tauri	—	Not eendemic
23	*C. biflorus* sub sp. albocoronatus	—	Endemic
24	*C. biflorus* sub sp. fibroannulatus	—	Endemic
25	*C. wattiorum*	—	Endemic
26	*C. adanensis*	CR	Endemic
27	*C. aerius*	VU	Endemic
28	*C. paschei*	—	Endemic
29	*C. leichtlinii*	CD	Endemic
30	*C. flavus* sub sp. flavus	—	Not eendemic
31	*C. flavus* sub sp. dissectus	VU	Endemic
32	*C. kerndorffiorum*	—	Endemic
33	*C. antalyensis*	NT	Endemic
34	*C. olivieri* sub sp. olivieri	—	Not eendemic
35	*C. olivieri* sub sp. balansae	NT	Endemic
36	*C. olivieri* sub sp. istanbulensis	—	Endemic
37	*C. candidus*	CD	Endemic
38	*C. graveolens*	—	Not eendemic

(continued)

TABLE 4.2
List of 62 Crocus Taxa Found in Turkey (Anonymous, 2019b).—cont'd

No.	Name of Taxon	Status According to the Red Book of Endangered Species	Endemizm
39	*C. vitellinus*	VU	Not eendemic
40	*C. scharojanii*	VU	Not eendemic
41	*C. vallicola*	—	Not eendemic
42	*C. kotschyanus* sub sp. kotschyanus	—	Not eendemic
43	*C. kotschyanus* sub sp. cappadocicus	—	Endemic
44	*C. kotschyanus* sub sp. suworowianus	—	Not eendemic
45	*C. kotschyanus* sub sp. hakkariensis	—	Endemic
46	*C. karduchorum*	EN	Endemic
47	*C. pallasii* sub sp. pallasi	—	Not eendemic
48	*C. pallasii* sub sp. turcicus	—	Not eendemic
49	*C. pallasii* sub sp. dispathaceus	—	Not eendemic
50	*C. mathewii*	—	Endemic
51	*C. sativus*	—	Not eendemic
52	*C. asumaniae*	EN	Endemic
53	*C. cancellatus* sub sp. cancellatus	—	Endemic
54	*C. cancellatus* sub sp. mazziaricus	—	Not eendemic
55	*C. cancellatus* sub sp. lycius	NT	Endemic
56	*C. cancellatus* sub sp. pamphylicus	—	Endemic
57	*C. cancellatus* sub sp. damascenus	—	Not eendemic
58	*C. speciosus* sub sp. speciosus	—	Not eendemic
59	*C. speciosus* sub sp. ilgazensis	NT	Endemic
60	*C. speciosus* sub sp. xantholaimos	—	Endemic
61	*C. pulchellus*	—	Not eendemic
62	*C. boissieri*	DD	Endemic

Source: Anonymous, 2019b, http://www.tubives.com/

erosion in the world biodiversity for its healthy transfer to future generations.

The genus *Crocus* can grow in areas ranging from 50m to 1900 m asl. In fact, there are reports on the existence of wild forms at an altitude of 3000 m in various countries (Anonymous, 2019b). It grows in all 7 agro-ecological zones of Turkey. Many domesticated and wild forms of *Crocus* are found and distributed in wide range of climates and geographies from America, Europe, and Australasia, which indicate that the *Crocus* species is least affected by the climatic or geographical effects (Humphries, 1996; McGimpsey et al., 1997; Negbie, 1999; Anonymous, 2019b).

To flower the plants, it is necessary to produce a certain level of cold shock for a certain period of time. Time and temperature vary from species to species (Molina et al., 2005a,b; Amooaghaie, 2007).

Generally, saffron and also most of the domesticated crocus species are planted during September—October, and their harvesting is done in June—July each year (López Rodríguez, 1989; Pérez Bueno, 1989, 1995). It remains in dormancy (sleep/slow growth) period during rest of the time. Therefore, the corms are dug and removed from the fields soon after harvest and are vernalized in a cool (4—12°C) dark or light-free environment until the time of planting (2—4 weeks to 3—4 months later). This practice helps to improve leaf formation and blossoming. Optimum temperature for saffron growth ranges from 15 to 25°C (Alarcón, 1986; López Rodríguez, 1989; Negbi et al., 1989; Plessner et al., 1989; Pérez Bueno, 1989, 1995).

METHODS OF SAFFRON MULTIPLICATION

  i. Natural conditions
  ii. Hybridization and seed multiplications
  iii. Cultivated conditions
  iv. *İn vitro* conditions
  v. *Ex vitro* conditions

NATURAL CONDITIONS

All corm species except *Crocus sativus* could be multiplied through seed or corm under natural conditions (Rubio, 1980; Alarcón, 1986; Tammaro, 1990; Sadeghi et al., 1992; Rees, 1992; Le Nard and De Hertogh, 1993).

HYBRIDIZATION AND SEED MULTIPLICATIONS

Although saffron (*C. Sativus*) is a self-sterile plant, it is possible to set seeds and mature capsules if pollen from *C. cartwrightianus* or *C. thomasii* is used to cross with *C. sativus* (Grilli Caiola, 2004). There is no report about successful cross and seed establishment from rest of the species in the genus *Crocus*. Some other crosses have also been reported by Chichiricco and Frizzi (1994), who has showed that it is possible to cross (1) *C. sativus* L. × *C. hadriaticus* Herb, (2) *C. sativus* L. × *C. oreocreticus* B.L: Burtt, (3) *C. sativus* L. × *C. thomasii* Ten., (4) *C. sativus* L. × *C. cartwrightianus* Herb, (5) *C. sativus* L. × *C. cancellatus* Herb, (6) *C. sativus* L. × *C. boryi* Gay, (7) *C. thomasii* Ten. × *C. hadriaticus* Herb, (8) *C. thomasii* Ten. × *C. boryi* Gay, (9) *C. hadriaticus* Herb × *C. boryi* Gay, (10) *C. cancellatus* Herb × *C. thomasii* Ten. (Table 4.3).

Haspolat et al. (2013) report seed germination of West Anatolian *Crocus olivieri* ssp. balansae, *C. chrysanthus*, *C. baytopiorum*, and *C. pallasii* ssp. Pallasii by sandwiching their seeds with Gibberellic acid (GA3) in moist blotting papers at 10ºC with seed germination of 73.8%, 14%, and 82.5% in the same order. At in vitro conditions, seeds were sown to MS (Murashige and Skoog 1962) medium without plant growth regulators with pretreatment of waiting seeds for 24 h in solutions of 250 and 500 mg/L GA3. The germination rate was higher at treatment of 500 mg/L GA3 than at 200 mg/L GA3. In vitro seed germination was started 8 months later, and the rates were 25% at Crocus olivieri ssp. balansae, 9.5% at Crocus chrysanthus, 80% at Crocus baytopiorum, and 90% at Crocus pallasii ssp. pallasii.

CULTIVATED CONDITIONS

Saffron (*C. sativus*) is propagated by corms, and the corms are selected by breeders or farmers to achieve maximum yield. This practice has led to selection of corms with improved populations including selection of corms for long red stigmas that make commercially important spice, when dried. This practice has enabled

TABLE 4.3
Cross breeding in saffron (Chichiricco and Frizzi, 1994)

Female	Male	Pollen germination	Percentage of of ovules with zygote and endosperm nuclei
C. sativus L. ×	*C. hadriaticus* Herb.[b]	++	0.6
C. sativus L. ×	*C. oreocreticus* B.L: Burtt[b]	++	11
C. sativus L. ×	*C. thomasii* Ten[b]	++	16.8
C. sativus L. ×	*C. cartwrighteanus* Herb[b].	++	10.2
C. sativus L. ×	*C. cancellatus* Herb	++	9
C. sativus L. ×	*C. boryi* Gay	++	9
C. thomasii Ten. ×	*C. hadriaticus* Herb.[b]	++	77
C. thomasii Ten. ×	*C. boryi* Gay	++	3.3
C. hadriaticus Herb. ×	*C. boryi* Gay[a]	++	0
C. cancellatus Herb. ×	*C. thomasii* Ten.[a]	++	0

[a] reciprocal crosses
[b] Crosses between related species

the farmers to keep the fidelity of the corms without depreciation in corm quality. Flow cytometry studies of saffron corms collected from different areas of the world show almost very low or meager genetic variability in morphological properties with very similar qualitative and quantitative characteristics (Brandizzi and Grilli Caiola, 1996).

Vegetative multiplication is beneficial and advantageous because it helps in maintaining true quality of the plants; however, any genetic improvement is not possible. Therefore, all corms in saffron which belong to same genotypes are clones of a single mother plant of the same species that has minor variations for morphological and biochemical characteristics only (Milyaeva and Azizbekova, 1978; Azizbekova and Milyaeva, 1999; Molina et al., 2005). Generally, the corms that have more than 2.5 cm diameter are preferred during selection. A flowering-size corm produce 10—12 buds, and theoretically every bud on a saffron corm has the ability to produce a new daughter corm; however, the environmental factors affect production of new corms on the mother corm (Pandey et al., 1974; Negbi et al., 1989; De Mastro and Ruta, 1993). The mother corms decay before producing three to four daughter corms during the second or subsequent year of production. The daughter corm formation occurs during vegetative growth (about October—March period) each year depending on the cultural conditions, environmental factors, and type of soil in fields. This growth cycle continues until the sixth or seventh year of production. The daughter corm production declined thereafter. Thus, a single corm produce 3—4, 20—22, and 18—20 corms in the second, third, and fourth years and onward period in the same order until seventh year if the mother corm is planted at a depth of about 7 cm (Negbie, 1999; McGimpsey et al., 1997; Gresta et al., 2008; Cavuosoglu and Erkel, 2009; Pers. Observations 2019). Each new mother corm ascends 1—2 cm each year after the production of daughter corms and decays. Saffron corms must be dug up thereafter, to avoid crowding with insufficient space and to obtain corms of desired size to enable good stigma yield and harvest by minimizing the chances of disease infestations. Every year, the corms are dug up or harvested from the soil in June—July and are vernalized in cold storages until October after screening them for size and possible defects (for diseases) to conserve the best corms for their phytochemical and morphological properties (Negbi, 1990; Pers. observations 2019). Generally, new corm formation starts soon after planting during October—November and continues up to March—April before drying of foliage. During a period starting soon after planting (winter—spring and summer), the corms begin to grow roots on the mother corm that ends up with production of daughter corms (Lopez et al., 2015; Pers. Observations 2019).

Yildirim et al. (2017) have noted variable effects of changing planting depths of saffron (*Crocus sativus* L.) corms under Mediterranean warm and temperate climate of Hatay in Turkey. It is reported that more number of corms could be produced by planting mother corms at a shallow depth (Negbi, 1990). Greenberg-Kaslasi (1991) reports that if corms are treated with gibberellins $_{4+7}$, they tend to decrease sprouting buds and increase apical dominance. Corms are produced on the tunics of corms. At the same time, Asil and Aynaoglu (2018) noted that corm treatment with GA3 improves flowering of saffron corms under cultivated conditions.

Every new daughter corm has one to two main buds at the top and 4—10 secondary buds in the lower portion at spir 1 that produces a cauline axis (Personal observations 2019). These corms are smaller in size (1/4—1/6) than those induced on apical buds. Therefore, the mother corms produce two to three daughter corms each on apical buds and many new corms on other lateral buds. It is also interesting to note that out of three types of saffron corm roots (absorbing, contractile, and contractile absorbing), daughter corms are also produced on contractile roots (Negbi, 1999; Pers. Observations 2019). These single roots are very short and thick and are produced in large number on shallow planted mother corms. Plurannual rather than annual saffron production is widely practiced world wide and in the Mediterranean countries that are characterized by a hot, dry summer climate (Negbi, 1999; Tammaro, 1999).

In Vitro Conditions

In vitro commercial production is desired, and the goal has to be achieved to attain virus-free corms (Homes et al., 1987; Isa and Ogasawara, 1988; Plessner et al., 1990; George et al., 1992; Dhar and Sapru, 1993, 1994; Milyaeva et al., 1978, 1995).

Saffron regeneration under tissue culture through embryogenesis and organogenesis has been reported by a number of workers (Ding et al., 1979, 1981; Chen and Huang, 1980; Chichiriccò and Grilli Caiola, 1987; Huang, 1987; Gui et al., 1988; Fakhrai and Evans, 1990; Dhar and Sapru, 1993; Ebrahimzadeh, 1996; Ebrahimzadeh et al., 2000a,b; Karamian, 2004; Karaoğlu et al., 2007; Darvishi et al., 2006a,b; Agayev et al., 2009; Husaini et al., 2010; Zeybek et al., 2012; Lapadatescu et al., 2013; Shahabzadeh et al., 2013; Sivanesan et al., 2014; Mir et al., 2010, 2014, 2015; Devi et al., 2011, 2014; Yasmin and Nehvi, 2014a,b; Abbas and Elahe, 2015; Gantait and Vahedi, 2015; Vahedi et al., 2014, 2015, Vatankhah et al., 2014; Yang et al., 2015).

However, all of them agree that in vitro tissue culture of saffron is not viable either because of unrepeatable methodologies or the longevity of cultures that are non-feasible for commercial production. There is a need to look for development of more refined tissue culture protocols for commercial saffron production (Husaini et al., 2010). Similar observations have been made in iris, tulip, Begonia evansiana, and Dioscorea sp. by Halevy and Shoub (1964), Rudnicki et al. (1976), Okagami (1972), and Okagami et al. (1977) using gibberellins in the same order.

Ex vitro Conditions

Although in vitro tissue culture has great importance and the goal is yet to be achieved, multiplication of saffron corms under ex vitro conditions has also been reported.

Azizbekova et al. (1982) were the first to report successful germination of saffron corm buds using gibberellin and found positive effects on functional activities of dormant buds of saffron. The results are also confirmed by Chrungoo and Farooq (1984). They report that GA3 had positive effects and 1-naphthaleneacetic acid (NAA) had negative effects on functional activities of buds on saffron corms. They noted that even single GA treatment to saffron corms in the apical notch has positive effects on promoting bud sprouting and growth with increased flowering on each corm with cumulative positive effects on saffron yield and the daughter corms' weights per mother corm plant. However, NAA treatments suppressed both blossoming and bud growth but released apical dominance. Bakhtavari et al. (2011) have also reported ex vitro regeneration of shoots from mother saffron corms, soon after harvesting them and treating them for 30, 60, 90, 120, and 150 min with 50 mg/L of IAA or 50 mg/L of Indole-3-acetic acid (IAA) + 10 mg/L of 1-Phenyl-3-(1,2,3-thiadiazol-5-yl) urea or Thidiazuron (TDZ).

Yildirim et al. (2016) noted that saffron treatment with 6-Benzylaminopurine (BAP) used singly or BAP + GA3 could improve daughter corm regeneration on saffron mother corms with induction of a number of new corms on the mother corm. Similarly, Yildirim and Hajyzadeh (2018) have reported feasibility to break mother corm dormancy, avoiding vernalization after harvest. Their results suggest that mother saffron corms could be multiplied under *ex vitro* conditions very rapidly. Using 20 mg L^{-1} of BAP or 20 mg·L^{-1} of BAP +300 mg·L^{-1} of GA3 pretreatment in a short period of 90 days for the first time. They reported 4, 6, 8, and 10 h of pretreatment of small mother corms of diameter 1.10−1.75 cm and large mother corms of diameter 1.75−2.40 cm. They figured out that both types of mother corms had maximum multiplication percentage of 80.00 and 86.67. These induced 6.17 and 5.55 daughter corms/mother corm with a diameter of 0.62 and 0.69 cm. However, 4 h rooting pretreatment induced variable number of roots depending on the corm diameter. The results further showed that pretreatment of saffron corms with BAP used singly or BAP + GA3 under greenhouse conditions in wooden boxes (Fig. 4.1A) could provide an opportunity for rapid ex vitro multiplication on economic scale without compromising any qualitative or quantitative parameter. The daughter corm sticks to mother corm and

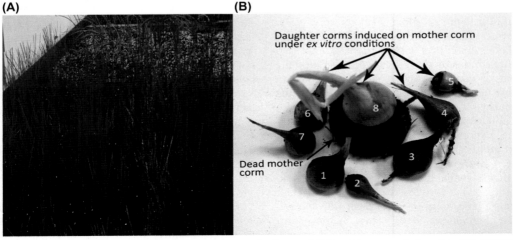

FIG. 4.1 **(A)** Ex vitro multiplication of saffron in wooden boxes. **(B)** Daughter corms induced on the mother corm.

consumes it completely at the time of harvest by converting it into a hard brown woody structure (Fig. 4.1B). The results will further help in designing multiplication of healthy daughter corms.

Yildirim et al. (2019) compared the effects of GA3 doses on saffron under different photoperiod conditions (light, temperature, and humidity control) under four categories namely 7–8 cm, 5–6 cm, 3–4 cm, and <3 cm circumference of saffron corms after treating each category of corms with 100, 250, 500, and 1000 mg/L of GA3 for 24 h and planting them in sand + peat moss + soil (1:1:1) under 8 h of light/16 h of dark and 12 h of light/12 h of dark photoperiod conditions. The results showed that photoperiod, corm circumference, and hormone doses interacted ($P < .05$) to induce leaf length, total number of leaves, and total weight of corms. The maximum weight of 2.08 g was noted on mother corms of 7–8 cm circumference using 250 mg/l of GA_3. The weight of corms decreased linearly with each unit decrease in the circumference of mother corms both under 8 and 12 h light photoperiods. Increased mean corm weight was noted on all treatments with 8 h light photoperiod compared with the corms treated with 12 h light photoperiod.

CONCLUSIONS

Vegetative multiplication of saffron offers advantages and maintains genetic fidelity of the plants without any genetic improvement. Attempts have been made to multiply different propagation techniques. Saffron is a very difficult plant, and there is scarcity of reports on saffron production. This study reports 5 methods of saffron propagation under natural, synthetic, cultivated, in vitro, and *ex vitro* conditions. There is no reliable report suggesting seed production in saffron. These propagation techniques offer only minor biochemical and morphological improvements in saffron properties. All techniques of multiplication are in vogue for the number of years, except ex vitro multiplication of saffron corms which is a relatively new and successful multiplication technique reported recently. More experiments are under way for refinement of this technique.

REFERENCES

Abbas, M.S., Elahe, P., 2015. Evaluation of callus formation and embryogenesis in saffron (*Crocus sativus* L.) for flower harvesting. J. Biodivers. Environ. Sci. 6, 127–131.

Agayev, Y.M., Fernandez, J.A., Zarifi, E., 2009. Clonal selection of saffron (*Crocus sativus* L.): the first optimistic experimental results. Euphytica 169, 81–99.

Alarcón, J., 1986. El azafrán. Servicio de Extensión Agraria del Ministerio de Agricultura, Pesca y Alimentación, Madrid, España.

Amooaghaie, R., 2007. Low temperature storage of corms extends the flowering season of saffron (*Crocus sativus* L.). Acta Hortic. 739, 41–47.

Anonymous 2019a. https://www.iucnredlist.org/search?query=Crocus&searchType=species.

Anonymous 2019b http://www.tubives.com/.

Anonymous 2019c. http://www.tehditaltindabitkiler.org.tr/v2/index.php?sayfa=listele&sinif=alfabetik.

Arslan, N., 1984. Safran Anbau in der Türkei (Saffron cultivation in Turkey.). HGK Mitteilungen 27 (9), 103–107. In German.

Arslan, N., 1984. Safran üzerine düşünceler. https://www.turktob.org.tr/dergi/makaleler/dergi20/66-69.pdf.

Arslan, N., 1984. Safran Anbau in der Türkei. HGK Mitteilungen 27 (9), 103–107 and genetic improvement of saffron. Agronomie 19: 603–610.

Asil, H., Ayanoglu, F., 2018. The Effects of Different Gibberellic Acid Doses and Corm Cutting Methods on Saffron (*Crocus Sativus* L.) Yield Components in Turkey.

Azizbekova, N.S., Milyaeva, E.L., 1999. Saffron cultivation in Azerbaijan. In: Negbi, M. (Ed.), Saffron: Crocus Sativus L. Harwood Academic Publishers, Amsterdam, The Netherlands, pp. 63–71.

Azizbekova, N.S., Milyaeva, E.L., Chailakhyan, M.K., 1982. Effect of gibberellin on functional activity of dormant saffron buds. Fiziol. Rast. 29 (6), 1164–1169.

Bakhtavari, A.S., Khawar, K.M., Arslan, N., 2011. Ex vitro shoot regeneration and lateral buds of freshly harvested saffron corms. Afr. J. Agric. Res. 6 (15), 3583–3588.

Brandizzi, F., Grilli Caiola, M., 1996. Quantitative DNA analysis in different *Crocus* species (Iridaceae) by means of flow cytometry. G. Bot. Ital. 130, 643–645.

Cavusoglu, A., Erkel, E., 2009. Saffron (*Crocus sativus* L.) growing without removing of mother corms under greenhouse condition. Turkish J. Field Crop. 14 (2), 170–180.

Chen, W., Huang, R.X., 1980. Tissue culture of *Crocus sativus* L. Plant Physiol. Commun. 1, 25–26.

Chichiricco, G., Frizzi, G., 1994. Cross-breeding in crocus L. (*Iridaceae*). G. Bot. Ital. 128 (1), 225. https://doi.org/10.1080/11263509409437075.

Chichiriccò, G., Grilli Caiola, M., 1987. *In vitro* development of parthenocarpic fruits of *Crocus sativus* L. Plant Cell Tissue Organ Cult. 11, 75–78.

Chrungoo, N.K., Farooq, S., 1984. Influence of gibberellic acid· and napthaleneacetic acid on the yield of saffron and on growth in saffron crocus (*Crocus sativus* L.). Indian J. Plant Physiol. XXVII (2), 201–205.

Darvishi, E., Zarghami, R., Mishani, C.A., Omidi, M., 2006a. Effects of different hormone treatments on non-embryogenic and embryogenic callus induction and time-term enzyme treatments on number and viability of isolated protoplasts in saffron (*Crocus sativus* L.). Acta Hortic. 739, 279–284.

Darvishi, E., Zarghami, R., Mishani, C.A., Omidi, M., Sarkhosh, 2006b. *In vitro* production of pathogen-free plantlets via meristem culture in saffron (*Crocus sativus* L.). Biotechnology 5, 292−295.

Davis, P.H., 1984,1988. Flora of Turkey, vols. 8 and 10. Edinburgh.

De Mastro, G., Ruta, C., 1993. Relations between corm size and saffron *(Crocus sativus* L.) flowering. Acta Hortic. 344, 512−517.

Devi, K., Sharma, M., Singh, M., Singh Ahuja, P., 2011. *In vitro* cormlet production and growth evaluation under greenhouse conditions in saffron (*Crocus sativus* L.) − a commercially important crop. Eng. Life Sci. 11, 189−194.

Devi, K., Sharma, M., Ahuja, P.S., 2014. Direct somatic embryogenesis with high frequency plantlet regeneration and successive cormlet production in saffron (*Crocus sativus* L.). South Afr. J. Bot. 93, 207−216.

Dhar, A.K., Sapru, R., 1993. Studies on Saffron (*Crocus Sativus*) in Kashmir. III. In Vitro.

Dhar, A.K., Sapru, R., 1994. Studies on saffron in Kashmir III. In vitro production of corm and shoot like structures. Indian J. Genet. Plant Breed. 53, 193−196.

Ding, B., Bai, S.H., Wu, Y., Wang, B.K., 1979. Preliminary report on tissue culture of corms of Crocus sativus. Acta Bot. Sin. 21, 387.

Ding, B.Z., Bai, S.H., Wu, Y., Wang, B.K., Fang, X.P., 1981. Induction of callus and regeneration of plantlets from corms of *Crocus sativus* L. Acta Bot. Sin. 23, 419−420 (in Chinese).

Ebrahimzadeh, H., Karamian, R., Noori-Daloii, M.R., 1996. *In vitro* regeneration of shoot and corm from the different explants of *Crocus sativus* L. J. Sci. Islam. Repub. Iran 7, 57−62.

Ebrahimzadeh, H., Karamian, R., Noori-Daloii, M.R., 2000a. Somatic embryogenesis and regeneration of plantlet in saffron, Crocus sativus L. J. Sci. Islam. Repub. Iran 11, 169−173.

Ebrahimzadeh, H., Radjabian, T., Karamian, R., 2000b. In vitro production of floral buds and stigma-like structures on floral organs of *Crocus sativus* L. Pak. J. Bot. 32, 141−150.

Fakhrai, F., Evans, P.K., 1990. Morphogenic potential of cultured floral explants of *Crocus sativus* L. for the *in vitro* production of saffron. J. Exp. Bot. 41, 47−52.

Frello, S., Ørgaard, M., Jacobsen, N., Heslop-Harrison, J.S., 2004. The genomic organization and evolutionary distribution of a tandemly repeated DNA sequence family in the genus *Crocus* (Iridaceae). Hereditas 141, 81−88.

Gadd, C.J., 1971. In: Edwards, I.E.S., Gadd, C.J., Hammand, N.G.L. (Eds.), The Dynasty of Agade and the Guitan Invasion. Cambridge University Press, Cambridge, pp. 417−463.

Gantait, S., Vahedi, M., 2015. *In vitro* regeneration of high value spice *Crocus sativus* L.: a concise appraisal. J. Appl. Res. Med. Aromatic Plants 2, 124−133.

George, P.S., Visvanath, S., Ravishankar, G.A., Venkataraman, L.V., 1992. Tissue culture of saffron (*Crocus sativus* L.): somatic embryogenesis and shoot regeneration. Food Biotechnol. 6, 217−223.

Greenberg-Kaslasi, D., 1991. Vegetative and Reproductive Development in Saffron Crocus (Crocus Sativus L.) (M.Sc. thesis). The faulty of Agriculture, the hebrew university of Jerasalem, Rehovot (Hebrew, English abstract).

Gresta, F., Lombardo, G.M., Siracusa, L., Ruberto, G., 2008. Effect of mother corm dimension and sowing time on stigma yield, daughter corms and qualitative aspects of saffron (*Crocus sativus* L.) in a Mediterranean environment. J. Sci. Food Agric. 88, 1144−1150.

Grilli Caiola, M., 2004. In: Saffron reproductive biology ISHS acta horticulturae 650: I International Symposium on Saffron Biology and Biotechnology. https://doi.org/10.17660/ActaHortic.2004.650-651.

Grisolia, S., 1974. Hypoxia, saffron and cardiovascular disease. Lancet 2, 41−42.

Gui, Y.L., Xu, T.Y., Gu, S.R., Liu, S.Q., Sun, G.D., Zhang, Q., 1988. Corm formation of saffron crocus *in vitro*. Acta Bot. Sin. 30, 338−340.

Halevy, A.H., Shoub, J., 1964. Tbe effect of cold storage and treatment with gibberellic acid on flowering and bulb yield of Duch iris. Hortic. Sci. 39, 123−129.

Haspolat, G., Ercan, M., Özzambak, E.M., Şık, L., 2013. Seed germination of some crocus species of western Anatolia. Anadolu, J. AARI 23 (2), 21−26. MFAL.

Homes, J., Legros, M., Jaziri, M., 1987. *In vitro* multiplication of *Crocus sativus* L. Acta Hortic. 212 (II), 675−676.

Huang, S.Y., 1987. A preliminary study on tissue culture of Crocus sativus. Plant Physiol. *Commun.* 6, 17−19 (in Chinese).

Humphries, J., 1996. The Essential Saffron Companion. Grub Street, London, 160 pp.

Husaini, A.M., Hassan, B., Ghani, M.Y., Teixeira da Silva, J.A., Kirmani, R.A., 2010. Saffron (*Crocus sativus* Kashmirianus) cultivation in Kashmir: practices and problems. Funct. Plant.

Isa, T., Ogasawara, T., 1988. Efficient regeneration from the callus of saffron (*Crocus sativus*). Jpn. J. Breed. 38, 371−374.

Karamian, R., 2004. Plantlet regeneration via somatic embryogenesis in four species of Crocus. Acta Hortic. 650, 253−259.

Karaoğlu, C., Çöcü, S., İpek, A., Parmaksız, I., Uranbey, S., Sarıhan, E., Arslan, N., Kaya, M.D., Sancak, C., Özcan, S., Gürbüz, B., Mirici, S., Er, C., Khawar, K.M., 2007. In vitro micropropagation of saffron. Acta Hortic. 739, 223−228.

Khorramdel, S., Mollafilabi, A., Hosseini, M., 2017. Evaluation of global warming potential of saffron agroecosystems (case study: khorasan, Iran). Acta Hortic. 1184, 259−262. https://doi.org/10.17660/ActaHortic.2017.1184.36. https://doi.org/10.17660/ActaHortic.2017.1184.36.

Lapadatescu, S., Petolescu, C., Furdi, F., Lazar, A., Velicevici, G., Danci, M., Bala, M., 2013. In vitro regeneration of *Crocus sativus* L. J. Hortic. For. Biotechnol. 17, 244−247.

Le Nard, M., De Hertogh, A.A., 1993. Bulb growth and development and flowering. In: Hertogh, A, De, Le Nard, M. (Eds.), The Physiology of Flower Bulbs. Elsevier Science Publishers, Amsterdam, The Netherlands, pp. 29−44.

López Rodríguez, F.N., 1989. Estudio histológico de Crocus sativus L. Tesina de Licenciatura. Universidad Pública de Pamplona, Pamplona, España.

Lopez-Corcoles, H., Brasa-Ramos, A., Montero-Garcia, F., Romero-Valverde, M., Montero-Riquelme, F., 2015. Phenological growth stages of saffron plant (Crocus sativus L) according to the BBCH Scale. Span. J. Agric. Res. 13 (3), e09SC01. ISSN 2171-9292. Available at: http://revistas.inia.es/index.php/sjar/article/view/7340 https://doi.org/10.5424/sjar/2015133-7340.

Mathew, B., 1982. The Crocus. A Revision of the Genus Crocus (Iridaceae). B.T. Ltd., Batsford, London.

Mathew, B., 1999. Botany, taxonomy, and cytology of C. sativus L. and its allies. In: Negbi, M. (Ed.), Saffron. Harwood Academic Publishers, The Netherlands, pp. 19−30.

Mathew, B., Brighton, C.A., Baytop, T., 1979. Taxonomic and Cytological Notes on Asiatic Crocus. Notes from the Royal Botanic Garden, Edinburgh, vol. 37, pp. 469−474.

McGimpsey, J.A., Douglas, M.H., Wallace, A.R., 1997. Evaluation of saffron (Crocus sativus L.) production in New Zealand. NZ J. Crop Hortic. Sci. 25, 159−168.

Milyaeva, E.L., Azizbekova, N.S., 1978. Cytophysiological changes in the course of development of stem apices of saffron crocus. Sov. Plant Physiol. 25 (2 part 1), 227−233.

Milyaeva, E.L., Azizbekova, N.S., Komarova, E.H., Akhundova, D.D., 1995. In vitro development of regenerating corms in Crocus sativus. Fiziol. Rast. 42, 127−134 (Russian).

Mir, J.I., Ahmed, N., Wani, S.H., Rashid, R., Mir, H., Sheikh, M.A., 2010. In vitro development of microcorms and stigma like structures in saffron (Crocus sativus L.). Physiol. Mol. Biol. Plants 16, 369−373.

Mir, J.I., Ahmed, N., Shafi, W., Rashid, R., Khan, M.H., Sheikh, M.A., Shah, U.N., Zaffar, S., Rather, I., 2014. In vitro development and regeneration of saffron (Crocus sativus L.). Afr. J. Biotechnol. 13, 2637−2640.

Mir, J.I., Ahmed, N., Singh, D.B., Shafi, W., Wani, S.H., Zaffer, S., 2015. In-vitro stigma like structure and stigma development in saffron. Vegetos 28, 55−58.

Molina, R.V., Valero, M., Navarro, Y., Garcia-Luis, A., Guardiola, J.L., 2005a. Low temperature storage of corms extends the flowering season of saffron (Crocus sativus L.). J. Hortic. Sci. Bitechnol. 80 (3), 319−326.

Molina, R.V., Valero, M., Navarro, Y., Guardiola, J.L., Garcia-Luis, A., 2005b. Temperature effects on flower formation in saffron (Crocus sativus L.). Sci. Hortic. 103, 361−379, 58.

Negbi, M., 1990. Physiological research on saffron crocus (Crocus sativus. In: Tammar, F., Marra, L. (Eds.), pp. 183−207.

Negbi, M., 1999. Saffron cultivation: past, present and future prospects. In: Negbi, M. (Ed.), Saffron: Crocus Sativus L. Harwood Academic Publishers, Australia, pp. 1−18.

Negbi, M., Dagan, D., Dror, A., Basker, D., 1989. Growth, flowering, vegetative reproduction and dormancy in the saffron crocus (Crocus sativus L.). Isr. J. Bot. 38, 95−113.

Negbie, M., 1999. Saffron: Crocus Sativus L. Medicinal and Aromatic Plants − Industrial Profiles. Harwood Academic Publishers, Amsterdam.

Okagami, N., 1972. The nature of gibberellin induced dormancy in aerial tubers of Begonia evansiana. Plant cell Physiol. 13, 763−771.

Okagami, N., Esashi, Y., Nagao, M., 1977. Gibberellin-induced inhibition and promotion of sprouting in aerial tubers of Begol~ia evans;ona Andr. in relation to photoperiodic treatment and tuber stage. Planta 136, 1−6.

Pandey, D., Pandey, V.S., Srivastava, A.P., 1974. A note on the effect of the size of corms on the sprouting and flowering of saffron. Progress. Hortic. 6, 89−92.

Pérez Bueno, M., 1989. El Azafrán. Mundi-Prensa, Madrid, España.

Pérez Bueno, M., 1995. El Azafrán, 2ª edición. Mundi-Prensa, Madrid, España.

Piqueras, A., Han, B.H., Escribano, J., Rubio, C., Hellin, E., Fernandez, J.A., 1999. Development of cormogenic nodules and microcorms by tissue culture, a new tool for the multiplication and genetic improvement of saffron. Agronomie 19, 603−610.

Plessner, O., Negbi, M., Ziv, M., Basker, D., 1989a. Effects of temperature on the flowering of the saffron crocus (Crocus sativus L.): induction of hysteranthy. Isr. J. Bot. 38, 1−7.

Plessner, O., Ziv, M., Negbi, M., 1990. In vitro corm production in the saffron (Crocus sativus L.). Plant Cell Tissue Organ Cult. 20, 89−94.

Rees, A.R., 1992. Ornamental Bulbs, Corms and Tubers. C.A.B. Internacional, Wallingford, UK.

Rubio, P., 1980. Estadística aplicada a la investigación agraria. Ministerio de Agricultura. Servicio de Publicaciones Agrarias, Madrid, España.

Rudnicki, R.M., Nowak, J., Saniewski, M., 1976. The dect of gibberel1ie acid OD sprouting and" flowering of some tulip cultivars. Selen. Hortic. 4, 389−397.

Sadeghi, B., Razavi, M., Mahajeri, M., 1992. The effect of mineral nutrients (N. P. K.) on saffron production. Acta Hortic. 306, 168−171.

Schnittler, M., Pfeiffer, T., Harter, D., Hamann, A., 2009. Bulbils contra seeds: reproductive investment in two species of Gagea (Liliaceae). Plant Syst. Evol. 279, 29−40.

Shahabzadeh, Z., Heidari, B., Dadkhodaie, A., 2013. Regenerating salt tolerant saffron (Crocus sativus) using tissue culture with increased pharmaceutical ingredients. J. Crop Sci. Biotechnol. 16, 209−217.

Sivanesan, I., Jana, S., Jeong, R.R., 2014. In vitro shoot regeneration and microcorm development in Crocus vernus (L.) Hill. Pak. J. Bot. 46, 693−697.

Tammaro, F., 1990. Crocus sativus L. cv. Piano di Navelli − L'Aquila (L'Aquila saffron): environment, cultivation, morphometric characteristics, active principles, uses. In: Tammaro, F., Marra, L. (Eds.), Proceedings of the International Conference on Saffron (Crocus Sativus L.) L' Aquila (Italy) October, 27−29 1989. Università degli Studi dell'Aquila, Academia Italiana della Cucina, L'Aquila, pp. 47−98.

Tammaro, F., 1999. Saffron (Crocus sativus L.) in Italy. In: Negbi, M. (Ed.), Saffron. Crocus Sativus L. Harwood Academic Publishers, Australia.

Vahedi, M., Kalantari, S., Salami, S.A., 2014. Factors affecting callus induction and organogenesis in saffron (*Crocus sativus* L.). Plant Tissue Cult. Biotechnol. 24, 1—9.

Vahedi, M., Kalantari, S., Salami, S.A., 2015. Effects of osmolytic agents on somatic embryogenesis of saffron (*Crocus sativus* L.). Not. Sci. Biol. 7, 57—61.

Vatankhah, E., Niknam, V., Ebrahimzadeh, E., 2014. Histological and biochemical parameters of *Crocus sativus* during *in vitro* root and shoot organogenesis. Biol. Plant. 58, 201—208.

Verma, S.K., Bordia, A., 1998. Antioxidant property of saffron on man. Indian J. Med. Sci. 52, 205—207.

Walia, E., Dattaa, A., Shresthac, R.P., Shresthad, S., 2016. Development of a land suitability model for saffron (*Crocus sativus* L.) cultivation in Khost Province of Afghanistan using GIS and AHP techniques. Arch. Agron Soil Sci. 62 (7), 921—934.

Yang, B.M., Huang, Y.L., Xu, W.J., Bao, L.X., 2015. Explant selection and cluster buds induction in vitro of saffron (*Crocus sativus* L.). Agric. Sci. Technol. Commun. 2, 106—108.

Yasmin, S., Nehvi, F.A., 2014a. *In vitro* microcorm formation in saffron (*Crocus sativus* L.). J. Cell Tissue Res. 14, 4463—4470.

Yasmin, S., Nehvi, F.A., 2014b. Effect of plant growth regulators on microcorm formation in saffron (*Crocus sativus* L.). Int. J. Curr. Microbiol. Appl. Sci. 3, 702—712.

Yildirim, M.U., Hayzadeh, M., 2018. Effects of mother corm diameter and plant growth regulators on ex vitro corm propagule regeneration in saffron (*Crocus sativus* L.). Rev. Fac. Agron. 35 (3), 318—342.

Yildirim, M.U., Özdemir, F.A., Kahriz, P.P., Nofouzi, F., Khawar, K.M., 2016. Safran (*Crocus sativus* L.) Bitkisinde Farklı Hormon Ön Muamele ve Sürelerinin Korm Çoğaltımı Üzerine Etkileri (Preconditioning Treatments Affect Regeneration on Different Sized Saffron (*Crocus sativus* L.) Corms). Tarla Bit. Merk. Araş. Enst. Derg 25, 301—305. (In Turkish with English Abstract).

Yildirim, M.U., Asil, H., Hajyzadeh, M., Sarihan, E.O., Khawar, K.M., 2017. Effect of changes in planting depths of saffron (*Crocus sativus* L.) corms and determining their agronomic characteristics under warm and temperate (Csa) climatic conditions of Turkish province of Hatay. Acta Hortic. 1184, 47—54.

Yildirim, M.U., Sarihan, E.O., Cetin, Y., 2019. In: Farklı Fotoperiyot Sürelerinin ve Gibberellik Asit (GA3) Uygulamalarının safran (*Crocus sativus* L.) bitkisinin bazı Tarımsal Özellikleri Üzerine Etkisi (the effect of different photoperiods and gibberellic acid (GA3) treatments on some agronomic characteristics of saffron (Crocus sativus L.). Erasmus Symposium, Erasmus Uluslararası Akademik Araştırmalar Sempozyumu. 5—6 Nisan/April 2019.Sayfa:143. İzmir, Türkiye.

Zargari, A., 1990. Medicinal Plant. Tehran University Press, Tehran, p. 574, 1990.

Zeybek, E., Önde, S., Kaya, Z., 2012. Improved in vitro micropropagation methods with adventitious corms and roots for endangered saffron. Cent. Eur. J. Biol. 7, 138—145.

CHAPTER 5

Molecular Approaches to Determine Phylogeny in Saffron

MORTAZA HAJYZADEH • FATIH OLMEZ • KHALID MAHMOOD KHAWAR

INTRODUCTION

The name "saffron" has its origin from the Arabic word *zafran* meaning yellow, which changed with the passage of time in pronunciation in English language to saffron (Caiola et al., 2004; Aytekin and Acikgoz, 2008). Saffron (*Crocus sativus* L.) is classified under the family Iridaceae (Crocus L.). No species in the Iridaceae family is used as an important food or vegetable crop of economic importance (Mathew, 1982; Harpke et al., 2013). Saffron is a general term used both for plant corms and dried, yellowish-red, three-lobed stigmas of a plant with a small yellow style (Mathew, 1982; Harpke et al., 2013). The commercial part of the saffron plant is the flower style that is composed of three stigmas and the corm itself. It is harvested manually to conserve a peculiar flavor and aroma, making saffron as the most expensive stigmas. The stigmas have wide range of applications including their use as spice (food dye or colorant for foodstuffs), in the manufacture of drugs used in folk and modern medicinal systems, and in natural dye industries (Abdullaev and Frankel, 1999; Mathew, 1982; Moraga et al., 2009a,b; Gómez et al., 2012, Harpke et al., 2013). The modern medicinal research has proven its significant effectiveness in reduction of cholesterol, and it has become the center of interest (Abdullaev and Frankel, 1999). The cultivation of saffron dates back to 1500—3000 B.C. in Iran, Greece, Kashmir, China, and the Mediterranean basin including Morocco, Turkey, Greece, Italy, and Eastern Europe (Fernández, 2004; Gresta et al., 2008; Fiore et al., 2010; Beiki et al., 2010). Different researchers report its center of diversity in a large area extending from the Balkan Peninsula to Asia Minor or Turkey (Larsen et al., 2015 - Fig. 5.1).

The saffron can grow and adapt on wide range of lands, photoperiods, and temperature ranges (Kafi et al., 2006; Moraga et al., 2009a,b). Now a days, saffron is cultivated in a large number of countries, including Pakistan, France (Babaei et al., 2014), Afghanistan, Israel, the United States, Australia, etc. as nonsignificant minor producers. Iran is the largest saffron producer with $\sim 80\%$ of the total production in the world (Ahmad et al., 2011).

There is a confusion about the center of diversity and also the origin of saffron. Saffron is a perennial triploid with $2n = 3$ $x = 24$ chromosomes derived from a *Crocus* grown as weed, probably by hybridization of two haploid sperm cells by a haploid sperm or hybridization of a haploid sperm cell by a diploid cell of unreduced egg (Chicchiricco, 1984; Caiola, 2004, 2005). Some researchers believe that saffron originated as a wild *Crocus* species (Negbi and Negbi, 2002). At the same time, other researchers based on morphological and molecular observations suggest different origins for the plant (Mathew, 1977; Chicchiricco, 1984; Caiola et al., 2004; Nemati et al., 2014). However, the exact picture is not clear yet about the origin of saffron. Its evolution may have involved number of unclear events as has been discussed in different studies. Some studies suggest that the saffron corm must have originated either by spontaneous natural hybridization—based allopolyploidy after a cross of two different *Crocus* species (Brighton, 1977; Ghaffari, 1986; Karasawa, 1940; Mathew, 1977; Caiola et al., 2004; Moraga et al., 2009b; Fluch et al., 2010), and the others believe that it must have originated by autopolyploidy (Tsaftaris et al., 2011; Harpke et al., 2013).

Saffron. https://doi.org/10.1016/B978-0-12-818462-2.00005-X

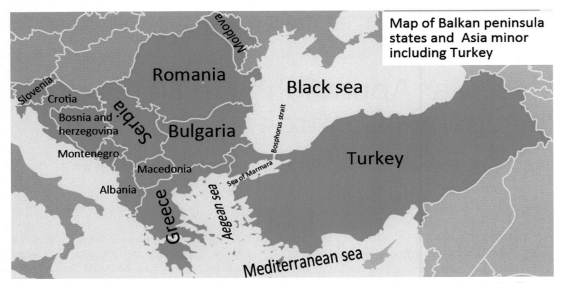

FIG. 5.1 Schematic representation of a large geographic area believed to be the center of diversity of saffron extending from the Balkan Peninsula to Asia Minor or Turkey.

It is a monocotyledonous herbaceous plant, grows as rosette, and owing to its incapacity to produce fertile pollen, it does not produce fertilizable gametes (Zanier and Caiola, 2000; Fiore et al., 2010; Jain et al., 2016; Serghini et al., 2017).

Saffron is a sterile male that is infertile, self-incompatible (Zanier and Caiola, 2000; Serghini et al., 2017; Caiola et al., 2000), and never set viable seeds. It propagates vegetatively through corms (Kafi et al., 2006; Petersen et al., 2008; Caiola and Canini, 2010). Therefore, its propagation is carried out vegetatively through corms that undergo a period of slow growth or dormancy (Fernández, 2004; Gresta et al., 2009). The sterility in saffron crocus is restricted, and there is a need to look for sources of genetic diversity in saffron. There is a need to conserve Crocus germplasm and its properties through individual or cumulative efforts at one place for breeding and improvement of the plant (Fernández, 2004).

Saffron is a male sterile plant and is propagated vegetatively. Therefore, it is understood that saffron is monomorphic. All the same morphological and phenotypic comparison in corms and flowers revealed a large variety in number of stamens and styles, with increased number in stigmas (Estilai, 1987), intensity of color, and existence of lobed tepals, other than differences in pollen size, leaves size and number, and viability percentage of samples collected from different areas in the world (Caiola et al., 2001; Nehvi et al., 2007; Agayev et al., 2009; Ghaffari and Bagheri, 2009). All these variations have shown some differences in accessions and were considered as a probable new variant of saffron. Preliminary characterization of the saffron and Crocus collection in the World Saffron and Crocus Collection (WSCC) has also emphasized the existence of phenotypic variations within and between saffron accessions for various morphologic and agronomic traits (De-Los-Mozos-Pascual et al., 2010; Fernández et al., 2011). Comparison of certain sharply different phenotypic characteristics among accessions is desired for plant breeding. The persistence of genetic variation through time and changing environments help plants to adapt to different growing conditions by addition of new or deletion of existing genes. This might have made saffron more or less able to survive, or the new alleles might have had no effect at all and the plants persisted over generations unaffected due to vegetative mode of propagation. Corms grow underground, and it is very difficult to mark their morphological changes; therefore, there is ambiguity and unclarity in data about the differences that are more or less dependent on corm size and the age of related genotypes. Therefore, unfruitful results could be due to limited available information about genetic diversity in saffron with failed selection during breeding (Alavi-Kia et al., 2008).

In clonal selection of saffron, differences in quality and phenotype are attributed to the effects of environments or to phenotypic effects (Agayev et al., 2009). The result of clonal selection has strongly suggested that there exists genetic variability in this species.

Cultivation in different environments may have induced numerous stresses during long time and may have undergone number of variant mutations. But these were not transformed/transferred among accessions because of sterility. So these variations were kept in genotype (Ahmad et al., 2011). The existence of phenotypic differences could be verified by molecular analysis, thereby confirming previous results obtained by Estilai (1978), Sik et al. (2008), and Beiki et al. (2010), and did not confirm the results obtained by Caiola (2004). Many researchers have considered evaluation of variations among saffron populations and accessions collected from different regions at phenotypic and genotypic levels. They have most often noted phenotypic variations under field conditions that are not stable and could change during different seasons. Some researchers believe that epigenetics could be a potential reason of expression of alternative phenotypes (Busconi et al., 2015). But this could not be accepted as a plausible potential reason because of the expression of alternative phenotypes; but, the plants belonging to same genetic background must express similar phenology under the same conditions. Alternative phenotypes among plants belonging to the same genetic background under the same conditions suggest the existence of genetic variations yet to be detected. Also, recent studies have strongly suggested a genetic polymorphic behavior among saffron accessions.

ORIGIN OF SAFFRON

It is postulated that greater knowledge about different variations in alleles across the genus *Crocus* has the potential to make new hybrids to increase the genetic base. It is well established that the genetic diversity in saffron (*C. sativus*) is limited and restricted; therefore, there is a need to look for sources of genetic diversity in saffron for breeding of the plant (Fernández, 2004) for specific traits, and this will address the issue of the origin of the detected phenotypic variabilities. The wild origin of species is the primary source of genetic diversity (Akhunov et al., 2010). The ancestral species, as a source of genetic variation, may play an important role in creation of biodiversity by transfer of genetic material; could introduce new genes and result in new chromosomal rearrangement of segments by crossing, integration, or manipulation; and could be exploited in crop-breeding programs (Vaughan et al., 2007; Heslop-Harrison et al., 2010). The origin of saffron is highly debatable and controversial. Different researchers have contrasting opinions, suggesting very different species responsible for its origin. No distinguishing distinct morphological characteristics could be easily seen in this genus because of wide range of emplacement, phenotypic diversity, and absence of net phylogenetic relationships between or within species of genus and series *Crocus* (Norbak, 2002). However, Mathew (1982, 1999) indicated many distinct characters to distinguish the members of this series. The researcher pointed out that most of the species included in this series have $2x = 2n$ but with different number of chromosomes. Furthermore, only *C. sativus* is triploid. There is a chance that these studies may have used single or insufficient number of markers or may have used insufficient number of samples of respective species. Petersen et al. (2008) have analyzed DNA sequences using five plastid regions in the series and genus *Crocus*. They were successful to resolve the issue of finding differences in different series (with a few ambiguities) and within the series where the resolution was poor.

The *Crocus* (former subgenus) has two sections *Crocus* and *Nudiscapus* (Norbak, 2002). The section *Crocus* is divided into six series, and among these series, saffron with nine other ally species take a place in the series *Crocus*. *C. sativus*, $2n = 3$ $x = 24$, *C. pallasii* (with four subspecies: *pallasii, turcicus, haussknechtii, dispathaceus*), *C. thomasii, C. mathewii, C. asumaniae, C. cartwrightianus, C. moabiticus, C. hadriaticus* (with three subspecies: *hadriaticus, parnonicus, parnassicus*), *C. oreocreticus,* and *C. naqabensis* are the members of the series *Crocus*.

Except for *C. sativus*, all other allies in the series *Crocus* are presumably diploid (Erol et al., 2014; Larsen et al., 2015). The common chromosome number in majority of the species of this series is $2n = 16$; *C. pallasii* subsp. *haussknechtii*, *C. thomasii*, *C. hadriaticus*, *C. oreocreticus*, and *C. cartwrightianus* have a chromosome number of $2n = 16$; *C. pallasii* subsp. *pallasii*, *C. pallasii* subsp. *dispathaceus*, *C. moabiticus*, and *C. naqabensis* have a chromosome number of $2n = 14$; and the highest of chromosome number with $2n = 70$ and $2n = 26$ are reported in *C. mathewii* and *C. asumaniae*, respectively. The lowest number of chromosomes with $2n = 12$ are reported in *C. pallasii* subsp *turcicus*. *C. sativus* is triploid among those in this genus with a chromosome number of $2n = 3$ $x = 24$ (Brighton et al., 1973, 1977; Mathew, 1982; Kerndorff and Pasche, 1994; Al-Eisawi, 2001; Mathew et al., 2009).

The most probable ancestor members that are morphologically distinct include *C. thomasii* (Chichiriccò, 1989) and *C. cartwrightianus* (Mathew, 1982), a progenitor of *C. sativus*.

In terms of phenotype, both these species have similar points; nevertheless, there are some confusing and unclear species that have diploid chromosome number and are fertile, while saffron is a sterile triploid plant with no similarity in size and color including quality of stigma (Negbi and Negbi, 2002; Nemati et al., 2019). Traditional morphological studies have revealed *C. cartwrightianus* to be the nearest relative of *C. sativus* (Maw, 1886; Mathew, 1982). Similarly, Mather (1932), Karasawa (1940), Pathak (1940), Mathew (1977), Heywood and Brighton (1983), Maw (1886), Brandizzi and Caiola (1998), Fernández (2004), and Caputo and Zanier (2004) have also approved that diploid *C. cartwrightianus* is more similar to *C. sativus* on a cytological and morphological basis, with confirmation of polymorphism among crocus species and low morphogenesis in *C. sativus*.

The cytofluorimetric techniques have revised the aforementioned division using nuclear DNA content, quality, and triploid DNA content of *C. sativus* in comparison with diploid content of *C. thomasii*, *C. cartwrightianus*, and *C. hadriaticus*. These results have indicated no difference in *C. sativus* DNA contents in spite of phenotypical variations. These studies also have confirmed more similarity between *C. cartwrightianus* and *C. sativus* compared with *C. thomasii* (Brandizzi and Caiola, 1998). Karyotype analyses have also revealed that *C. cartwrightianus* is one of the potential ancestors of *C. sativus* (in case of autotriploidy) (Mathew, 1982; Caiola et al., 2004).

Caiola et al. (2010) have described obtaining the seeds of *C. sativus* ×, a hybrid of *Crocus sativus* as the female and *C. cartwrightianus* as the male parent along with the seeds of allopollinated *C. cartwrightianus*, *C. hadriaticus*, and *C. thomasii*. Conclusively, the microstructure similarities in the surface of seeds of *C. cartwrightianus* and *C. sativus* × are proved, but these structures were different from the seed structure of *C. thomasii* and *C. hadriaticus*.

The molecular genetic base marker on phylogeny of the *Crocus* genus remains the topic of major interest (Caiola and Canini, 2010; Erol et al., 2013; Nemati et al., 2014). More of such research was carried out by using different or novel molecular markers to understand the parental and evolutional status of saffron. Molecular phenotypic studies of this group (genus *Crocus*) showed that all members of the *Crocus* genus were monophyletic (Erol et al., 2014; Harpke et al., 2014; Larsen et al., 2015, Rukšans, 2017). However, others have interestingly found *C. hadriaticus* and *C. pallasii* subsp. *pallasii* seem polyphyletic (Nemati et al., 2018). Harpke et al. (2014, 2016) suggests that several *Crocus* subspecies could

present independent evolutionary lineages. Both Erol et al. (2014) and Larsen et al. (2015) point out that all these *C. pallasii* subspecies have a very large genetic diversity. This information helped Rukšans (2017) to rank *C. haussknechtii*, *C. dispathaceus*, and *C. turcicus* as species from being subspecies.

Frello et al. (2004) noted small or no differences between *C. sativus* DNA and allied species namely *C. thomasii*, *C. cartwrightianus*, and *C. hadriaticus* in a study, using tandemly repeated DNA sequence in their phylogenetic relationships from five plastid regions. They, in confirmation to the wok of Tsoktouridis et al. (2009), used ITS1 and ITS2 (internal transcribed nuclear ribosomal regions) and internal trnH and psbA genes of cpDNA, along with 5.8S and 16S ribosomal genes to investigate the phylogeny among species of the genus *Crocus* and had inconclusive evidence about the origin of the *C. sativus*. Similar studies using chloroplast, ribosomal, and nuclear single-copy gene sequences focused on phylogeny could not find any clear evidence for the site of domestication or ancestral species of saffron (Petersen et al., 2008; Erol et al., 2014). The result of DNA barcode genes application in different *Crocus* species showed that evolution of *C. sativus* species occurred after independent events, under the influence of several Agro ecogeographical pressures. Additionally, the results showed *C. thomasii* and *C. hadriaticus* species to be more closely related to one another (Gismondi et al., 2013). Randomly Amplified Polymorphism DNA (RAPD) data analysis findings suggested *C. cartwrightianus* and *C. thomasii* as the nearest and *C. pallasii* and *C. asumaniae* more distant relatives of saffron (Caiola et al., 2004). Zubor et al. (2004) have also approved close relationship of *C. thomasii* and *C. cartwrightianus* with *C. sativus* by using Amplified fragment length polymorphism (AFLP) markers without identifying genomic differences. AFLP and inter-simple sequence repeat (ISSR) data also have analyzed the species in the *Crocus* genus by introducing the most close species of *C. sativus* (Sik et al., 2008; Caiola and Canini, 2010).

These results are in agreement with the work of Petersen et al. (2008), who analyzed five plastid of barcode regions. Their result showed too low genetic distance by DNA sequence analyzing. They proved that *C. cartwrightianus* was the nearest wild relative or progenitor of saffron and related to *C. sativus* followed by *C. thomasii*. The potential of *C. cartwrightianus* as an ancestor of *C. sativus* has also been confirmed in other studies (Caiola and Caniani, 2010; Gismondi et al., 2013). Similarly, Gedik et al. (2017) used 83 interprimer binding site (iPBS) markers in 17 different species of the *Crocus* genus, and their result showed *C. pallasii* subsp. pallasii and *C. cartwrightianus* were a close relative to *C. sativus*. The same result was reported using inter-retroelement amplified polymorphism (IRAP) data (Alsayied et al., 2015). Contrarily, Harpke et al. (2013) used ribosomal, chloroplast, and nuclear barcode gene sequences with a suggestion of *C. cartwrightianus* and *C. pallasii* as ancestors and parent species of *C. sativus*. These results are in agreement according to the AFLP analysis result of Erol et al. (2014).

Some other researchers have found that different species such as *C. hadriaticus* and *C. thomasii* are the ancestors of *C. sativus* (Caiola et al., 2004; Tsaftaris et al., 2011).

Some studies ascertain that *C. hadriaticus* species grown on continental Greece are distinctly separate from *C. cartwrightianus*, *C. oreocreticus*, and *C. hadriaticus* species and categorized with *C. sativus* species (Larsen et al., 2015).

Frizzi et al. (2007) checked allozyme-based variations in the genome of Crocus species. They reported that phylogenetically *C. sativus* seemed nearer to *C. cartwrightianus* without finding definite evidence. Contrary to this study, Moraga et al. (2010) used ISSR and suggested *C. cartwrightianus* cv. albus as more closely related to *C. sativus* instead of *C. cartwrightianus*.

On the contrary, Alavi-Kia et al. (2008) used IRAP markers and found that *C. almehensis* and *C. michelosnii* to be the possible ancestral species of *C. sativus*. Beiki et al. (2010) using RAPD detected that *C. hausskntchii* species is too closely related to saffron and it seems to be one of saffron's wild ancestors.

Nemati et al. (2014), using 27 microsatellite markers in phylogenetic analyses for 67 accessions from four species of the genus *Crocus* collected from Iran, suggested that *C. sativus* was more closer to *C. speciosus* and *C. hausknechtii*. However, the results are inconsistent about the contribution of potential parental taxa because of lack or absence of a link with a number of other similar species in the study with possible or potential contribution. Results of this study have shown similarity with RAPD, ISSR, and AFLP data. This has further revealed that genetic distances are autonomous of geographical origin (Moraga et al., 2009b; Erol et al., 2014). Sheidai et al. (2018) analyzed five different species including 90 plant samples in the *Crocus* genus using inter simple sequence repeat (ISSR) and was supported with Internal Transcribed Spacer (ITS) data that showed close genetic relationship of *C. pallisii* with *C. sativus* (in both data). Multilocus and Single Nucleotide Polymorphisms (SNP) through Genotyping by Sequencing (GBS) (genotyping by sequencing) data have identified that *C. sativus* took a place within *C. cartwrightianus* only without any allies (Nemati et al., 2018). In another, more advanced study by Nemati et al. (2019), they analyzed nuclear single-copy loci, GBS data, chloroplast genomes, and genome size. Their results have revealed and confirmed that wild *C. cartwrightianus* population in the south of Athens (Greece) is very similar to *C. sativus* and the single progenitor of saffron. Besides identifying the potential ancestors of *C. sativus*, the barcoding genes method revealed intraspecific variation in different accessions of *C. pallasii*, *C. cartwrightianus*, and *C. sativus*. Possible reasons for such variations could be related to a difference in geographical distribution or nursery practices that may have caused heritable epigenetic changes (Hyten et al., 2006).

AUTOPLOIDY AND ALLOPLOIDY SITUATION IN SAFFRON

Polyploid formation is widely accepted as a significant mechanism in the evolution of many plants, responsible for speciation and adaptation (Ramsey and Schemske, 1998; Madlung, 2013). This is due to the presence of repetition through genome during the process; the chromosomes are doubled, and this may involve a single genome (autopolyploidy) or a combination of two or more genomes of hybrid origin (allopolyploidy) and lead to diversity of novel genome or phenotypes (Harper et al., 2012; Buggs, 2010; Byfield and Wendel, 2014). Polyploid origins are an important investigation in determining phylogenetic relationships among the species (Kalendar et al., 2011; Estep et al., 2013). Previous studies have revealed allopolyploidization in *C. sativus* involving two parental species (Tsaftaris et al., 2011; Caiola and Canini, 2010; Harpke et al., 2013). In the case of allopolyploid saffron, *C. hadriaticus*, *C. cartwrightianus*, and *C. oreocreticus* are proposed as potential ancestral species (https://www.ncbi.nlm.nih.gov/pmc/articles/PMC4549961/, Jacobsen and Orgaard, 2004; Agayev et al., 2009), or *C. thomasii* and *C. pallasii* or *C. cartwrightianus* and *C. pallasii* (Fig. 5.1) (https://www.ncbi.nlm.nih.gov/pmc/articles/PMC4549961/, Tammaro, 1990), with each contributing the basic set of $x = 8$ chromosomes. Similarly, Alsayied et al. (2015) do not support the concept of autopolyploidy of saffron in another study. They used IRAP markers and concluded that *C. sativus* appears an allotriploid of *C. cartwrightianus* and *C. pallasii* subsp. pallasii (Fig. 5.2). The researchers could not observe any unique banding pattern, whereby the origin of bands could be related to any one of the diploid species. Also Beiki et al. (2010)

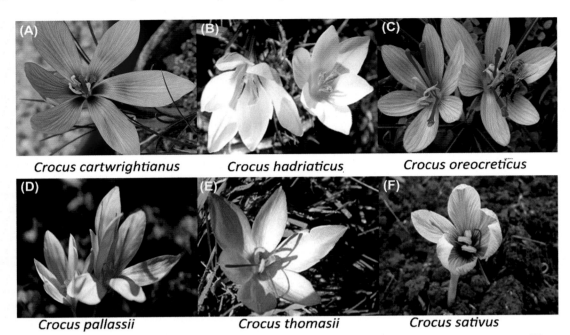

FIG. 5.2 Crocus sativus and potential parent species. (A) *C. cartwrightianus*, (B) *C. hadriaticus*, (C) *C. oreocreticus*, (D) *C. pallasii*, (E) *C. thomasii*, (F) *C. sativus* (https://www.flickr.com/).

have detected using RAPD that saffron is an alloploid plant.

The result is in contrast to the findings of cytofluorimetric studies that are in agreement to direct autopolyploid origin of *C. sativus* similar to that of *C. cartwrightianus* (Karasawa, 1940; Brandizzi and Caiola, 1998). Extensive studies have reported the origin of *C. sativus* to be through autopolyploidy of a single progenitor (Brighton, 1977; Mathew, 1982; Ghaffari, 1986; Caiola et al., 2004). The researchers have identified that *C. cartwrightianus* alone might have contributed to the hypothesized evolution of *C. sativus* by forming autotriploids. The authors have defined *C. oreocreticus*, the closest relative of both *C. cartwrightianus* and *C. sativus* (Nemati et al., 2018). Izadpanah et al. (2015) also support the idea of autotriploidy in *C. sativus* at genetic level. Nemati et al. (2019) used nuclear single-copy loci, chloroplast genomes GBS data to notify and identify that *C. cartwrightianus* populations growing naturally in southern regions of Athens as the single autotriploid progenitor of saffron.

Variation Level in Saffron

Saffron is a significantly important economic plant; therefore, there is a need to know the extent of diversity of accessions to select new genotypes and populations in crop-improvement programs. All these need management of germplasm and conservation of biodiversity for species. New studies have generated and detected variations in a triploid species (Odong et al., 2011). Saffron only blooms after a cold treatment of a few weeks to months after passing through a certain vegetative phase in the spring season and is planted once a year from corms. The origin of this plant would be compatible with that condition. Saffron is a cloned species, with insufficient genetic variation for utilization in selection programs. This confirms and proposes an intrinsic variability among saffron clones with potential variance at the genetic level and further increases chances of selection. Beygy et al. (2010) reported the precise properties of saffron corms such as weight, diameter, height, and volume for the first time. The researchers did not detect variations in corms from any region of east Iran.

However, the presence and extent of genetic variation in saffron *Crocus* corm is being debated, to reach a clear conclusion to deduce controversy about the monomorphic or polymorphic status of the plant species (Abdullaev and Espinosa-Aguirre, 2004).

Some researchers have proposed the creation of a saffron gene or germplasm bank including wild relatives for more research on the subject. The loss of land surface for saffron cultivation in many European countries has resulted in genetic erosion of the *Crocus* species.

Hence, the creation of a germplasm bank to conserve and use this species for genetic improvement and conservation (Fernández et al., 2011; Poczai, 2011) is necessary for genetic breeding purposes.

It will be a great achievement in breeding of saffron and the *Crocus* species. Identification of methods to determine genetic erosion will help in extensive uniform selection to prevent erosion and maintain genetic variation (Poczai, 2011). Over the past centuries, the genetic erosion issue in the *Crocus* genus due to land erosion−based losses has reduced saffron and crocus species crop in large areas, which furthermore reduced the genetic variation in saffron (Abdullaev and Espinosa-Aguirre, 2004). Therefore, it is desired as an urgent need to find, evaluate, and identify genetic variations to stop genetic erosion. Broad selection and proper breeding practices can help in reducing genetic erosion and restricting genetic variability (Poczai, 2011). Saffron, as a cloned species, does not have sufficient genetic variability for use in plant-selection programs.

Cytofluorimetric analyses of nuclear DNA of *C. sativus* accessions, from Holland, Israel, Italy, and Spain, have also shown morphological variations without any variation in base compositions and DNA content (Brandizzi and Caiola, 1998). Moraga et al. (2009b) also did not confirm any clear polymorphic differences in various accessions of saffron from 11 countries and declared *C. sativus* as a monomorphic species. Macchia et al. (2013) have explained using RAPD and ISSR data that *C. sativus* is a monomorphic species and did not find any polymorphic signals after analyzing accessions from various countries.

Differences in quality and phenotype are attributed to the effects of environments, resulting in different phenotypes (Agayev et al., 2009). Phenotypic and genotypic variations within and between accessions for agronomic and morphologic traits with a number of phenotypes have been reported by the WSCC among some *Crocus* populations and accessions of different regions (De-Los-Mozos-Pascual et al., 2010; Fernández et al., 2011).

They suggested that this was due to epigenetic effects (Busconi et al., 2015). Bagheri and Vesal (2002) have defined that *C. haussknechtii* is the closest relative of saffron (*C. sativus*) based on morphological properties.

So far, no correlation has been detected between phenotypes and genetic variability (Siracusa et al., 2013). Genetic differences were identified using AFLP markers among samples taken from European and Asian regions. They found no evidence for any significant phenotypic variation among the samples. They also detected intraaccession variations after analysis of four plants from each accession without any clear evidence of genetic variation (Siracusa et al., 2013).

Siracusa et al. (2013) found genetic differences using AFLP markers among samples taken from European and Asian regions. They found no evidence for any significant phenotypic variation among the samples. They also detected intraaccession variations after analysis of four plants from each accession without any clear evidence of genetic variation (Siracusa et al., 2013).

SAFFRON GENETIC VARIATION

Genetic diversity in *C. sativus* is very limited or largely unknown (Fernández, 2004; Harpke et al., 2013). This restricted genetic diversity may be partly connected to its sterile nature and self-incompatibility, yet it could be crossed using the pollen of *C. thomasii* (Chichiricco, 1984) or *C. cartwrightianus* (Caiola et al., 2004) to induce maturing capsules with seeds set (Tammaro, 1990). It has also been observed in field and in vitro studies on intraovarian and stigmatic pollination that embryo development of *C. sativus* and *C. cartwrightianus*, *C. thomasii*, or *C. hadriaticus* has no relationship with somatic embryogenesis or apomixes. Caiola et al. (2004) also found that *C. pallasii* and *C. asumaniae* are the more distantly related species of saffron. Therefore, they suggest the need to carry out more studies on sexual reproduction in saffron before taking steps about saffron breeding more precisely.

This clade consists of *C. vernus*, *C. tommasinianus*, *C. kotschyanus*, *C. versicolor*, *C. goulimyi*, *C. niveus*, *C. speciosus*, *C. angustifolius*, *C. flavus*, *C. laevigatus*, and *C. boryi*. Notably, *C. sativus* (saffron) is placed in between the recognized diploid species *C. pallasii* and "*C. sativus cartwrightianus*", while *C. mathweii* (series Crocus) is the second closest species of *C. pallasii*.

Environmental parameters such as day length and sunshine growth degree days affect vegetative and generative growth. These parameters also create phenotypic diversity including growth of saffron corms, blooming, and stigmas in terms of size and quality (Gresta et al. 2008, 2009; Hajyzadeh et al., 2017; Yildirim and Hajyzadeh, 2018). They showed that colder environments influenced to produce higher number of flowers but with poor stigma quality. Large-sized corms induce more flowers with a greater stigma yield (Ordoudi and Tsimidou, 2004; Maggi et al., 2011). These observations have also been approved by nuclear DNA cytofluorimetric analyses of *C. sativus* accessions, from the Netherland, Italy, Israel, and Spain. These studies have emphatically shown that morphological variations may result without any variation in base compositions and DNA content (Brandizzi and Caiola, 1998; Moraga et al., 2009b). Moraga et al. (2009) also did not confirm any clear polymorphic differences in saffron accessions from 11 countries and declared them a monomorphic species.

Molecular markers are not influenced by environment and plant-developmental processes, and the interpretations could be more valuable and reliable than morphological markers (Kumar et al., 2009). Therefore, contradictory reports about genetic diversity of saffron are very astonishing.

These studies have considered examination of some polymorphisms or low variations detected among saffron populations or accessions in different regions at genotypic levels.

In this context, chloroplast and nuclear gene region sequences have revealed a very low variations within the saffron (C. sativus) samples taken from various areas of the world for their sequence (https://www.sciencedirect.com/science/article/pii/S1055790317308229, Petersen et al., 2008). In similarity, Fernández (2004) and Harpke et al. (2013) detected narrow and restricted genetic diversity in C. sativus. According to Fluch et al. (2010), Ranieri et al. (2013), Bayat et al. (2016), and Namayandeh et al. (2013) using simple sequence repeat (SSR) and Babaei et al. (2014) using SRAP markers, low genetic differences are identified using SSR data. Similarly, Alsayied et al. (2015) found that according to the sequenced regions of IRAP data, the C. sativus had the minimum genetic variation. Most of these studies show that S. crocus is a monomorphic plant (Alavi-Kia et al., 2008; Caiola et al., 2004; Moraga et al., 2009b).

On contrary, Nemati et al. (2012, 2014) have observed a good level of polymorphism for extensive genetic diversity among C. sativus (Iranian) using microsatellite markers. Beiki et al. (2010) and Keify and Beiki (2012) also noted genetic diversity among six cultivated accessions of different origins using SRAP and RAPD markers. Similarly, Busconi et al. (2015) screened 112 accessions with methyl-sensitive AFLP and AFLP markers. The experiment ended up in two defined clusters of group accessions, each from the east and west, respectively, Cuenca/Teruel and Toledo/Ciudad. Javan and Gharari (2018) used SSR and SNP markers to define genetic diversity in C. sativus plants in Iranian saffron. Bayat et al. (2018), using iPBS, detected genetic variations among saffron accessions collected from various geographical areas of Spain, Iran, and Turkey.

The existence of genetic variation in phenotypic samples from plants of different origins is confirmed by the results of Estilai (1978) and Sik et al. (2008) with the help of ISSR and RAPD and by the results of Beiki et al. (2010) using RAPD, but they did not confirm the results of Caiola (2004). Izadpanah et al. (2015) noted molecular diversity, confirmed by morphological analysis among 29 C. sativus Iranian accessions. They noted 108 polymorphic bands using 17 RAPD primers. However, complete polymorphism was noted with 12 primers only, with a maximum genetic similarity of 0.92 and minimum genetic similarity of 0.42, in the same order. Siracusa et al. (2013) also found genetic differences using AFLP markers among samples taken from European and Asian regions. They found no evidence for any significant phenotypic variation among the samples. They also detected intraaccession variations after analysis of four plants from each accession without any clear evidence of genetic variation. This study confirmed the results of Estilai (1978), Sik et al. (2008), and Beiki et al. (2010) but did not confirm the results of Caiola (2004).

The results of these reports suggest that there is a need to identify more precise molecular markers to identify more genetic diversity in saffron (C. sativus).

CONCLUSION

Consistent with results from different studies carried out through out world, the existing literature suggests that

a. Some morphological variations due to the effect of environment and size of corm circumference could be observed in saffron stigmas and blooming, but these morphological variations have not been testified by any molecular technique.

b. Most of the studies are very informative. It has been proposed that saffron is either an allotriploid species that was introduced through a cross of C. cartwrightianus and C. pallasii subsp. pallasii or C. cartwrightianus cv. Albus and C. thomasii or through autotriploidy at the genetic level with wild C. cartwrightianus growing in the southern regions of Athens (Greece) as a single progenitor. All phylogenetic studies indicate that the origin of saffron is yet to be decided as no distinct relationships among the taxa of series are established within a single analysis. Origin of saffron is controversial, and different researchers have proposed different theories of the origin of the plant due to number of reasons. More technological advances in molecular techniques could open new insights into taxonomic analysis. The problem of intense genetic erosion in Crocus and identifying new techniques in molecular biology and cytology to sequence data about these species could lead to more precise results about the origin of the ancestors of *Crocus sativus*.

c. All studies establish very low morphogenesis and limited and narrow genetic diversity in saffron (*C. sativus*) using different morphologic and molecular studies (using different schemes of molecular markers). The persistence of genetic variation through time and changing environments help plants to adapt to different growing conditions. These changes in alleles might have no effect at all, or these might have persisted over long time because of vegetative or asexual propagation of the plant. Asexual propagation might have prevented segregation for favorable or unfavorable traits. This could be a reason why assumed addition or subtraction of a new allele or alleles to saffron probably had made it more or less able to survive for so many years with low interaction with environment. Moreover, genetic diversity and population structure are poorly understood and defined for saffron *C. sativus*, and more research is needed.

d. There exists a significant genetic variability among the species in the genus *Crocus* as testified by so many researchers using morphological, cytological, and molecular biology techniques. Using much larger panels of genetic markers, more studies would definitely uncover more practical information.

e. It is expected that the future research will address these unanswered issues more precisely to draw future pathway/s to saffron breeding.

REFERENCES

Abdullaev, F., Frankel, G., 1999. Saffron in biological and medicinal research. In: Negbi, M. (Ed.), Saffron: Crocus Sativus L. Harwood Academic Publishers, Amsterdam, pp. 103–113.

Abdullaev, F.I., Espinosa-Aguirre, J.J., 2004. Biomedical properties of saffron and its potential use in cancer therapy and chemoprevention trials. Cancer Detect. Prev. 28 (6), 426–432. https://doi.org/10.1016/j.cdp.2004.09.002.

Agayev, Y.M., Fernández, J.A., Zarifi, E., 2009. Clonal selection of saffron (*Crocus sativus* L.): the first optimistic experimental results. Euphytica 169, 81–99.

Ahmad, M., Zaffar, G., Mir, S.D., Razvi, S.M., Rather, M.A., Mir, M.R., 2011. Saffron (Crocus sativus L.) strategies for enhancing productivity. Res. J. Med. Plant 5 (6), 630–649. ISSN 1819-3455.

Akhunov, E.D., Akhunova, A.R., Anderson, O.D., Anderson, J.A., Blake, N., Clegg, M.T., et al., 2010. Nucleotide diversity maps reveal variation in diversity among wheat genomes and chromosomes. BMC Genomics 11, 702. https://doi.org/10.1186/1471-2164-11-702.

Alavi-Kia, S.S., Mohammadi, S.A., Aharizad, S., Moghaddam, M., 2008. Analysis of genetic diversity and phylogenetic relationships in crocus genus of Iran using InterRetrotransposon amplified polymorphism. Biotechnol. Biotechnol. Equip. 22 (3), 795–800. https://doi.org/10.1080/13102818.2008.10817555.

Al-Eisawi, D., 2001. Two new species of Iridaceae, Crocus naqabensis and Romulea petraea from Jordan. Arab Gulf J. Sci. Res. 19, 167–169.

Alsayied, N.F., Fernández, J.A., Schwarzacher, T., Heslop-Harrison, J.S., 2015. Diversity and relationships of Crocus sativus and its relatives analysed by inter-retroelement amplified polymorphism (IRAP). Ann. Bot. 116 (3), 359–368. https://doi.org/10.1093/aob/mcv103.

Aytekin, A., Acikgoz, A.O., 2008. Hormone and microorganism treatments in the cultivation of saffron (*Crocus sativus* L.) plants. Molecules 13, 1135–1147.

Babaei, S., Talebi, M., Bhara, M., Zeinali, H., 2014. Analysis og genetic diversity among saffron (*Crocus sativus*) accessions from different regions og Iran as revealed by SRAP maerkers. Sci. Hortic. 171, 27–31.

Bagheri, A.R., Vesal, S.R., 2002. In: Kafi, M. (Ed.), Saffron, Producing and Processing Technology. Zaban-o-Adab Press, Mashad, Iran, pp. 149–173 (In Persian).

Bayat, M., Amirinia, R., Tanyolac, B., Rahimi, M., 2016. Molecular phylogenetic among saffron (*Crocus sakus* L.) accessions from Iran, Spain and Turkey by SSR marker. J. Med. Spice Plants 21 (4), 168–173.

Bayat, M., Amirnia, R., Ozkan, H., Gedik, A., Ates, D., Tanyulac, B., Rahimi, M., 2018. Diversity and Phylogeny of Saffron (*crocus sativus* L.) Accessions based on ıpbs markers. Genetika 50. https://doi.org/10.2298/gensr1801033b.

Beiki, A.H., Keifi, F., Mozafari, J., 2010. Genetic differentiation of Crocus species by random amplified polymorphic DNA. Genet. Eng. Biotechnol. J. 18, 1–10.

Beygy, S.R.H., Ghanbarian, D., Kianmehr, M.H., Farahmand, M., 2010. Some physical properties of saffron crocus corm. Cercetări Agronomice în Moldova XLIII (1), 141.

Brandizzi, F., Caiola, M.G., 1998. Flow cytometric analysis of nuclear DNA in Crocus sativus and allies (Iridaceae). Plant Syst. Evol. 211, 149–154.

Brighton, C.A., 1977. Cytology of *Crocus sativus* and its allies (iridaceae). Plant Syst. Evol. 128, 137–157.

Brighton, C.A., Mathew, B., Marchant, C.J., 1973. Chromosome counts in the genus Crocus (iridaceae). Kew Bull. 28, 451–464.

Buggs, R.J., Chamala, S., Wu, W., Gao, L., May, G.D., Schnable, P.S., Soltıs, D.E., et al., 2010. Characterization of duplicate gene evolution in the recent natural allopolyploid tragopogon miscellus by nextgeneration sequencing and sequenom iPLEX MassARRAY genotyping. Mol. Ecol. 19, 132–146.

Busconi, M., Colli, L., Sánchez, R.A., Santaella, M., De-Los-Mozos Pascual, M., Santana, O., et al., 2015. AFLP and MS-AFLP analysis of the variation within saffron crocus (*Crocus sativus* L.) germplasm. PLoS One 10 (4), e0123434. https://doi.org/10.1371/journal.pone.0123434.

Byfield, S.R., Wendel, J.F., 2014. Doubling down on genomes: polyploidy and crop plants. Am. J. Bot. 101 (10) https://doi.org/10.3732/ajb.1400119.

Caiola, M., 2004. Saffron reproductive biology. Acta Hortic. 650, 25–37. https://doi.org/10.17660/ActaHo rtic.2004.650.1.

Caiola, M., 2005. Embryo origin and development in Crocus sativus L. (Iridaceae). Plant Biosyst. 139, 335–343.

Caiola, M., Canini, A., 2010. Looking for Saffron's (*Crocus sativus* L.) Parents. In: Functional Plant Science and Biotechnology, vol. 4. Global Science Books (Special Issue 2).

Caiola, M., Caputo, P., Zanier, R., 2004. RAPD analysis in *Crocus sativus* L. accessions and related *Crocus* species. Biol. Plant. 48, 375–380. https://doi.org/10.1023/B:BIOP.0000041089.9255 9.84.

Caiola, M., Di-Somma, D., Lauretti, P., 2001. Comparative study of pollen and pistil in *Crocus sativus* L. (Iridaceae) and allied species. Ann. Bot. 1, 93–103.

Caiola, M., Leonardi, D., Canini, A., 2010. Seed structure in *Crocus sativus* L.×, C. cartwrightianus Herb., C. thomasii Ten., and C. hadriaticus Herb. at SEM. Plant Syst. Evol. 285 (1–2), 111–120.

Caiola, M.G., Di Somma, D., Lauretti, P., 2000. Comparative study of pollen and pistil in *Crocus sativus* L. (Iridaceae) and allied species. Ann. Bot. 58 (1), 73–82.

Caputo, P., Zanier, R., 2004. RAPD analysis in *Crocus sativus* L. and related Crocus species. Biol. Plant. 48, 375–380.

Chicchiricco, G., 1984. Karyotype and meiotic behaviour of the triploid *Crocus sativus* L. Caryologia 37, 233–239.

Chichiriccò, G., 1989. Microsporogenesis and pollen development in Crocus sativus. LCaryologia 42, 249–257.

De-Los-Mozos-Pascual, M., Santana-Méridas, O., Rodríguez-Conde, M.F., Sánchez-Vioque, R., PastorFérriz, T., Fernández, J.A., et al., 2010. A preliminary characterization of saffron germplasm from the CROCUSBANK collection. Acta Hortic. 850, 35–40.

Erol, O., Kaya, H., Şik, L., Tuna, M., Can, L., Tanyolaç, M., 2013. The genus Crocus, series Crocus (Iridaceae) in Turkey and 2 East Aegean islands: a genetic approach. Turk. J. Biol. 38, 48–62.

Erol, O., Kaya, H.B., Şık, L., Tuna, M., Can, L., Tanyolaç, M.B., 2014. The genus Crocus, series Crocus (Iridaceae) in Turkey and 2 East Aegean islands: a genetic approach. Turk. J. Biol. 276, 543. https://dx.doi.org/10.3906/biy-1305-14.

Estep, M.C., DeBarry, J.D., Bennetzen, J.L., 2013. The dynamics of LTR retrotransposon accumulation across 25 million years of panicoid grass evolution. Heredity 110, 194–204.

Estilai, A., 1978. Variability in saffron (*Crocus sativus* L.). Experientia 34, 725.

Fernández, J.A., 2004. Biology, biotechonolgy and biomedicine of saffron. Recent Res. Dev. Plant Sci. 2, 127–159.

Fernández, J.A., Santana, O., Guardiola, J.L., Molina, R.V., Heslop-Harrison, P., Borbely, G., et al., 2011. The World Saffron and *Crocus* collection: strategies for establishing, management, characterisation and utilisation. Genet. Resour. Crop Evol. 58, 125–137.

Fiore, A., Pizzichini, D., Diretto, G., Scossa, F., Spano, L., 2010. Gnenomics and Transcriptomics of Saffron: New Tools to Unravel the Secrets of an Attractive Spice. In: Functional Plant Science and Biotechnology ©2010. Global Science Books, pp. 25–30.

Fluch, S., Hohl, K., Stierschneider, M., Kopecky, D., 2010. *Crocus sativus* L. Molecular evidence on its clonal origin. Acta Hortic. 850, 41–46. https://doi.org/10.17660/ActaHortic. 850.4.

Frello, S., Ørgaard, M., Jacobsen, N., Heslop- Harrison, J.S., 2004. The genomic organization and evolutionary distribution of a tandemly repeated DNA sequence family in the genus Crocus (Iridaceae). Hereditas 141, 81–88.

Frizzi, G., Miranda, M., Pantani, C., Tammaro, F., 2007. Allozyme differentiation in four species of the Crocus cartwrightianus group and in cultivated saffron (*Crocus sativus*). Biochem. Syst. Ecol. 35 (12), 859–868.

Gedik, A., Ates, D., Erdogmus, S., Comertpay, G., Tanyolac, M.B., Ozkan, H., 2017. Genetic diversity of crocus sativus and its close relative species analyzed by iPBS-retrotransposons. Turk. J. Field Crops 22 (2), 243–252. https://doi.org/10.17557/tjfc.357426.

Ghaffari, S.M., 1986. Cytogenetic studies of cultivated *Crocus sativus* (Iridaceae). Plant Syst. Evol. 153, 199–204.

Ghaffari, S.M., Bagheri, A., 2009. Stigma variability in saffron (*Crocus sativus* L.). Afr. J. Biotechnol. 8, 601–604.

Gismondi, A., Fanali, F., Labarga, J.M.M.N., Caiola, M.G., Canini, A., 2013. *Crocus sativus* L. genomics and different DNA barcode applications. Plant Syst. Evol. 299, 1859–1863. https://doi.org/10.1007/s00606-013-0841-7.

Gómez, L.G., Trapero-Mozos, A., Gómez, M.D., Rubio-Moraga, A., Ahrazem, O., 2012. Identification and possible role of a MYB transcription factor from saffron (*Crocus sativus*). J. Plant Physiol. 169 (5), 509–515. https://doi.org/10.1016/j.jplph.2011.11.021.

Gresta, F., Avola, G., Lombardo, G.M., Siracusa, L., Ruberto, G., 2009. Analysis of flowering, stigmas yield and qualitative traits of saffron (*Crocus sativus* L.) as affected by environmental conditions. Sci. Hortic. 119, 320–324.

Gresta, F., Lombardo, G.M., Siracusa, L., Ruberto, G., 2008. Saffron, an alternative crop for sustainable agricultural systems. A review. Agron. Sustainable Dev. 28, 95–112.

Hajyzadeh, M., Asil, H., Yildirim, M.U., Sarihan, E.O., Ayanoglu, F., Khawar, K.M., 2017. Evaluating effects of corm circumference and storage temperatures on yield and yield components of saffron at different elevations. Acta Hortic. 1184, 39–46, 1184.6. https://doi.org/10.17660/ActaHortic.

Harper, A.L., Trick, M., Higgins, J., Fraser, F., Clissold, L., Wells, R., Hattori, C., Werner, P., Bancroft, I., 2012. Associative transcriptomics of traits in the polyploid crop species Brassica napus. Nat. Biotechnol. 30, 798–802.

Harpke, D., Kerndorff, H., Pasche, E., Peruzzi, L., 2016. Neotypification of the name Crocus biflorus Mill. (Iridaceae) and its consequences in the taxonomy of the genus. Phytotaxa 260, 131–143. https://doi.org/10.11646/phytotaxa.260.2.3.

Harpke, D., Meng, S., Rutten, T., Kerndorff, H., Blattner, F.R., 2013. Phylogeny of *Crocus* (Iridaceae) based on one chloroplast and two nuclear loci: ancient hybridization and chromosome number evolution. Mol. Phylogenet. Evol. 66, 617−627.

Harpke, D., Peruzzi, L., Kerndorff, H., Karamplianis, T., Constantinidis, T., Ranđelović, V., Ranđelović, N., Juškovič, M., Pasche, E., Blattner, F.R., 2014. Phylogeny, geographic distribution and new taxonomic circumscription of the Crocus reticulatus species group (Iridaceae). Turk. J. Bot. 38, 1182−1198.

Heslop-Harrison, J.P., 2010. Genes in evolution: the control of diversity and speciation. Ann. Bot. 106, 437−438.

Heywood, V.A., Brighton, C.A., 1983. Meiosis in some species and cultivars of Crocus (Iridaceae). Plant Syst. Evol. 143, 207−225.

Hyten, D.L., Song, Q., Zhu, Y., Choi, I.Y., Randall, L.N., Costa, J.M., et al., 2006. Impacts of genetic bottlenecks on soybean genome diversity. Proc. Natl. Acad. Sci. U.S.A. 105, 16667−16671.

Izadpanah, F., Kalantari, S., Hassani, M.E., Naghavi, M.R., Shokrpour, M., 2015. Molecular and morphological variation in some Iranian saffron (Crocus sativus L.) accessions. Genetika 47 (2), 711−722. https://doi.org/10.2298/GENSR15027111.

Jacobsen, N., Orgaard, M., 2004. Crocus cartwrightianus on the attica peninsula. Acta Hortic. https://doi.org/10.17660/ActaHortic.2004.650.6.

Jain, M., Srivastava, P.L., Verma, M., Ghangal, R., Garg, R., 2016. De novo transcriptome assembly and comprehensive expression profiling in Crocus sativus to gain insights into apocarotenoid biosynthesis. Sci. Rep. 6, 22456. https://doi.org/10.1038/srep22456.

Javan, I.Y., Gharari, F., 2018. Genetic diversity in saffron (Crocus sativus L.) cultivars grown in Iran using SSR and SNP markers. J. Agric. Sci. Technol. 20, 1213−1226.

Kafi, M., Koocheki, A., Rashed, M.H., Nassiri, M. (Eds.), 2006. Saffron (Crocus sativus) Production and Processing, vol. 8. Science Publishers, Enfield, NH.

Kalendar, R., Flavell, A.J., Ellis, T.H.N., Sjakste, T., Moisy, C., Schulman, A.H., 2011. Analysis of plant diversity with retrotransposon based molecular markers. Heredity 106, 520−530.

Karasawa, K., 1940. Karyological studies in crocus: II. Jap. J. Bot. 11, 129−140.

Keify, F., Beiki, A.H., 2012. Exploitation of random amplified polymorphic DNA (RAPD) and sequence-related amplified polymorphism (SRAP) markers for genetic diversity of saffron collection. J. Med. Plants Res. 6, 2761−2768.

Kerndorff, H., Pasche, E., 1994. Crocus methewii. A new Autumn flowering Crocus from Turkey. N. Plantsman 1 (2), 102−106.

Kumar, P., Gupta, V., Misra, A., Modi, D., Pandey, B., 2009. Potential of molecular markers in plant biotechnology. Plant Omics 2 (4), 141.

Larsen, B., Orabi, J., Pedersen, C., Orgaard, M., 2015. Large intraspecific genetic variation within the saffron-crocus group (Crocus L., series crocus; iridaceae). Plant Syst. Evol. 301 (1), 425−437.

Macchia, M., Ceccarini, L., Molfetta, I., Cioni, P.L., Flamini, G., 2013. Studies on saffron (Crocus sativus L.) from Tuscan Maremma (Italy): effects of geographical origin, cultivation environment and drying method on volatile emission. Int. J. Food Sci. Technol. 48, 2370−2375.

Madlung, A., 2013. Polyploidy and its effect on evolutionary success: old questions revisited with new tools. Heredity 110, 99−104.

Maggi, L., Carmona, M., Kelly, S.D., Marigheto, N., Alonso, G.L., 2011. Geographical origin differentiation of saffron spice (Crocus sativus L. stigmas) Preliminary investigation using chemical and multi-element (H, C, N) stable isotope analysis. Food Chem. 128, 543−548.

Mather, K., 1932. Chromosome variation in crocus. Genetics 26, 129−142.

Mathew, B., 1977. Crocus studies and its allies (Iridaceae). Plant Syst. Evol. 128, 137−157.

Mathew, B., 1982. The Crocus. A Revision of the Genus Crocus (Iridaceae). Timber Press, Portland. Batsford, B.T. Ltd., London.

Mathew, B., 1999. Botany, taxonomy and cytology of C. sativus L. and its allies. In: Negbi, M. (Ed.), Saffron: Crocus sativus L. Harwood Acad Publ., Amsterdam, pp. 19−30.

Mathew, B., Petersen, G., Seberg, O., 2009. A reassessment of Crocus based on molecular analysis. Plantsman 8, 50−57.

Maw, G., 1886. A Monograph of the Genus Crocus. Dulau & Co., London, p. 238.

Moraga, A.R., Castillo-López, R., Gómez-Gómez, L., Ahrazem, O., 2009b. Saffron is a monomorphic species as revealed by RAPD, ISSR and microsatellite analyses. BMC Res. Notes 2, 189. https://doi.org/10.1186/1756-0500-2-189.

Moraga, Á.R., Rambla, J.L., Ahrazem, O., Granell, A., Gómez-Gómez, L., 2009a. Metabolite and target transcript analyses during Crocus sativus stigma development. Phytochemistry 70 (8), 1009−1016.

Moraga, A.R., Trapero-Mozos, A., Gómez-Gómez, L., Ahrazem, O., 2010. Intersimple sequence repeat markers for molecular characterization of Crocus cartwrightianus cv. albus. Ind. Crop Prod. 32 (2), 147−151.

Namayandeh, A., Nemati, Z., Kamelmanesh, M.M., Mokhtari, M., Mardi, M., 2013. Genetic relationships among species of Iranian crocus (Crocus spp.). Crop Breed. J. 3 (1).

Negbi, M., Negbi, O., 2002. The painted plaster floor of the Tell Kabri palace: reflections on saffron domestication in the Aegean Bronze Age. In: Oren, E.D., Ahituv, S. (Eds.), Aharon Kempinski Memorial Volume. Beer-Sheva: Ben-Gurion Univ Press, pp. 325−340.

Nehvi, F.A., Wani, S.A., Dar, S.A., Makhdoomi, M.I., Allie, B.A., Mir, Z.A., 2007. Biological interventions for enhancing saffron productivity in Kashmir. Acta Hortic. 739, 25−32.

Nemati, Z., Blattner, F.R., Kerndorff, H., Erol, O., Harpke, D., 2018. Phylogeny of the saffron-crocus species group, Crocus series Crocus (Iridaceae). Mol. Phylogenet. Evol. 127, 891−897. https://doi.org/10.1016/j.ympev.2018.06.036.

Nemati, Z., Harpke, D., Gemicioglu, A., Kerndorff, H., Blattner, F.R., 2019. Saffron (Crocus Sativus) Is an Autotriploid that Evolved in Attica (Greece) from Wild Crocus Cartwrightianus bioRxiv. https://doi.org/10.1101/537688.

Nemati, Z., Mardi, M., Majidian, P., Zeinalabedini, M., Pirseyedi, S.M., Bahadori, M., 2014. Saffron (*Crocus sativus* L.), a monomorphic or polymorphic species? Span. J. Agric. Res. 12 (3), 753−762. https://doi.org/10.5424/sjar/2014123-5564 ISSN: 1695-971X eISSN: 2171-9292.

Nemati, Z., Zeinalabedini, M., Mardi, M., Pirseyediand, S.M., Marashi, S.H., Nekoui, S.M.K., 2012. Isolation and characterization of a first set of polymorphic microsatellite markers in saffron, *Crocus sativus* (Iridaceae). Am. J. Bot. 99 (9), e340−e343. https://doi.org/10.3732/ajb.1100531.

Norbak, R., Brandt, K., Nielsen, J.K., Orgaard, M., Jacobsen, N., 2002. Flower pigment composition of Crocus species and cultivars used for a chemotaxonomic investigation. Biochem. Syst. Ecol. 30, 763−791.

Odong, T.L., van Heerwaarden, J., Jansen, J., van Hintum, T.J.L., van Eeuwijk, F.A., 2011. Determination of genetic structure of germplasm collections: are traditional hierarchical clustering methods appropriate for molecular marker data? Theor. Appl. Genet. 123, 195−205.

Ordoudi, S.A., Tsimidou, M.Z., 2004. Saffron quality: effect of agricultural practices, processing and storage. In: Production Practices and Quality Assessment of Food Crops, vol. 1. Springer, Netherlands, pp. 209−260.

Pathak, G.N., 1940. Studies in the cytology of crocus. Botany 14, 227−256.

Petersen, G., Seberg, O., Thorsøe, S., Jørgensen, T., Mathew, B., 2008. A phylogeny of the genus *Crocus* (Iridaceae) based on sequence data from five plastid regions. Taxon 57 (2), 487−499.

Poczai, P.K., 2011. Molecular Genetic Studies on Complex Evolutionary Processes in Archaesolanum (Solanum, Solanaceae) (Ph. D. thesis). University of Pannonia, Keszthely, Hungary.

Ramsey, J., Schemske, W.D., 1998. All rights reserved pathways, mechanisms, and rates of polyploid formation in flowering plants. Annu. Rev. Ecol. Syst. 29, 467−501.

Ranieri, E., Alsayaid, N., Heslop-Harrison, J.S., Falistocco, E., 2013. Analysis of an EST-SSR to find the genome composition and candidate ancestors of saffron, the sterile triploid species Crocus sativus. In: Prooceedings of the 57th Italian Society of Agricultural Genetics Annual Congress. Foggia September 16− 19.

Rukšans, J., 2017. The World of Crocuses. Latvian Acad. Sci., Riga.

Serghini, M.A., Lagram, K., Ben, M., Caid El, Lachheb, M., Atyane, L.H., Salaka, L., Karra, Y., 2017. Saffron (Crocus sativus): current state of scientific research. Acta Hortic. https://doi.org/10.17660/ActaHortic.2017.1184.12, 1184. ISHS.

Sheidai, M., Tabasi, M., Mehrabian, M.R., Koohdar, F., Ghasemzadeh-Baraki, S., Noormohammadi, Z., 2018. Species delimitation and relationship in crocus L. (Iridaceae). Acta Bot. Croat. 77 (1), 10−17. https://doi.org/10.1515/botcro-2017-0015. ISSN 0365-0588 eISSN 1847-8476.

Sik, L., Candan, F., Soya, S., Karamenderes, C., Kesercioglu, T., Tanyyolc, B., 2008. Genetic variation among Crocus L. species from western Turkey as revealed by RAPD and ISSR marker. J. Appl. Biol. Sci. 2, 73−78.

Siracusa, L., Gresta, F., Avola, G., Albertini, E., Raggi, L., Marconi, G., et al., 2013. Agronomic, chemical and genetic variability of saffron (*Crocus sativus* L.) of different origin by LC-UV−vis-DAD and AFLP analyses. Genet. Resour. Crop Evol. 60, 711−721.

Tammaro, F., 1990. Saffron (*Crocus sativus* L.) in Italy. In: Negbi, M. (Ed.), Saffron (Crocus Sativus L.). Hareard Academic Publishers, Australia, pp. 53−61.

Tsaftaris, A., Pasentsis, K., Makris, A., Darzentas, N., Polidoros, A., Kalivas, A., Argiriou, A., 2011. The study of the E-class Sepallata3-like MADS-box genes in wild-type and mutant flowers of cultivated saffron crocus (*Crocus sativus* L.) and its putative progenitors. Plant Physiol. 168, 1675−1684.

Tsoktouridis, G., Krigas, N., Karamplianis, T., Constantinidis, T., Maloupa, E., 2009. Genetic differences among wild Greek Crocus taxa and cultivated saffron (*Crocus sativus* L.). In: 3rd International Symposium on Saffron Forthcoming Challenges in Cultivation Research and Economics. Krokos, Kozani, Greece Book of Abstracts, p. 37.

Vaughan, D.A., Balázs, E., Heslop-Harrison, J.S., 2007. From crop domestication to superdomestication. Ann. Bot. 100, 893−901.

Yildirim, M.U., Hajyzadeh, M., 2018. Effects of mother corm diameter and plant growth regulators on ex vitro corm propagule regeneration in saffron (*Crocus sativus* L.). Rev. Fac. Agron. 35, 318−342.

Zanier, R., Caiola, M.G., 2000. Self Incompatibility Mechanisms in the Crocus sativus Aggregate (Iridaceae): a Preliminary Investigation, pp. 83−90 (Roma) 1(2).

Zubor, A.A., Suranyi, G., Gyori, Z., Borbely, G., Prokish, J., 2004. Molecular biological approach of the systematics of *Crocus sativus* L. and its allies. Acta Hortic. 650, 85−93.

determined in Iranian saffron. Safranal was reported to form the majority of volatile compounds with its relative amount in all the samples, as expected. Although the main compounds were found common in both Italian and Iranian samples, it was indicated that some peculiarities exist between samples affected from the growth region.

In one of the recent studies, the effects of various drying conditions on volatile compounds of Italian saffron were investigated with the application of SPME-coupled GC-MS by Urbani et al. (2015). As drying process is crucial in the aroma formation of saffron, the authors tried to recreate the optimum conditions with the aim of obtaining desired aroma. The samples were dried with various combinations of time and temperature, and safranal was reported to maintain its majority regardless of the procedure. Isophorone, 4-ketoisophorone, and 2,2,6-trimethyl-1,4-cyclohexanedione followed safranal and contributed highly on overall volatiles. New compounds such as 2,4,4-trimethyl-1-pentene and 1,3,3-trimethyl-7-oxabicyclo[4.1.0]heptane-2,5-dione formed due to drastic drying conditions. In brief, the authors concluded that the drying conditions exceedingly affected saffron's volatile profile.

Apart from SPME, SBSE method is also a clean procedure without the need of solvent usage. This technique allows sorptive enrichment with the application of polydimethylsiloxane-coated stir bars. Coated stir bars are submerged into the aqueous sample, and extraction takes place during stirring (Baltussen et al., 1999). The procedure acquires higher surface area and includes much coating than an SPME fiber. Hence, the method has increased efficiency in comparison with SPME. Yet still, the duration of analysis requires more than 60 min including the extraction and desorption (He et al., 2014).

For the first time, SBSE technique was applied on saffron to investigate the ability to use the herb as a bioindicator by determining the contamination of polycyclic aromatic hydrocarbons (PAHs) (Maggi et al., 2009). The authors aimed to obtain quantitative information about PAHs contamination in saffron to check if this spice could be used as a biomarker or vice versa. The study investigated 27 saffron samples obtained from different regions and found out that some of the samples had higher values of contamination than allowed limits from European Commission for spices.

Ultrasound-Assisted Extraction

This technique may be attributed as an alternative to the LLE method as both of them carry out an extraction with the use of organic solvents (Cabredo-Pinillos et al.,

2006). Extraction by ultrasound involves application of increased intensity and frequency of sound waves, and the energy created from the vibrations helps to release specific compounds from the sample matrix (Romanik et al., 2007; Sereshti et al., 2014). Ultrasound-assisted methods have been used in a broad array of analyzes including extraction of toxic elements and herbicides in soil samples (Väisänen et al., 2002; Caballo-López and de Castro, 2003), metal extraction and determination in products (García-Rey et al., 2003; Moreno-Cid et al., 2003; Moreno-Cid and Yebra, 2004), and volatile extractions from food matrices (Kimbaris et al., 2006; Sereshti et al., 2013).

This technique was also used for the extraction of saffron volatiles in several studies. Maggi et al. (2010) used UAE to comparatively investigate the effects of storage time on saffron volatile compounds. The authors elucidated volatiles from 77 of Spanish saffron in three storage times that is distributed as: 50 samples stored less than a year, 13 samples stored approximately for 4 years, and the rest is for 8 to 9 years of storage. A total of 19 volatiles were extracted from the samples with the application of UAE-GC-MS, and the main eight of these compounds represented approximately 90% of total volatiles. Safranal constituted the majority of the whole profile, and it was expressed to have fluctuation in concentration during long storage times. In accordance with the literature, the authors stated that an increment in safranal amount takes place in the first 2 years of storage, then it displays a reverse situation. Safranal was followed by 4-hydroxy-2,6,6-trimethyl-3-oxocyclohexa1,4-diene-1-carboxaldehyde, HTCC, isophorone, and 2,2,6-trimethyl-1,4-cyclohexanedione. These compounds had a decrease in their amounts continually in comparison with safranal; hence, authors underlined the possibility of these compounds to behave as a precursor in safranal production throughout aging. Eventually, the duration of storage was reported to result in quantitative changes in volatile compounds of saffron.

Sereshti et al. (2014) designed a combined extraction procedure to assess the volatile profile of Iranian saffron. A novel experiment of UAE coupled with dispersive liquid—liquid microextraction (DLLME) was applied, and a total of 27 compounds were determined in saffron samples. Hexadecanoic acid was reported to have the highest peak area in GC chromatogram followed by safranal and tetradecanoic acid. It was expressed that the sonication facilitated the volatile release via breaking the cell walls of saffron cells and subsequently DLLME procedure enhanced the sensitivity and the efficiency of the whole technique.

A broad array of procedures in addition to the abovementioned techniques are still tried to be created and applied on plants to gather comprehensive knowledge about aroma compounds. In these circumstances, the problem of selecting the appropriate extraction method arises expectedly. The selection of suitable procedures with optimum conditions plays a substantial role in obtaining an aromatic extract with the closest odor properties to the original samples.

REPRESENTATIVENESS OF THE AROMATIC EXTRACT FOR OLFACTOMETRIC ANALYSIS

Saffron is one of the most consumed spices in the worldwide because of its valuable nutritional and highly appreciated sensory (flavor) properties. The secret of the flavor of saffron mainly lies in its key odorants' fraction. GC with olfactometric detection (GC-O) is considered as a powerful technique to characterize the key odorant compound in food samples. One of the most important problems in olfactometric researches is that of the odor representativeness of the aromatic extract. Odor representativeness can be defined as a similarity between the extract odor and the original sample odor, and test of representativeness is based on the sensory evaluation using similarity, intensity, and descriptive tests of original sample and its aromatic extract by a trained panel. GC-O can be used after the assessment of the odor representativeness of the aromatic extract. To perform a precise GC-O analysis, it is essential to first recover aromatic extract as a representative of the product as possible. Indeed, this step is of vital importance before all quantitative, qualitative, and olfactometric analyses to guarantee that the aromatic extract smells as the odor of the original studied food sample. Several aroma extraction techniques have been studied for saffron volatile compounds. These include microsimultaneous hydrodistillation–extraction, vacuum headspace (Tarantilis and Polissiou, 1997; Amanpour et al., 2015), stir bar sorptive extraction (Maggi et al., 2008), supercritical fluid extraction (Zougagh et al., 2006), LLE (Tarantilis and Polissiou, 1997; Amanpour et al., 2015), solid–phase microextraction (D'Auria et al., 2004), ultrasonic solvent extraction (Jalali-Heravi et al., 2009), the SDE, and solvent-assisted flavor extraction (Amanpour et al., 2015). Up to now, numerous investigations have been performed aimed at determining the representativeness of the different spices and aromatic herb extracts including wild thyme (*Thymus serpyllum*) (Sonmezdag et al., 2016), shade-dried aerial parts of Iranian dill (*Anethum graveolens* L.), and savory (*Satureja sahendica* Bornm.)

(Amanpour et al., 2017), black cumin (*Nigella sativa* L.) (Kesen et al., 2018), shade-dried aerial parts of basil (*Ocimum basilicum*) (Sonmezdag et al., 2018), and Iranian endemic (*Echium amoenum*) herbal tea (Amanpour et al., 2018); but only one research has investigated on the representativeness of the saffron aromatic extract, which was by Amanpour et al. (2015). In this study, the aromatic extracts of Iranian saffron obtained by four different extract techniques (solvent-assisted flavor extraction [SAFE], solid phase extraction [SPE], LLE, and SDE were compared to saffron (reference) odor using descriptive, similarity, and intensity tests by panelists.

On the basis of the descriptive test results of this study, odor descriptors of reference and its extracts were defined as saffron, flowery, spicy, fresh-cut grass/grass, vegetable, citrus, caramel-like, mushroom earthy, vinegary odor notes (Fig. 6.2). Among these, saffron, spicy, flowery, and vegetable were the highest scores, while mushroom earthy, caramel-like, fresh-cut grass/grass, citrus, and vinegary reached the lowest scores. Authors reported that the sensory properties of the SAFE technique are very similar to that of the reference (saffron) rather than the other techniques (SPE, LLE, and SDE). With regard to similarity and intensity test results, the similarity scores of the saffron extracts from SAFE, SPE, LLE, and SDE techniques were found to be 71.8, 61.1, 55.4, and 37.8 mm, while intensity scores 63.9, 69.1, 53.5, and 58.7 mm on a 100-mm unstructured scale, respectively. According to similarity and intensity scores, the most representative extract was achieved with the SAFE technique. Therefore, this technique was used for the characterization of aroma-active compounds in saffron sample using GC-MS-O. In recent years, SAFE technique has been used for the extraction of volatile compounds of different food matrix such as white mustard seeds (*Sinapis alba* L.) and rapeseeds (*Brassica napus* L.) (Ortner et al., 2016), raw licorice (*Glycyrrhiza glabra* L.) (Wagner et al., 2016), dill (*Anethum graveolens* L.), and savory (*Satureja sahendica* Bornm.) (Amanpour et al., 2017), raw and cooked red mullet (*Mullus barbatus*) (Salum et al., 2017), and pistachio oil (Sonmezdag et al., 2018) before olfactometric analysis.

KEY ODORANTS OF SAFFRON

GC or GC- MS with olfactometric detection (GC-O or GC-MS-O) has become the most widely used technique for elucidation of food flavor complexity because this technique directly provides important information about the presence of compounds with different aromatic properties in food samples. This technique has

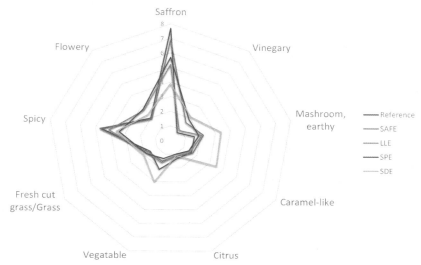

FIG. 6.2 Representativeness results of Iranian saffron (Amanpour et al., 2015).

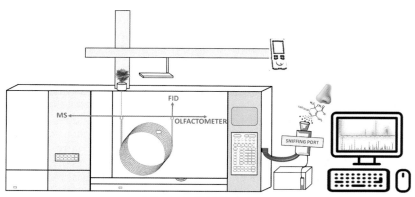

FIG. 6.3 GC-MS-O system.

been expansively used in aroma studies and permits the direct elucidation of powerful odorants in samples. Characterization of the analyte odor is possible, thanks to the presence of a special olfactometric port, connected in parallel to the FID or mass spectrometer (MS) (Fig. 6.3). The flow of the aromatic extract is split in such a way that the volatiles reach both detectors simultaneously, owing to which both signals can be elucidated. Using GC-MS-O is particularly advantageous as it helps not only with the assessment of odor properties of a compound with receptors in human olfactory bulbs but also with the direct identification of a key odorant with mass spectral characteristics. There are a few different olfactometric ports currently in use, and their design is very similar. The aromatic extract

delivered to the port through a dedicated transfer line (deactivated silica capillaries) is sniffed in a glass conical port fitted to the shape of a nose. During the olfactometric analysis, the transfer line is heated to avoid the condensation of semivolatile compounds on the walls of the capillary. Auxiliary gas (humid air) is added to the eluate to prevent the drying of the nose mucous membranes of the evaluating sniffer, as this could cause discomfort in sniffing analyses.

Olfactometric techniques can be classified into three groupings: dilution methods, time-intensity methods, and detection frequency methods (Serot et al., 2001). In time-intensity GC-O method, a human evaluator defines the odor quality of the aromatic extract, specifies the time and period when an aroma is noticed, and/

or assesses aroma intensity (Hognadottir et al., 2003). In detection frequency, GC-O method makes it possible to characterize key odorants in food samples within a minimum time, with no tiring and detailed training of the sniffers. The 6–12 number of sniffers detecting an aroma-active compound at the olfactometric port simultaneously (detection frequency) is used as a measure for the intensity of an aroma-active compound (Le Guen et al., 2001; van Ruth, 2001, 2004). In dilution analysis, combined hedonic aroma response measurement (CharmAnalysis) and aroma extract dilution analysis (AEDA) are frequently used (Acree et al., 1984; Debonneville et al., 2002; Grosch, 2001). Both analyses are based on the evaluation of the odor activity of single aroma compounds by sniffing the GC effluent of a series dilutions (usually 1:2, 1:3, or more dilutions) of the original aromatic extract, and each diluted aromatic extract is sniffed by sniffers until no odor is detected in the sniffing port. Within dilution analysis, AEDA is the most frequently applied method for GC-MS-O analysis in food samples because of its simplicity. In CharmAnalysis, sniffers determine the duration of odors (records the beginning and the end of each odorant perception) and creates chromatographic peaks. As a result of this technique, the aromagram is obtained by plotting the duration of the odor sensation against the dilution. $C = R^{n-1}$ formula is used to calculate the Charm value of the odorant where n is the number of coincident odor responses detected at a single retention index and R is the dilution level of the aromatic extract (Blank, 1996; Brattoli et al., 2013). In AEDA, the dilution factor (FD value) is simply the last dilution at which an odor active compound is detected. Several injections are required to reach a dilution of the aromatic extract in which odorous regions are no longer detected. The AEDA results are given as the logarithm of the factor of dilution (log FD) versus the linear retention index or by listing the FD values of the odorant. It is used to evaluate the key odorants according to their importance in the studied sample aromatic extract, hence providing a better understanding of the role individual key odorant plays in the general flavor of the food samples (Grosch, 1993).

Up to now, numerous studies have been performed at identifying the volatile compounds in different saffron samples (Kanakis et al., 2004; Bononi et al., 2015; Amini et al., 2017; Kosar et al., 2017; D'Archivio et al., 2018). As far as we are aware, only three olfactometric studies were conducted so far to characterize aroma-active compounds in saffron (one Iranian and two Spanish) samples (Amanpour et al., 2017; Cadwallader et al., 2001; Cullere et al., 2011).

Aroma-active compounds of saffron samples and their odor descriptions and olfactometric analysis techniques are given in Table 6.1. The saffron key odorants were determined using AEDA for the determination of FD factors and combined detection intensity and frequency technique (DIF) in these studies.

A total of 37 aroma-active compounds were detected in the aromatic extract by application of AEDA and DIF. Among these, nine unknown compounds detected by GC-O but not identified by GC-MS. These findings demonstrate that the characteristic aroma of saffron actually comprises a complex combination of various different odorants, rather than being any individual aroma-active compound. On the basis of the FD factor, the most powerful key odorants were safranal (2,2,6-trimethyl-1,3-cyclohexadiene-1-carboxaldehyde; saffron odor), 4-ketoisophorone (saffron odor), and dihydrooxophorone (3,5,5-trimethyl-1,4-cyclohexanedione; saffron odor) in an Iranian saffron sample (Amanpour et al., 2015) and 2-hydroxy-4,4,6-trimethyl-2,5-cyclohexadien-1-one (saffron, dried hay-like), safranal (saffron, tea-like), and an unknown-2 compound (a saffron, dried hay-like odor) in Spanish saffron (Cadwallader et al., 2001). Regarding to DIF technique, safranal (modified frequency value [MF] 93%), followed by 2,3-butanedione, hexanal, (E)-2-nonenal, and one unknown-9 compound were the most important aroma active compounds in Spanish saffron providing saffron, butter-cream, grass, and burnt-curry odor notes, respectively (Cullere et al., 2011). Safranal has been identified as the most dominant aroma-active compound in all three studies, and this compound is obtained from the picrocrocin in saffron (Lozano et al., 2000). Except safranal, two isophorone compounds have been reported as strong aroma-active compounds in Iranian saffron. Isophorones are the main volatile compounds of the saffron essential oil and are responsible for the typical saffron aroma (Iborra et al., 1992).

There were a number of positively identified aroma-active compounds with moderate intensities including 3-hexen-2-one (grass, geranium), octanal (lemon), 6-methyl-5-hepten-2-one (clove, spicy), acetic acid (vinegar), (E,Z)-2,6-nonadienal (cucumber), isovaleric acid (cheese), linaool (floral, honeysuckle), 3-methyl butanoic acid (rotten, sour, dried fruit), and 2-phenylethanol (floral, rose) in Spanish saffron samples (Cullere et al., 2011; Cadwallader et al., 2001), whereas linalool (floral), isophorone (saffron) and 2-phenylethanol (floral, rose) in Iranian saffron sample (Amanpour et al., 2015).

TABLE 6.1
Key Odorants of Saffron Reported According to GC-O Analyzes.

Key odorants	ODOR DESCRIPTION			Olfactometry techniques[d]
	Iranian saffron[a]	Spanish saffron[b]	Spanish saffron[c]	
Safranal	Saffron	Saffron	Saffron, tea	AEDA, DIF
Isophorone (3,5,5-trimethyl-2-cyclohexen-1-one)	Saffron, herbal	Saffron	nd	AEDA, DIF
2,3-Butanedione	nd	Butter, cream	Buttery, cream cheese	AEDA, DIF
Unknown-1	Buttery, oily	nd	nd	AEDA
Linalool	Floral	nd	Floral, honeysuckle	AEDA
(E,Z)-2,6-Nonadienal	nd	Cucumber	Sweet, cucumber	AEDA, DIF
Hexanal	nd	Grass	nd	DIF
3-(Methylthio)propanal	nd	nd	Baked potato	AEDA
Unknown-2	nd	nd	Saffron, dried hay	AEDA
4-Ketoisophorone	Saffron	nd	nd	AEDA
3-Hexen-2-one	nd	Grass, geranium	nd	DIF
Octanal	nd	Lemon	nd	DIF
Unknown-3	nd	nd	Green onion	AEDA
Dihydrooxophorone	Saffron	nd	nd	AEDA
Phenylethyl alcohol	Floral, rose	nd	nd	AEDA
6-Methyl-5-hepten-2-one	nd	Clove, spicy	nd	DIF
2-Acetyl-1-pyrroline	nd	nd	Nutty, popcorn	AEDA
3-Methylbutanoic acid	nd	Cheese	Rotten, sour, dried fruit	AEDA, DIF
Unknown-4	nd	nd	Green onion	AEDA
Acetic acid	nd	Vinegar	Vinegar, acidic	AEDA, DIF
4-Hydroxy-2,6,6-trimethyl-1-cyclohexene-1-carboxaldehyde	Green	nd	nd	AEDA
(Z)-2-nonenal	nd	Green, metallic	nd	DIF
Unknown-5	nd	nd	Fruity, stale	AEDA
(E)-2-nonenal	nd	Melon, aldehydic	nd	DIF
1-Octen-3-one	nd	Mushroom	Mushroom, earthy	AEDA, DIF
2-Hydroxy-4,4,6-trimethyl-2,5-cyclohexadien-1-one	nd	nd	Saffron, stale, dried hay	AEDA
Unknown-6	nd	nd	Stale, soapy	AEDA
Butyric acid	nd	Cheese	nd	DIF
3,5,5-Trimethyl-3-cyclohexen-1-one	nd	nd	Saffron, floral, hay	AEDA
Unknown-7	nd	nd	Floral, rose, saffron	AEDA
(E,E)-2,4-Nonadienal	nd	Rancid oil	nd	DIF
(E,E)-2,4-Decadienal	nd	Fatty, deep-fried	Fatty, fried fat	AEDA, DIF

Continued

TABLE 6.1
Key Odorants of Saffron Reported According to GC-O Analyzes.—cont'd

| Key odorants | ODOR DESCRIPTION | | | Olfactometry techniques[d] |
	Iranian saffron[a]	Spanish saffron[b]	Spanish saffron[c]	
β-phenylethanol	nd	Roses	Floral, rose	AEDA, DIF
Furaneol	nd	Cotton candy	Cotton candy, strawberries	AEDA, DIF
Unknown-8	Burnt, buttery	nd	nd	AEDA
Homofuraneol	nd	Cotton candy	nd	DIF
Unknown-9	nd	Burnt, curry	nd	DIF

[a] Amanpour et al. (2015).
[b] Cullere et al. (2011).
[c] Cadwallader et al. (2001).
[d] AEDA, aroma extract dilution analysis; DIF, combined detection intensity and frequency technique; nd, not detected.

A total of nine unknown compounds may contribute to the overall aroma of saffron samples. These compounds could not be identified by GC-MS because of their low concentrations in saffron samples. Two and six unknown compounds were detected in Iranian and Spanish saffron samples by the application of AEDA, respectively, whereas one unknown compound in Spanish saffron by the application DIF technique (Table 6.1). Unknown-1 was the most intense with a high FD (64) values in the Iranian saffron sample. The odor of this compound was buttery-oily note. Regarding Spanish saffron samples, unknown-2 compound (a saffron, dried hay-like odor) using AEDA and unknown-9 compound (burnt curry—like odor) using DIF techniques were found to be the important overall aroma contributors as unknown compounds. The other unknown compounds detected in all samples had moderate intensities.

CONCLUSIONS

The aroma and key odorant profiles of different saffron samples were elucidated in this chapter. Saffron aroma is composed of a wide variety of aroma groups with different chemical properties and carbonyl compounds (aldehydes and ketones) that are one of the major saffron compounds that contribute to saffron's aroma. GC-O methods are used to elucidate the key odorants in saffron samples. A total of 37 key odorants appear to contribute to the characteristic aroma profile in saffron samples. Among them, nine unknown compounds have not been identified by GC-MS. Results of GC-O showed that the complex combination of several aroma-active compounds contributed to the characteristic aroma of saffron samples, with safranal, 4-ketoisophorone,

dihydrooxophorone, and 2-hydroxy-4,4,6-trimethyl-2, 5-cyclohexadien-1-one being primarily responsible for the typical aroma of saffron samples providing a strong saffron odor. The outcomes from the present work might be considered as supplying useful information concerning the presence of aroma and key odorant profiles of saffron samples.

REFERENCES

Acree, T.H., Barnard, J., Cunningham, D.G., 1984. A procedure for the sensory analysis of gas chromatographic effluents. Food Chem. 14, 273—286.

Akhondzadeh, S., Sabet, M.S., Harirchian, M.H., Togha, M., Cheraghmakani, H., Razeghi, S., Rezazadeh, S.A., 2010. A 22-week, multicenter, randomized, double-blind controlled trial of *Crocus sativus* in the treatment of mild-to-moderate Alzheimer's disease. Psychopharmacology 207 (4), 637—643.

Alonso, G.L., Zalacain, A., Carmona, M., 2012. Saffron. In: Handbook of Herbs and Spices. Woodhead Publishing, pp. 469—498.

Amanpour, A., Sonmezdag, A.S., Kelebek, H., Selli, S., 2015. GC-MS-Olfactometric characterization of the most aroma-active components in a representative aromatic extract from Iranian saffron (*Crocus sativus* L.). Food Chem. 182, 251—256.

Amanpour, A., Kelebek, H., Selli, S., 2017. Aroma constituents of shade-dried aerial parts of Iranian dill (*Anethum graveolens* L.) and savory (*Satureja sahendica* Bornm.) by solvent-assisted flavor evaporation technique. J. Food Meas. Charact. 11, 1430—1439.

Amanpour, A., Kelebek, H., Selli, S., 2018. GLC/HPLC methods for saffron (*Crocus sativus* L.). Bioact. Mol. Food 1—49.

Amini, M., Ghoranneviss, M., Abdijadid, S., 2017. Effect of cold plasma on crocin esters and volatile compounds of saffron. Food Chem. 235, 290—293.

Assimopoulou, A.N., Sinakos, Z., Papageorgiou, V.P., 2005. Radical scavenging activity of *Crocus sativus* L. extract and its bioactive constituents. Phytother Res. 19, 997−1000.

Augusto, F., e Lopes, A.L., Zini, C.A., 2003. Sampling and sample preparation for analysis of aromas and fragrances. TrAC Trends Anal. Chem. 22 (3), 160−169.

Azenha, M.A., Nogueira, P.J., Silva, A.F., 2006. Unbreakable solid-phase microextraction fibers obtained by sol− gel deposition on titanium wire. Anal. Chem. 78 (6), 2071−2074.

Baghalian, K., Sheshtamand, M.S., Jamshidi, A.H., 2010. Genetic variation and heritability of agro-morphological and phytochemical traits in Iranian saffron (*Crocus sativus* L.) populations. Ind. Crops Prod. 31 (2), 401−406.

Baltussen, E., Sandra, P., David, F., Cramers, C., 1999. Stir bar sorptive extraction (SBSE), a novel extraction technique for aqueous samples: theory and principles. J. Microcolumn Sep. 11 (10), 737−747.

Blanch, G.P., Reglero, G., Herraiz, M., Tabera, J., 1991. A comparison of different extraction methods for the volatile components of grape juice. J. Chromatogr. Sci. 29 (1), 11−15.

Blank, I., 1996. Gas chromatography-olfactometry in food aroma analysis. In: Marsili, R. (Ed.), Techniques for Analyzing Food Aroma. CRC Press, Rockford, IL, USA.

Bononi, M., Milella, P., Tateo, F., 2015. Gas chromatography of safranal as preferable method for the commercial grading of saffron (*Crocus sativus* L.). Food Chem. 176, 17−21.

Brattoli, M., Cisternino, E., Dambruoso, P.R., de Gennaro, G., Giungato, P., Mazzone, A., Palmisani, J., Tutino, M., 2013. Gas chromatography analysis with olfactometric detection (GC-O) as a useful methodology for chemical characterization of odorous compounds. Sensors 13, 16759−16800.

Caballo-López, A., de Castro, M.L., 2003. Continuous ultrasound-assisted leaching of phenoxyacid herbicides in soil and sediment with in-situ sample treatment. Chromatographia 58 (5−6), 257−262.

Caballero-Ortega, H., Pereda-Miranda, R., Abdullaev, F.I., 2007. HPLC quantification of major active components from 11 different saffron (*Crocus sativus* L.) sources. Food Chem. 100 (3), 1126−1131.

Cabredo-Pinillos, S., Cedrón-Fernández, T., González-Briongos, M., Puente-Pascual, L., Sáenz-Barrio, C., 2006. Ultrasound-assisted extraction of volatile compounds from wine samples: optimisation of the method. Talanta 69 (5), 1123−1129.

Cadwallader, K.R., Baek, H.H., Cai, M., 1997. Characterization of saffron flavor by aroma extract dilution analysis. ACS Symp. Ser. 660, 66−79.

Cadwallader, K.R., 2001. Flavor Chemistry of Saffron. Carotenoid-Derived Aroma Compounds, ACS Symp. Ser. 220−239.

Carmona, M., Zalacain, A., Sánchez, A.M., Novella, J.L., Alonso, G.L., 2006. Crocetin esters, picrocrocin and its related compounds present in *Crocus sativus* stigmas and *Gardenia jasminoides* fruits. Tentative identification of seven new compounds by LC-ESI-MS. J. Agric. Food Chem. 54 (3), 973−979.

Chen, Y., Guo, Z., Wang, X., Qiu, C., 2008. Sample preparation. J. Chromatogr. A 1184, 191−219.

Christodoulou, E., Kadoglou, N.P., Kostomitsopoulos, N., Valsami, G., 2015. Saffron: a natural product with potential pharmaceutical applications. J. Pharm. Pharmacol. 67 (12), 1634−1649.

Condurso, C., Cincotta, F., Tripodi, G., Verzera, A., 2017. Bioactive volatiles in Sicilian (South Italy) saffron: safranal and its related compounds. J. Essent. Oil Res. 29 (3), 221−227.

Cosano, I., Pintado, C., Acevedo, O., Novella, J.L., Alonso, G.L., Carmona, M., Rotger, R., 2009. Microbiological quality of saffron from the main producer countries. J. Food Prot. 72 (10), 2217−2220.

Cot'e, F., Cormier, F., Dufresne, C., Willemont, C., 2001. A highly specific glucotransferase is involved in the synthesis of crocetin glycosylesteres in *Crocus sativus* cultured cells. J. Plant Physiol. 158, 553−560.

Culleré, L., San-Juan, F., Cacho, J., 2011. Characterisation of aroma active compounds of Spanish saffron by gas chromatography−olfactometry: quantitative evaluation of the most relevant aromatic compounds. Food Chem. 127 (4), 1866−1871.

D'Auria, M., Mauriello, G., Racioppi, R., Rana, G.L., 2006. Use of SPME-GC-MS in the study of time evolution of the constituents of saffron aroma: modifications of the composition during storage. J. Chromatogr. Sci. 44, 18−21.

D'Auria, M., Mauriello, G., Rana, G.L., 2004. Volatile organic compounds from saffron. Flavour Fragrance J. 19 (1), 17−23.

D'Archivio, A.A., Di Pietro, L., Maggi, M.A., Rossi, L., 2018. Optimization using chemometrics of HS-SPME/GC−MS profiling of saffron aroma and identification of geographical volatile markers. Eur. Food Res. Technol. 244 (9), 1605−1613.

Debonneville, C., Orsier, B., Flament, I., Chaintreau, A., 2002. Improved hardware and software for quick gas chromatography− olfactometry using CHARM and GC-"SNIF" analysis. Anal. Chem. 74 (10), 2345−2351.

Deo, B., 2003. Growing saffron−the World's most expensive spice. N Z Ins. Crop Food Res. 20, 1−4.

Díaz-Maroto, M.C., Díaz-Maroto Hidalgo, I.J., Sánchez-Palomo, E., Pérez-Coello, M.S., 2005. Volatile components and key odorants of Fennel (*Foeniculum vulgare* Mill.) and Thyme (*Thymus vulgaris* L.) oil extracts obtained by simultaneous distillation− extraction and supercritical fluid extraction. J. Agric. Food Chem. 53 (13), 5385−5389.

Du, H., Wang, J., Hu, Z., Yao, X., 2008. Quantitative structure-retention relationship study of the constituents of saffron aroma in SPME-GC−MS based on the projection pursuit regression method. Talanta 77 (1), 360−365.

Engel, W., Bahr, W., Schieberle, P., 1999. Solvent assisted flavor evaporation−a new and versatile technique for the careful and direct isolation of aroma compounds from complex food matrices. Eur. Food Res. Technol. 209 (3−4), 237−241.

Fancello, F., Petretto, G., Sanna, M.L., Pintore, G., Lage, M., Zara, S., 2018. Isolation and characterization of microorganisms and volatiles associated with Moroccan saffron during different processing treatments. Int. J. Food Microbiol. 273, 43−49.

García-Rey, R.M., Quiles-Zafra, R., de Castro, M.L., 2003. New methods for acceleration of meat sample preparation prior to determination of the metal content by atomic absorption spectrometry. Anal. Bioanal. Chem. 377 (2), 316−321.

Gohari, A.R., Saeidnia, S., Mahmoodabadi, M.K., 2013. An overview on saffron, phytochemicals, and medicinal properties. Pharmacogn. Rev. 7 (13), 61.

Golumbic, C., 1951. Liquid-liquid extraction analysis. Anal. Chem. 23, 1210−1217.

Grosch, W., 1993. Dedection of potent odorants in foods by aroma extract dilution analysis. Trends Food Sci. Technol. 4, 68−71.

Grosch, W., 2001. Evaluation of the key odorants of foods by dilution experiments, aroma models and omission. Chem. Senses 26, 533−545.

He, M., Chen, B., Hu, B., 2014. Recent developments in stir bar sorptive extraction. Anal. Bioanal. Chem. 406 (8), 2001−2026.

Hognadottir, A., Russell, L., Rouseff, R.L., 2003. Identification of aroma active compounds in orange essence oil using gas chromatography−olfactometry and gas chromatography-mass spectrometry. J. Chromatogr. A 998, 201−211.

Iborra, J.L., Castellar, M.R., Cánovas, M., Manjón, A., 1992. TLC preparative purification of picrocrocin, HTCC and crocin from saffron. J. Food Sci. 57, 714−716.

Jalali-Heravi, M., Parastar, H., Ebrahimi-Najafabadi, H., 2009. Characterization of volatile components of Iranian saffron using factorial-based response surface modeling of ultrasonic extraction combined with gas chromatography−mass spectrometry analysis. J. Chromatogr. A 1216 (33), 6088−6097.

Kanakis, C.D., Daferera, D.J., Tarantilis, P.A., Polissiou, M.G., 2004. Qualitative determination of volatile compounds and quantitative evaluation of safranal and 4-hydroxy-2, 6, 6-trimethyl-1-cyclohexene-1-carboxaldehyde (HTCC) in Greek saffron. J. Agric. Food Chem. 52 (14), 4515−4521.

Kesen, S., Amanpour, A., Tsouli Sarhir, S., Sevindik, O., Guclu, G., Kelebek, H., Selli, S., 2018. Characterization of aroma-active compounds in seed extract of black cumin (*Nigella sativa* L.) by aroma extract dilution analysis. Foods 7, 4−10.

Kesen, S., Kelebek, H., Sen, K., Ulas, M., Selli, S., 2013. GC−MS−olfactometric characterization of the key aroma compounds in Turkish olive oils by application of the aroma extract dilution analysis. Food Res. Int. 54 (2), 1987−1994.

Kimbaris, A.C., Siatis, N.G., Daferera, D.J., Tarantilis, P.A., Pappas, C.S., Polissiou, M.G., 2006. Comparison of distillation and ultrasound-assisted extraction methods for the isolation of sensitive aroma compounds from garlic (*Allium sativum*). Ultrason. Sonochem. 13 (1), 54−60.

Kosar, M., Demirci, B., Goger, F., Kara, I., Baser, K.H.C., 2017. Volatile composition, antioxidant activity, and antioxidant

components in saffron cultivated in Turkey. Int. J. Food Prop. 20 (Suppl. 1), S746−S754.

Koulakiotis, N.S., 2009. Development of a Liquid Chromatography Methodology for the Quantification of Bioactive Components of *Crocus sativus* and Other Endemic Taxa (M.Sc. thesis). University of Patra-Greece.

Kumar, R., Singh, V., Devi, K., Sharma, M., Singh, M.K., Ahuja, P.S., 2008. State of art of saffron (*Crocus sativus* L.) agronomy: a comprehensive review. Food Rev. Int. 25 (1), 44−85.

Lee, S.J., Ahn, B., 2009. Comparison of volatile components in fermented soybean pastes using simultaneous distillation and extraction (SDE) with sensory characterisation. Food Chem. 114 (2), 600−609.

Le Guen, S., Carole Prost, P., Demaimay, M., 2001. Evaluation of the representativeness of the odor of cooked mussel extracts and the relationship between sensory descriptors and potent odorants. J. Agric. Food Chem. 49, 1321−1327.

Lozano, P., Delgado, D., Gomez, D., Rubio, M., Iborra, J.L., 2000. A non-destructive method to determine the safranal content of saffron (*Crocus sativus* L.) by supercritical carbon dioxide extraction combined with high-performance liquid chromatography and gas chromatography. J. Biochem. Biophys. Methods 43, 367−378.

Macchia, M., Ceccarini, L., Molfetta, I., Cioni, P.L., Flamini, G., 2013. Studies on saffron (*Crocus sativus* L.) from Tuscan Maremma (Italy): effects of geographical origin, cultivation environment and drying method on volatile emission. Int. J. Food Sci. Technol. 48 (11), 2370−2375.

Maggi, L., Carmona, M., del Campo, C.P., Zalacain, A., de Mendoza, J.H., Mocholí, F.A., Alonso, G.L., 2008. Multi-residue contaminants and pollutants analysis in saffron spice by stir bar sorptive extraction and gas chromatography−ion trap tandem mass spectrometry. J. Chromatogr. A 1209, 55−60.

Maggi, L., Carmona, M., Zalacain, A., Alonso, G.L., Martínez Tomé, M., Murcia, M.A., García Diz, L., 2009. Saffron as environmental biomarker of diffuse contamination. In: III International Symposium on Saffron: Forthcoming Challenges in Cultivation, vol. 850. Research and Economics, pp. 265−270.

Maggi, L, Carmona, M, Zalacain, A, Alonso, G.L, Martínez Tomé, M., Murcia, M.A, García Diz, L, 2010. Saffron as environmental biomarker of diffuse contamination. In: In III International Symposium on Saffron: Forthcoming Challenges in Cultivation, 850. Research and Economics, pp. 265−270.

Maggi, L., Sánchez, A.M., Carmona, M., Kanakis, C.D., Anastasaki, E., Tarantilis, P.A., Alonso, G.L., 2011. Rapid determination of safranal in the quality control of saffron spice (*Crocus sativus* L.). Food Chem. 127 (1), 369−373.

Moraga, A.R., Nohales, P.F., Fernandez-Perez, J.A., Gomez-Gomez, L., 2004. Glucosilation of the saffron apocarotenoid crocetin by a glucotransferase isolated from *Crocus sativus* stigmas. Planta 219 (6), 955−966.

Moreno-Cid, A., Yebra, M.C., Cancela, S., Cespón, R.M., 2003. Flow injection on-line ultrasound-assisted extraction of iron in meat samples coupled to a flame atomic absorption spectrometric system. Anal. Bioanal. Chem. 377 (4), 730–734.

Moreno-Cid, A., Yebra, M.C., 2004. Continuous ultrasound-assisted extraction coupled to a flow injection-flame atomic absorption spectrometric system for calcium determination in seafood samples. Anal. Bioanal. Chem. 379 (1), 77–82.

Noorbala, A.A., Akhondzadeh, S.H., Tahmacebi-Pour, N., Jamshidi, A.H., 2005. Hydro-alcoholic extract of *Crocus sativus* L. versus fluoxetine in the treatment of mild to moderate depression: a double-blind, randomized pilot trial. J. Ethnopharmacol. 97 (2), 281–284.

Ortner, E., Granvogl, M., Schieberle, P., 2016. Elucidation of thermally induced changes in key odorants of white mustard seeds (*Sinapis alba* L.) and rapeseeds (*Brassica napus* L.) using molecular sensory science. J. Agric. Food Chem. 64, 8179–8190.

Papandreou, M.A., Kanakis, C.D., Polissiou, M.G., Efthimiopoulos, S., Cordopatis, P., Margarity, M., Lamari, F.N., 2006. Inhibitory activity on amyloid-β aggregation and antioxidant properties of *Crocus sativus* stigmas extract and its crocin constituents. J. Agric. Food Chem. 54 (23), 8762–8768.

Pawliszyn, J., 1997. Solid Phase Microextraction: Theory and Practice. John Wiley & Sons.

Premkumar, K., Thirunavukkarasu, C., Abraham, S.K., Santhiya, S.T., Ramesh, A., 2006. Protective effect of saffron (*Crocus sativus* L.) aqueous extract against genetic damage induced by anti-tumor agents in mice. Hum. Exp. Toxicol. 25 (2), 79–84.

Romanik, G., Gilgenast, E., Przyjazny, A., Kamiński, M., 2007. Techniques of preparing plant material for chromatographic separation and analysis. J. Biochem. Biophys. Methods 70 (2), 253–261.

Rödel, W., Petrzika, M., 1991. Analysis of the volatile components of saffron. J. High Resolut. Chromatogr. 14 (11), 771–774.

Salum, P., Guclu, G., Selli, S., 2017. Comparative evaluation of key aroma-active compounds in raw and cooked red mullet (*Mullus barbatus*) by aroma extract dilution analysis. J. Agric. Food Chem. 65, 8402–8408.

Sanchez, A.M., Winterhalter, P., 2013. Carotenoid cleavage products in saffron (*Crocus sativus* L.). In: ACS Symposium Series, vol. 1134, pp. 45–63.

Selli, S., Cayhan, G.G., 2009. Analysis of volatile compounds of wild gilthead sea bream (*Sparus aurata*) by simultaneous distillation–extraction (SDE) and GC–MS. Microchem. J. 93 (2), 232–235.

Selli, S., Kelebek, H., Ayseli, M.T., Tokbas, H., 2014. Characterization of the most aroma-active compounds in cherry tomato by application of the aroma extract dilution analysis. Food Chem. 165, 540–546.

Sereshti, H., Heidari, R., Samadi, S., 2014. Determination of volatile components of saffron by optimised ultrasound-assisted extraction in tandem with dispersive liquid–liquid

microextraction followed by gas chromatography–mass spectrometry. Food Chem. 143, 499–505.

Sereshti, H., Samadi, S., Jalali-Heravi, M., 2013. Determination of volatile components of green, black, oolong and white tea by optimized ultrasound-assisted extraction-dispersive liquid–liquid microextraction coupled with gas chromatography. J. Chromatogr. A 1280, 1–8.

Serot, T., Prost, C., Visan, L., Burcea, M., 2001. Identification of the main odor-active compounds in musts from French and Romanian hybrids by three olfactometric methods. J. Agric. Food Chem. 49 (4), 1909–1914.

Shahi, T., Assadpour, E., Jafari, S.M., 2016. Main chemical compounds and pharmacological activities of stigmas and tepals of 'red gold'; saffron. Trends Food Sci. Technol. 58, 69–78.

Smolskaite, L., Talou, T., Fabre, N., Venskutonis, P.R., May 2011. Valorization of saffron industry by-products: bioactive compounds from leaves. In: Baltic Conference on Food Science and Technology FoodBalt-2011, vol. 6.

Soeda, S., Ochiai, T., Shimeno, H., Saito, H., Abe, K., Tanaka, H., Shoyama, Y., 2007. Pharmacological activities of crocin in saffron. J. Nat. Med. 61 (2), 102–111.

Sonmezdag, A.S., Amanpour, A., Kelebek, H., Selli, S., 2018a. The most aroma-active compounds in shade-dried aerial parts of basil obtained from Iran and Turkey. Ind. Crops Prod. 124, 692–698.

Sonmezdag, A.S., Kelebek, H., Selli, S., 2016. Characterization of aroma-active and phenolic profiles of wild thyme (*Thymus serpyllum*) by GC-MS-Olfactometry and LC-ESI-MS/MS. J. Food Sci. Technol. 53 (4), 1957–1965.

Sonmezdag, A.S., Kelebek, H., Selli, S., 2018b. Pistachio oil (*Pistacia vera* L. cv. Uzun): characterization of key odorants in a representative aromatic extract by GC-MS-olfactometry and phenolic profile by LC-ESI-MS/MS. Food Chem. 240, 24–31.

Straubinger, M., Bau, B., Eckstein, S., Fink, M., Winterhalter, P., 1998. Identification of novel glycosidic aroma precursors in saffron (*Crocus sativus* L.). J. Agric. Food Chem. 46 (8), 3238–3243.

Sujata, V., Ravishankar, G.A., Venkataraman, L.V., 1992. Methods for the analysis of the saffron metabolites crocin, crocetins, picrocrocin and safranal for the determination of the quality of the spice using thin-layer chromatography, high-performance liquid chromatography and gas chromatography. J. Chromatogr. A 624 (1–2), 497–502.

Tarantilis, P.A., Polissiou, M.G., 1997. Isolation and identification of the aroma components from saffron (*Crocus sativus* L.). J. Agric. Food Chem. 45, 459–462.

Urbani, E., Blasi, F., Chiesi, C., Maurizi, A., Cossignani, L., 2015. Characterization of volatile fraction of saffron from central Italy (Cascia, Umbria). Int. J. Food Prop. 18 (10), 2223–2230.

Väisänen, A., Suontamo, R., Silvonen, J., Rintala, J., 2002. Ultrasound-assisted extraction in the determination of arsenic, cadmium, copper, lead, and silver in contaminated soil samples by inductively coupled plasma atomic emission spectrometry. Anal. Bioanal. Chem. 373 (1–2), 93–97.

van Ruth, S.M., 2001. Methods for gas chromatography-olfactometry: a review. Biomol. Eng. 17, 121–128.

van Ruth, S.M., 2004. Evaluation of two gas chromatography–olfactometry methods: the detection frequency and perceived intensity method. J. Chromatogr. A 1054, 33–37.

Wagner, J., Granvogl, M., Schieberle, P., 2016. Characterization of the key aroma compounds in raw licorice (*Glycyrrhiza glabra* L.) by means of molecular sensory science. J. Agric. Food Chem. 64, 8388–8396.

Zarghami, N.S., Heinz, D.E., 1971. Monoterpene aldehydes and isophorone-related compounds of saffron. Phytochemistry 10 (11), 2755–2761.

Zougagh, M., Ríos, A., Valcárcel, M., 2006. Determination of total safranal by in situ acid hydrolysis in supercritical fluid media: application to the quality control of commercial saffron. Anal. Chim. Acta 578 (2), 117–121.

CHAPTER 7

Biosynthesis and Derivatization of the Major Phytoconstituents of Saffron

NEERUPMA DHIMAN • HARSHA KHARKWAL

Saffron is obtained from the dried stigmas of colored flowers of *Crocus sativus* L., belonging to the Iridaceae family. The thin filament-like stigmas of the saffron flower contains a large number of metabolites which are responsible for the organoleptic qualities, i.e., carotenoids (crocin, crocetin-imparts color), picrocrocin (bitterness), and terpenes aldehyde (safranal, for odor). The metabolite of the saffron, i.e., crocin, crocetin, and safranal, have shown to possess antitumor, antioxidation, antihypertension, antiatherosclerotic, and antidepressant activities. In addition, it has potential applications in food and textile industry. However, the solubility issue of crocetin acts as a road block and hampers its use in the medical field. The present chapter highlights the biosynthesis and derivatization aspect of metabolites of saffron giving an insight for developing new bioactives from this highly relevant and less researched medicinal plant.

INTRODUCTION

Saffron crocus (*Crocus sativus Linnaeus*) is the perennial flowering plant and is the costliest spice (Saffron) in the world. Saffron is utilized in different industries, i.e., as a dyeing agent in textiles, for painting walls and books, food colorant, and as a medicine. Iran has been listed as the major producer of saffron (Bathaie et al., 2014). Eighty Kilos of flowers are required to obtain 1 kg of dried saffron. It contains various components including fat, moisture, minerals, proteins, crude fibers, and sugars (Mollazadeh et al., 2015). The important phytochemical constituents of saffron include carotenoids, monoterpene aldehydes, monoterpenoids, isophorones, and flavonoids (Hosseinzadeh et al., 2013). The unique organoleptic properties imparted by saffron which categorizes it under the most expensive material in the world is basically due to the presence of following components: (1) crocins (which

make up the 10% of dry weight of stigma) are water-soluble colored compounds (imparts red orange color), and chemically these are glycosides of the crocetin; (2) picrocrocin is responsible for saffron's bitter taste, and chemically, it is a monoterpene glycoside; (3) safranal imparts characteristic fragrance (Cossignani et al., 2014; Nescatelli et al., 2017).

Saffron and related major constituents have significant pharmacological properties and are used in the treatment of cardiovascular (Imenshahidi et al., 2014; Mehdizadeh et al., 2013), central nervous system (CNS) (Ghasemi et al., 2015; Vahdati et al., 2014; Mehri et al., 2015; Rashedinia et al., 2015), cancer (Amin et al., 2015; Rastgoo et al., 2013; Ghaeni et al., 2014), urine calculi formation (Ghaeni et al., 2014), inflammation, and pain (Amin et al. 2012, 2014; Sahebari et al., 2011). The other pharmacological activities are genoprotective (Hosseinzadeh et al., 2008a, b), antidotal (Razavi et al., 2016; Lari et al., 2015; Razavi et al., 2015; Moallem et al., 2014; Ardebil et al., 2015.), antisolar (Golmohammadzadeh et al., 2011), and aphrodisiac properties (Hosseinzadeh et al., 2008a, b). The indispensable pharmacological effects of the phytochemical constituents of saffron have made them to study extensively in many fields. Many researchers have investigated its role in pharmaceutical formulations and enhancing its efficacy by intervention with nanotechnology (Mehrnia et al., 2017; Faridi Esfanjani et al., 2017; Khazaei et al., 2016; Jafari et al., 2016).

Along with stigma of the flower of the saffron plant, the tepals also serve as an economical source of primary and secondary metabolites (Shahi et al., 2016). The extracts of tepals have shown antidepressant (Moshiri et al., 2006), antioxidant (Sánchez-Vioque et al., 2012), antiproliferative (Sánchez-Vioque et al., 2016), antinociceptive, and antiinflammatory effects (Hosseinzadeh et al., 2002). The extracts can lower

Saffron. https://doi.org/10.1016/B978-0-12-818462-2.00007-3

blood pressure and contractile responses (Fatehi et al., 2003). This chapter provides an insight into phytochemical constituents, their biosynthesis, and derivatization for pharmaceutical applications.

PHYTOCHEMICAL CONSTITUENTS OF SAFFRON

Saffron stigmas contain more than 150 volatile and aromatic compounds, but only few of them could be completely validated. Bathie and Mousavi were able to completely characterize few isolated metabolites from saffron extract (Bathaie and Mousavi, 2010), and the structure of these compounds is shown in Fig. 7.1.

Carotenoids

Carotenoids, also called as tetraterpenoids are the lipid-soluble colorful pigments which have omnipresence (El-Agamey et al., 2004; Tapiero et al., 2004). A large

number of carotenoids are present in the human body and their diet (Rao and Rao, 2007). Carotenoids are responsible for the different colors such as yellow, orange, and red of various parts of the plants, i.e., fruits, flowers, and leaves. The carotenoids which are responsible for the colors belong to the tetraterpenes family (C40-based isoprenoid) (Kaulmann and Bohn, 2014; Tapiero et al., 2004). The carotenoids are classified into carotenes, xanthophylls, and lycopene (Jomova and Valko, 2013; Rutz et al., 2016). For example, (1) carotenes and xanthophylls are present in the green vegetable; (2) lycopene is a liposoluble pigment imparting color in tomatoes; (3) β-carotene is responsible for the orange color of carrots; (4) pepper gets its color from capsanthin; and (5) source for color of crustaceans is astaxanthin (Astorg, 1997). The unique feature of carotenoids is that chemically these contain a carbon chain with conjugated double bonds and have cyclic or acyclic end groups (Stahl and Sies, 2005). Chemically most

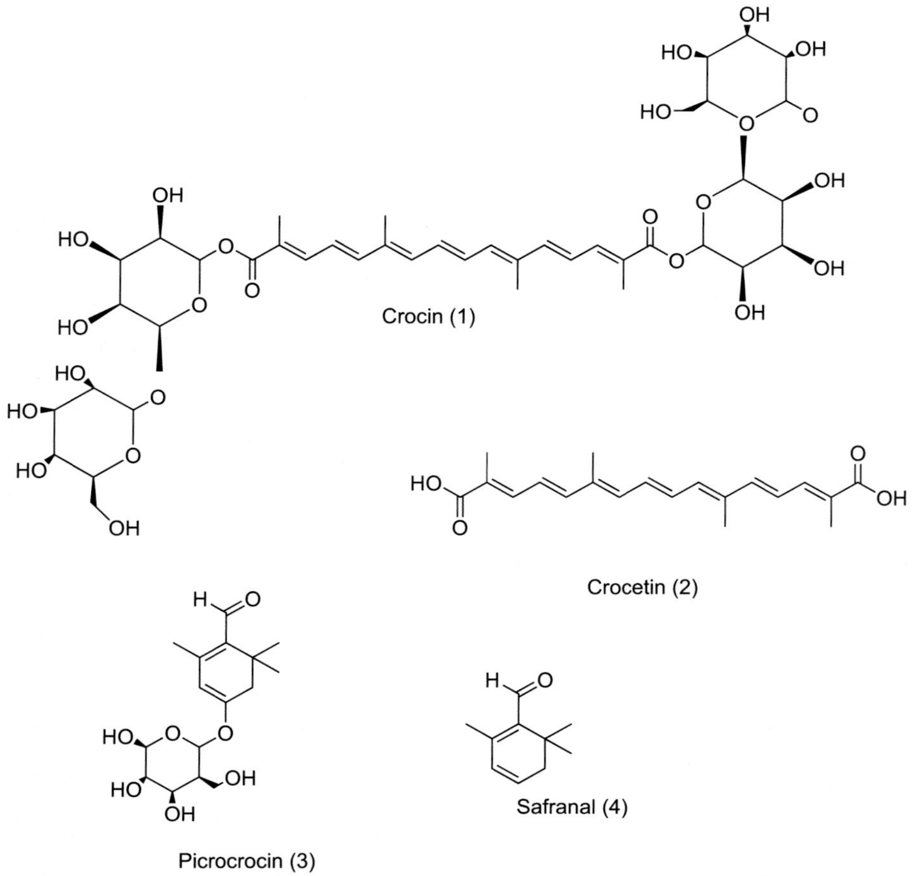

FIG. 7.1 Major phytochemical of saffron.

naturally available carotenoids have more than 20 carbon atoms and are lipophilic in nature and hence soluble in nonpolar solvents. A few carotenoids, i.e., lycopene, are acyclic, majority having an alicyclic ring in either end of molecule, e.g., β carotene. The crocin that belongs to the carotenoid family is unusual because these are water soluble, and this hydrophilicity of the crocin is due to the presence of the terminal glycosyl units (Iborra et al. 1992; Bathaie and Mousavi, 2010).

Crocins

Crocins are chemically crocetin glycosides that are water-soluble carotenoids (Nam et al., 2010), and almost 30% of the dry matter of saffron is composed of the crocins (Nassiri-Asl and Hosseinzadeh (2015).; Melnyk et al., 2010). Crocins (C) are the mixture of C-1 or α-C, C-2 (tricrocin), C-3, C-4, and C-5 or dicrocin (Poma et al., 2012; Fig. 7.2).

The nonionic crocin-1, or α-crocin, is responsible for water solubility and imparts reddish yellow color to the saffron (Bolhasani et al., 2005). Crocin-1 is hydrophilic in nature; therefore, it is insoluble in most of the organic solvents (O' Neil et al., 2001). The most abundant ester is di-β-D-gentiobiosyl, which is highly polar due to the presence of sugar molecule. Crocin-3 is a small compound, and chemically it is a gentiobiose monoester that possesses a hydrophilic anion. Crocetin is obtained when the crocins are hydrolyzed by dilute alkali.

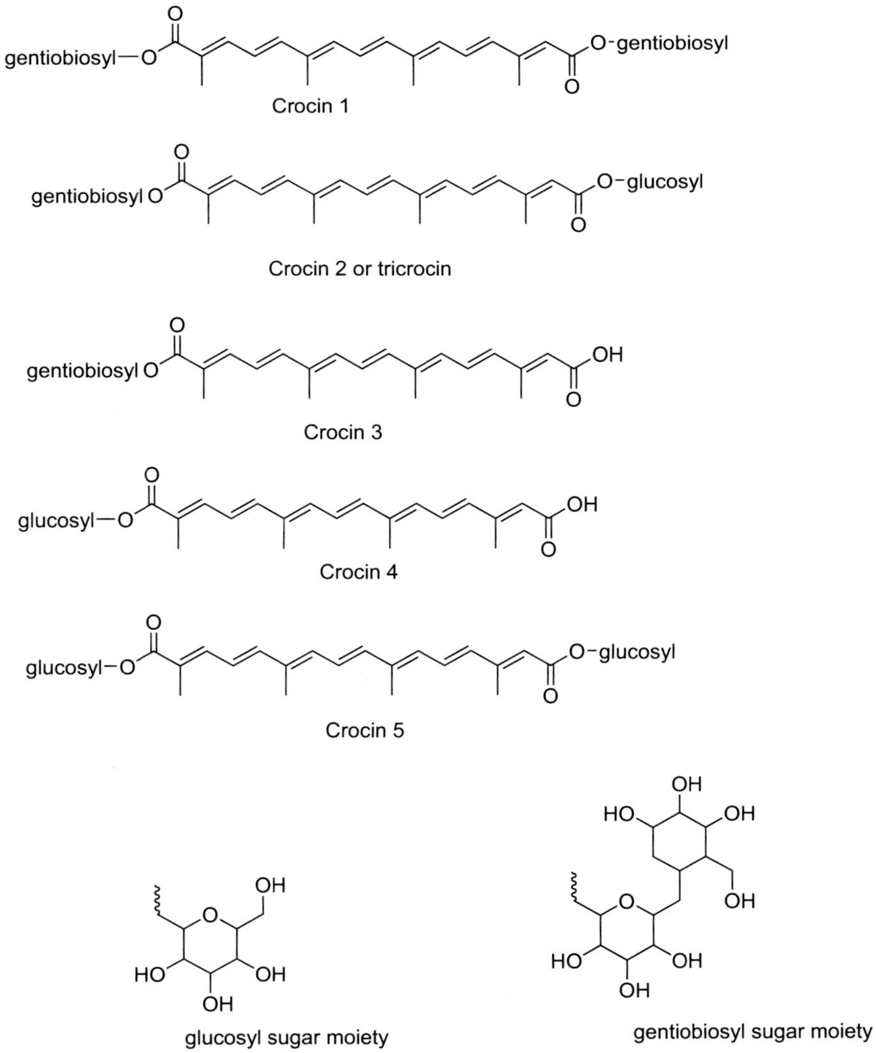

FIG. 7.2 Types of crocin.

Crocetin

It is a apocarotenoid dicarboxylic acid obtained from saffron and is also responsible for the red saffron color in combination with other phytoconstituents (Martin et al., 2002). It is obtained by addition of hydroxyl group to the crocin. Crocetin contains a polyene chain which has a carboxyl group at both the ends. The trans form of crocetin is mostly present in saffron. Crocetin can also function as an acid (anionic) dye for biological staining in its ionized form (Lillie 1977). At pH nine, crocetin dissolves in aqueous alkali solution, or in other words, the crocetin is highly water soluble in the anionic form.

Monoterpene Glycoside

Picrocrocin is accountable for the bitter taste of saffron, which is a colorless glycoside. The metabolism of the precursor zeaxanthin is responsible for the bitterness of spice. The more the metabolism of the zeaxanthin, the more the bitterness. The drying process is the key factor which influences the ratio between aroma and bitterness (Carmona et al., 2005).

Monoterpene Aldehyde

Safranal is the example of monoterpene aldehyde. Safranal is formed from picrocin after dehydration during the saffron drying process. The optimal temperature required for safranal generation is above 80°C (Gregory et al., 2005). Saffron when dried at 80°C leads to formation of 4-β-hydroxy-cyclocitral and safranal which is the main component of *C. sativus* essential oil and responsible for saffron's distinctive fragrance (Rezaee and Hosseinzadeh et al., 2013). Safranal, the essential oil obtained from saffron, constitutes more than 50% of the total yield of oil (Abdullaev and Espinosa-Aguirre, 2004).

BIOSYNTHESIS OF CROCIN, PICROCROCIN, AND SAFRANAL

The precursor for the biosynthesis of crocin and other important compounds in *C. sativus* stigmas is zeaxanthin. The biosynthesis of crocin is initiated through Zeaxanthin's symmetric oxidative cleavage at the 7,8/7′,8′ positions, yielding a cyclocitral and dialdehyde. This cyclocitral compound, after series of reactions, is converted to safranal. Diacid crocetin formation by NADP+-dependent oxidoreductase is trigged by the instability of crocetin dialdehyde. The enzymatic process attaching glycans by crocetin constitutes the final phase of crocin biosynthesis catalyzed by uridine diphosphate glycosyltransferase.

The multistepped enzyme catalyzed pathway of crocin (Fig. 7.3) occurs in a series of subcellular compartments: the zeaxanthin, which is the precursor of this biosynthesis, is located in plastids and crocins, the end product, accumulates in vacuoles (Bouvier et al., 2003b; Gómez-Gómez et al., 2017).

Frusciante et al. identified the key enzyme, i.e., carotenoid cleavage dioxygenase (CCD) which is responsible for the initiation of the biosynthesis of carotenoids in *C. sativus*. They also showed that CCD catalyzes the cleavage of the zeaxanthin so that crocin will be biosynthesized (Frusciante et al., 2014). Ahrazem et al. reported that the CCD is present in the plastid (Ahrazem et al., 2016). In comparison, the presence of other intermediates responsible for the biosynthesis of crocin and the enzymes catalyzing the synthesis of those intermediates remain indescribable.

Gómez-Gómez et al. proposed a model for multistepped enzyme catalyzed reaction of crocin, in which the sequestration process is responsible for the transport of crocin to vacuoles, and this was validate by microscopic studies and data generation through proteomics (Gómez-Gómez et al., 2017). This model projected that plastid is the only site where crocins are biosynthesized, preceding to gathering in plastid-localized vesicles and finally transferring vacuoles. Demurtas et al. (2018) have shown that biosynthesis of the carotenoids is basically located at three subcellular locations, i.e., chromoplasts, the ER surface, and the cytosol. It also represents that the ER membrane functions as a hydrophobic pathway that joins the synthesis of lipophilic compounds in the chromoplast, followed by the formation of hydrophilic glycosylated products which gets accumulated in the vacuole.

DERIVATIVES OF CROCETIN AND SAFRANAL

The derivatives of compounds are usually synthesized either to enhance the solubility of the parent compound or to increase the bioavailability or efficacy of the parent compound. As discussed, the main constituents of saffron, crocin, crocetin, picrocrocin, and safranal, have shown one or more pharmacological activity; hence, they are important in pharmaceutical as well as in medical world. Therefore, saffron derivatives were synthesized.

Derivatives of Crocetin

Crocetin is a polyene dicarboxylic acid with two lipophobic free carboxylic groups and lipophilic polyene structure, which are responsible for the poor solubility

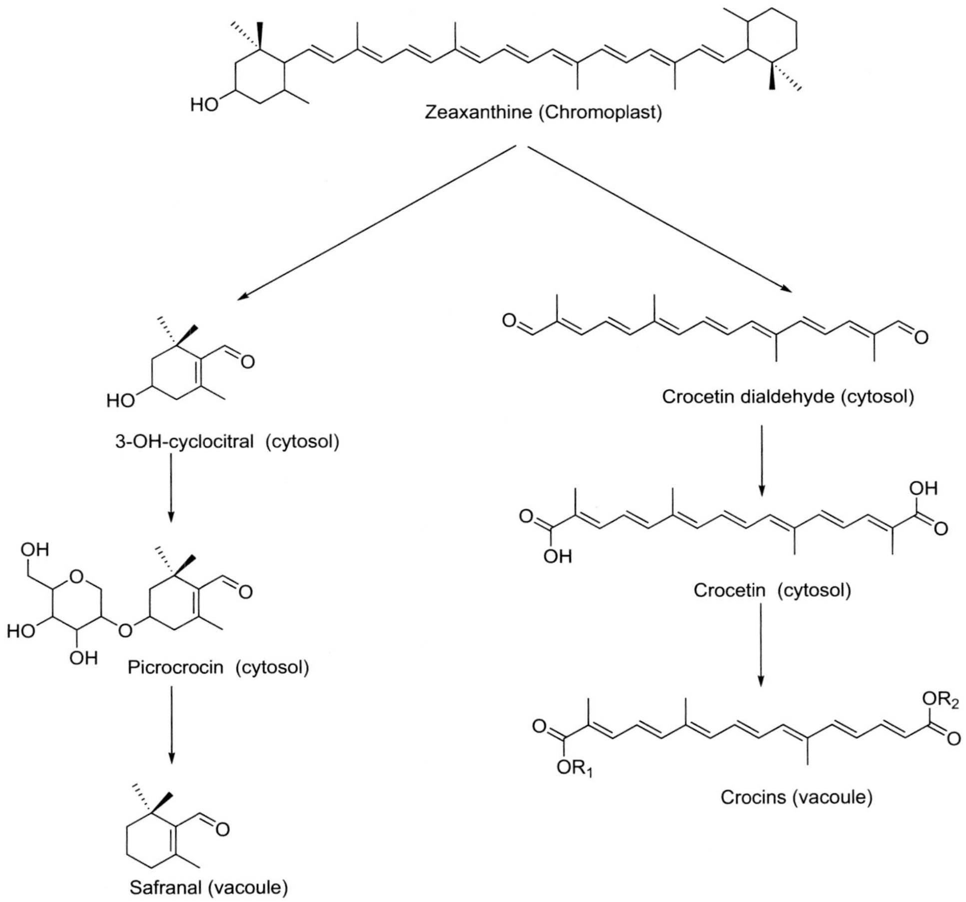

FIG. 7.3 Biosynthesis of crocin, crocetin, picrocrocin, and safranal.

in various solvents. Crocetin has a great prospective in the treatment of many life-threatening diseases (Zheng et al., 2006). The poor solubility of the crocetin greatly restricts its dose-dependent effects and bioavailability (Bijttebier et al., 2014; Foss et al., 2005).To enhance the solubility of crocetin, many scientific groups had either used various types of solubilizer or incorporated the compound in other drug-delivery vehicles (Mages et al., 2009; Ohba et al., 2016). The use of solubilizers and other compounds to enhance the solubility of cro-cetin did not reveal the exact results of crocetin and the biological safety of the drug formulation. As a result, de-rivatives of the crocetin were made to enhance its solu-bility and are useful for its efficacy and application. Till date, fewer studies have been reported on the influence of chemical modification on the solubility and biolog-ical effect of crocetin (Chua et al., 2018; Gao et al., 2017). It has been described in literature that the

replacement of the acid group by amide group increases lipophilicity and that the permeability of the com-pounds could be enhanced by incorporating alkyl chain to amino moiety (Conradi, 1991; Ihnat, 2000). Howev-er, large compounds having an amide group play an important role in the synthesis of many biological as well as pharmaceutical products (Wang et al., 2011; Montalbetti et al., 2005; Boonen et al., 2012; Ghosh and Brindisi et al., 2015; Lee et al., 2016).

Chua et al. (2018) had made some chemical modi-fications to the crocetin to enhance its solubility and augment its pharmacological properties. During the synthesis of the crocetin derivatives, the pharmaco-phore, which is important for pharmacological activi-ties, had been retained. Chu et al. synthesized the derivatives by the exchange of the carboxy group of cro-cetin with piperidine, diethylene, and benzylamine groups (Fig. 7.4).

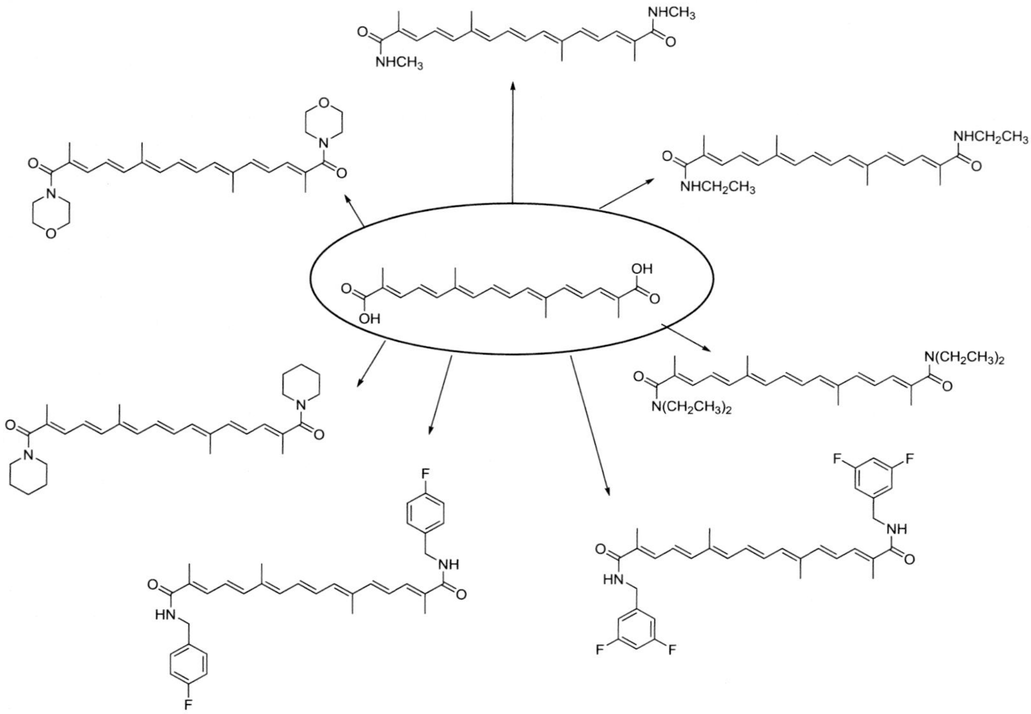

FIG. 7.4 Derivatives of crocetin.

The crocetin piperidine and diethylene derivatives became more water soluble and also showed strong anticancer and antiinflammatory activity. The benzylamine derivative of crocetin had less solubility than the piperidyl and diethylene but had a significant tumor inhibition effect. The conjugation of crocetin with the heteroatomic compounds showed improved solubility and enhanced antitumor action of the crocetin. The piperidyl derivative showed the maximum inhibitory action on A549 and MCF-7 cell lines, whereas the diethylene derivative showed a potent antitumor effect on B16F10 and SKOV3 cell lines. The benzylamine derivative of crocetin has a strong inhibitory action on A549, MCF-7, and B16F10 cell lines than piperidyl and diethylene derivatives with the same amount of derivatives (Chua et al. 2018).

Gao et al., (2017) reported the crocetin amide derivatives and the cardioprotective activity of the synthesized derivatives. The result of their studies showed that the N-ethyl derivative and N,N-diethyl derivative displayed stronger cardioprotective activity than the crocetin and other derivatives. The structural activity relationship of the derivatives synthesized revealed that the substitution of ethyl group with piperidine or morpholine rings decreased the potency. Decreasing the carbon number in the alkyl chain from ethyl to methyl also reduced the potency. The addition of benzene rings with fluorine group substitution into crocetin showed a marked decrease in the cardioprotective activity (Gao et al., 2017).

Derivative of Safranal

Safranal is a cyclic terpenic aldehyde which is responsible for the aroma of the saffron. Safranal was shown to have a protective action against gentamicin-induced nephrotoxicity (Boroushaki and Sadeghnia, 2009) as well as against hexachlorobutadiene-induced nephron toxicity in rats (Sadeghnia et al., 2005; Boroushaki et al., 2007). Monoterpenes showed to have chemopreventive and anticancer activity for various types of tumors in animals at cellular level and also in clinical trials (Crowell, 1999; Carnesecchi, 2001). Khayyat et al. (2018) had carried out the oxidation of safranal to get monoepoxy and diepoxy derivatives of safranal. The oxidation of the safranal was performed either by thermal or photochemical process. The thermal

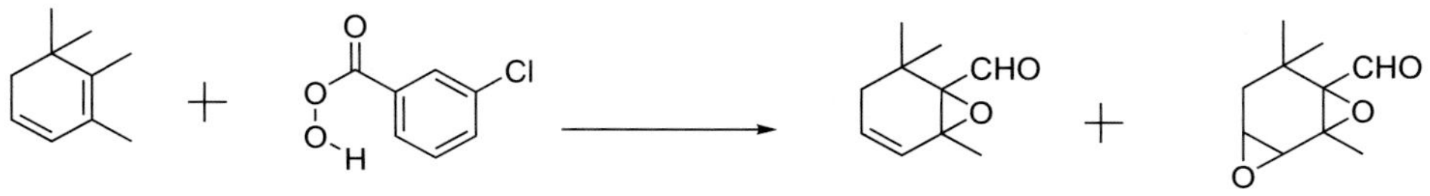

FIG. 7.5 Epoxide of safranal.

oxidation was done by using m-chloroperbenzoic acid, and photo chemical oxidation reaction was done with hydrogen peroxide (Fig. 7.5).

The epoxide derivatives of safranal showed DNA alkylation to a moderate extent, whereas the diepoxide derivative had shown high antimicrobial activity against methicillin-resistant *Staphylococcus aureus* as compared with monoepoxide derivatives (Khayyat and Elgendy, 2018).

CONCLUSION

It can be concluded that saffron and its derivatives play an important role in the treatment of life-threatening diseases. Solubility and bioavailability remain an issue and act as hindrance for its application, which can be further resolved by the derivatization of the chemical constituents of saffron. The results introduced the possibility that saffron, its phytoconstituents, and the derivatives of chemical constituents might be used as an alternative for different pharmacological activities, either alone or in combination with synthetic compounds. It is reasonable to say at this point that we have just begun to study the potential applications of saffron in human health and disease. But this chapter will open new avenues in drug discovery.

REFERENCES

Abdullaev, F.I., Espinosa-Aguirre, J.J., 2004. Biomedical properties of saffron and its potential use in cancer therapy and chemoprevention trials. Cancer Detect. Prev. 28, 426—432.

Ahrazem, O., Rubio-Moraga, A., Berman, J., Capell, T., Christou, P., Zhu, C., Gómez-Gómez, L., 2016. The carotenoid cleavage dioxygenase CCD2 catalysing the synthesis of crocetin in spring crocuses and saffron is a plastidial enzyme. New Phytol. 209, 650—663.

Amin, B., Hosseinzadeh, H., 2012. Evaluation of aqueous and ethanolic extracts of saffron, *Crocus sativus* L., and its constituents, safranal and crocin in allodynia and hyperalgesia induced by chronic constriction injury model of neuropathic pain in rats. Fitoterapia 83, 888—895.

Amin, B., Abnous, K., Motamedshariaty, V., Hosseinzadeh, H., 2014. Attenuation of oxidative stress, inflammation and apoptosis by ethanolic and aqueous extract of *Crocus sativus* L. stigma after chronic constriction injury of male rats. An Acad. Bras Ciências 86, 1821—1832.

Amin, B., Malekzadeh, M., Heidari, M.R., Hosseinzadeh, H., 2015. Effect of Crocus sativus extracts and its active constituent safranal on the harmaline-induced tremor in mice. Iran. J. Basic Med. Sci. 18, 449—458.

Astorg, P., 1997. Food carotenoids and cancer prevention: an overview of current research. Trends Food Sci. Technol. 8, 406—413.

Bathaie, S.Z., Mousavi, S.Z., 2010. New applications and mechanisms of action of saffron and its important ingredients. Crit. Rev. Food Sci. Nutr. 50, 761—786.

Bathaie, S.Z., Farajzade, A., Hoshyar, R., 2014. A review of the chemistry and uses of crocins and crocetin, the carotenoid natural dyes in saffron, with particular emphasis on applications as colorants including their use as biological stains. Biotech. Histochem. 6, 401—411.

Bijttebier, S., D'Hondt, E., Noten, B., Hermans, N., Apers, S., Voorspoels, S., 2014. Ultra high performance liquid chromatography versus high performance liquid chromatography: stationary phase selectivity for generic carotenoid screening. J. Chromatogr. A 1332, 46—56.

Bolhasani, A., Bathaie, S.Z., Yavari, I., Moosavi-Movahedi, A.A., Ghaffari, M.M., 2005. Separation and purification of some components of Iranian saffron. Asian J. Chem. 17, 725—729.

Boonen, J., Bronselaer, A., Nielandt, J., Veryser, L., Tre, D.G., Spiegeleer, D.B., 2012. J. Ethnopharmacol. 142, 563—590.

Boroushaki, M., Sadeghnia, H., 2009. Protective effect of safranal against gentamicin-induced nephrotoxicity in rat. Iran. J. Med. Sci. 34, 285—288.

Boroushaki, M., Mofidpour, H., Sadeghnia, H., 2007. Protective effect of safranal against hexachlorobutadiene-induced nephrotoxicity in rat. Iran. J. Med. Sci. 32, 173—176.

Bouvier, F., Suire, C., Mutterer, J., Camara, B., 2003. Oxidative remodeling of chromoplast carotenoids: identification of the carotenoid dioxygenase CsCCD and CsZCD genes involved in Crocus secondary metabolite biogenesis. Plant Cell 15, 47—62.

Carmona, M., Zalacain, A., Pardo, J.E., Lopez, E., Alvarruiz, A., Alonso, G.L., 2005. Influence of different drying and aging conditions on saffron constituents. J. Agric. Food Chem. 53, 3974—3979.

Carnesecchi, S., Schneider, Y., Ceraline, J., Duranton, B., Gosse, F., Seller, N., Raul, F., 2001. Geraniol, a component of plant essential oils inhibit growth and polyamine synthesis in human colon cancer cells. J. Pharmacol. Exp. Ther. 298, 197—200.

Chua, Y., Gao, J., Huanga, Y., Chenb, M., Wanga, M., Shang, Q., Luc, W., Penga, L., Jiang, Z., 2018. Synthesis, characterization and inhibitory effects of crocetin derivative compounds in cancer and inflammation. Biomed. Pharmacother. 98, 157−164.

Conradi, R.A., Hilgers, A.R., Ho, N.F., Burton, P.S., 1991. The influence of peptide structure on transport across Caco-2 cells. Pharm. Res. 8, 1453−1460.

Cossignani, L., Urbani, E., Simonetti, M.S., Maurizi, A., Chiesi, C., Blasi, F., 2014. Characterisation of secondary metabolites in saffron from central Italy (Cascia, Umbria). Food Chem. 143, 446−451.

Crowell, P., 1999. Prevention and therapy of cancer by dietary monoterpenes. J. Nutr. 129, 775s−778s.

Demurtas, O.C., Frusciante, S., Ferrante, P., Diretto, G., Azad, N.H., Pietrella, M., Aprea, G., Taddei, A.R., Romano, E., Mi, J., 2018. Candidate enzymes for saffron crocin biosynthesis are localized in multiple cellular compartments. Plant Physiol. 177, 990−1006.

El-Agamey, A., Lowe, G.M., McGarvey, D.J., Mortensen, A., Phillip, D.M., Truscott, T.G., 2004. Carotenoid radical chemistry and antioxidant/pro-oxidant properties. Arch. Biochem. Biophys. 430, 7−48.

Faridi Esfanjani, A., Jafari, S.M., Assadpour, E., 2017. Preparation of a multiple emulsion based on pectin whey protein complex for encapsulation of saffron extract nanodroplets. Food Chem. 221, 1962−1969.

Fatehi, M., Rashidabady, T., Fatehi-Hassanabad, Z., 2003. Effects of Crocus sativus petals' extract on rat blood pressure and on responses induced by electrical field stimulation in the rat isolated vas deferens and Guinea-pig ileum. J. Ethnopharmacol. 84, 199−203.

Foss, B.J., Sliwka, H.R., Partali, V., Naess, S.N., Elgsaeter, A., Melø, T.B., Naqvi, K.R., 2005. Hydrophilic carotenoids: surface properties and aggregation behavior of a highly unsaturated carotenoid lysophospholipid. Chem. Phys. Lipids 134, 85−96.

Frusciante, S., Diretto, G., Bruno, M., Ferrante, P., Pietrella, M., Prado-Cabrero, A., Rubio-Moraga, A., Beyer, P., Gomez-Gomez, L., Al-Babili, S., 2014. Novel carotenoid cleavage dioxygenase catalyzes the first dedicated step in saffron crocin biosynthesis. Proc. Acad. Sci. USA 111, 12246−12251.

Gao, J., Chen, M., Ren, X., Xiao-Bo Zhou, X., Shanga, Q., Luc, W., Luo, P., Jianga, Z., 2017. Synthesis and cardiomyocyte protection activity of crocetin diamide derivatives. Fitoterapia 121, 106−111.

Ghaeni, F.A., Amin, B., Hariri, A.T., 2014. Antilithiatic effects of crocin on ethylene glycol-induced lithiasis in rats. Urolithiasis 42, 549−558.

Ghasemi, T., Abnous, K., Vahdati, F., 2015. Antidepressant effect of Crocus sativus aqueous extract and its effect on CREB, BDNF, and VGF transcript and protein levels in rat hippocampus. Drug Res. 65, 337−343.

Ghosh, A.K., Brindisi, M.J., 2015. Organic carbamates in drug design and medicinal chemistry. J. Med. Chem. 58, 2895−2940.

Golmohammadzadeh, S., Imani, F., Hosseinzadeh, H., 2011. Preparation, characterization and evaluation of sun protective and moisturizing effects of nanoliposomes containing safranal. Iran. J. Basic Med. Sci. 14, 521−533.

Gómez-Gómez, L., Parra-Vega, V., Rivas-Sendra, A., Seguí-Simarro, J.M., Molina, R.V., Pallotti, C., Rubio-Moraga, Á., Diretto, G., Prieto, A., Ahrazem, O., 2017. Unraveling massive crocins transport and accumulation through proteome and microscopy tools during the development of saffron stigma. Int. J. Mol. Sci. 18, E76.

Gregory, M.J., Menary, R.C., Davies, N.W., 2005. Effect of drying temperature and air blow on the production and retention of secondary metabolites in saffron. J. Agric. Food Chem. 53, 5969−5975.

Hosseinzadeh, H., Nassiri-Asl, M., 2013. Avicenna's (Ibn Sina) the canon of medicine and saffron (Crocus sativus):A review. Phytother Res. 27, 475−483.

Hosseinzadeh, H., Younesi, H.M., 2002. Antinociceptive and anti-inflammatory effects of Crocus sativus L. stigma and petal extracts in mice. BMC Pharmacol. 2, 7.

Hosseinzadeh, H., Abootorabi, A., Sadeghnia, H.R., 2008a. Protective effect of Crocus sativus stigma extract and crocin (trans-crocin 4) on methyl methanesulfonate-induced DNA damage in mice organs. DNA Cell Biol. 27, 657−664.

Hosseinzadeh, H., Ziaee, T., Sadeghi, A., 2008b. The effect of saffron, Crocus sativus stigma, extract and its constituents, safranal and crocin on sexual behaviors in normal male rats. Phytomedicine 15, 491-49.

Iborra, J.L, Castellar, M.R, Cánovas, M, Manjón, A, 1992. TLC preparative purification of picrocrocin, HTCC and crocin from saffron. J. Food Sci 3, 714−716.

Ihnat, P.M., Vennerstrom, J.L., Robinson, D.H., 2000. Synthesis and solution properties of deferoxamine amides. J. Pharmceutical Sci. 89, 1525−1536.

Imenshahidi, M., Razavi, B.M., Faal, A., 2014. Effects of chronic crocin treatment on desoxycorticosterone acetate (doca)-salt hypertensive rats. Iran. J. Basic Med. Sci. 1, 9−13.

Jafari, S.-M., Mahdavi-Khazaei, K., Hemmati-Kakhki, A., 2016. Microencapsulation of saffron petal anthocyanins with cress seed gum compared with Arabic gum through freeze drying. Carbohydr. Polym. 140, 20−25.

Jomova, K., Valko, M., 2013. Health protective effects of carotenoids and their interactions with other biological antioxidants. Eur. J. Med. Chem. 70, 102−110.

Kaulmann, A., Bohn, T., 2014. Carotenoids, inflammation, and oxidative stress-implications of cellular signaling pathways and relation to chronic disease prevention. Nutr. Res. 34, 907−929.

Khayyat, S., Elgendy, E., 2018. Safranal epoxide − a potential source for diverse therapeutic applications. Saudi Pharm. J. 26, 115−119.

Khazaei, K.M., Jafari, S.M., Ghorbani, M., 2016. Optimization of anthocyanin extraction from saffron petals with response surface methodology. Food Anal. Methods 9, 1993−2001.

Lari, P., Abnous, K., Imenshahidi, M., 2015. Evaluation of diazinon-induced hepatotoxicity and protective effects of crocin. Toxicol. Ind. Health 31, 367−376.

Lee, E.C., Futatsugi, K., Arcari, J.T., Bahnck, K., Coffey, S.B., Derksen, D.R., Kalgutkar, A.S., Lillie, R.D., 1977. Conn's

Biological Stains: A Handbook on the Nature and Uses of the Dyes Employed in the Biological Laboratory. Williams & Wilkins, Baltimore, MD.

Lillie RD. Conn's Biological Stains: a Handbook on the Nature and Uses of the Dyes Employed in the Biological Laboratory , 9 th ed. Baltimore, MD: Williams & Wilkins; 1977. p. 459

Magesh, V., Durgabhavani, K., Senthilnathan, P., Rajendran, P., Sakthisekaran, D., 2009. In vivo protective effect of crocetin on benzo(a)pyrene-induced lung cancer in Swiss albino mice. Phytother Res. 23, 533–539.

Martin, G., Goh, E., Neff, A., 2002. Evaluation of the developmental toxicity of crocetin on Xenopus. Food Chem. Toxicol. 40, 959–964.

Mehdizadeh, R., Parizadeh, M.R., Khooei, A.R., 2013. Cardioprotective effect of saffron extract and safranal in isoproterenol-induced myocardial infarction in wistar rats. Iran. J. Basic Med. Sci. 16, 56–63.

Mehri, S., Abnous, K., Khooei, A., 2015. Crocin reduced acrylamide-induced neurotoxicity in wistar rat through inhibition of oxidative stress. Iran. J. Basic Med. Sci. 18, 902–908.

Mehrnia, M.-A., Jafari, S.-M., Makhmal-Zadeh, B.S., 2017. Rheological and release properties of double nanoemulsions containing crocin prepared with Angum gum, Arabic gum and whey protein. Food Hydrocolloid 66, 259–267.

Melnyk, J.P., Wang, S.N., Marcone, M.F., 2010. Chemical and biological properties of the world's most expensive spice saffron. Food Res. Int. 43, 1981–1989.

Moallem, S.A., Hariri, A.T., Mahmoudi, M., 2014. Effect of aqueous extract of Crocus sativus L. (saffron) stigma against subacute effect of diazinon on specific biomarkers in rats. Toxicol. Ind. Health 30, 141–146.

Mollazadeh, H., Emami, S.A., Hosseinzadeh, H., 2015. Razi's Al-Hawi and saffron (Crocus sativus): a review. Iran. J. Basic Med. Sci. 18, 1153–1166.

Montalbetti, C.A.G.N., Falque, V., 2005. Amide bond formation and peptide coupling. Tetrahedron 61, 10827–10852.

Moshiri, E., Basti, A.A., Noorbala, A.-A., 2006. Crocus sativus L. (petal) in the treatment of mild-to moderate depression: a double-blind, randomized and placebo-controlled trial. Phytomedicine 3, 607–611.

Nam, K.N., Park, Y.M., Jung, H.J., Lee, J.Y., Min, B.D., Park, J.J., Jung, W.S., Cho, K.H., Park, J.H., Kang, I., Hong, J.W., Lee, E.H., 2010. Anti-inflammatory effects of crocin and crocetin in rat brain microglial cells. Eur. J. Pharmacol. 648, 110–116.

Nassiri-Asl, M., Hosseinzadeh, H., 2015. Neuropharmacology effects of saffron (Crocus sativus) and its active constituents. Brain Dis. 3, 29–39.

Nescatelli, R., Carradori, S., Marini, F., Caponigro, V., Bucci, R., De Monte, C., Mollica, A., Mannina, L., Ceruso, M., Supuran, C.T., Secci, D., 2017. Geographical characterization by MAE-HPLC and NIR methodologies and carbonic anhydrase inhibition of Saffron components. Food Chem. 221, 855–863.

O 'Neil, M.J., Smith, A., Heckelman, P.E., Budavari, S., 2001. The Merck Index: An Encyclopedia of Chemicals, Drugs, and Biologicals. Merck & Co, New York.

Ohba, T., Ishisaka, M., Tsujii, S., Tsuruma, K., Shimazawa, M., Kubo, K., Umigai, N., Iwawaki, T., Hara, H., 2016. Crocetin protects ultraviolet A-induced oxidative stress and cell death in skin in vitro and in vivo. Eur. J. Pharmacol. 789, 244–253.

Poma, A., Fontecchio, G., Carlucci, G., Chichiricco, G., 2012. Antiinflammatory properties of drugs from saffron crocus. Antiinflamm. Antiallergy Agents Med. Chem. 11, 37–51.

Rao, A.V., Rao, L.G., 2007. Carotenoids and human health. Pharmacol. Res. 55, 207–216.

Rashedinia, M., Lari, P., Abnous, K., Hosseinzadeh, H., 2015. Protective effect of crocin on acrolein-induced tau phosphorylation in the rat brain. Acta Neurobiol. Exp. J. 75, 208–219.

Rastgoo, M., Hosseinzadeh, H., Alavizadeh, H., 2013. Antitumor activity of PEGylated nanoliposomes containing crocin in mice bearing C26 colon carcinoma. Planta Med. 79, 447–451.

Razavi, B.M., Hosseinzadeh, H., Abnous, K., 2016. Protective effect of crocin against apoptosis induced by subchronic exposure of the rat vascular system to diazinon. Toxicol. Ind. Health 32, 1237–1245.

Razavi, B.M., Hosseinzadeh, H., Imenshahidi, M., 2015. Evaluation of protein ubiquitylation in heart tissue of rats exposed to diazinon (an organophosphate Insecticide) and crocin (an active saffron ingredient): role of HIF-1α. Drug Res. 65, 561–566.

Rezaee, R., Hosseinzadeh, H., 2013. Safranal: from an aromatic natural product to a rewarding pharmacological agent. Iran. J. Basic Med. Sci. 16, 12–26.

Rutz, J.K., Borges, C.D., Zambiazi, R.C., da Rosa, C.G., da Silva, M.M., 2016. Elaboration of microparticles of carotenoids from natural and synthetic sources for applications in food. Food Chem. 202, 324–333.

Sadeghnia, H., Boroushaki, M., Mofidpour, H., 2005. Effect of safranal, a constituent of saffron (Crocus Sativus L.), on lipid peroxidation level during renal Ischemia- reperfusion injury in rats. Iran. J. Basic Med. Sci. 8, 179–185.

Sahebari, M., Mahmoudi, Z., Rabe, S.Z.T., 2011. Inhibitory effect of aqueous extract of Saffron (Crocus sativus L.) on adjuvant-induced arthritis in Wistar rat. Pharmacology 3, 802–808.

Sánchez-Vioque, R., Rodríguez-Conde, M.F., Reina-Ureña, J.V., 2012. In vitro antioxidant and metal chelating properties of corm, tepal and leaf from saffron (Crocus sativus L.). Ind. Crops Prod. 39, 149–153.

Sánchez-Vioque, R., Santana-Méridas, O., Polissiou, M., 2016. Polyphenol composition and in vitro antiproliferative effect of corm, tepal and leaf from Crocus sativus L. on human colon adenocarcinoma cells (Caco-2). J. Funct. Foods 24, 18–25.

Shahi, T., Assadpour, E., Jafari, S.M., 2016. Main chemical compounds and pharmacological activities of stigmas and tepals of 'red gold'; saffron. Trends Food Sci. Technol. 58, 69–78.

Stahl, W., Sies, H., 2005. Bioactivity and protective effects of natural carotenoids. Biochim. Biophys. Acta 101–107.

Tapiero, H., Townsend, D.M., Tew, K.D., 2004. The role of carotenoids in the prevention of human pathologies. Biomed. Pharmacother. 58, 100–110.

Vahdati Hassani, F., Naseri, V., Razavi, B.M., Mehri, S., Abnous, K., Hosseinzadeh, H., 2014. Antidepressant effects of crocin and its effects on transcript and protein levels of CREB, BDNF, and VGF in rat hippocampus. Daru 22, 16.

Wang, T., Shu, J., Zheng, L., Xiong, L., Wang, J., Jin, L., Wu, Q., Zou, H., Zhang, C., 2011. Lat. Am. J. Pharm. 30, 1355–1359.

Zheng, S., Qian, Z., Sheng, L., Wen, N., 2006. Crocetin attenuates atherosclerosis in hyperlipidemic rabbits through inhibition of LDL oxidation. J. Cardiovasc. Pharmacol. 47, 70–76.

CHAPTER 8

Saffron as a Neuroprotective Agent

DHONDUP NAMGYAL • MARYAM SARWAT

INTRODUCTION

Neurological disorders are one of the major challenges that we are facing in today's world. Beginning from the time of Hippocrates, these disorders have evolved dramatically and assumed different features. On the other hand, advancements in the field of surgical knowledge, radiation therapy, and chemotherapy have improved the survival rates of people afflicted with neurological disorders and also enhanced their quality of life. However, there is a need to shift our focus from radical ablation toward curative and restorative efforts (Seitz, 2004; Yirka and Gollo, 2018).

Neurodegenerative disorders are age-related degeneration of neurons or progressive loss of structure and functions of neurons in the central nervous system and peripheral nervous system (Przedborski and Lewis, 2003).

Currently, there are countless numbers of different types of neurological disorders starting from the most common age-related neurodegenerative disorders such as AD to most complicated neurological disorder such as phantom limb syndrome. As the knowledge and research tools have advanced, researchers have found many similarities between these disorders at a subcellular level. The similarities at the subcellular level in these diseases offer hope for therapeutic advancements that could ameliorate many neurological disorders simultaneously. Most of these neurodegenerative disorders have been found to be caused by age-related cellular changes (Hung et al., 2010), mitochondria DNA mutation which lead to mitochondria dysfunction (Lin and Beal, 2006; Johri and Beal, 2012), or increase of prooxidant level and decrease of antioxidant level which leads to oxidative stress (Li et al., 2013).

In 1993, the World Bank, WHO, and Harvard school of public health carried out a field study to assess the global burden of disease (GBD) for the year 1990, and they found that neurological disorders contribute 6.3% to GBD. About 92 million of the population was found to be struggling with neurological disorders in 2005, and researchers have predicted that this will be increased to 103 million of the population by 2030. Among the neurological disorders, 50% is contributed by cerebrovascular disease, 12% by AD and dementia, and 8% by epilepsy migraine (Murray et al., 1996). Neurological disorders had affected to varying extents in different classes of the population. About 10.9% contributed from high-class population, 6.7% contributed from upper-middle-class population, 8.7% contributed from lower-middle-class population, and 4.5% contributed from low-income countries. Most of the high-class population and developed countries are highly exploited by the electronic gadgets and robotic lifestyle, and this leads to poor mental health. Neurological disorders constitute approximately 12% of total death globally and within this cerebrovascular disease contribute 85% (Murray et al., 1996).

During the last 4 decades, the growth and development of neuroepidemiology in India has been documented highlighting the historical milestone. The prevalence rates of the spectrum of neurological disorders from different regions of the country ranged from 976 to 4070 with a mean of 2394 per 1,00,000 population, providing a rough estimate of over 30 million people with neurological disorders (excluding neuroinfections and traumatic injuries). Technological advancements and industrialization had made our day-to-day life easier, but at the same time, it has a tremendous negative effect on our mental health. Many researchers have suggested that populations living in cities have higher risk of suffering mental disorders than the people living in rural. This is due to the fact that environmental pollution and electronic pollution are higher in the cities (Gourie-Devi M, 2014).

In today's world, people are forgetting the importance of mental health and social life. Each time we purchase a new electronic gadget, we subsequently tend to isolate ourselves from social life. Advancements in technology have had many applications toward our livelihood, yet the overexploitation of electronic gadgets such as mobile phones and computers are insidiously affecting our physical and mental well-being. Accumulated evidence suggests that exposure to artificial dim light at night has deleterious effect on our mental health as these electronic gadgets carries strong electromagnetic radiations which damages and alters our brain physiology.

Although there are many synthetic drugs available at different pharmacies for the treatment of neurodegenerative diseases, most of them are only effective in relieving the symptoms of the disease while bringing along a volley of side effects. For instance, the most commonly used and effective synthetic drugs for the treatment of Parkinson's disease (PD) is L-Dopa. The treatment using L-Dopa for PD is accepted as it improves the motor symptoms, but the effects on cognitive performance are more complex, as both positive and negative effects were observed (Pandey and Srivanitchapoom, 2017). Owing to limitations associated with synthetic drugs, we need to look toward finding natural therapeutic approaches, especially from plant products that are embedded with natural antioxidant, anti-inflammatory, antiangiogenesis, antiapoptosis, and potential neuroprotective properties.

Our search for such a novel therapeutic plant-based alternative leads us to this bright orange spice known as saffron. It is derived from the Crocus sativus, which is a plant species belonging to the Iridaceae family and has been widely used as a herbal medicine, spice, food coloring, and flavoring agent since times immemorial. It is a perennial, bulbous plant that grows 8- to 10-cm high, and it has a large squat tuber surrounded by reticulate and fibrous sheath. The leaves of saffron plants are splayed, narrow, and have a ciliated margin and keel. The lily-like flowers have two bracts at the base. There is a pale violet-veined calyx, yellow anthers, and white filament. The thread-like style of the plant is 10-mm long, and the stigma is bright orange. The stigmas are harvested and dried for use. It can require up to 75,000 saffron flowers to produce a pound of saffron spice, thus rendering it as one of the most expensive spices in the world (Fig. 8.1).

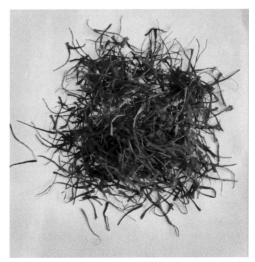

FIG. 8.1 Image showing dried saffron after being collected from field.

Saffron has been widely used as medicinal plant for promoting human health since ancient times, especially in Asian and middle eastern countries (Javadi and Emami, 2013). Most of the saffron extract belongs to the category of carotenoids including crocin and crocetin. The median lethal dose (LD_{50}) of saffron is 200 mg/mL in in vitro and 20.7 g/kg in animal model (Bostan and Hosseinz, 2017).

It has been suggested that saffron and its extracts were being effective in the treatment of a wide range of disorders including coronary artery disease (Kamalipour and Akhondzadeh, 2011), hypertension (Nasiri et al., 2015), stomach disorder (Khorasany and Hosseinzadeh, 2016), dysmenorrhea (Mirabi et al., 2014), learning, and memory impairment (Ghaffari and Dehghan, 2015). Apart from that, many researchers have reported that saffron has properties such as antiinflammatory (Poma et al., 2012), antioxidant (Verma and Bordia, 1998), antiatherosclerotic (Kakisis, 2018), antigenotoxic (Abdullaev et al., 2003; Premkumar et al., 2006), and anticytotoxic effects (Abdullaev et al., 2003). Saffron also has oxytoxic properties, and traditionally it has been prescribed to facilitate difficult labors. Razi has mentioned that "Ingestion of 6–7 g of saffron induces the labor. I myself prescribed it many times and the results were always a success".

Saffron has been also used to treat urogenital disorders as different doses of saffron extract has dose-dependent effects on the management of premenstrual syndromes, dysmenorrhea, and irregular menstruation (Agha-Hosseini et al., 2008). One of the well-known effects of saffron and its extracts were exhilarant and antidepressant activity which leads to a sense of happiness and laughter. Jrojani has stated that "Saffron is astringent and resolvent and its fragrance can strengthen these two effects. Hence, its action on enlivening the essence of the spirit and inducing happiness is great" (Agha-Hosseini et al., 2008).

Saffron has also aphrodisiac properties as there is clinical and experimental evidences indicating that saffron and its bioactive extract crocin could improve sexual behavior, and it could also lead to amelioration of semen quality (Heidary et al., 2008). Saffron and its extracts crocetin and crocin are effective for the enhancement of retinal blood flow, and it was found to be protective against tunicamycin and hydrogen peroxide (H_2O_2)-induced retinal damage. Saffron and its extracts were widely used to prepare a special formulation called collyrium to treat a range of ophthalmic disorders such as cataract and conjunctivitis and to improve vision (Bisti and Falsini, 2014).

Saffron has been used to enhance the cardiovascular functions and treatment of palpitation. Many researchers have supported the cardioprotective and anti-atherosclerotic effects of saffron-derived bioactive components such as crocin and crocetin. The mechanism underlying the antiatherosclerotic effect of saffron-derived bioactive components include antihyperlipidemic and insulin-sensitizing effect and oxidized low-density lipoprotein uptake as well as lipid absorption (Melnyk and Marcone, 2010).

Saffron has been used to treat tumor and malignancies since a long time ago. Ibn Sina has noted that local application of saffron with beeswax or egg yolk and olive oil is effective to treat uterus malignancies (Aciduman et al., 2009). There are a number of in vitro and in vivo studies with evidence indicating the assurance anticarcinogenic effects of saffron and its bioactive extract such as crocin, crocetin, dimethyl-crocetin, and diglucosylcrocetin against different types of cancer.

The broad spectrum anticancer properties of saffron and its extract were due to its modulatory effect on gene expression, induction of changes in DNA, induction of apoptosis, scavenging of free radicals, and inhibition of topoisomerase II (Magesh et al., 2006). The major challenge faced by pharmacies and researchers are the bioavailability and absorption rates of novel drugs. There are many studies that have reported that saffron and its bioactive components can increase the bioavailability and enhance the absorption rate of novel drugs (Magesh et al., 2006).

Recently, many researchers have reported that saffron and its constituents have protective effects on many age-related neurodegenerative disorders such as AD, PD (Rao et al., 2016), Schizophrenia disease (Pitsikas, 2016), neuronal injury and apoptosis (Wang et al., 2015), neuroinflammation (Khazdair and Hosseini, 2015), brain neurotransmitter concentration (Ettehadi et al., 2013), and stress and depression-like behavior (Jelodar et al., 2018). Researchers have discovered over 150 compounds in saffron which have neuroprotective effects (Fig. 8.2).

In this chapter, we will discuss the neuroprotective effect of saffron in detail.

IN VITRO NEUROPROTECTIVE FUNCTIONS OF SAFFRON

Saffron Extract Crocin Prevents Oxidative Stress and PC-12 Cell Apoptosis by Increasing Intracellular Antioxidant Glutathione (GSH) in Serum-/Glucose-Free Media

Oxidative stress is a state of imbalanced free radicals and antioxidants in the cell which can lead to cell and tissue damage by oxidative stress. Our body's cells produce free radicals and reactive oxygen species (ROS) during normal metabolic processes. At the same time, cells also produce antioxidants that neutralize these free radicals. In general, our body is able to maintain the balance between antioxidants and free radicals. Free radicals are molecules with unpaired electron in their outer orbit. Some of the free radicals play an important role in origin of life and biological evolution (McCord, 2000). For instance, oxygen radicals are involved in many biochemical activities of cells such as signal transduction, gene transcription, and regulation of guanylate cyclase activity (Uttara et al., 2009). We are constantly exposed to free radicals created by electromagnetic radiation from the man-made sources such as environmental pollutants and natural sources such as cosmic radiation and cellular metabolism (enzymatic reaction). The most common cellular free radicals are hydroxyl (OH), superoxide (O^{2-}), and nitric monoxide (NO). Our body produces oxygen free radicals and other ROS through numerous physiological and biochemical processes. At the same time, antioxidants such as glutathione, arginine, taurine, creatine, vitamin E, vitamin C, and vitamin A along with antioxidant enzymes such as superoxide dismutase (SOD), glutathione reductase (GSH), and catalase were constantly produced by our body's cells. But, under certain circumstances, the production of antioxidants

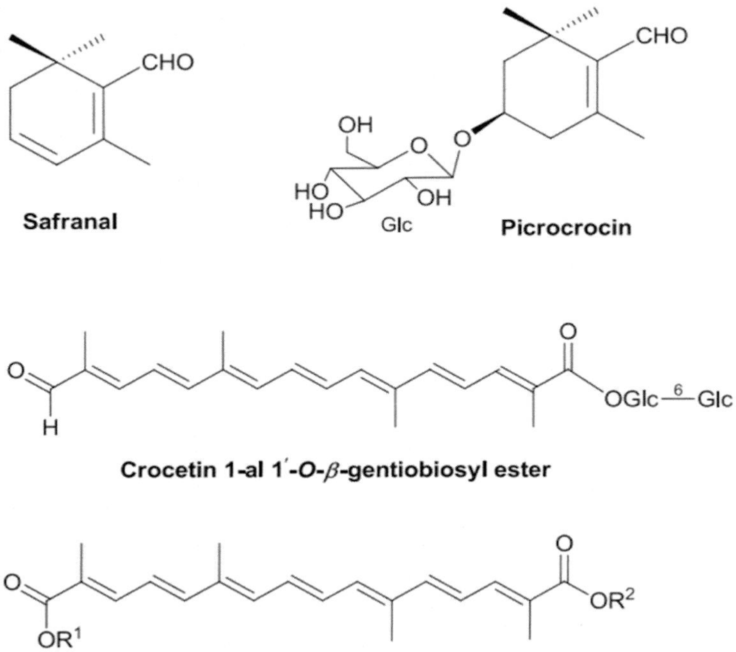

FIG. 8.2 Major constituents of saffron (crocin, safranal, and picrocrocin).

from our body cell does not meet the required amount to neutralize the ROS and free radicals, thereby leading to protein and DNA injury, inflammation, tissue damage, and subsequent cellular apoptosis (Gilgum-Sherki, 2001).

Neurodegenerative disease is a progressive loss of nerve cells from the brain and spinal cord and leads to either functional loss (ataxia) or sensory dysfunction (dementia). There were numerous physiological and environmental factors that cause neurodegeneration, and one of the major factors is abnormal metal metabolism. Oxidative stress and free radicals generation catalyzed by redox metals have been shown to play a major role in regulating redox reaction in *in vivo* contributing ROS, which were the main factors in neurodegeneration (Emerit and Bricaire, 2004).

Researchers have analyzed the effect of crocin on PC-12 cells cultured in serum-/glucose-free media in comparison with those of α-tocopherol. Deprivation of serum/glucose in PC-12 cell culture had caused changes in morphology and the prooxidant level in the cells (Soeda et al., 2016). There is a significant increase in the prooxidant malondialdehyde (MDA) levels and the number of phosphatidylserine externalization, which later can be used as an early marker of apoptotic induction (Mukhopadhyay et al., 2007). They have also

reported that deprivation of serum/glucose had decreased the SOD activity by 14% of that in the control cell. However, crocin (0.1−10 μM), an extract from saffron had significantly decreased the prooxidant MDA level and increased the SOD activity as compared to α-tocopherol activity. The restoration of SOD activity and MDA level suggests that crocin had an important role in modulating oxidative stress in the PC-12 cell line (Mukhopadhyay et al., 2007).

The level of total glutathione (GSH) in the PC-12 cells subjected to 3 h in serum-/glucose-free Dulbecco's Modified Eagle Medium (DMEM) had significantly decreased to half than that found in the normal control cells and thereafter remained constant. However, the addition of crocin to the medium increases the intracellular GSH level dose dependently. Saffron-extract crocin had a maximum effect in PC-12 cell culture at a concentration of 10 μM. The mechanism by which GSH activity increased in cell culture with crocin is not completely understood, but researchers have reported that c-glutamylcysteinyl synthase (cGCS) mRNA expression is involved in the regulation of GSH activity (Soeda et al., 2016). Nakajima (2002) had reported that nerve growth factor (NGF) had an ability to increase the activity of c-GCS at the transcriptional level by extending the half-life of c-GCS mRNA. However, addition of crocin

(10 μM) doubles cGCS mRNA expression in PC-12 cells cultured in serum-/glucose-free DMEM, while it had no effect on the mRNA levels in control PC-12 cells (Nakajima et al., 2002).

It was well known that serum or NGF deprivation induces apoptosis in PC-12 cells (Matrone et al., 2008). When PC-12 cells were cultured in serum/glucose containing DMEM (DMEM+), they had a normal morphological structure at 24 h, while those cultured in serum-/glucose-free DMEM medium for 24 h were showing the characteristic properties of necrotic or apoptotic cells, and approximately 60% of cell death had occurred in the culture medium deprived of serum/glucose (Soeda et al., 2016). In their previous study, they have reported that saffron extract crocin increased the production of antioxidant GSH level through upregulation of γ-glutamylcysteinyl synthase (γ-GCS), which is involved in the GSH synthesis (Ochiai et al., 2007).

A recent study has reported evidence that dietary saffron can modulate the brain transcriptome and upregulate a specific stress-inducible pathway. Saffron exerts its neuroprotection by acting as a mild biological stressor with nonlinear dose-response relationship (Skladnev and Johnstone, 2017). In addition, the activation of magnesium-dependent N-SMase in PC-12 cell membrane leads to cell apoptosis through elevation of intracellular ROS and protein kinase C / c-Jun NH2-terminal kinase pathway. However, treatment with saffron-extract crocin of 10 μM had no direct effect on N-SMase activation, but it increases the intracellular antioxidant GSH level, thereby protecting the cells from apoptosis and promoting survival of PC-12 cells (Soeda et al., 2016) (Fig. 8.3).

NEUROPROTECTIVE ACTIVITY OF CROCIN IN *IN VIVO*
Crocin Reduces the Infarcted Areas Caused by Occultation of the Middle Cerebral Artery in Mice Brian

Infarction is tissue death or necrosis due to inadequate blood supply to the affected area. It may be caused by artery blockage, rupture, mechanical compression, or vasoconstriction. Infarction care is divided based on histopathology (white infarction and red infarction) and location (heart, brain, lung, etc.). Researchers

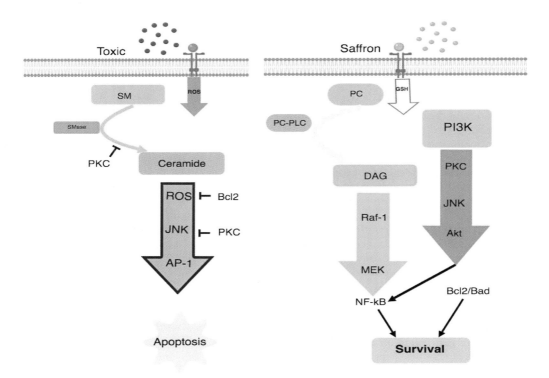

FIG. 8.3 Neuroprotective effects of saffron through upregulation of intracellular antioxidant GSH level and through activation of protein kinase C (PKC) and diglyceride (DAG), it promotes cell survival.

have investigated the effect of crocin on an infarcted area caused by occlusion of the middle cerebral artery (MCA) in mice. They have administrated crocin (10 mg/kg) immediately 3 h before and 3 h after the MCA occlusion. The administration of crocin had effectively reduced the infarct volume significantly compared with the vehicle control group (Soeda et al., 2016). Vakili and colleague (2014) have reported that the protective effect of crocin against cerebral ischemia occurs in a dose-dependent manner in rat model. These evidences suggest that crocin is a novel therapeutic compound against infarction induced by occlusion of the MCA.

Neuroprotective Effects of Saffron Extract on Neurodegenerative Disorders

Age-related neurological disorder is one of the major challenges that we are facing in today's world. Even though there are many synthetic drugs available for neurodegenerative disorders, most of them are only relieving the symptoms and do very little for the root causes of degeneration. Many researchers have reported the tremendous side effects of these synthetic drugs on both mental and physical health. So, it is very important to look for an alternative novel and natural product of plant for these neurodegenerative disorders. Saffron is one of the best candidates for this purpose as it has a long history of being used in traditional medicine and it has many medical benefits with minimal known side effects. In traditional medicine, saffron extract crocin has been frequently used as herbal sedative, antispasmodic, aphrodisiac, diaphoretic, expectorant, anticatarrhal, and eupeptic (Nemati and Vostakolaei, 2008). An in vitro study conducted by Papandreous and colleague have reported that saffron and its extract crocin has an inhibitory activity on amyloid beta peptide fibrillogenesis and protective action against hydrogen peroxide (H_2O_2)-induced toxicity in human neuroblastoma cells (Papandreous et al., 2006).

In Iranian traditional medicine, saffron and its extracts have been used as an anticonvulsant herb, and researchers have confirmed its anticonvulsant effect in rats and mice (Skladnev and Johnstone, 2017). Saffron and its extract crocin at a dose of 400 mg/kg and 800 mg/kg showed antiepileptic activity in pentylenetetrazole-induced seizure model in a dose-dependent manner (Sunanda et al., 2014). AD is described as an age-related condition and pathologically as deposition of amyloid beta peptide. The saffron extract of C. sativus stigma has strong antioxidant properties in a concentration and time-dependent manner,

which was accompanied by inhibition of amyloid beta (Aβ) fibrillogenesis (Papandreous et al., 2006).

Researchers have revealed that treatment of C. sativus extract 30 mg/kg for 3 weeks could significantly improve cognitive deficits in AD mice model (Khalili et al., 2008). In clinical study, administration of saffron 30 mg/day was found to be as effective as donepezil for treatment of mild to moderate AD in subjects aged 55 years and older (Akhondzadeh et al., 2010). In another study, 46 patients with mild to moderate AD were treated by saffron for 16 weeks, and the result shows that the cognitive functions in the saffron-treated group were significantly better than those of placebo (Akhondzadeh et al., 2010).

Depression is a mood disorder characterized by persistently low mood and feeling of sadness and loss of interest. Prolonged depression has a tremendous effect on our brain's function and structure. Many researchers have reported that saffron and its extract has a significant antidepressant effect. A clinical study conducted by Noorbala and colleague has revealed that administration of saffron extract 30 mg/day for 6 weeks had significantly improved depression regardless of whether it was mild or moderate in severity (Noorbala et al., 2005). Many researchers have thus reported the effectiveness of C. sativus as a treatment for depression in mice model.

AD and PD are two major neurodegenerative diseases that are affecting the people older than 60 years. Formation of a toxic amyloid structure is a major cause of this neurodegenerative disease (Ebrahim-Habibi et al., 2010). Researchers have suggested the neuroprotective effect of saffron extract crocetin (25, 50, and 75 µg/kg of body weight, i.p.) against 6-hydroxyldopamine (6-OHDA, 10 µg intrastriatal) induced in a PD rats model, and the reduction of dopamine utilization by tissue was suggested as a possible mechanism (Ahmad et al., 2005). Purushothuman et al. have reported that pretreatment with saffron (0.01w/v) had saved many dopaminergic cells in substantia nigra pars compacta (SNc) and retina in mice model of acute 1-methyl-4-phenyl-1,2,3,6-tetrahydropyridine (MPTP) induced PD by increasing tyrosine hydrolase (TH+) cells (Purushothuman et al., 2013).

Saffron Extract Crocin Improves Learning and Memory Capacity

Normal aging is associated with a decline in various memory abilities and cognitive tasks. Learning and memory are a vital part of our life. The analysis of anatomical and physical bases of learning and memory is one of the greatest successes of modern neuroscience. According to the literature review, Zhang and colleagues had reported that the alcohol extract of pistils of C. sativus leaf improves learning and memory in mice (Zhang. Y et al., 1994). This finding was further supported by others finding. However, some other researchers have reported that oral administration of saffron extract crocin alone had no effect on learning behavior of mice in passive avoidance test, but it improves significantly in ethanol-induced impairment of memory acquisition. They have also reported that crocin can significantly antagonize the inhibitory effect of ethanol on long-term potential (LTP) in both in vivo and in vitro studies (Sugiura et al., 1995). LTP is a mechanism underlying memory formation. Since dentate gyrus and hippocampal regions of the brain are involved in learning and memory acquisition, researchers have reported that alcohol extract of C. sativus leaves can prevent adverse effects induced by ethanol and its metabolite on neuronal activity in the dentate gyrus (Suugiura et al., 1995). On the basis of these results, researchers have suggested that saffron and its crocin extracts are capable of antagonizing the blocking effect of ethanol for memory acquisition. From neuroscience point of view, LTP is a persistent strengthening of synapses based on a recent pattern of activity. These are the patterns of synaptic activity that produce a long-lasting increase in signal transmission between two neurons and facilitate the neuroplasticity and memory acquisition. The opposite of LTP is long-term depression (Ltd.), which produces long-lasting decrease in synaptic strength and leads to neuronal apoptosis, and the most common neurotransmitters for Ltd. is L-glutamate. Since memory and learning are thought to be encoded by modification of synaptic strength, LTP is widely considered as one of the major cellular mechanisms that control learning and memory (Cooke and Bliss, 2006). Administration of saffron 60 mg/kg to normal and aged mice for 1 week had significantly improved learning and memory (Papandreous et al., 2011). Researchers have investigated the effect of saffron extract crocin on LTP, and they have reported that the blocking effect of ethanol on LTP decrease dose dependently. When 50 mg/kg dose of crocin was injected 5 min before administration of ethanol, LTP was induced at 84% compared with control. This result suggesting the LTP-blocking effect of ethanol was improved dose dependently with the administration of crocin (Sugiura et al., 1995).

Saffron Promotes Neurogenesis through Regulation of Sleep

Neurogenesis is the process of continuous production of new neurons in the brain, particularly in the dentate gyrus of the hippocampus and subventricular zone of the lateral ventricles. Once new neurons are produced, they will migrate, differentiate, and proliferate based on their neuronal fate. Researchers have reported that the integration of new neurons into the existing neuronal circuitry in the hippocampus might be involved in memory process and the regulation of emotion and thoughts (Meerlo et al., 2009). Recently, various studies have reported that the production of new neurons is affected by sleep and disruption for a short time appears to have a deleterious effect on the basal rate of cell proliferation, cell survival, and neurogenesis. As sleep is not a continuous process but a circular process with different stages (rapid eye movement and nonrapid eye movement), the effect of sleep on neurogenesis might be dependent on different stages of sleep. The deprivation of sleep is one of the major problems of people who work during night time. Since our body and mind are innately tuned by the natural light and dark cycle, deprivation of sleep will affect both nonrapid eye movement (NREM) and rapid eye movement sleep (REM). Accumulated evidence suggest that a decrease in cell proliferation is related to a reduction in REM sleep, whereas decrease in the number of neurons that developed into mature neurons may relate to reduction in both NREM and REM sleep (Guzman-Marin R 2005). It is well known that saffron and traditional Japanese Kampo medicine promote the sleep activity in patients with a mental disorder. Recently, researchers have investigated the sleep-promoting effect of saffron and its extract crocin in mice, and they have reported that administration of crocin 100 mg/kg in mice caused a significant increase in NREM sleep from 2 to 4 h, but there was no observable change in REM sleep after administration (Masaki et al., 2012). Another study has reported that administration of crocin (30 mg/kg and 100 mg/kg) had significantly increased the total amount of NREM sleep by 160% and 270%, respectively (Soeda et al., 2016).

CONCLUSION

We know that from the ancient times, people have used different herbs and procedure in treatment of different mental disorders. But, during the last century, numerous scientific discoveries and industrial growth had contributed tremendous medicinal development and significantly improved the quality of the life of patients with a mental disorder. However, we have neglected the traditional method and procedure of treating mental disorders and unnecessarily thrown out some of the natural drugs used step by step. Saffron has been used from approximately 3000 years ago as a spice, food colorant, and medicine. In fact, saffron is known well as safety food because oral administration of saffron extract at concentrations of up to 50 g/kg is still nontoxic in mice.

As we discussed earlier, saffron is one of the most effective herbal medicine that have been used since the ancient period. It was widely used in the Middle East countries for different treatment purposes. Many medical scripts of ancient times have mentioned the medical uses of saffron and its extract. Saffron has been used to treat different illness such as cancer, mental disorders, inflammation, blood disorders, cerebral ischemia, neurodegenerative disorders, depression, and memory impairment. After modern science and technology came to exist, many ancient medical philosophic and knowledge had been vanished along with saffron and other herbs. However, after more than two centuries of modern scientist debate and struggle on synthetic drugs to tackle various diseases, now we are focusing back the ancient knowledge and philosophic of medicine.

Mental health issue is one of the major challenges in today's world. There are countless spectrums of neurological disorders, and the preventive and treatment measures are still in a naive state. We had discussed the therapeutic effects of saffron on different neurological disorders, and still there are many more to uncover, mysterious health benefits of saffron. In summary, saffron has antiinflammatory, antioxidant, antiapoptosis, anticarcinogenic, and antiatherosclerosis effect, and it also protects neuronal cells from degeneration; it has a neuroprotective effect on different neurodegenerative disorders such as PD, AD, and memory impairment. Saffron also acts as an antidepressant, and during ancient times, scholars called it a happy drug.

Even though, we have the general knowledge of saffron's benefits toward neurological disorders, there are many mysterious and secret benefits of saffron that we were struggling to uncover. Although modern technology had helped us to learn detailed mechanisms of saffron's neuroprotective functions, still the exact cellular and subcellular mechanisms of saffron and extract's neuroprotections were not completely understood. In future, apart from proteomic and genomic study of saffron's benefit, we should focus more on the cellular and subcellular signaling pathways so that we could draw the complete map of saffron's neuroprotection.

REFERENCES

Abdullaev, F.I., Riveron-Negrete, L., Caballero-Ortega, H., Hernández, J.M., Perez-Lopez, I., Pereda-Miranda, R., Espinosa-Aguirre, J.J., 2003. Use of in vitro assays to assess the potential antigenotoxic and cytotoxic effects of saffron (Crocus sativus L.). Toxicol. In Vitro 17 (5–6), 731–736.

Aciduman, A., Arda, B., Özaktürk, F.G., Telatar, Ü.F., 2009. What Does Al-Qanun Fi Al-Tibb (The Canon of Medicine) Say on Head Injuries?.

Agha-Hosseini, M., Kashani, L., Aleyaseen, A., Ghoreishi, A., Rahmanpour, H.A.L.E.H., Zarrinara, A.R., Akhondzadeh, S., 2008. Crocus sativus L.(saffron) in the treatment of premenstrual syndrome: a double-blind, randomised and placebo-controlled trial. Int. J. Obstet. Gynaecol. 115 (4), 515–519.

Ahmad, A.S., Ansari, M.A., Ahmad, M., Saleem, S., Yousuf, S., Hoda, M.N., Islam, F., 2005. Neuroprotection by crocetin in a hemi-parkinsonian rat model. Pharmacol. Biochem. Behav. 81 (4), 805–813.

Akhondzadeh, S., Sabet, M.S., Harirchian, M.H., Togha, M., Cheraghmakani, H., Razeghi, S., Hejazi, S.S., Yousefi, M.H., Alimardani, R., Jamshidi, A., Zare, F., 2010. Saffron in the treatment of patients with mild to moderate Alzheimer's disease: a 16-week, randomized and placebo-controlled trial. J. Clin. Pharm. Ther. 35 (5), 581–588.

Bisti, S., Maccarone, R., Falsini, B., 2014. Saffron and retina: neuroprotection and pharmacokinetics. Vis. Neurosci. 31 (4–5), 355–361.

Bostan, H.B., Mehri, S., Hosseinzadeh, H., 2017. Toxicology effects of saffron and its constituents: a review. Iran. J Basic Med Sci. https://doi.org/10.22038/ijbms.2017.8230.

Cooke, S.F., Bliss, T.V.P., 2006. Plasticity in the human central nervous system. Brain 129 (Pt 7), 1659–1673. https://doi.org/10.1093/brain/awl082. England.

Ebrahim-Habibi, M.B., Amininasab, M., Ebrahim-Habibi, A., Sabbaghian, M., Nemat-Gorgani, M., 2010. BFibrillation of α-lactalbumin: effect of crocin and safranal, two natural small molecules from Crocus sativus. Biopolymers 93 (10), 854–865.

Emerit, J., Edeas, M., Bricaire, F., 2004. Neurodegenerative diseases and oxidative stress. Biomed. Pharmacother. 58 (1), 39–46. France.

Ettehadi, H., Mojabi, S.N., Ranjbaran, M., Shams, J., Sahraei, H., Hedayati, M., Asefi, F., 2013. Aqueous extract of saffron (Crocus sativus) increases brain dopamine and glutamate concentrations in rats. J. Behav. Brain Sci. 3 (3), 315–319.

Ghaffari, S., Hatami, H., Dehghan, G., 2015. Saffron ethanolic extract attenuates oxidative stress, spatial learning, and memory impairments induced by local injection of ethidium bromide. Res. Pharmaceut. Sci. 10 (3), 222–232. Iran.

Gilgun-Sherki, Y., Melamed, E., Offen, D., 2001. Oxidative stress induced-neurodegenerative diseases: the need for antioxidants that penetrate the blood brain barrier. Neuro-pharmacology 40 (8), 959—975. England.

Gourie-Devi, M., 2014. Epidemiology of neurological disorders in India: review of background, prevalence and incidence of epilepsy, stroke, Parkinson's disease and tremors. Neurol. India 62 (6), 588.

Guzman-Marin, R., Suntsova, N., Methippara, M., Greiffenstein, R., Szymusiak, R., McGinty, D., 2005. Sleep deprivation suppresses neurogenesis in the adult hippocampus of rats. Eur. J. Neurosci. 22 (8), 2111—2116.

Heidary, M., Vahhabi, S., Nejadi, J.R., Delfan, B., Birjandi, M., Kaviani, H., Givrad, S., 2008. Effect of saffron on semen parameters of infertile men. Urol. J. 5 (4), 255—259.

Hung, C.W., Chen, Y.C., Hsieh, W.L., Chiou, S.H., Kao, C.L., 2010. Ageing and neurodegenerative diseases. Ageing Res. Rev. 9, S36—S46.

Javadi, B., Sahebkar, A., Emami, S.A., 2013. A survey on saffron in major islamic traditional medicine books. Iran. J. Basic Med. Sci. 16 (1), 1—11. https://doi.org/10.22038/IJBMS.2013.243.

Jelodar, G., Javid, Z., Sahraian, A., Jelodar, S., 2018. Saffron improved depression and reduced homocysteine level in patients with major depression: a Randomized, double-blind study. Avicenna J. Phytomed. 8 (1), 43.

Johri, A., Beal, M.F., 2012. Mitochondrial dysfunction in neurodegenerative diseases. pharmacol. Exp. Ther. 342 (3), 619—630. https://doi.org/10.1124/jpet.112.192138.

Kakisis, J.D., 2018. Saffron: from Greek mythology to contemporary anti-atherosclerotic medicine. Atherosclerosis 193—195. https://doi.org/10.1016/j.atherosclerosis.2017.11.021. Ireland.

Kamalipour, M., Akhondzadeh, S., 2011. Cardiovascular efects of Saffron : an evidence-based review. J. Tehran Heart Cent. 59—61.

Khalili, M., Roghani, M., Ekhlasi, M., 2008. The effect of aqueous crocus sativus L. Extract on intracerebroventricular streptozotocin-induced cognitive deficits in rat: a behavioral analysis. Iran. J. Pharm. Res. 8.

Khazdair, M.R., Boskabady, M.H., Hosseini, M., Rezaee, R., Tsatsakis, A.M., 2015. The effects of *Crocus sativus* (saffron) and its constituents on nervous system: a review. Avicenna J. Phytomed. 5 (5), 376.

Khorasany, A.R., Hosseinzadeh, H., 2016. Therapeutic effects of saffron (*Crocus sativus* L.) in digestive disorders : a review. Iran. J. Basic Med. Sci. https://doi.org/10.22038/ijbms.2016.6929.

Li, J., Li, W., Jiang, Z.G., Ghanbari, H., 2013. Oxidative stress and neurodegenerative disorders. Int. J. Mol. Sci. 14 (12), 24438—24475.

Lin, M.T., Beal, M.F., 2006. Mitochondrial dysfunction and oxidative stress in neurodegenerative diseases. Nature 443, 787. Available at: https://doi.org/10.1038/nature05292.

Magesh, V., Singh, J.P.V., Selvendiran, K., Ekambaram, G., Sakthisekaran, D., 2006. Antitumour activity of crocetin in accordance to tumor incidence, antioxidant status, drug metabolizing enzymes and histopathological studies. Mol. Cell. Biochem. 287 (1—2), 127—135.

Masaki, M., Aritake, K., Tanaka, H., Shoyama, Y., Huang, Z.L., Urade, Y., 2012. Crocin promotes non-rapid eye movement sleep in mice. Mol. Nutr. Food Res. 56 (2), 304—308.

Matrone, C., Di Luzio, A., Meli, G., D'Aguanno, S., Severini, C., Ciotti, M.T., Cattaneo, A., Calissano, P., 2008. Activation of the amyloidogenic route by NGF deprivation induces apoptotic death in PC12 cells. J. Alzheimer's Dis. 13 (1), 81—96.

McCord, J.M., 2000. The evolution of free radicals and oxidative stress. Am. J. Med. 108 (8), 652—659. United States.

Meerlo, P., Mistlberger, R.E., Jacobs, B.L., Heller, H.C., McGinty, D., 2009. New neurons in the adult brain: the role of sleep and consequences of sleep loss. Sleep Med. ev. 13 (3), 187—194.

Melnyk, J.P., Wang, S., Marcone, M.F., 2010. Chemical and biological properties of the world ' s most expensive spice : Saffron. Food Res. Int. 43 (8), 1981—1989. https://doi.org/10.1016/j.foodres.2010.07.033. Elsevier Ltd.

Mirabi, P., Alamolhoda, S.H., Esmaeilzadeh, S., Mojab, F., 2014. Effect of medicinal herbs on primary dysmenorrhoea-a systematic review. Iran. J. Pharm. Res. 13 (3), 757.

Mukhopadhyay, P., Rajesh, M., Haskó, G., Hawkins, B.J., Madesh, M., Pacher, P., 2007. Simultaneous detection of apoptosis and mitochondrial superoxide production in live cells by flow cytometry and confocal microscopy. Nat. Protoc. 2 (9), 2295.

Murray, C.J.L., Lopez, A.D., World Health Organization, World Bank & Harvard School of Public Health, 1996. In: Murray, C.J.L., Lopez, A.D. (Eds.), The Global Burden of Disease: A Comprehensive Assessment of Mortality and Disability from Diseases, Injuries, and Risk Factors in 1990 and Projected to 2020: Summary. World Health Organization, Geneva. http://www.who.int/iris/handle/10665/41864.

Nakajima, A., Yamada, K., Zou, L.B., Yan, Y., Mizuno, M., Nabeshima, T., 2002. Interleukin-6 protects PC12 cells from 4-hydroxynonenal-induced cytotoxicity by increasing intracellular glutathione levels. Free Radic. Biol. Med. 32 (12), 1324—1332.

Nasiri, Z., Sameni, H.R., Vakili, A., Jarrahi, M., Khorasani, M.Z., 2015. Dietary saffron reduced the blood pressure and prevented remodeling of the aorta in L-NAME-induced hypertensive rats. Iran. J. Basic Med. Sci. 18 (11), 1143.

Nemati, H., Boskabady, M.H., Ahmadzadef Vostakolaei, H., 2008. Stimulatory effect of Crocus sativus (saffron) on beta2-adrenoceptors of Guinea pig tracheal chains. Phytomedicine 15 (12), 1038—1045. https://doi.org/10.1016/j.phymed.2008.07.008. Germany.

Noorbala, A.A., Akhondzadeh, S.H., Tahmacebi-Pour, N., Jamshidi, A.H., 2005. Hydro-alcoholic extract of *Crocus sativus* L. versus fluoxetine in the treatment of mild to moderate depression: a double-blind, randomized pilot trial. J. Ethnopharmacol. 97 (2), 281—284.

Ochiai, T., Shimeno, H., Mishima, K.I., Iwasaki, K., Fujiwara, M., Tanaka, H., Shoyama, Y., Toda, A., Eyanagi, R., Soeda, S., 2007. Protective effects of carotenoids from saffron on neuronal injury in vitro and in vivo. Biochim. Biophys. Acta Gen. Subj. 1770 (4), 578—584.

Pandey, S., Srivanitchapoom, P., 2017. Levodopa- induced dyskinesia: clinical features, pathophysiology, and medical management. Ann. Indian Acad. Neurol. 20 (3), 190−198. https://doi.org/10.4103/aian.AIAN_239_17. India.

Papandreou, M.A., Kanakis, C.D., Polissiou, M.G., Efthimiopoulos, S., Cordopatis, P., Margarity, M., Lamari, F.N., 2006. Inhibitory activity on amyloid-β aggregation and antioxidant properties of Crocus sativus stigmas extract and its crocin constituents. J. Agric. Food Chem. 54 (23), 8762−8768.

Papandreou, M.A., Tsachaki, M., Efthimiopoulos, S., Cordopatis, P., Lamari, F.N., Margarity, M., 2011. Memory enhancing effects of saffron in aged mice are correlated with antioxidant protection. Behav. Brain Res. 219 (2), 197−204.

Pitsikas, N., 2016. Constituents of saffron (*Crocus sativus* L.) as potential candidates for the treatment of anxiety disorders and schizophrenia. Molecules 21 (3), 303.

Poma, A., Fontecchio, G., Carlucci, G., Chichiricco, G., 2012. Anti-inflammatory properties of drugs from saffron crocus. Antiinflamm. Antiallergy Agents Med. Chem. 11 (1), 37−51. United Arab Emirates.

Przedborski, S., Vila, M., Jackson-Lewis, V., 2003. Series Introduction: neurodegeneration: what is it and where are we? J. Clin. Investig. 111 (1), 3−10.

Purushothuman, S., Nandasena, C., Johnstone, D.M., Stone, J., Mitrofanis, J., 2013. The impact of near-infrared light on dopaminergic cell survival in a transgenic mouse model of parkinsonism. Brain Res. 1535, 61−70.

Rao, S.V., Yenisetti, S.C., Rajini, P.S., 2016. Evidence of neuroprotective effects of saffron and crocin in a Drosophila model of parkinsonism. Neurotoxicology 52, 230−242.

Seitz, R.J., 2004. Concepts on neurological disease evolution. Pharmacopsychiatry 37 (Suppl. 2), S120−S125. https://doi.org/10.1055/s-2004-832665. Germany.

Skladnev, N.V., Johnstone, D.M., 2017. Neuroprotective properties of dietary saffron: more than just a chemical scavenger? Neural Regen. Res. 12 (2), 210.

Soeda, S., Aritake, K., Urade, Y., Sato, H., Shoyama, Y., 2016. Neuroprotective activities of saffron and crocin. In: The Benefits of Natural Products for Neurodegenerative Diseases. Springer, Cham, pp. 275−292.

Sugiura, M., Shoyama, Y., Saito, H., Nishiyama, N., 1995. Crocin improves the ethanol-induced impairment of learning behaviors of mice in passive avoidance tasks. Proc. Jap. Acad. B 71 (10), 319−324.

Sunanda, B.P.V., Rammohan, B., Kumar, A., Kudagi, B.L., 2014. The effective study of aqueous extract of crocus sativus linn in chemical induced convulsants in rats. World J. Pharm. Pharmacuet. Sci. 3 (3), 1175−1182.

Uttara, B., Singh, A.V., Zamboni, P., Mahajan, R.T., 2009. Oxidative stress and neurodegenerative diseases: a review of upstream and downstream antioxidant therapeutic options. Curr. Neuropharmacol. 7 (1), 65−74.

Vakili, A., Einali, M.R., Bandegi, A.R., 2014. Protective effects of crocin against cerebral ischemia in a dose-dependent manner in a rat model of ischemic stroke. J. Stroke Cerebrovasc. Dis. 23 (1), 106−113. https://doi.org/10.1016/j.jstrokecerebrovasdis.2012.10.008. Elsevier Ltd.

Verma, S.K., Bordia, A., 1998. Antioxidant property of Saffron in man. Indian J. Med. Sci. 52 (5), 205−207. India.

Wang, K., Zhang, L., Rao, W., Su, N., Hui, H., Wang, L., Peng, C., Tu, Y., Zhang, S., Fei, Z., 2015. Neuroprotective effects of crocin against traumatic brain injury in mice: involvement of notch signaling pathway. Neurosci. Lett. 591, 53−58. https://doi.org/10.1016/j.neulet.2015.02.016. Ireland.

Yirka, B., Gollo, L.L., 2018. Are neurological disorders the result of brain evolution mistakes? Neurosci. Nat. 2018−2019. https://doi.org/10.1038/s41593-018-0188-z.

Zhang, Y., Shoyama, Y., Sugiura, M., Saito, H., 1994. Effects of Crocus sativus L. on the ethanol-induced impairment of passive avoidance performances in mice. Biol. Pharm. Bull. 17 (2), 217−221.

CHAPTER 9

Saffron and Neurological Disorders

SAEED SAMARGHANDIAN • TAHEREH FARKHONDEH

BACKGROUND

Medicinal herbs are considered as important sources for synthesis of novel plant-derived drugs with high efficiency (Farkhondeh et al., 2019; Samarghandian et al., 2016a). Several of them including saffron are composed of main constituents that are responsible for their neuroprotective impacts (Samarghandian et al., 2013, 2016b; Samarghandian and Borji, 2014; Farahmand et al., 2013; Menghini et al., 2018; Farkhondeh et al., 2016; Rahiman et al., 2018; Samini et al., 2013). Chemical analysis of the saffron has found that safranal, crocins, crocetin, and picrocrocin are the important constituents of this plant (Samini et al., 2013; Caballero-Ortega et al., 2007). Saffron is applied as an eupeptic, sedative, expectorant, emmenagogue, anticatarrhal, and antispasmodic in traditional medicine (Samarghandian et al., 2016a). Additionally, saffron has been applied in folk medicine for cognitive dysfunction and memory (Samarghandian et al., 2016b).

Several pharmacological impacts of saffron and its main constituent have been found in animal and clinical trials studies, such as antiinflammatory (Menghini et al., 2018; Farkhondeh et al., 2016), antioxidant (Menghini et al., 2018), anticonvulsant (Samarghandian et al., 2016b; Samarghandian and Borji, 2014), antidepressant (Samarghandian et al., 2013; Farahmand et al., 2013), anti-Alzheimer disease (AD) (Samini et al., 2013; Caballero-Ortega et al., 2007; Boskabady and Farkhondeh, 2016), and antitumor (Rahiman et al., 2018).

It has been found that Crocus sativus and its main constituents act as a potent management tool for neurodegenerative disorders by modulating oxidative stress, inflammation, and apoptosis pathways (Boskabady and Farkhondeh, 2016). The controlled clinical trial studies have approved the safety of this plant in patients with chronic neurodegenerative diseases (Boskabady and Farkhondeh, 2016; Hemmati et al., 2015). According to the experimental and clinical studies, this chapter discusses the impact of Crocus sativus and its main components on neurological diseases.

NEUROPROTECTIVE IMPACT

Impact of Crocus sativus and Its Main Components on Oxidative Stress-Induced Neurotoxicity

Oxidative stress is defined as an imbalance between the oxidant and antioxidant system, which causes various neurodegenerative diseases (Tsantarliotou et al., 2013). Numerous studies have been investigated on plants containing ingredients with antioxidant activities, among which saffron has been recognized as a potent natural antioxidant (Tsantarliotou et al., 2013). In this regards, Crocus sativus (50, 100, and 200 mg/kg) modulates oxidative stress indices in the rat's brain that induced by diazinon (Moallem et al., 2014). Saffron extract decreases the nitric oxide (NO) and malondialdehyde (MDA) levels, however, increases the activities of glutathione peroxidase (GPx), catalase (CAT), and superoxide dismutase (SOD) as well as the levels of Glutathione (GSH) in the hippocampus of aged rats (Samarghandian et al., 2016c). The preadministration of rats exposed to middle cerebral artery occlusion with saffron (100 mg/kg, p.o., 7 days) showed a reduction of cerebral ischemia by enhancing the antioxidant content (Saleem et al., 2006). The other study has indicated the coadministration of honey (500 mg/kg) with Crocus sativus extract (200 mg/kg) decreases neurotoxicity induced by aluminum chloride in mice (Shati et al., 2011). Studies have shown that saffron extract decreases the activity of monoamine oxidase A and B as well as the level of lipid peroxidation in cerebellum and the brain of rats exposed to aluminum (Linardaki et al., 2013). Crocin (10 μM) is shown to prevent the activity of lipid peroxidation in the PC12 cells and preserve neuron morphology by increasing the SOD. Some of the crocin concentrations have indicated high-potent antioxidant activity comparing with α-tocopherol as a known antioxidant.

Saffron. https://doi.org/10.1016/B978-0-12-818462-2.00009-7

Crocin (10 and 50 μM) and *Crocus sativus* (25 and 5 mg/mL) can also reduce the neurotoxic affect of glucose, as shown in a in vitro study. Additionally, crocin enhances significantly the GPx and SOD activities and also decreases the MDA level in the cortex of ischemic stroke model (Vakili et al., 2014). Motaghinejad et al. have shown that crocin inhibits oxidative damage induced by alcohol in the brain through amelioration of Cyclic adenosine monophosphate (cAMP) response element-binding protein/brain-derived neurotrophic factor (BDNF) and Akt/phosphatidylinositol 3-kinase (PI3K) signaling pathways (Motaghinejad et al., 2019). Crocin (25–500 μM, 24 h) can also inhibit D-galactose-induced reactive oxygen species (ROS) and Advanced Glycosylated End-products (AGEs) production in SH-SY5Y cells (Heidari et al., 2018). Altinoz et al. has indicated that crocin inhibits oxidative damage in the brain induced by CCl4. The increasing total antioxidant status (TAS), GSH levels, and also CAT activity as well as decreasing MDA level confirm the neuroprotective effect of crocin (Altinoz et al., 2018). Crocin and saffron extract ameliorate memory and learning dysfunction caused through chronic stress by modifying the oxidant-antioxidant system in the hippocampus (Ghadrdoost et al., 2011). Studies have indicated that treatment with crocetin ameliorates oxidative damage in the brain induced by 6OHDA (Ahmad et al., 2005). Safranal administration (0.5 mg/kg) ameliorates an imbalance induced by age in the oxidant-antioxidant systems in the rats' brain (Samarghandian et al., 2015). Administration of safranal has a protective impact on oxidative damage in the hippocampal of ischemic rats (Hosseinzadeh and Sadeghnia, 2005) and hippocampus of rats exposed to quinolinic acid (QA) (Sadeghnia et al., 2013).

Impact of *Crocus sativus* and Iits Main Components on Apoptosis-Induced Neurotoxicity

Neuronal death is the leading mechanism connected with the pathogenesis of several neurodegeneration disorders (Samarghandian et al., 2014; Mehrpour et al., 2014). The known pathways that induce apoptosis are oxidative stress, mitochondrial dysfunction, disruption of calcium homeostasis, and activation of caspases (Samarghandian and Shabestari, 2013). Identification of medicinal plants that prevent apoptosis in nervous system may be a suitable approach for preventing and treating neurological diseases (Samarghandian and Shabestari, 2013). The antiapoptotic impact of *Crocus sativus* and its main components is confirmed by several studies. Crocin is recognized as a fruitful chemical against apoptosis by its impact on the both internal

and external pathways (Soeda et al., 2001). Crocin (60 mg/kg) is known as an effective treatment component on cerebral edema and ischemia/reperfusion injury in the stroke rat model through inhibiting apoptosis (Vakili et al., 2014). Studies have shown that crocin (50 mg/kg) shows a protective aspect on apoptosis of retinal ganglion cells (RGCs) caused by retinal ischemia/reperfusion. It has been indicated that crocin reduces apoptosis in the RGCs through phosphatidylinositol 3-kinase/AKT (PI3K/AKT) pathway. Furthermore, crocin also leads to an elevation in the Bcl-2 to BAX ratio (Qi et al., 2013). It seems that crocin (10 μM) decreases the tumor necrosis factor alpha (TNF-α) expression, resulting in the inhibition of mRNA expression of proapoptotic genes. An *in vitro* study has shown that crocin suppresses the activation of caspase-3 and caspase-8 induced via *in vitro* ischemia in PC12 (Ochiai et al., 2004a). The neuroprotective impact of crocetin, another ingredient of saffron, is also found for its regulatory effect on apoptosis pathways in the brain of animal model (Bie et al., 2011). Crocetin has also indicated effective aspects against apoptosis caused by H_2O_2 in the RGC-5 cells via preventing the activities of caspase-3 and caspase-9 (Yamauchi et al., 2011).

Impact of *Crocus sativus* and Its Main Components on Inflammation-nduced Neurotoxicity

The central nervous system (CNS) neuroinflammation is determined through the activation of resident immune cells called microglia (Mehrpour et al., 2012; Alinejad et al., 2018). It is suggested that microglia form the first line for defending retina and the brain (Li et al., 2017; Bussi et al., 2017). Recent studies have shown that the pathological damage of microglia activates the initiation or aggravation of neurodegenerative disorders (Li et al., 2017). Long-term activation of microglia decreases neuronal survival through inducing inflammatory mediators (Bussi et al., 2017). Flavonoids including saffron have been selected as an effective treatment for neurological diseases in folk medicine (Costa et al., 2016; Cirmi et al., 2016). Documents have indicated that crocin inhibits the NF-κB activation and decreases the TNF-α, IL-1β, and NO levels, as well as intracellular ROS in rat brain microglial cells exposed to lipopolysaccharide (LPS) (Nam et al., 2010). α-Crocin can also inhibit TNF-α–induced apoptotic components in the rat brain microglial cells (Yamauchi et al., 2011). It seems that the effect of crocin on inflammation is mostly related to its inhibitory effect on NF-κB signaling pathway (Lv et al., 2016). Crocetin and safranal are also suitable for controlling neuroinflammation in the various pathological conditions in the CNS. The modulating aspects of *Crocus sativus* and its constituents on inflammation are caused by a reduction in the levels of inflammatory cytokines including IL-1β and TNF-α (Wang et al., 2017; Li Puma et al., 2019).

Impact of *Crocus sativus* and Its Main Components on Neurotransmitters

Saffron (250, 150, 100, and 50 mg/kg, IP) elevates the dopamine levels in the brain (Ettehadi et al., 2013). However, the extract has no impact on the levels of serotonin and norepinephrine in the brain. Additionally, the findings indicate that the saffron aqueous extract (250 mg/kg) elevates the release of glutamate and dopamine in the rat brain (Ettehadi et al., 2013). The impact of saffron on morphine-induced conditioning place preference (CPP) has been indicated as potent as the impact of antagonists of N-methyl-D-aspartate (NMDA) receptor (Liu et al., 2010). Research has shown that the analgesic impact of saffron decreases with NMDA receptor antagonists (IA, 2011). The NMDA receptors have been found to be connected with posttraining memory function in the hippocampus and amygdala (IA, 2011). They function in morphine state-dependent learning (IA, 2011; Zarrindast et al., 2006). The recent findings indicate that saffron and its main constituents modulate memory function through NMDA receptors (Liu et al., 2010). The protective impacts of *Crocus sativus* on memory function may modulate through the cholinergic system (Ghadami and Pourmotabbed, 2009).

Impact of *Crocus sativus* and Its Main Components on Opioids System

Ethanolic (400–800 mg/kg) and aqueous (80–320 mg/kg) extracts of saffron decrease morphine withdrawal symptoms in mice (Hosseinzadeh and Jahanian, 2010). Additionally, crocin (600 and 200 mg/kg) can decrease withdrawal symptoms without decreasing the locomotor function (Hosseinzadeh and Jahanian, 2010; Amin and Hosseinzadeh, 2012). Research has shown that safranal (1, 5, and 10 mg/kg) and saffron ethanolic extract (100, 50, and 10 mg/kg) decrease the morphine-induced attainment of CPP (Ghoshooni et al., 2011). However, preadministration of crocin (600 and 400 mg/kg, i.p.) reduces the reinstatement and attainment of morphine-caused CPP in mice (Imenshahidi et al., 2011). Administration of saffron ethanolic extract (10 and 5 μg/rat) 5 min after injection of morphine (10 mg/kg) to the rats' nucleus accumbens decreases the drug-paired side spent time. Studies have indicated that administration of saffron to the rats treated with morphine (10 mg/kg) reduce

the morphine-induced CPP (Yaribeygi et al., 2014). Saffron aqueous extract (50, 100, 150, and 250 mg/kg) increases dopamine secretion in the rat brain. Additionally, saffron extract (250 mg/kg) also increases glutamate release (Ettehadi et al., 2013). Researchers have also shown that *Crocus sativus* decreases morphine-induced memory deficit (Naghibi et al., 2012; Haghighizad et al., 2008).

Alzheimer's Disease

AD is a neurological disorder which is known as the accumulation of amyloid β peptide (Aβ) plaques in the brain (Ghaderi et al., 2015). AD is accompanied by neuronal death, resulting in cognitive and memory deficiency (Alhebshi et al., 2013). The AD prevalence is related to increasing age and is caused after chronic neurodegeneration (Alhebshi et al., 2013). The neurodegeneration results in a disturbance in cognitive function, causing memory impairment, confusion, and difficulties in doing the daily activities (Alhebshi et al., 2013). Conventional therapy is not currently used to treat AD (Pitsikas, 2015). Present therapeutic approaches for AD are mostly focused on increasing cerebral circulation, modulating the cholinergic system and cleaning free radicals. Although, acetylcholine esterase (AChE) inhibitors are routinely used in the management of AD (Pitsikas, 2015; Hsiung and Feldman, 2008), these drugs have shown a low to moderate efficacy and cause serious side effects (Forchetti, 2005). Many studies confirm the protective effects of saffron against AD because of the presence of its flavonoids with potent antioxidant effects (Forchetti, 2005). Saffron extract and its main ingredients can inhibit Aβ fibrillogenesis in the experimental models of AD (Papandreou et al., 2006). The protective effect of this plant is also indicated by intracerebroventricular administration of streptozotocin (STZ) to rodents (Labak et al., 2010; Khalili and Hamzeh, 2010). One of the mechanism by which saffron prevents AD is inhibition of acetylcholinesterase (AChE) activity (Geromichalos et al., 2012). Modulation of oxidative stress, apoptosis, and inflammation are the other main mechanisms targeted by saffron and its ingredients. Saffron extract (125–500 mg/kg, orally) ameliorates ethanol-induced memory deficit in the passive avoidance paradigm in mice (Zhang et al., 1994). Crocin (50–200 mg/kg, orally) also can combat against ethanol-induced performance impairment in the mice (Sugiura et al., 1995). A single dose of saffron extract (30 and 60 mg/kg, IP) helps ameliorate the scopolamine-induced impairment on the passive avoidance function and recognition memory in the rats (Pitsikas and Sakellaridis, 2006). Crocin (15 and 30 mg/kg, IP) also improves the scopolamine-induced memory impairment, as evident through the novel object recognition test and in the radial water maze task in rats (Pitsikas et al., 2007). Studies have also shown that chronic administration of crocin (15 and 30 mg/kg, IP) ameliorates memory impairment induced by STZ in rats (Khalili and Hamzeh, 2010). Crocin may be effective against organophosphate pesticides (OPs)-induced cognitive dysfunction in the animal models by decreasing oxidative stress, apoptosis, inflammation, and TAU protein hyperphosphorylation (Mohammadzadeh et al., 2019). It has also shown that crocin can prevent the AD-like behavior in mice exposed to D-galactose and aluminum trichloride via decreasing the oxidative stress–related apoptosis pathway (Wang et al., 2019). Crocin is able to ameliorate the dysfunction in memory and long-term potentiation by reducing c-Fos in the hippocampus of AD rat model (Hadipour et al., 2018). Studies have shown that crocetin inhibits Aβ deposit-induced memory disorders in the Alzheimer transgenic mice by modulating inflammation and apoptosis (Zhang et al., 2018). The research has shown that crocetin ameliorates the memory and learning disorders through the NF-κB and P53 pathways (Ai et al., 1997). Safranal can also combat against Aβ and hydrogen peroxide (H2O2)-induced AD cell damage in PC12 by regulating MAPK (ERK1/2), PI3 kinase P85, Phospho-PI3 kinase P85, and SAPK/JNK pathways (Rafieipour et al., 2019). Clinical studies have confirmed the safety and efficacy of *Crocus sativus* against AD. Saffron 15 mg, twice daily, is as effective as donepezil for treating cognitive functions of middle-aged patients with AD (Akhondzadeh et al., 2010a, 2010b). However, the comparison study between safety and efficacy of saffron (30 mg/day, PO) and the NMDA receptor antagonist memantine (20 mg/day, PO) in patients with severe to moderate AD do not indicate any difference (Farokhnia et al., 2014).

Parkinson's Disease

Parkinson's disease (PD) is known via alpha-synuclein (αS) aggregation in the brain and also the damage of dopaminergic neurons in the substantia nigra (Venda et al., 2010). Inflammation and oxidative stress act as a main function in the pathogenesis of PD (Neuroinflammation et al., 2019). The protective impact of *Crocus sativus* and its ingredients (safranal, crocetin, and crocin) on oxidative damage in dopamine neurons in the mesencephalic induced by N-methyl-4-phenyl-1, 2, 3, 6-tetrahydropyridine hydrochloride (MPPþ) has been shown in the animals models (Ebrahim-Habibi et al., 2010). Crocin and safranal inhibit fibrillation in an amyloidogenic condition that crocin has a more

potent inhibitory effect than safranal. It has been confirmed that amyloidogenesis is involved in the pathogenesis of PD (Mohammadzadeh et al., 2018). Studies have proved that crocin administration prevent OP-induced Parkinson-like behaviors in rats. This effect of crocin is related to the inhibitory effect on lipid peroxidation and inflammation (Delkhosh-Kasmaie et al., 2018). Crocetin combats 6-OHDA–caused PD in animal by reducing dopamine levels (Delkhosh-Kasmaie et al., 2018). It is suggested that the combination of crocin administration and exercise may be effective for treating both motor and memory dysfunction induced by 6-OHDA in rats (Delkhosh-Kasmaie et al., 2018).

Anxiety and Depression

Depression and anxiety are important health threats all over the world (Hamner et al., 2004). Anxiety and depression are mental diseases that affect normal activities such as thinking, working, feeling, eating, and sleeping (Hamner et al., 2004; Van Ameringen et al., 2004). Anxiety is characterized by particular behavioral fear responses to a stressful situation and threatening stimuli. γ-Aminobutyric acid (GABA), serotonergic neurotransmitter, serotonergic 5-HT$_{1A}$ receptor, and serotonin reuptake are targeted for treating anxiety (Van Ameringen et al., 2004; Cryan and Sweeney, 2011). Owing to low efficacy and safety of the available drugs, finding alternative medicine strategies is necessary (Kell et al., 2017). Saffron, as a medicinal plant, has shown a potential for ameliorating depression and anxiety problems in the human and animal models. Research has shown that standardized saffron extract (affron, 26 mg/day, for 5 weeks) improves stress, mood, sleep, and anxiety quality in the normal adults (Lopresti and Drummond, 2017). Administration of affron® for 8 weeks has indicated an antidepressant and anxiolytic impact in young patients with moderate to mild depression (Mazidi et al., 2016). *Crocus sativus* 50 mg twice daily for 12 weeks ameliorates anxiety and depression diseases in adult patients (Ghajar et al., 2017). *Crocus sativus* (40 mg/day, for 6 weeks) has also an antidepressant impact in the major depression patients (Milajerdi et al., 2018). The other researchers have indicated that saffron (30 mg/day for 9 weeks) improves anxiety and sleep disturbance in patients with mild to moderate Comorbid Depression- Anxiety (CDA) (Bangratz et al., 2018).The combination of saffron and Rhodiola (one tablet containing 154 mg of Rhodiola and 15 mg of saffron; two tablets per day for 6 weeks) can be more potent than saffron for the management of depression (mild–moderate) and make better the symptoms of anxiety and depressive in the adult (Karimi et al.,

2001). Administration of *Crocus sativus* (16 mg, for 10 weeks) plus curcumin has shown a great potential for decreasing anxiolytic and depressive behavior in the major depressive disease (Mazidi et al., 2016). The extracts of ethanolic and aqueous *Crocus sativus*, crocin, and safranal are found to show an antidepressant impact in the animal models (Hosseinzadeh et al., 2003). Forced swimming test has indicated that crocin (600−50 mg/kg) elevates climbing time and decreases immobility time in the rat model of depression (Akhondzadeh et al., 2005). Saffron (30 mg/day) administration improves the mood of patients with depression (Noorbala et al., 2005). Administration of saffron extract (40 mg/day, for 8 weeks) has indicated saffron is as effective as imipramine (100 mg/day) and fluoxetine (Akhondzadeh et al., 2004) for treating moderate to mild depression (Akhondzadeh Basti et al., 2007). Protective effect of the petals of *Crocus sativus* in the management of depression (moderate to mild) has also been discovered (Shahmansouri et al., 2014). Treatment with *Crocus sativus* (30 mg/day) has shown that saffron is as potent as fluoxetine (40 mg/day) in ameliorating symptoms of depression in the major depressive disorder (MDD patients [Shahmansouri et al., 2014]. Saffron (5 mg/kg) administration accompanied with deep brain stimulation in a posttraumatic stress disorder animal model inhibits anxiety-like behavior by decreasing amygdala c-Fos protein expression (Hashtjini et al., 2018). Saffron and safranal administration improve anxiolytic activity, locomotor activity, and motor coordination in the mice model of anxiety (Hosseinzadeh and Noraei, 2009). Treatment with crocin ameliorates behavioral and morphological deficits induced by chronic stress in adulthood rats (Ghalandari-Shamami et al., 2019; Pitsikas et al., 2008). Crocin causes an anxiolytic impact in the rat model of anxiety (Farkhondeh et al., 2018). Crocetin (20, 40, 60 mg/kg) administration for 21 days in the animals submitted to the chronic stress ameliorates depression-like behavior by modulating oxidative damage in the brain (Samarghandian et al., 2017). Research has shown that safranal (0.75 mg/kg) improves depressant-like effects caused by chronic stress through regulating the oxidative stress indices in the brain (Zhang et al., 2018). It is suggested that crocin can improve anxiety and depressive-like behaviors in the animal model by inhibiting NLRP3 inflammasome and NF-κB and promoting the conversion of phenotype microglia M1 to M2 (Ai et al., 1997). The exact mechanisms of saffron and its main constituents responsible for their anxiolytic impact are fully understood. Some flavonoids have high affinity to binding to γ-Aminobutyric acid type A (GABAA) receptors similar to benzodiazepine (Marder et al., 2001; Miller and O'Callaghan, 2002). It is suggested that saffron and its constituents act as an agonist of benzodiazepine that interacts with the GABAA receptor—binding site (Marder et al., 2001; Miller and O'Callaghan, 2002). Numerous evidences show that stress induces the axis that increases the plasma levels of corticosterone (Halataei et al., 2011). Crocin may interact with the hypothalamus-pituitary-adrenal axis and decrease the corticosterone levels caused under stress condition (Liu et al., 2010; Lechtenberg et al., 2008). Saffron prevents opioid receptors and NMDA (Liu et al., 2010). Crocin and saffron decrease corticosterone release in the stressed mice through sigma opioid receptors and by blocking NMDA in the adrenal cortex (Lechtenberg et al., 2008).

Epilepsy

Epilepsy is a neurodegenerative disease that features unusual behavior and also a loss of consciousness and sensations (Khosravan, 2002). Oxidative stress has a main function in the epilepsy pathogenesis (Khosravan, 2002). There are several approaches for treating seizures, including using medicinal plants. Saffron has been found as an anticonvulsant plant (Sunanda et al., 2014). The experimental studies have also confirmed that saffron act as an anticonvulsant agent in the animal models (Sunanda et al., 2014; Hosseinzadeh and Talebzadeh, 2005). Studies have proved that saffron (800 and 400 mg/kg) has an antiepileptic effect in a model for seizure caused by pentylenetetrazole (Hosseinzadeh and Talebzadeh, 2005). The anticonvulsant effects of saffron extracts have been indicated in the mice model of maximal electroshock seizure (Sunanda et al., 2014). Safranal (0.35 and 0.15 mL/kg) decreases occurrence of pentylenetetrazole-caused seizure and postpones the beginning of tonic convulsion and protects death in the mice (Hosseinzadeh and Sadeghnia, 2007). Safranal (291, 145.5, and 72.75 mg/kg) can reduce the incidence of minimal clonic seizures and induced tonic-clonic seizures (Sadeghnia et al., 2008). Safranal ameliorates the acute experimental seizures, resulting in alteration of binding sites of benzodiazepine in the GABA receptor (Tamaddonfard et al., 2012). Crocin shows an anticonvulsant impact in the animal model exposed to penicillin. Crocin (100, 50, and 25 μg) administration increases the latency time of the first spike wave onset and decreases the amplitude of spike waves. The modification of GABA (A)-benzodiazepine receptor acts as a main function in the anticonvulsant impact of crocin (Xiting et al., 2017). Crocin (20 mg/kg) also attenuates behavioral seizure and decreases cumulative afterdischarge duration during hippocampus rapid kindling acquisition in mice (Xiting et al., 2017). Crocin at the concentrations of 200 and 100 mg/kg reduces the occurrence of the generalized seizure and decreases average stages of seizure in kindled mice (Gilgun-Sherki et al., 2004). The inhibitory impact of crocin on epilepsy progression is caused by inducing the hippocampus BDNF expression and potentiating the TrkB receptor function (Gilgun-Sherki et al., 2004). Additionally, the preventive effect of crocin on epilepsy is also related to the inflammatory indexes such as IL-1β, TNF-α, and IL-6 (Gilgun-Sherki et al., 2004).

Encephalomyelitis

Encephalomyelitis is a loss of myelinated fibers disorder in the brain and spinal cord. Research has indicated that oxidative stress and inflammation are involved in its pathogenesis (Ghazavi et al., 2009). Researchers have considered the experimental autoimmune encephalomyelitis (EAE) as a suitable model for investigating on multiple sclerosis (MS) (Ghazavi et al., 2009). Saffron administration improves EAE symptoms in the mice via inhibiting oxidative damage and inflammation in the brain and may be effective for MS treatment (Christensen, 2005). Crocin inhibits astrocyte and oligodendrocyte toxicities induced by syncytin-1 and NO and also decreases neurological impairments in the EAE model. Syncytin-1 can lead to neuroinflammation and oligodendrocyte death (Barnett and Prineas, 2004). The expression of syncytin-1 is increased in the glial cells of the MS models' astrocytes and microglia (Marciniak et al., 2004). Endoplasmic reticulum (ER) stress is the one of the known inflammatory pathways (Marciniak et al., 2004). EAE induces the ER stress gene expression such as XBP-1/s (Deslauriers et al., 2011). Crocin decreases inflammatory genes and the expression of ER stress in the spinal cord and suppresses the ER stress genes XBP-1/s expression on day 7 after EAE induction (Fathimoghadam et al., 2019). Glutamic acid (GA) and QA lead to inflammation and demyelination in neurological disorders such as MS (Fathimoghadam et al., 2019). They act mostly through the activation of oligodendrocytes and overproduction of free radicals (Fathimoghadam et al., 2019). Crocin (100 mg/kg) can also be effective against demyelination induced by ethidium bromide by modulating the levels of oxidative parameters (MDA, GPx, SOD) in the brain of animal model (Alavi et al., 2018).

Safranal (0.1, 1, 10, 50, 100, and 200 μM) has a protective effect on OLN-93 oligodendrocytes injury induced by GA or QA through inhibiting oxidative stress (Lieberman et al., 2005).

Schizophrenia

Schizophrenia is the serious cognitive illness that influences nearly 1% of people in the world (Georgiadou et al., 2014). This illness diminishes individual, social, and occupational operating capacities and decreases the life quality of patients (Georgiadou et al., 2014). Schizophrenia is characterized by three groups of symptoms: positive symptoms (delusions, hallucinations, burble assessment processing, and catatonic behavior), negative indicators (anhedonia, abolition, social withdrawal), and mental deficiency (Georgiadou et al., 2014). The abnormalities in neurotransmitter systems including dopaminergic, cholinergic, glutamatergic, serotonergic, and the GABAergic system are involved in the pathogenesis of this disease (Georgiadou et al., 2014). Medicinal plants with the antipsychotic effect have been indicated useful in treating symptoms of schizophrenia (Pitsikas and Tarantilis, 2017). Crocin (16−31 mg/kg) ameliorates learning disorders caused via applying ketamine (3 mg/kg) in animals (Pitsikas and Tarantilis, 2017). Additionally, crocin (50 mg/kg) improves the psychotomimetic impact which is induced by ketamine (25 mg/kg) in the rat. Studies have also shown that crocin (50 mg/kg) improves the social isolation caused by ketamine (8 mg/kg) in rats (Pitsikas and Tarantilis, 2017). Crocin (15 and 30 mg/kg) administration is effective against apomorphine (1 mg/kg)-caused performance deficits in rats (Hosseinzadeh et al., 2008). The effect of crocin on the DAergic system may be effective against schizophrenia-like behavior (Hosseinzadeh et al., 2008). Clinical trial studies have also confirmed the efficacy and safety of crocin and saffron in treating schizophrenia (Mousavi et al., 2015). Administration of saffron or crocin (15 mg, twice daily) is fine and effective in the treatment of patients with schizophrenia (Mousavi et al., 2015).

Safranal administration decreases extracellular glutamate levels in the hippocampus of rats exposed to kainic acid (Berger et al., 2011). Saffron extracts prevent glutamatergic synaptic transmission in the cortical of rats (Ochiai et al., 2004b). The protective impact of crocin on schizophrenia is related to its antioxidant activities (Ghadrdoost et al., 2011; Papandreou et al., 2011). Saffron extracts and crocin have been shown to have protective effects versus spatial learning impairment and oxidative stress after long-term stress in the animal models (Bitanihirwe and Woo, 2011). Although schizophrenia pathogenesis is not clear, a close link between oxidative stress and schizophrenia has been indicated (de Oliveira et al., 2009). Subanesthetic concentrations of ketamine administration elevate oxidative damage, which is evident by an elevation in protein oxidation, lipid peroxidation, and a reduction in antioxidant enzymes in the animal model of schizophrenia (de Oliveira et al., 2009). It is supposed that the protective impact of crocin on ketamine-induced behavioral impairments is related to their antioxidant activities (de Oliveira et al., 2009).

Ischemia

Ischemia induces delayed and a selective death in neuronal cells (Bramlett and Dietrich, 2004). Inflammation, oxidative stress, and apoptosis are main mechanisms involved in the pathogenesis of cerebral ischemia (Bramlett and Dietrich, 2004). Flavonoids are effective agents to protect the brain in the ischemic condition and ameliorate behavioral alterations (Zhao et al., 2016; Sadeghnia et al., 2017). Safranal is an effective agent versus cerebral damages in the brain ischemia model in rats. Safranal (145 and 72.5 mg/kg) decreases total sulfhydryl content and increases thiobarbituric acid reactive substances (TBARS) as well as the TAS in the hippocampal tissue. The protective effects of safranal on ischemic reperfusion injury are mainly caused by decreasing free radicals generation in the rat (Ahmad et al., 2017). Administration of safranal mucoadhesive nanoemulsion has shown that safranal has a protective effect in the neurobehavioral function and enhances antioxidant capacity in the brain damage caused by brain ischemia-reperfusion in rats (Zheng et al., 2007). Crocin is able to protect against I-R injury—caused oxidative and nitrosative stress in the cerebral microvessels of the mice. Crocin reverses the elevated levels of MDA, NO synthase, and NO as well as reduced the activities of GPx and SOD in the cortical microvascular of mice (Sarshoori et al., 2014). Crocin reduces the extracellular signal—regulated kinase 1/2 ERK1/2 phosphorylation and the expression of matrix metalloproteinase (MMP)-9 as well as inhibits the translocation of G protein—coupled receptor kinase 2 from the cytosol to the membrane in the cortical microvessels (Sarshoori et al., 2014). Crocin (120, 60, 30, and 15 mg/kg) has a therapeutic impact on cerebral edema and ischemic reperfusion injury by reducing MDA level and elevating the activities of GPx and SOD in

the brain of rat model of stroke (Vakili et al., 2014). The therapeutic effects of crocin on the four-vessel occlusion ischemia have been confirmed (Vakili et al., 2014). Oral administration of 40 mg/kg/day of crocin for 10 days reduces caspase-3, hypoxia-inducible factor-1 alpha, and oxidative stress markers Terminal deoxynucleotidyl transferase dUTP nick end labeling (TUNEL)-positive cells in four-vessel occlusion ischemic rat model—induced brain damage (Samarghandian and Shabestari, 2013). The protective effect of crocin on blood-brain barrier (BBB) injury in aged rats after cerebral ischemia has also been found (Unterberg et al., 2004). Crocin ameliorates the loss of tight junction proteins and increases NADPH oxidase in the brains of rat model of traumatic brain injury (TBI) (Unterberg et al., 2004). Additionally, crocin decreases the MMP-2 and MMP-9 expressions in the aged rat model of ischemia (Unterberg et al., 2004). Indeed, crocin has a protective effect against cerebral ischemia by preserving the integrity of BBB in the aged rats via decreasing the activation of matrix metalloproteinase pathway (Unterberg et al., 2004).

Traumatic Injury
Brain injury
TBI after external force injuries on the brain is the important reason for mortality all over the world (Wang et al., 2015). After TBI, a series of biochemical changes including lipid peroxidation, free radical generation, and inflammation are caused that lead to neurological dysfunction (Wang et al., 2015). Studies have clearly shown the protective aspects of crocin on cerebral injury after TBI in mice (Rubin, 2014). The researchers have indicated that crocin (20 mg/kg) protects versus TBI by modulating brain edema and decreasing microglial activation, inflammatory mediators, as well as apoptosis (Rubin, 2014). Research has indicated that crocin shows a protective impact against TBI in mice through activation of Notch signaling (Rubin, 2014).

Spinal injury
A spinal cord injury (SCI) is a temporary or permanent damage to spinal cord (Sabapathy et al., 2015; Karami et al., 2013). The protective impact of crocin on chronic pain induced by SCI is related to a decrease in the levels of calcitonin-gene—related peptide and inflammatory cytokines [156]. Studies have shown that crocin (150 mg/kg) ameliorates locomotive, mechanical, and behavioral functions in the SCI rat model [156] (Table 9.1).

TABLE 9.1
Summary of Saffron Effects on Alzheimer's Disease, Anxiety, and Depression in Patients

First Author	Year of Publication	Subject	Intervention	Period	Effect
Akhondzadeh	2010	Patients with AD (mild-moderate)	Two capsule of saffron/day (containing 15 mg)	16 weeks	Improvement of AD
Akhondzadeh	2010	Patients with AD (mild-moderate symptoms)	Two capsule of saffron/day (15 mg/capsule)	22 weeks	Improvement of AD
Farokhnia	2014	Patients with AD (mild-moderate)	Capsule saffron 30 mg/day	12 months	Improvement of AD
Akhondzadeh	2004	Depressive patients (mild-moderate)	Capsule saffron 30 mg/day	6 weeks	Improvement of depression similar to imipramine
Akhondzadeh	2005	Depressive patients (severe)	Capsule saffron 30 mg/day	6 weeks	Improvement of depression
Noorbala	2005	Patients with major depression	Capsule saffron 30 mg/day	6 weeks	Improvement of depression similar to fluoxetine
Akhondzadeh Basti	2007	Depressive patients (severe)	2 capsule of saffron petal/day (15 mg/capsule)	8 weeks	Improvement of depression similar to fluoxetine
Shahmansouri	2014	Patients with mild to moderate depression	Capsule saffron 30 mg/day	3 & 6 weeks	Improvement of depression similar to fluoxetine
Mazidi	2016	Depressive and anxious patients	Capsule saffron 50 mg/day	12 weeks	Improvement of anxiety and depression
Kell	2017	Patients with low mood without depression	affron, a standardized stigmas extract from Crocus sativus 28 mg/kg	4 weeks	Improvement of mood, anxiety, and stress
Lopresti	2017	Patients with major depression	15 mg of saffron extract plus curcumin extract	3 months	Improvement of anxiety and depression
Ghajar	2017	Patients with major depression	Capsule saffron 30 mg/day	6 weeks	Improvement of depression
Milajerdi	2018	Diabetic patients with comorbid depression—anxiety	Saffron capsule contained 15 mg of saffron hydroalcoholic extracts	4 weeks	Improvement of moderate to mild comorbid depression—anxiety
Bangratz	2018	Depressive patients (mild-moderate)	One tablet /day containing saffron extract (15 mg) plus rhodiola extract (154 mg)	6 weeks	Improvement of depressive and anxious symptoms

REFERENCES

Ahmad, A.S., Ansari, M.A., Ahmad, M., Saleem, S., Yousuf, S., Hoda, M.N., Islam, F., 2005. Neuroprotection by crocetin in a hemi-parkinsonian rat model. Pharmacol. Biochem. Behav. 81 (4), 805–813.

Ahmad, N., Ahmad, R., Abbas Naqvi, A., Ashafaq, M., Alam, M.A., Ahmad, F.J., Al-Ghamdi, M.S., 2017. The effect of safranal loaded mucoadhesive nanoemulsion on oxidative stress markers in cerebral ischemia. Artif. Cells, Nanomed. Biotechnol. 45 (4), 775–787.

Ai, J., Dekermendjian, K., Wang, X., Nielsen, M., Witt, M.R., 1997. 6-Methylflavone, a benzodiazepine receptor ligand with antagonistic properties on rat brain and human recombinant GABAA receptors in vitro. Drug Dev. Res. 41 (2), 99–106.

Akhondzadeh Basti, A., Moshiri, E., Noorbala, A.A., Jamshidi, A.H., Abbasi, S.H., Akhondzadeh, S., 2007. Comparison of petal of Crocus sativus L. and fluoxetine in the treatment of depressed outpatients: a pilot double-blind randomized trial. Prog. Neuropsychopharmacol. Biol. Psychiatry 31, 439–442.

Akhondzadeh, S., Fallah-Pour, H., Afkham, K., Jamshidi, A.-H., Khalighi-Cigaroudi, F., 2004. Comparison of Crocus sativus L. and imipramine in the treatment of mild to moderate depression: a pilot double-blind randomized trial. BMC Complement. Altern. Med. 4, 1.

Akhondzadeh, S., Tahmacebi-Pour, N., Noorbala, A.A., Amini, H., Fallah-Pour, H., Jamshidi, A.H., Khani, M., 2005. Crocus sativus L. in the treatment of mild to moderate depression: a double-blind, randomized and placebo-controlled trial. Phytother Res. 19, 148–151.

Akhondzadeh, S., Sabet, M.S., Harirchian, M.H., Togha, M., Cheraghmakani, H., Razeghi, S., Zare, F., 2010. Saffron in the treatment of patients with mild to moderate Alzheimer's disease: a 16-week, randomized and placebo-controlled trial. J. Clin. Pharm. Ther. 35 (5), 581–588.

Akhondzadeh, S., Sabet, M.S., Harirchian, M.H., Togha, M., Cheraghmakani, H., Razeghi, S., Hejazi, S.S., Yousefi, M.H., Alimardani, R., Jamshidi, A., 2010. A 22-week, multicenter, randomized, double-blind controlled trial of Crocus sativus in the treatment of mild-to-moderate Alzheimer's disease. Psychopharmacology 207, 637643.

Alavi, M.S., Fanoudi, S., Fard, A.V., Soukhtanloo, M., Hosseini, M., Barzegar, H., Sadeghnia, H.R., 2018. Safranal Attenuates Excitotoxin-Induced Oxidative OLN-93 Cells Injury. Drug research.

Alhebshi, A.H., Gotoh, M., Suzuki, I., 2013. Thymoquinone protects cultured rat primary neurons against amyloid β-induced neurotoxicity. Biochem. Biophys. Res. Commun. 433 (4), 362–367.

Alinejad, S., Aaseth, J., Abdollahi, M., Hassanian-Moghaddam, H., Mehrpour, O., 2018. Clinical aspects of opium adulterated with lead in Iran: a review. Basic Clin. Pharmacol. Toxicol. 122 (1), 56–64.

Altinoz, E., Erdemli, M.E., Gul, M., Aksungur, Z., Gul, S., Bag, H.G., Turkoz, Y., 2018. Neuroprotection against CCl4 induced brain damage with crocin in Wistar rats. Biotech. Histochem. 93 (8), 623–631.

Amin, B., Hosseinzadeh, H., 2012. Evaluation of aqueous and ethanolic extracts of saffron, Crocus sativus L., and its constituents, safranal and crocin in allodynia and hyperalgesia induced by chronic constriction injury model of neuropathic pain in rats. Fitoterapia 83 (5), 888–895.

Bangratz, M., Abdellah, S.A., Berlin, A., Blondeau, C., Guilbot, A., Dubourdeaux, M., Lemoine, P., 2018. A preliminary assessment of a combination of rhodiola and saffron in the management of mild–moderate depression. Neuropsychiatr. Dis. Treat. 14, 1821.

Barnett, M.H., Prineas, J.W., 2004. Relapsing and remitting multiple sclerosis: pathology of the newly forming lesion. Ann. Neurol. 55 (4), 458–468.

Berger, F., Hensel, A., Nieber, K., 2011. Saffron extract and trans-crocetin inhibit glutamatergic synaptic transmission in rat cortical brain slices. Neuroscience 180, 238–247.

Bie, X., Chen, Y., Zheng, X., Dai, H., 2011. The role of crocetin in protection following cerebral contusion and in the enhancement of angiogenesis in rats. Fitoterapia 82 (7), 997–1002.

Bitanihirwe, B.K., Woo, T.U.W., 2011. Oxidative stress in schizophrenia: an integrated approach. Neurosci. Biobehav. Rev. 35 (3), 878–893.

Boskabady, M.H., Farkhondeh, T., 2016. Antiinflammatory, antioxidant, and immunomodulatory effects of Crocus sativus L. and its main constituents. Phytother Res. 30 (7), 1072–1094.

Bramlett, H.M., Dietrich, W.D., 2004. Pathophysiology of cerebral ischemia and brain trauma: similarities and differences. J. Cereb. Blood Flow Metab. 24 (2), 133–150.

Bussi, C., Ramos, J.M.P., Arroyo, D.S., Gaviglio, E.A., Gallea, J.I., Wang, J.M., Iribarren, P., 2017. Autophagy down regulates pro-inflammatory mediators in BV2 microglial cells and rescues both LPS and alpha-synuclein induced neuronal cell death. Sci. Rep. 7, 43153.

Caballero-Ortega, H., Pereda-Miranda, R., Abdullaev, F.I., 2007. HPLC quantification of major active components from 11 different saffron (Crocus sativus L.) sources. Food Chem. 100 (3), 1126–1131.

Christensen, T., 2005. Association of human endogenous retroviruses with multiple sclerosis and possible interactions with herpes viruses. Rev. Med. Virol. 15 (3), 179–211.

Cirmi, S., Ferlazzo, N., Lombardo, G., Ventura-Spagnolo, E., Gangemi, S., Calapai, G., Navarra, M., 2016. Neurodegenerative diseases: might citrus flavonoids play a protective role? Molecules 21 (10), 1312.

Costa, S.L., Silva, V.D.A., dos Santos Souza, C., Santos, C.C., Paris, I., Munoz, P., Segura-Aguilar, J., 2016. Impact of plant-derived flavonoids on neurodegenerative diseases. Neurotox. Res. 30 (1), 41–52.

Cryan, J.F., Sweeney, F.F., 2011. The age of anxiety: role of animal models of anxiolytic action in drug discovery. Br. J. Pharmacol. 164 (4), 1129–1161.

de Oliveira, L., Spiazzi, C.M.D.S., Bortolin, T., Canever, L., Petronilho, F., Mina, F.G., Zugno, A.I., 2009. Different sub-anesthetic doses of ketamine increase oxidative stress in the brain of rats. Prog. Neuropsychopharmacol. Biol. Psychiatry 33 (6), 1003–1008.

Delkhosh-Kasmaie, F., Farshid, A.A., Tamaddonfard, E., Imani, M., 2018. The effects of safranal, a constitute of saffron, and metformin on spatial learning and memory impairments in type-1 diabetic rats: behavioral and hippocampal histopathological and biochemical evaluations. Biomed. Pharmacother. 107, 203–211.

Deslauriers, A.M., Afkhami-Goli, A., Paul, A.M., Bhat, R.K., Acharjee, S., Ellestad, K.K., Power, C., 2011. Neuroinflammation and endoplasmic reticulum stress are coregulated by crocin to prevent demyelination and neurodegeneration. J. Immunol. 187 (9), 4788–4799.

EbrahimHabibi, M.B., Amininasab, M., Ebrahim-Habibi, A., Sabbaghian, M., Nemat-Gorgani, M., 2010. Fibrillation of α-lactalbumin: effect of crocin and safranal, two natural small molecules from Crocus sativus. Biopolymers 93 (10), 854–865.

Ettehadi, H., Mojabi, S.N., Ranjbaran, M., Shams, J., Sahraei, H., Hedayati, M., Asefi, F., 2013. Aqueous extract of saffron (Crocus sativus) increases brain dopamine and glutamate concentrations in rats. J. Behav. Brain Sci. 3, 315–319.

Farahmand, S.K., Samini, F., Samini, M., Samarghandian, S., 2013. Safranal ameliorates antioxidant enzymes and suppresses lipid peroxidation and nitric oxide formation in aged male rat liver. Biogerontology 14 (1), 63–71.

Farkhondeh, T., Samarghandian, S., Samini, F., 2016. Antidotal effects of curcumin against neurotoxic agents: an updated review. Asian Pac. J. Trop. Biomed. 9 (10), 947–953.

Farkhondeh, T., Samarghandian, S., Samini, F., Sanati, A.R., 2018. Protective effects of crocetin on depression-like behavior induced by immobilization in rat. CNS Neurol. Disord. Drug Targets 17 (5), 361–369.

Farkhondeh, T., Samarghandian, S., Pourbagher-Shahri, A.M., 2019. Hypolipidemic effects of Rosmarinus officinalis L. J. Cell. Physiol. 234 (9), 14680–14688.

Farokhnia, M., ShafieeSabet, M., Iranpour, N., Gougol, A., Yekehtaz, H., Alimardani, R., Akhondzadeh, S., 2014. Comparing the efficacy and safety of Crocus sativus L. with memantine in patients with moderate to severe Alzheimer's disease: a double-blind randomized clinical trial. Hum. Psychopharmacol. Clin. Exp. 29 (4), 351–359.

Fathimoghadam, H., Farbod, Y., Ghadiri, A., Fatemi, R., 2019. Moderating effects of crocin on some stress oxidative markers in rat brain following demyelination with ethidium bromide. Heliyon 5 (2), e01213.

Forchetti, C.M., 2005. Treating patients with moderate to severe Alzheimer's disease: implications of recent pharmacologic studies. Prim. Care Companion J. Clin. Psychiatry 7 (4), 155.

Georgiadou, G., Grivas, V., Tarantilis, P.A., Pitsikas, N., 2014. Crocins, the active constituents of Crocus sativus L., counteracted ketamine–induced behavioural deficits in rats. Psychopharmacology 231 (4), 717–726.

Geromichalos, G.D., Lamari, F.N., Papandreou, M.A., Trafalis, D.T., Margarity, M., Papageorgiou, A., Sinakos, Z., 2012. Saffron as a source of novel acetylcholinesterase inhibitors: molecular docking and in vitro enzymatic studies. J. Agric. Food Chem. 60 (24), 6131–6138.

Ghadami, M.R., Pourmotabbed, A., 2009. The effect of Crocin on scopolamine induced spatial learning and memory deficits in rats. Physiol. Pharmacol. 12 (4), 287–295.

Ghaderi, A., Vahdati-Mashhadian, N., Oghabian, Z., Moradi, V., Afshari, R., Mehrpour, O., 2015. Thallium exists in opioid poisoned patients. Daru 23 (1), 39.

Ghadrdoost, B., Vafaei, A.A., Rashidy-Pour, A., Hajisoltani, R., Bandegi, A.R., Motamedi, F., Pahlvan, S., 2011. Protective effects of saffron extract and its active constituent crocin against oxidative stress and spatial learning and memory deficits induced by chronic stress in rats. Eur. J. Pharmacol. 667 (1–3), 222–229.

Ghajar, A., Neishabouri, S.M., Velayati, N., Jahangard, L., Matinnia, N., Haghighi, M., Akhondzadeh, S., 2017. Crocus sativus L. versus citalopram in the treatment of major depressive disorder with anxious distress: a double-blind, controlled clinical trial. Pharmacopsychiatry 50 (04), 152–160.

Ghalandari-Shamami, M., Nourizade, S., Yousefi, B., Vafaei, A.A., Pakdel, R., Rashidy-Pour, A., 2019. Beneficial effects of physical activity and crocin against adolescent stress induced anxiety or depressive-like symptoms and dendritic morphology remodeling in prefrontal cortex in adult male rats. Neurochem. Res. 1–13.

Ghazavi, A., Mosayebi, G., Salehi, H., Abtahi, H., 2009. Effect of ethanol extract of saffron (Crocus sativus L.) on the inhibition of experimental autoimmune encephalomyelitis in C57bl/6 mice. Pak. J. Biol. Sci. 12 (9), 690–695.

Ghoshooni, H., Daryaafzoon, M., Sadeghi-Gharjehdagi, S., Zardooz, H., Sahraei, H., Tehrani, S.P., Sadraei, S.H., 2011. Saffron (Crocus sativus) ethanolic extract and its constituent, safranal, inhibits morphine-induced place preference in mice. Pak. J. Biol. Sci. 14 (20), 939–944.

Gilgun-Sherki, Y., Melamed, E., Offen, D., 2004. The role of oxidative stress in the pathogenesis of multiple sclerosis: the need for effective antioxidant therapy. J. Neurol. 251 (3), 261–268.

Hadipour, M., Kaka, G., Bahrami, F., Meftahi, G.H., Pirzad Jahromi, G., Mohammadi, A., Sahraei, H., 2018. Crocin improved amyloid beta induced long-term potentiation and memory deficits in the hippocampal CA1 neurons in freely moving rats. Synapse 72 (5), e22026.

Haghighizad, H., Pourmotabbed, A., Sahraei, H., Ghadami, M.R., Ghadami, S., Kamalinejad, M., 2008. Protective effect of Saffron extract on morphine–induced inhibition of spatial learning and memory in rat. Physiol. Pharmacol. 12 (3), 170–179.

Halataei, B.A.S., Khosravi, M., Arbabian, S., Sahraei, H., Golmanesh, L., Zardooz, H., Ghoshooni, H., 2011. Saffron (Crocus sativus) aqueous extract and its constituent crocin reduces stress-induced anorexia in mice. Phytother. Res. 25 (12), 1833–1838.

Hamner, M.B., Robert, S., Frueh, B.C., 2004. Treatment-resistant posttraumatic stress disorder: strategies for intervention. CNS Spectrums 9 (10), 740–752.

Hashtjini, M.M., Jahromi, G.P., Meftahi, G.H., 2018. Aqueous extract of saffron administration along with amygdala deep brain stimulation promoted alleviation of symptoms in post-traumatic stress disorder (PTSD) in rats. Avicenna J. Phytomed. 8 (4), 358.

Heidari, S., Mehri, S., Shariaty, V., Hosseinzadeh, H., 2018. Preventive effects of crocin on neuronal damages induced by D-galactose through ages and oxidative stress in human neuroblastoma cells (SH-SY5Y). J. Pharmacopuncture 21 (1), 18.

Hemmati, M., Zohoori, E., Mehrpour, O., Karamian, M., Asghari, S., Zarban, A., Nasouti, R., 2015. Anti-atherogenic potential of jujube, saffron and barberry: anti-diabetic and antioxidant actions. EXCLI J. 14, 908.

Hosseinzadeh, H., Jahanian, Z., 2010. Effect of Crocus sativus L.(saffron) stigma and its constituents, crocin and safranal, on morphine withdrawal syndrome in mice. Phytother. Res. 24 (5), 726–730.

Hosseinzadeh, H., Noraei, N.B., 2009. Anxiolytic and hypnotic effect of Crocus sativus aqueous extract and its constituents, crocin and safranal, in mice. Phytother. Res. 23 (6), 768–774.

Hosseinzadeh, H., Sadeghnia, H.R., 2005. Safranal, a constituent of Crocus sativus (saffron), attenuated cerebral ischemia induced oxidative damage in rat hippocampus. J. Pharm. Pharm. Sci. 8 (3), 394–399.

Hosseinzadeh, H., Sadeghnia, H.R., 2007. Protective effect of safranal on pentylenetetrazol-induced seizures in the rat: involvement of GABAergic and opioids systems. Phytomedicine 14 (4), 256–262.

Hosseinzadeh, H., Talebzadeh, F., 2005. Anticonvulsant evaluation of safranal and crocin from Crocus sativus in mice. Fitoterapia 76 (7–8), 722–724.

Hosseinzadeh, H., Karimi, G., Niapoor, M., 2003. Antidepressant effect of Crocus sativus L. stigma extracts and their constituents, crocin and safranal, in mice. In: I International Symposium on Saffron Biology and Biotechnology, vol. 650, pp. 435–445.

Hosseinzadeh, H., Sadeghnia, H.R., Rahimi, A., 2008. Effect of safranal on extracellular hippocampal levels of glutamate and aspartate during kainic acid treatment in anesthetized rats. Planta Med. 74 (12), 1441–1445.

Hsiung, G.Y.R., Feldman, H.H., 2008. Pharmacological treatment in moderate-to-severe Alzheimer's disease. Expert Opin. Pharmacother. 9 (15), 2575–2582.

IA, J., 2011. Inhibition of pain and inflamation induced by formalin in male mice by ethanolic extract of saffron (crocus sativus) and its constituents; crocin and safranal. Kowsar Med. J. 15 (4), 189–195.

Imenshahidi, M., Zafari, H., Hosseinzadeh, H., 2011. Effects of crocin on the acquisition and reinstatement of morphine-induced conditioned place preference in mice. Pharmacologyonline 1, 1007–1013.

Karami, M., Bathaie, S.Z., Tiraihi, T., Habibi-Rezaei, M., Arabkheradmand, J., Faghihzadeh, S., 2013. Crocin improved locomotor function and mechanical behavior in the rat model of contused spinal cord injury through decreasing calcitonin gene related peptide (CGRP). Phytomedicine 21 (1), 62–67.

Karimi, G.R., Hosseinzadeh, H., Khalegh, P.P., 2001. Study of antidepressant effect of aqueous and ethanolic extract of Crocus sativus in mice. Iran. J. Basic Med. Sci. 4, 11–15.

Kell, G., Rao, A., Beccaria, G., Clayton, P., Inarejos-García, A.M., Prodanov, M., 2017. Saffron a novel saffron extract (Crocus sativus L.) improves mood in healthy adults over 4 weeks in a double-blind, parallel, randomized, placebo-controlled clinical trial. Complement. Ther. Med. 33, 58–64.

Khalili, M., Hamzeh, F., 2010. Effects of active constituents of Crocus sativus L., crocin on streptozocin-induced model of sporadic Alzheimer's disease in male rats. Iran. Biomed. J. 14 (1–2), 59.

Khosravan, V., 2002. Anticonvulsant effects of aqueous and ethanolic extracts of Crocus sativus L. stigmas in mice. Arch. Iran. Med. 5, 44.

Labak, M., Foniok, T., Kirk, D., Rushforth, D., Tomanek, B., Jasiński, A., Grieb, P., 2010. Metabolic changes in rat brain following intracerebroventricular injections of streptozotocin: a model of sporadic Alzheimer's disease. In: Brain Edema XIV. Springer, Vienna, pp. 177–181.

Lechtenberg, M., Schepmann, D., Niehues, M., Hellenbrand, N., Wünsch, B., Hensel, A., 2008. Quality and functionality of saffron: quality control, species assortment and affinity of extract and isolated saffron compounds to NMDA and σ1 (sigma-1) receptors. Planta Medica 74 (07), 764–772.

Li, D.C., Bao, X.Q., Wang, X.L., Sun, H., Zhang, D., 2017. A novel synthetic derivative of squamosamide FLZ inhibits the high mobility group box 1 protein-mediated neuroinflammatory responses in murine BV2 microglial cells. Naunyn-Schmiedeberg's Arch. Pharmacol. 390 (6), 643–650.

Li Puma, S., Landini, L., Macedo Jr., S.J., Seravalli, V., Marone, I.M., Coppi, E., De Logu, F., 2019. TRPA 1 mediates the antinociceptive properties of the constituent of Crocus sativus L., safranal. J. Cell Mol. Med. 23 (3), 1976–1986.

Lieberman, J.A., Stroup, T.S., McEvoy, J.P., Swartz, M.S., Rosenheck, R.A., Perkins, D.O., Severe, J., 2005. Effectiveness of antipsychotic drugs in patients with chronic schizophrenia. N. Engl. J. Med. 353 (12), 1209–1223.

Linardaki, Z.I., Orkoula, M.G., Kokkosis, A.G., Lamari, F.N., Margarity, M., 2013. Investigation of the neuroprotective action of saffron (Crocus sativus L.) in aluminum-exposed adult mice through behavioral and neurobiochemical assessment. Food Chem. Toxicol. 52, 163–170.

Liu, J., Wang, A., Li, L., Huang, Y., Xue, P., Hao, A., 2010. Oxidative stress mediates hippocampal neuron death in rats after lithium–pilocarpine-induced status epilepticus. Seizure 19 (3), 165–172.

Lopresti, A.L., Drummond, P.D., 2017. Efficacy of curcumin, and a saffron/curcumin combination for the treatment of major depression: a randomised, double-blind, placebo-controlled study. J. Affect. Disord. 207, 188–196.

Lv, B., Huo, F., Zhu, Z., Xu, Z., Dang, X., Chen, T., Yang, X., 2016. Crocin upregulates CX3CR1 expression by suppressing NF-κB/YY1 signaling and inhibiting lipopolysaccharide-induced microglial activation. Neurochem. Res. 41 (8), 1949–1957.

Marciniak, S.J., Yun, C.Y., Oyadomari, S., Novoa, I., Zhang, Y., Jungreis, R., Ron, D., 2004. Chop induces death by promoting protein synthesis and oxidation in the stressed endoplasmic reticulum. Genes Dev. 18 (24), 3066–3077.

Marder, M., Estiú, G., Blanch, L.B., Viola, H., Wasowski, C., Medina, J.H., Paladini, A.C., 2001. Molecular modeling and QSAR analysis of the interaction of flavone derivatives with the benzodiazepine binding site of the GABAA receptor complex. Bioorg. Med. Chem. 9 (2), 323–335.

Mazidi, M., Shemshian, M., Mousavi, S.H., Norouzy, A., Kermani, T., Moghiman, T., Ferns, G.A., 2016. A double-blind, randomized and placebo-controlled trial of Saffron (Crocus sativus L.) in the treatment of anxiety and depression. J. Complement. Integr. Med. 13 (2), 195–199.

Mehrpour, O., Karrari, P., Abdollahi, M., 2012. Chronic Lead Poisoning in Iran; a Silent Disease.

Mehrpour, O., Abdollahi, M., Sharifi, M.D., 2014. Oxidative stress and hyperglycemia in aluminum phosphide poisoning. J. Res. Med. Sci. 19 (2), 196.

Menghini, L., Leporini, L., Vecchiotti, G., Locatelli, M., Carradori, S., Ferrante, C., Brunetti, L., 2018. Crocus sativus L. stigmas and byproducts: qualitative fingerprint, antioxidant potentials and enzyme inhibitory activities. Food Res. Int. 109, 91–98.

Milajerdi, A., Jazayeri, S., Shirzadi, E., Hashemzadeh, N., Azizgol, A., Djazayery, A., Akhondzadeh, S., 2018. The effects of alcoholic extract of saffron (Crocus satious L.) on mild to moderate comorbid depression-anxiety, sleep quality, and life satisfaction in type 2 diabetes mellitus: a double-blind, randomized and placebo-controlled clinical trial. Complement. Ther. Med. 41, 196–202.

Miller, D.B., O'Callaghan, J.P., 2002. Neuroendocrine aspects of the response to stress. Metab. Clin. Exp. 51 (6), 5–10.

Moallem, S.A., Hariri, A.T., Mahmoudi, M., Hosseinzadeh, H., 2014. Effect of aqueous extract of Crocus sativus L.(saffron) stigma against subacute effect of diazinon on specific biomarkers in rats. Toxicol. Ind. Health 30 (2), 141–146.

Mohammadzadeh, L., Hosseinzadeh, H., Abnous, K., Razavi, B.M., 2018. Neuroprotective potential of crocin against malathion-induced motor deficit and neurochemical alterations in rats. Environ. Sci. Pollut. Control Ser. 25 (5), 4904–4914.

Mohammadzadeh, L., Abnous, K., Razavi, B.M., Hosseinzadeh, H., 2019. Crocin-protected malathion-induced spatial memory deficits by inhibiting TAU protein hyperphosphorylation and antiapoptotic effects. Nutr. Neurosci. 1–16.

Motaghinejad, M., Safari, S., Feizipour, S., Sadr, S., 2019. Crocin may be useful to prevent or treatment of alcohol induced neurodegeneration and neurobehavioral sequels via modulation of CREB/BDNF and Akt/GSK signaling pathway. Med. Hypotheses 124, 21–25.

Mousavi, B., Bathaie, S.Z., Fadai, F., Ashtari, Z., 2015. Safety evaluation of saffron stigma (Crocus sativus L.) aqueous extract and crocin in patients with schizophrenia. Avicenna J. Phytomed. 5 (5), 413.

Naghibi, S.M., Hosseini, M., Khani, F., Rahimi, M., Vafaee, F., Rakhshandeh, H., Aghaie, A., 2012. Effect of aqueous extract of Crocus sativus L. on morphine-induced memory impairment. Adv. Pharmacol. Sci. 2012.

Nam, K.N., Park, Y.M., Jung, H.J., Lee, J.Y., Min, B.D., Park, S.U., Hong, J.W., 2010. Anti-inflammatory effects of crocin and crocetin in rat brain microglial cells. Eur. J. Pharmacol. 648 (1–3), 110–116.

Neuroinflammation, oxida- tive stress, and the pathogenesis of Parkinson's disease Haeri, P., Mohammadipour, A., Heidari, Z., Ebrahimzadeh-bideskan, A., 2019. Neuroprotective effect of crocin on substantia nigra in MPTP-induced Parkinson's disease model of mice. Anat. Sci. Int. 94 (1), 119–127.

Noorbala, A., Akhondzadeh, S., Tahmacebi-Pour, N., Jamshidi, A., 2005. Hydro-alcoholic extract of Crocus sativus L. versus fluoxetine in the treatment of mild to moderate depression: a double-blind, randomized pilot trial. J. Ethnopharmacol. 97, 281–284.

Ochiai, T., Ohno, S., Soeda, S., Tanaka, H., Shoyama, Y., Shimeno, H., 2004. Crocin prevents the death of rat pheochromyctoma (PC-12) cells by its antioxidant effects stronger than those of α-tocopherol. Neurosci. Lett. 362 (1), 61–64.

Ochiai, T., Soeda, S., Ohno, S., Tanaka, H., Shoyama, Y., Shimeno, H., 2004. Crocin prevents the death of PC-12 cells through sphingomyelinase-ceramide signaling by increasing glutathione synthesis. Neurochem. Int. 44 (5), 321–330.

Papandreou, M.A., Kanakis, C.D., Polissiou, M.G., Efthimiopoulos, S., Cordopatis, P., Margarity, M., Lamari, F.N., 2006. Inhibitory activity on amyloid-β aggregation and antioxidant properties of Crocus sativus stigmas extract and its crocin constituents. J. Agric. Food Chem. 54 (23), 8762–8768.

Papandreou, M.A., Tsachaki, M., Efthimiopoulos, S., Cordopatis, P., Lamari, F.N., Margarity, M., 2011. Memory enhancing effects of saffron in aged mice are correlated with antioxidant protection. Behav. Brain Res. 219 (2), 197–204.

Pitsikas, N., 2015. The effect of Crocus sativus L. and its constituents on memory: basic studies and clinical applications. Evid. Based Complement Altern. Med. 2015.

Pitsikas, N., Sakellaridis, N., 2006. Crocus sativus L. extracts antagonize memory impairments in different behavioural tasks in the rat. Behav. Brain Res. 173 (1), 112–115.

Pitsikas, N., Tarantilis, P.A., 2017. Crocins, the active constituents of Crocus sativus L., counteracted apomorphine-induced performance deficits in the novel object recognition task, but not novel object location task, in rats. Neurosci. Lett. 644, 37–42.

Pitsikas, N., Zisopoulou, S., Tarantilis, P.A., Kanakis, C.D., Polissiou, M.G., Sakellaridis, N., 2007. Effects of the active constituents of Crocus sativus L., crocins on recognition and spatial rats' memory. Behav. Brain Res. 183 (2), 141–146.

Pitsikas, N., Boultadakis, A., Georgiadou, G., Tarantilis, P.A., Sakellaridis, N., 2008. Effects of the active constituents of *Crocus sativus* L., crocins, in an animal model of anxiety. Phytomedicine 15 (12), 1135−1139.

Qi, Y., Chen, L., Zhang, L., Liu, W.B., Chen, X.Y., Yang, X.G., 2013. Crocin prevents retinal ischaemia/reperfusion injury-induced apoptosis in retinal ganglion cells through the PI3K/AKT signalling pathway. Exp. Eye Res. 107, 44−51.

Rafieipour, F., Hadipour, E., Emami, S.A., Asili, J., Tayarani-Najaran, Z., 2019. Safranal protects against beta-amyloid peptide-induced cell toxicity in PC12 cells via MAPK and PI3 K pathways. Metab. Brain Dis. 34 (1), 165−172.

Rahiman, N., Akaberi, M., Sahebkar, A., Emami, S.A., Tayarani-Najaran, Z., 2018. Protective effects of saffron and its active components against oxidative stress and apoptosis in endothelial cells. Microvasc. Res. 118, 82−89.

Rubin, M., October 2014. Overview of Spinal Cord Disorders. Merck Manuel, Retrieved.

Sabapathy, V., Tharion, G., Kumar, S., 2015. Cell therapy augments functional recovery subsequent to spinal cord injury under experimental conditions. Stem Cells Int. 2015, 132172.

Sadeghnia, H., Cortez, M., Liu, D., Hosseinzadeh, H., Snead, O.C., 2008. Antiabsence effects of safranal in acute experimental seizure models: EEG and autoradiography. J. Pharm. Pharm. Sci. 11 (3), 1−14.

Sadeghnia, H.R., Kamkar, M., Assadpour, E., Boroushaki, M.T., Ghorbani, A., 2013. Protective effect of safranal, a constituent of *Crocus sativus*, on quinolinic acid-induced oxidative damage in rat hippocampus. Iran. J. Basic Med. Sci. 16 (1), 73.

Sadeghnia, H.R., Shaterzadeh, H., Forouzanfar, F., Hosseinzadeh, H., 2017. Neuroprotective effect of safranal, an active ingredient of *Crocus sativus*, in a rat model of transient cerebral ischemia. Folia Neuropathol. 55 (3), 206−213.

Saleem, S., Ahmad, M., Ahmad, A.S., Yousuf, S., Ansari, M.A., Khan, M.B., Islam, F., 2006. Effect of saffron (*Crocus sativus*) on neurobehavioral and neurochemical changes in cerebral ischemia in rats. J. Med. Food 9 (2), 246−253.

Samarghandian, S., Borji, A., 2014. Anticarcinogenic effect of saffron (*Crocus sativus* L.) and its ingredients. Pharmacogn. Res. 6 (2), 99.

Samarghandian, S., Shabestari, M.M., 2013. DNA fragmentation and apoptosis induced by safranal in human prostate cancer cell line. Indian J. Urol. 29 (3), 177.

Samarghandian, S., Borji, A., Delkhosh, M.B., Samini, F., 2013. Safranal treatment improves hyperglycemia, hyperlipidemia and oxidative stress in streptozotocin-induced diabetic rats. J. Pharm. Pharm. Sci. 16 (2), 352−362.

Samarghandian, S., Shoshtari, M.E., Sargolzaei, J., Hossinimoghadam, H., Farahzad, J.A., 2014. Anti-tumor activity of safranal against neuroblastoma cells. Pharmacogn. Mag. 10 (Suppl. 2), S419.

Samarghandian, S., Azimi-Nezhad, M., Samini, F., 2015. Preventive effect of safranal against oxidative damage in aged male rat brain. Exp. Anim. 64 (1), 65−71.

Samarghandian, S., Azimi-Nezhad, M., Borji, A., Farkhondeh, T., 2016. Effect of crocin on aged rat kidney through inhibition of oxidative stress and proinflammatory state. Phytother Res. 30 (8), 1345−1353.

Samarghandian, S., Azimi-Nezhad, M., Borji, A., Farkhondeh, T., 2016. *Crocus sativus* L.(saffron) extract reduces the extent of oxidative stress and proinflammatory state in aged rat kidney. Prog. Nutr. 18 (3), 299−310.

Samarghandian, S., Azimi-Nezhad, M., Samini, F., Farkhondeh, T., 2016. The role of saffron in attenuating age-related oxidative damage in rat hippocampus. Recent Pat. Food, Nutr. Agric. 8 (3), 183−189.

Samarghandian, S., Samini, F., Azimi-Nezhad, M., Farkhondeh, T., 2017. Anti-oxidative effects of safranal on immobilization-induced oxidative damage in rat brain. Neurosci. Lett. 659, 26−32.

Samini, F., Samarghandian, S., Borji, A., Mohammadi, G., 2013. Curcumin pretreatment attenuates brain lesion size and improves neurological function following traumatic brain injury in the rat. Pharmacol. Biochem. Behav. 110, 238−244.

Sarshoori, J.R., Asadi, M.H., Mohammadi, M.T., 2014. Neuroprotective effects of crocin on the histopathological alterations following brain ischemia-reperfusion injury in rat. Iran. J. Basic Med. Sci. 17 (11), 895.

Shahmansouri, N., Farokhnia, M., Abbasi, S.-H., Kassaian, S.E., Noorbala Tafti, A.-A., Gougol, A., Yekehtaz, H., Forghani, S., Mahmoodian, M., Saroukhani, S., 2014. A randomized, double-blind, clinical trial comparing the efficacy and safety of Crocus sativus L. with fluoxetine for improving mild to moderate depression in post percutaneous coronary intervention patients. J. Affect. Disord. 155, 216−222.

Shati, A.A., Elsaid, F.G., Hafez, E.E., 2011. Biochemical and molecular aspects of aluminium chloride-induced neurotoxicity in mice and the protective role of *Crocus sativus* L. extraction and honey syrup. Neuroscience 175, 66−74.

Soeda, S., Ochiai, T., Paopong, L., Tanaka, H., Shoyama, Y., Shimeno, H., 2001. Crocin suppresses tumor necrosis factor-α-induced cell death of neuronally differentiated PC-12 cells. Life Sciences 69 (24), 2887−2898.

Sugiura, M., Shoyama, Y., Saito, H., Nishiyama, N., 1995. Crocin improves the ethanol-induced impairment of learning behaviors of mice in passive avoidance tasks. Proc. Jap. Acad. B 71 (10), 319−324.

Sunanda, B.P.V., Rammohan, B., Kumar, A., Kudagi, B.L., 2014. The effective study of aqueous extract of crocus sativus linn in chemical induced convulsants in rats. World J. Pharm. Pharm. Sci. 3 (3), 1175−1182.

Tamaddonfard, E., Gooshchi, N.H., Seiednejad-Yamchi, S., 2012. Central effect of crocin on penicillin-induced epileptiform activity in rats. Pharmacol. Rep. 64 (1), 94−101.

Tsantarliotou, M.P., Poutahidis, T., Markala, D., Kazakos, G., Sapanidou, V., Lavrentiadou, S., Sinakos, Z., 2013. Crocetin administration ameliorates endotoxin-induced disseminated intravascular coagulation in rabbits. Blood Coagul. Fibrinolysis 24 (3), 305−310.

Unterberg, A.W., Stover, J., Kress, B., Kiening, K.L., 2004. Edema and brain trauma. Neuroscience 129 (4), 1019–1027.

Vakili, A., Einali, M.R., Bandegi, A.R., 2014. Protective effect of crocin against cerebral ischemia in a dose-dependent manner in a rat model of ischemic stroke. J. Stroke Cerebrovasc. Dis. 23 (1), 106–113.

Van Ameringen, M., Mancini, C., Pipe, B., Bennett, M., 2004. Optimizing treatment in social phobia: a review of treatment resistance. CNS Spectrums 9 (10), 753–762.

Venda, L.L., Cragg, S.J., Buchman, V.L., Wade-Martins, R., 2010. α-Synuclein and dopamine at the crossroads of Parkinson's disease. Trends Neurosci. 33 (12), 559–568.

Wang, K., Zhang, L., Rao, W., Su, N., Hui, H., Wang, L., Fei, Z., 2015. Neuroprotective effects of crocin against traumatic brain injury in mice: involvement of notch signaling pathway. Neurosci. Lett. 591, 53–58.

Wang, X., Zhang, G., Qiao, Y., Feng, C., Zhao, X., 2017. Crocetin attenuates spared nerve injury-induced neuropathic pain in mice. J. Pharmacol. Sci. 135 (4), 141–147.

Wang, C., Cai, X., Hu, W., Li, Z., Kong, F., Chen, X., Wang, D., 2019. Investigation of the neuroprotective effects of crocin via antioxidant activities in HT22 cells and in mice with Alzheimer's disease. Int. J. Mol. Med. 43 (2), 956–966.

Xiting, W.A.N.G., Oufeng, T.A.N.G., Yilu, Y.E., Mingzhi, Z.H.E.N.G., Jue, H.U., Zhong, C.H.E.N., Kai, Z.H.O.N.G., 2017. Effects of crocin on hippocampus rapid kindling epilepsy in mice. J. Zhejiang Univ. 46 (1), 7–14.

Yamauchi, M., Tsuruma, K., Imai, S., Nakanishi, T., Umigai, N., Shimazawa, M., Hara, H., 2011. Crocetin prevents retinal degeneration induced by oxidative and endoplasmic reticulum stresses via inhibition of caspase activity. Eur. J. Pharmacol. 650 (1), 110–119.

Yaribeygi, H., Sahraei, H., Mohammadi, A.R., Meftahi, G.H., 2014. Saffron (Crocus sativus L.) and morphine dependence: a systematic review article. Am. J. Biol. Life Sci. 2 (2), 41–45.

Zarrindast, M.R., Jafari-Sabet, M., Rezayat, M., Djahanguiri, B., Rezayof, A., 2006. Involvement of nmda receptors in morphine state–dependent learning in mice. Int. J. Neurosci. 116 (6), 731–743.

Zhang, Y., Shoyama, Y., Sugiura, M., Saito, H., 1994. Effects of Crocus sativus L. on the ethanol-induced impairment of passive avoidance performances in mice. Biol. Pharm. Bull. 17 (2), 217–221.

Zhang, L., Previn, R., Lu, L., Liao, R.F., Jin, Y., Wang, R.K., 2018. Crocin, a natural product attenuates lipopolysaccharide-induced anxiety and depressive-like behaviors through suppressing NF-kB and NLRP3 signaling pathway. Brain Research Bulletin 142, 352–359.

Zhao, S., Gao, X., Dong, W., Chen, J., 2016. The role of 7, 8-dihydroxyflavone in preventing dendrite degeneration in cortex after moderate traumatic brain injury. Mol. Neurobiol. 53 (3), 1884–1895.

Zheng, Y.Q., Liu, J.X., Wang, J.N., Xu, L., 2007. Effects of crocin on reperfusion-induced oxidative/nitrative injury to cerebral microvessels after global cerebral ischemia. Brain Research 1138, 86–94.

FURTHER READING

Akhondian, J., Kianifar, H., Raoofziaee, M., Moayedpour, A., Toosi, M.B., Khajedaluee, M., 2011. The effect of thymoquinone on intractable pediatric seizures (pilot study). Epilepsy Research 93 (1), 39–43.

CHAPTER 10

Therapeutic Benefits of Saffron in Brain Diseases: New Lights on Possible Pharmacological Mechanisms

BHUPESH SHARMA • HARIOM KUMAR • PRACHI KAUSHIK • ROOHI MIRZA • RAJENDRA AWASTHI • G.T. KULKARNI

INTRODUCTION

Saffron belongs to the family Iridaceae and is majorly cultivated in Central Asia, China, India, Turkey, Iran, Algeria, and Europe. Saffron is derived from the flower of *Crocus sativus*. Saffron has about 150 chemical components in stigmas, which include minerals, sugars, vitamins, fats, and various secondary metabolites such as anthocyanins, terpenes, carotenoids, and flavonoids. Crocins are trans-crocetin (β-D-glucosyl)-(β-D-gentiobiosyl) ester (named trans-3-Gg), trans-crocetin di-(β-D-glucosyl) ester (named trans-2-gg), trans-crocetin di-(β-D-gentiobiosyl) ester (named trans-4-GG), trans-crocetin (β-D-gentiobiosyl) ester (named trans-2-G), cis-crocetin (β-D-glucosyl)-(β-D-gentiobiosyl) ester (named cis-3-Gg), and cis-crocetin di-(β-D-gentiobiosyl) ester (named cis-4-GG) (Gismondi, 2012).

Saffron has a brick red color because of crocetin having a 285°C of melting point and crocin with a melting point of 186°C (Bolhasani et al., 2005; Dar et al., 2012). Saffron has many applications because of its main active constituents such as safranal, picrocrocin, and crocin. Saffron' color is generally because of the glycoside carotenoid structure of crocin (Mohamadpour et al., 2013). Picrocrocin is responsible for the bitter taste of saffron (Javadi et al., 2013; Mohamadpour et al., 2013). Zeaxanthin carotenoid and monoterpene glycoside precursors of safranal degrades to produce picrocrocin (Bolhasani et al., 2005). Safranal is an aromatic aldehyde, which is the main component of plant volatile oil (Javadi et al., 2013). Safranal contains about 70% of volatiles from flowers of saffron. The extracts of *C. sativus* can also synthesize dimethyl crocetin (DMC) and many more.

ROLE OF SAFFRON IN THE TREATMENT OF BRAIN CONDITIONS

Saffron and its active moieties have been tested for their therapeutic benefits in different brain conditions such as Alzheimer's disease (Adalier and Parker, 2016; Finley and GAO, 2017), Parkinson's disease (Rao et al., 2016; Pan et al., 2016), depression, cerebral ischemia (Sadeghnia et al., 2017), vascular dementia, posttraumatic stress disorder (MokhtariHasht jini et al., 2018), mood and anxiety disorders (Ravindran et al., 2016), aging (Mohammadi et al., 2018), seizure (Sadeghnia et al., 2008), insomnia and sleep disorder (Sarris et al., 2011; Masaki et al., 2012), brain tumor (Nam et al., 2010), multiple sclerosis (Mojaverrostami et al., 2018), and opioid withdrawal (Hosseinzadeh and Jahanian, 2010).

Saffron is a neuroprotective agent that shows the neuromodulatory effects on various neuropathological processes and mechanisms. Saffron possess not only the free radical antioxidant and antiapoptotic property but also the modulatory action on brain cellular pathways such as dendritic morphology remodeling and brain infraction (Pan et al., 2016; Skladnev and Johnstone, 2017; Sadeghnia et al., 2017; Ghalandari-Shamami et al., 2019). Saffron has the ability to protect the nerve cells from disturbed acetylcholinesterase activity, amyloid β (Aβ) plaques, and neurofibrillary tangles (Adalier and Parker,

Saffron. https://doi.org/10.1016/B978-0-12-818462-2.00010-3

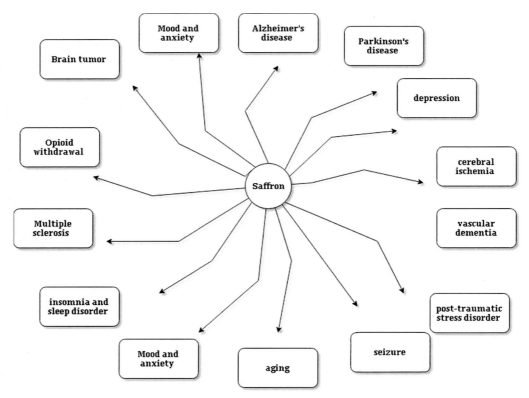

FIG. 10.1 Possible role of saffron in different brain diseases.

2016). Furthermore, Saffron has pleotropic activity because of its different active constituents. It is suggested that saffron has a diverse range for therapeutic management approaches for different neurological conditions (Fig. 10.1).

POSSIBLE MECHANISM OF ACTION FOR MODULATORY EFFECTS OF SAFFRON AND ITS ACTIVES

Many molecular and cellular mechanisms have been reported by researchers working on saffron. The major mechanisms that have been found for possible benefits of saffron and its chemical constituents, including nuclear factor-κB (NF-κB) signaling, B-cell lymphoma and B-cell lymphoma–associated X protein regulation, C- Fos protein regulation, p53 signaling pathway, Kelch-like Enoyl-CoA hydratase (ECH)-associated protein 1–nuclear factor (erythroid-derived 2)-like two signaling, cytosine-cytosine-adenosine-adenosine-thymidine (CCAAT)-enhancer–binding protein homologous protein/Wnt/β-catenin pathway, mitogen-activated protein kinase (MAPK) signaling,

phosphatidylinositol-3-kinase (PI3K) signaling, Notch signaling pathway, G protein–coupled receptor kinase 2 (GRK) pathway, cyclic adenosine monophosphate (cAMP) response element-binding protein, Brain-derived neurotropic factor, vascular growth factor (VGF) nerve growth factor inducible, glutamate signaling, GABAergic-benzodiazepine receptor regulation, serotonergic signaling, dopaminergic signaling, acetyl-cholinergic signaling, hypothalamic pituitary adrenal axis regulation, and Aβ.

Nuclear Factor-κB (NF-κB) Signalling

The NF-κB regulates many of the cellular signaling pathways related to inflammatory process such as modulation of chemokine, cytokines, proinflammatory enzymes and adhesion molecules, and proinflammatory transcription factors within the neurons, glial cells, and cerebral blood vessels. The activation of NF-κB is found in Parkinson's disease (PD), Alzheimer's disease (AD), and epilepsy. Therefore, it may suggest that NF-κB regulation and dysregulation play a major role in neuroinflammation of diseases (Shih et al., 2015).

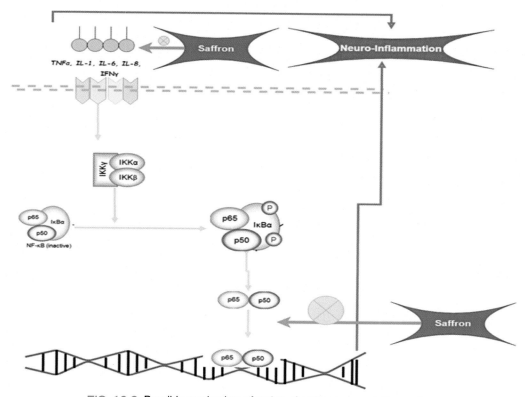

FIG. 10.2 Possible mechanism of action of saffron in neuroinflammation.

Crocetin is a neuroprotective agent having antioxidant, antiinflammatory, and antiapoptotic properties. There are several brain disorders such as AD, PD, and epilepsy that have characteristic features of neuroinflammation and NF-κB. Saffron has an active component called crocetin, which leads to generation of NF-κB, induction of nitric oxide synthase, and inhibition of inflammatory cytokines. It has been observed that crocetin reduces the extent of proinflammatory cytokines, such as, IL-6, IL-8, IL-1β, and TNF-α. In this way, crocetin may inhibit the upregulation of NF-κB in the brain. It has been studied that crocetin reversed the upregulation of NF-κB—mediated cellular signaling, which are responsible for learning and memory impairments in AD and PD. Furthermore, crocetin enhances learning and memory deficit in cases of AD possibly by its modulation of neuroinflammation (Zhang et al., 2018). Crocin treatment suppressed NF-κB pathway activation and neuronal damage, leading to improved cognitive function in cases of epilepsy (Mazumder et al., 2017). Interaction of active carotenoid crocin with cellular NF-κB pathway has also been reported. Interestingly, activation of NF-κB is

also correlated with learning and memory processes via excitatory synaptic transmission. On the basis of the aforementioned line, a conclusion could be drawn that saffron and its actives modulate the NF-κB responsible for AD-, PD-, and epilepsy-related pathogenesis (Fig. 10.2).

B-Cell Lymphoma (Bax) and B-Cell Lymphoma—Associated X Protein (Bcl-2) Regulation

Bax is responsible for apoptosis in normal cells. However, Bcl-2 is responsible for cell survival by suppressing apoptosis. In inherent pathways, mitochondria discharges cytochrome c by enlistment of Bax and Bak, and at that point, cytochrome c ties with apoptotic protease activating factor-1 (APAF-1) to make a complex with procaspase-9, prompting actuation of caspase-9 and inevitably enactment of divided caspase-3. Bcl-2 can inhibit this pathway. By measuring Bcl-2 and Bax levels, it reveals the inhibition and activation of intrinsic pathway, respectively. Bax is a proapoptotic protein, whereas Bcl-2 is an antiapoptotic protein that relates to the Bcl family. Thus, for measuring the

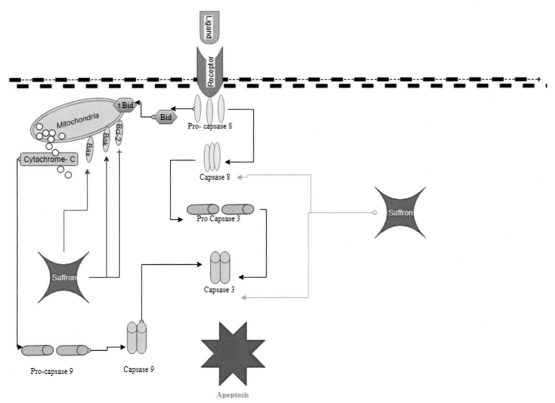

FIG. 10.3 Possible mechanism of action of saffron in apoptosis.

apoptosis level, the Bax/Bcl-2 ratio is an important indicator (Asadi et al., 2015) (Fig. 10.3).

Administration of crocin significantly decreased the Bax/Bcl-2 ratio to restore the balance of Bax and Bcl-2 to impart antiapoptotic activity. Intrahippocampal administration of Aβ decreased the Bcl-2 level and increased Bax, thus resulting in significant increase of Bax/Bcl-2 ratio. Generally, the ratio of Bax/Bcl-2 was increased by about 32% in Aβ-exposed animals in comparison to control animals. Crocin administration significantly restored the ratio on different doses. This shows, crocin inhibits Aβ-associated apoptosis (Asadi et al., 2015). Moreover, crocin has also been noted for protecting PC12 cells against potent neurotoxic effects of acrylamide through downregulation of Bcl-2 and the upregulation of Bax and decreasing apoptosis (Shafiee et al., 2018). PC12 cells treated with acrylamide (ACR) significantly upregulated the expression of Bax and downregulated the expression of Bcl-2 protein compared with the control group, which resulted in a high Bax/Bcl-2 ratio. Pretreatment with crocin decreased the Bax levels in PC12 cells, and crocin mitigated Bax/Bcl-2 ratio (Mehri et al., 2011).

C-Fos Protein Regulation

c-Fos is an immediate early response gene associated in cell separation and proliferation after extracellular stimulus, while its deregulation has been associated with progression of oncogenic. As other members of the FOS family proteins and proteins of the ATF family, c-Fos can heterodimerize with members of the JUN family to form the transcription factor activator protein 1 (AP-1). c-Fos can be used as a marker of neuronal action and associated with a number of neurobehavioral responses to acute stimuli expression (Velazquez et al., 2015). In addition, c-Fos protein expression in the amygdala increases during stressful situations and induces corticotropin-releasing hormone (CRH) release. Deep brain stimulation (DBS) treatment and combination therapy of saffron with DBS reduced c-Fos expression, which further reduced CRH release to normal (Mokhtari Hashtjini et al., 2018). It has been documented that activation of c-Fos and c-Fos mRNA overexpression leads to Aβ protein–associated neurotoxicity in the AD. The main reason for memory impairment is believed to be Aβ neurotoxicity in the AD. Aβ neurotoxicity has been shown to induce neurodegeneration via the DNA fragmentation and activation of c-Fos. c-Fos levels were recorded by Western blot tests of Aβ-exposed animals. Crocin significantly reduced the levels of hippocampal c-Fos in animals (Mohammadi et al., 2018). Immunohistochemical study showed that safranal increased c-Fos expression in the ventrolateral preoptic nucleus (VLPO), which is one of the putative sleep centers, as well as decreased it in the arousal histaminergic tuber mammillary nuclei. It indicated that safranal increases non-rapid eye movement (NREM) sleep in pentobarbital-treated mice. It has been documented that the VLPO contains a high number of sleep-promoting neurons, which are more active during sleep, as indicated by the expression of c-Fos (Liu et al., 2012).

p53 Signaling Pathway

The intrinsic and extrinsic type of cell stresses may act upon p53 pathway. Activation of the p53 pathway may disrupt the integrity of DNA template and initiates a process of cell cycle arrest and apoptosis (Harris and Levine, 2005). Apoptosis is basically a programmed cell death. Morphological changes such as cell shrinkage and degradation of DNA are characteristics of apoptosis (Papaliagkas et al., 2007).

In transgenic AD mouse models, elevated levels of p53 were found in the hippocampus of mice, indicating process of apoptosis can be enhanced. This elevated p53 level is known to be inhibited in the brain of AD transgenic mice by crocetin, which is an active constituent of saffron. The levels of p53 have been measured by Western blot analysis. This result proves that crocetin may have some neuroprotective and antiapoptotic effects (Zhang et al., 2018).

Kelch-like ECH-Associated Protein 1 (Keap1)–Nuclear Factor Erythroid-Derived two like 2 (Nrf2) Signaling

The regulation of various antioxidant and some of the cytoprotective genes is done by Nrf2 which prevent oxidative stress. Nrf2 is controlled by Keap1, which further binds to Nrf2 and promotes Nrf2 degradation. Keap1 releases Nrf2 and activates the transcription of antioxidant enzymes including glutathione S transferase, glutamate-cysteine ligase catalytic subunit, NADPH-quinone oxidoreductase 1, and heme oxygenase 1. A recent study has suggested that the Keap1/Nrf2 signaling plays an important role in neurodegenerative diseases (NDDs) including PD, depression, AD, and Huntington disease. p8, p60, p61, and p60 Nrf2 levels are known to reduce in patients with AD. Thus, the activation of Nrf2 could be a therapeutic target for AD and PD (Pan et al., 2016; Deshmukh et al., 2017; Hashimoto et al., 2018).

To investigate whether Keap1/Nrf2 signaling is involved in the protective effect of safranal against rotenone-induced neurotoxicity, we detected the expression of Keap1 and Nrf2 in rotenone-induced dopaminergic neurons. The results showed that rotenone treatment significantly upregulated Keap1 expression and decreased the nuclear Nfr2 expression. However, the pretreatment with safranal to rotenone markedly decreased the Keap1 expression and upregulated the nuclear Nfr2 expression. The results implied that Keap1/Nrf2 signaling may be involved in the protective effect of safranal against rotenone-induced neurotoxicity. To further investigate whether Keap1/Nrf2 signaling is associated with the defensive effect of safranal, we blocked the Keap1/Nrf2 signaling by knockdown of Nrf2 and then detected the protective effect of safranal against rotenone-induced neurotoxicity. The results showed that transfection of Nrf2 siRNA significantly decreased the protein expression and mRNA of Nrf2. The knockdown of Nrf2 significantly abolished the protective effect on safranal against rotenone-induced cell death, cell apoptosis, and ROS generation. These results suggest that safranal protects dopaminergic neurons against rotenone-induced neurotoxicity at least in part through Keap1/Nrf2 signaling. Safranal has shown a protective effect as it activates the Nrf2 signaling, which further inhibits the oxidative stress and cell apoptosis. As Safranal has been found to report to inhibit Keap1 expression and promoted Nrf2 nuclear accumulation, this led to transcription of antioxidant gene expression, by which safranal alleviated rotenone-induce neurotoxicity in dopaminergic neurons. In all, Safranal has been found to inhibit Keap1 and activate Nrf2 signaling against oxidative stress (Pan et al., 2016).

CCA AT-Enhancer–Binding Protein Homologous Protein (CHOP)/Wnt/β-Catenin (Wnt) Pathway

Wnt signaling pathways play an important role in many of cellular processes which includes development, cell proliferation, cell fate, motility, and synaptic plasticity. As it has been found that many of the components of this pathway are found in the adult brain, Wnt/β-catenin signaling found to be important to maintain and protect neural connections (Maguschak and Ressler, 2012). CHOP is induced by ER stress, and the prolonged ER stress activates the apoptosis signaling

(Nishitohet al., 2012). Overexpressed CHOP could alert cells to ER stress by stimulating ROS formation, decreased glutathione activity, as well as differently regulating Bcl-2 family proteins. The impairment in ER functioning is said to be associated with neuronal dysfunction in PD or we can say there is upregulation of ER stress in PD.

Zhang et al. demonstrated that crocin found the inhibitory effects on CHOP/Wnt signaling on 1-methyl-4-phenylpyridinium (MPP+)-induced cyto-toxicity and thus provided new lights on the benefits of crocin in PD. To find out the potential molecular mechanism that underlies crocin-induced protection and MPP+-induced injury, β catenin was examined in PC12 cells. MPP+ considerably decreases the β catenin nuclear localization and also minimizes the top flash action which reversely correlate with CHOP. By giving crocin treatment, there is markedly an increase in top flash action as compared with the MPP+ group. In all it was reported that crocin defend PC12 cells from MPP+-associated cytotoxicity through CHOP associate destruction of Wnt expression. Crocin reduces the communication of CHOP, which is required for coun-teracting the function of prosurvival Wnt/β-catenin signaling. Crocin also constrains the proapoptotic factor caspase-12 activation. It also has been found that crocin treatment attenuates morphological changes of ER and eventually prevents caspase-3 activation and apoptosis in PC12 cells (Zhang et al., 2015).

MAPK Pathway

MAPKs are serine-threonine kinases that regulate many of the intracellular signaling which are associated with cellular activities such as cell proliferation, differentiation, survival, death, and transformation. MAPKs include extracellular signal-regulated kinase, p38, and c-Jun NH2-terminal ki-nase (JNK), with each MAPK signaling pathway consisting of at least three components, a MAPK kinase (MAP3K), a MAPK kinase (MAP2K), and a MAPK. Intracellular and diverse extracellular stimuli which includes cytokines, pep-tide growth factors, hormones, endoplasmic reticulum stress, and various cellular stressors such as oxidative stress activate the MAPK pathways. Disruption in MAPK signaling pathways has been found to implicate many dis-eases such as PD, AD, and amyotrophic lateral sclerosis along with cancer (Kim and Choi, 2010). Safranal de-creases the ratio of phospho-stress-activated protein kinase/c (SAPK)/JNK to SAPK/JNK and reduces the cell loss where Aβ is activating JNK and increase in the ratio of phospho-p44/42MAPK to p44/42MAPK where Aβ is reducing the ratio of phospho-p44/42MAPK to p44/42MAPK (Rafieipour et al., 2019).

PI3K Signaling

PI3K signaling is also involved in cell differentiation, proliferation, growth, motility, intracellular trafficking, and cellular survival. PI3K is classified as the family of three different classes: class I, II, and III (Koh and Lo, 2015). It has been reported that in AD and PD and other neurodegenerative disorders, the PI3K/AKT pathway is altered, which leads to autophagy disrup-tion. The activation of the PI3K/AKT/mTOR pathway inhibits the autophagic process and provides neuropro-tection. In NDDs having cognitive deficits, PI3K/AKT/mTOR pathway activation is important for synaptic ac-tivity and normal neuronal functions (Rai et al., 2019). It has been reported that along with antiapoptotic activ-ity of safranal, safranal can reduce the ratio of phospho-PI3 kinase p85/p55 to PI3 kinase p85/p55 (Rafieipour et al., 2019).

Notch Signaling Pathway

Notch signaling has a role in the regulation of migra-tion, morphology, synaptic plasticity, and survival of immature as well as mature neurons. Notch signaling is a master regulator of neural stem cells (NSCs) and neural development. Abnormal Notch expression levels are found in Down's syndrome and AD. (Jessica et al., 2011). In various brain injury models, the activation of Notch signaling occurred, but some conflicting ef-fects are also reported. Like, blocking Notch improves the functional outcome in stroke mouse model, whereas Notch activation was protective in transient ce-rebral ischemia by decreasing neuronal apoptosis (Wang et al., 2015) p52. Notch is operative in diverse brain pathologies including tumor genesis, stroke, and neurological disorders such as Alzheimer's disease, Down syndrome, and multiple sclerosis (Mathieu et al., 2013). Crocin was found to activate the Notch signaling in rodent after traumatic brain injury (TBI). Crocin has been reported to activate Notch signaling and provide neuroprotection in mice model. Crocin inhibited neuroinflammation after TBI via activation of Notch signaling. However, Notch signaling inhibi-tion significantly decreased the defensive effects of cro-cin on proinflammatory cytokines release, microglial response, and neuronal apoptosis. This outcome sug-gested that Notch signaling activation is considered as an important therapeutic strategy for the treatment of TBI (Kai et al., 2015).

GRK Pathway

GRK2 is a member of the GRK family which was initially identified as serine/threonine kinases and plays a central role in signal transduction cascades. GRKs perform diverse cellular functions and are multidomain proteins. Among various isoforms of GRK, GRK2 has an emerging role in signal transduction pathways. GRK2 has been proposed to gene expression and regulation related to different brain conditions such as neuroimmune dysfunction and cerebral ischemia (Penela et al., 2010). Weinaokang (WNK), the active compounds extracted from saffron, Ginkgo, and Ginseng, exhibits protective effects that appear to inhibit GRK2 pathways in the ischemic brain. The level of GRK2 was found to be significantly decreased in the soluble fraction (cytosol) and enlarged in the particulate fraction (membrane) after global cerebral ischemia—reperfusion. WNK pretreatment in vivo not only reduced membrane (functional) GRK2 expression but also increased cytosol GRK2 expression, suggesting its ability to inhibit GRK2 translocation from the cytosol to the membrane. WNK modulates subcellular distribution of GRK2. GRK2 may be considered as one of the most important targets of crocin, which was concluded by the effect of WNK on GRK2 subcellular division (Zheng et al., 2010).

cAMP Response Element-Binding Protein (CREB)

Superfamily of transcription factors includes CREB, cAMP response element modulator, activating transcription factor-1 (ATF-1), etc. CREB family binds to specific DNA sequences which immediately initiate the new gene transcription. Many of the processes such as neuronal proliferation, differentiation, learning, memory, synaptic plasticity, neuronal plasticity, and some neuropathological conditions are appeared to be modulated by CREB family transcription factors/signaling (Yu and Rasenick, 2012). cAMP-dependent protein kinase (PKA) CREB signaling has involved in the pathogenesis of depression as reduction in expression of CREB in depression patients. The systemic perturbations of the PKA/CREB signal pathway could induce cascade reactions of neuropathology in depression, including abnormalities in regional brain activity, alterations in synaptic function, and impaired neurogenesis (Jiang et al., 2017).

Saffron aqueous extract at the dose of 80 mg/kg/day was administered intraperitoneally for 21 days to rats. The levels of P-CREB and CREB in the cerebellum were evaluated using Western blot technique. Aqueous extract of saffron was found to significantly increase the levels of P-CREB in long-term treatment of cerebellum (Asrari et al., 2018). Crocin was administered intraperitoneal for 21 days to rats. CREB and phospho-CREB (P-CREB) protein and mRNA levels in the rat cerebellum

were evaluated using quantitative reverse transcription-polymerase chain reaction (qRT-PCR) and Western blot. Chronic administration of saffron aqueous extract and crocin in the rat hippocampus exhibited significant increases in CREB and P-CREB protein levels. These changes were associated with elevation in CREB mRNA level (Razavi et al., 2017). Crocin was administered intraperitoneal to male Wistar rats for 21 days. Protein expression and transcript levels of CREB and p-CREB in the rat hippocampus were evaluated using Western blot and qRT-PCR, respectively. In the results of Western blot analysis, it was showed that there is a significant and dose-dependent increase in the levels of CREB by crocin. Levels of p-CREB increased significantly at 50 mg/kg of crocin (Vahdati et al., 2014). Cellular mechanism for depression through saffron and its effect on the levels of p-CREB were assessed. The transcript levels of brain-derived neurotrophic factor (BDNF) and protein expression in rat hippocampus were evaluated using Western blot and qRT-PCR. All doses of saffron drastically increase CREB levels. High dose of saffron increased the level of CREB up to 24% compare with control. The saffron at doses of 40 and 160 mg/kg raised the levels of p-CREB up to 28% and 32%, respectively. The effects of aqueous extract of saffron at doses of 40 and 160 mg/kg on levels of p-CREB were more than those of synthetic imipramine (Shafiee et al., 2018).

Brain-Derived Neurotrophic Factor

BDNF (a member of the neurotrophin family) is a small dimmer neuroprotective protein that involves in maintenance and cell survival of nervous system (Dorri et al., 2015; Asrari et al., 2018). BDNF is also involved in the management of many of the physiological brain functions (Sangiovanni et al., 2017). Alteration in BDNF expression is involved in the development of many central nervous system diseases, including neurodegenerative disorders such as AD, PD, Huntington's disease, and amyotrophic lateral sclerosis, as well as psychiatric disorders such as depression and schizophrenia (Sangiovanniet al., 2017). BDNF is considered as a potential therapeutic agent as many of the NDDs result from the insufficient supply of neurotropic factors. Reduction in brain BDNF mRNA levels have been found to cause depression, AD (hippocampus), and PD (SN). Thus, new pharmacological strategies are focused on neuroprotective role, particularly antidepressant activity of BDNF (Binder et al., 2004).

Crocin (12.5, 25, and 50 mg/kg) was administered intraperitoneal to male Wistar rats for 21 days. Transcript levels of BDNF and protein expression were evaluated using qRT-PCR and Western blot. Western blot analysis showed that crocin increased the levels of BDNF significantly and dose dependently. The crocin caused BDNF transcription level increase (Vahdati et al., 2014). Male Wistar rats were exposed to malathion alone or in combination with crocin, imipramine, and vitamin E. The forced swimming test was performed. The protein level of BDNF was evaluated using Western blot analysis. Malathion significantly decreased protein level of BDNF in rat hippocampus. Both imipramine and crocin could increase the protein level of BDNF in comparison with malathion in rat hippocampus (Dorri et al., 2015). Molecular mechanism of antidepressant effect of aqueous extract of saffron and its effect on the levels of BDNF in rat hippocampus were investigated. The aqueous extract of saffron was injected intraperitoneal. The protein expression and transcript levels of BDNF in rat hippocampus were evaluated using Western blot and qRT-PCR. Aqueous extract of saffron in all doses significantly increased protein levels of BDNF. The aqueous extract of saffron significantly increased transcript levels of BDNF (Ghasemi et al., 2015; Shafiee et al., 2018).

VGF Nerve Growth Factor Inducible

The VGF gene (nonacronymic) is highly conserved and was identified on the basis of its rapid induction in vitro by nerve growth factor, although it can also be induced by BDNF and glial-derived growth factor. The VGF gene and peptides are widely expressed throughout the brain, particularly in the hypothalamus and hippocampus. Subsequent studies demonstrated that VGF is similarly upregulated by numerous neurotrophins, including neurotrophin-3, BDNF, in neuronal targets such as hippocampal or cortical neurons. However, levels of VGF mRNA increased by interleukin-6, fibroblast growth factor, insulin, and epidermal growth factor (Lewis et al., 2015). VGF implicated in neurite growth, neurogenesis, and synaptic plasticity of the brain. Patients diagnosed with depression and bipolar disorders have lower-than-normal VGF levels, while patients with schizophrenia and depression have higher-than-normal values. VGF knockout mice show behavioral abnormalities such as higher depressive behavior and memory dysfunction. However, it is unclear whether upregulation of VGF affects brain function (Mizoguchi et al., 2017). Hippocampal VGF expression is decreased in animal models of depression (Jiang et al., 2018).

Crocin was administered intraperitoneal to male Wistar rats. Transcript levels of VGF and protein expression and the rat hippocampus were evaluated using qRT-PCR and Western blot. Western blot analysis showed that crocin at all doses, as compared to saline, significantly and dose-dependently increases the VGF levels in a dose-dependent manner. Crocin could increase the VGF levels similar to that of imipramine (Vahdati et al., 2014). Molecular mechanism of antidepressant effect of aqueous extract of saffron and its effect on the levels of BDNF in rat hippocampus were investigated. The saffron was injected intraperitoneal for 21 days to rats. The protein expression and transcript levels of VGF in rat hippocampus was evaluated using qRT-PCR and Western blot. Although the aqueous extracts of saffron increased the levels of VGF, the increase was not significant.

Glutamate Signaling

Glutamate is an excitatory neurotransmitter and a nonessential amino acid that proliferates normal and neoplastic cells and keenly involved in bioenergetic, biosynthetic, metabolic, and oncogenic pathways. It also participates in many of the neural functions such as synaptic plasticity, learning, and memory and long-term potentiation. Glutamate signaling activates two of the receptors, ionotropic glutamate receptors and metabotropic glutamate receptors, which have been implicated in brain conditions such as Schizophrenia, multiple sclerosis, AD, PD. An increase in the level of Glu can cause excitotoxicity and neural cell death and implicates Glu toxicity in NDDs. Glu signaling mechanisms facilitate the development of treatments for Glu-related NDDs such as multiple sclerosis, AD, and PD (Willard et al., 2013). Inhibition of glutamatergic synaptic transmission by interaction with N-methyl-D-aspartate (NMDA) and kainate receptors have shown by hydroethanolic saffron extract in a concentration-dependent manner (Berger et al., 2011). Safranal pretreatment along with kainic acid (KA) administration significantly and dose-dependently decreased hippocampal glutamate concentration. Safranal attenuated cerebral ischemia-induced oxidative damage in the rat hippocampus, in vivo, and also has antioxidant properties, in vitro. These effects may be involved in the safranal-mediated decrease of glutamate release after KA administration (Hosseinzadeh et al., 2008).

GABAergic Benzodiazepine Receptor Regulation

The GABAA/benzodiazepine receptor complex, which is also known as the central benzodiazepine receptor, is a heteromeric protein complex containing binding sites for classes of compounds such as GABA and benzodiazepines (Andersson and Halldin, 2013). GABAergic-benzodiazepine mechanisms have a special role in the neurophysiology of seizure, anxiety, and other psychiatric conditions. A research finding has been found that when saffron was administered peripherally, it results in prevention of PTZ-induced minimal clonic seizures (MCS) and tonic-clonic seizures (GTCS) in a dose-dependent manner. Researcher claimed the dose-dependent decrease in MCS and GTCS was induced by PTZ by safranal. This has been assumed that anticonvulsant effects of safranal are through GABAA-benzodiazepine receptor complex (Hosseinzadeh and Sadeghnia, 2007).

Serotonergic Signaling

Serotonin (5-hydroxytrympamine) regulates the many physiological functions through ligand-gated ion channels and G protein-coupled receptors (GPCRs). Serotonin is occupied in different aspects of neural development, such as growth cone motility, neurite outgrowth, synaptogenesis, somatic morphology regulation, and control of dendritic spine density and shape. Serotonergic neurons are widely distributed throughout the brain. Disproportion in serotonergic signaling is found to be involved in many of the pathophysiological conditions, including Alzheimer's disease, schizophrenia, anxiety, and depression. In particular, 5-HT1AR is linked to the pathogenesis of stress-related disorders and depression (Wirth et al., 2017).

It has been postulated that safranal affects the serotonergic system. Saffron is characterized by the inhibition of serotonin reuptake by which mental conditions can be improved (Nemat Shahi et al., 2017). Saffron extract may inhibit serotonin reuptake in synapses (Sophia Esalatmanesh et al., 2017). Serotonergic mechanisms have been influenced by crocin by showing antagonistic action at the 5-HT2c receptor site (Lopresti et al., 2014).

Dopaminergic Signaling

Dopamine is an important receptor, which is also a key neurotransmitter. D_1-like receptor comprises of D_1 and D_5 receptor subtypes, and the D_2-like receptor class comprises of the D_2, D_3, and D_4 receptor subtypes. All classes of the dopamine receptors are GPCRs, and signaling of these receptors is regulated by interaction with and activation of heterotrimeric GTP-binding proteins (G proteins) (Neve et al., 2004). Impaired dopamine receptor signaling results into many of the neurological and neuropsychiatric disorders, including schizophrenia, attention-deficit hyperactivity disorder, obsessive-compulsive disorder, PD, Huntington's disease, and drug addiction (Neve, 2004).

Ettehadi et al (2013) showed that the aqueous extract of saffron increases the release of important neurotransmitters, such as dopamine and glutamate, in rat brains. The study demonstrated that the effect of the extract on dopamine release was dose dependent (Hosseinali et al., 2013). Aqueous saffron extract is reported to increase the brain dopamine concentration in a dose-dependent manner. (Khazdair et al., 2015). In a model of a 6OHDA toxicity, crocetin reduced the increase in dopamine utilization by the tissue. So, it has been found that crocetin pretreatment protected against 6OHDA-induced Parkinsonism. Crocetin also has the ability to save the degeneration of nigrostriatal dopaminergic neurons up to some extent and maintain the dopamine level closer to basal level. It has been reported that the protective effect of crocetin might be due to decrease in autooxidation of dopamine by activity of antioxidant enzymes, mainly GPx, which have a higher level of activity in striatum and substantia nigra than in other brain regions. (Ahmad et al., 2005).

Acetyl-Cholinergic Signaling

Acetylcholine receptors (AChRs) belong to a member of a protein's superfamily called pentameric ligand gated ion channels (Prinston et al., 2017). Neuronal excitability, synaptic transmission, and synaptic plasticity all these activities are altered by acetylcholine in the brain. ACh comprises of two classes of receptors: metabotropic muscarinic receptors (mAChRs) and ionotropic nicotinic receptors (nAChRs) (Picciotto et al., 2012). AChE inhibitors or anticholinesterase plays an important role as they inhibit the breaking down of ACh by AChE and disrupt the level and duration of the neurotransmitter action at neuromuscular junctions and cholinergic brain synapses (Colovic et al., 2013). Acetylcholine (ACh) signaling affects cognitive functions and behaviors, including attention, learning, memory, and motivation. Alterations in ACh signaling are involved in the pathophysiology of multiple neuropsychiatric disorders including Alzheimer's disease, schizophrenia, and drug addiction (Luchicchi et al., 2014).

Saffron aqueous methanol extract administration has shown significant enhancement in learning and memory, antioxidant protection, and inhibition of AChE in brain. Saffron infusion can significantly decrease cerebral AChE activity and also can lower the activity of whole-brain AChE isoforms. Crocetin inhibits AChE by binding at two different loci, the catalytic center, and the peripheral anionic sites (Linardaki et al., 2017). Saffron coadministration with Al also caused significant reduction in cerebral AChE isoforms activity. Al + saffron inhibited DS-AChE in whole brain at a high rate as compared to the SS-AChE isoform, which suggests greater susceptibility of DS isoform of

AChE toward saffron (Linardaki et al., 2013). In adult mice, saffron administration resulted in a significant decrease in AChE-specific activity in both fractions, i.e., salt- and detergent-soluble fractions of brain homogenates as a marker of central cholinergic status with the percentage of inhibition ranging between 38% and 52% (Papandreou et al., 2011).

Hypothalamo-Pituitary-Adrenocortical (HPA) Axis

The HPA axis is required for stress adaptation. Activation of the HPA axis causes secretion of glucocorticoids, and it represents a primary hormonal response to homeostatic challenge. Some changes in the HPA axis is a hallmark of the physiological reaction to stress (James et al., 2016). Depression patients exhibit HPA hyperactivity, elevated cortisol levels, and impairment in negative feedback response to glucocorticoids, a phenomenon which is known as glucocorticoid resistance. Increase in size and activity of the pituitary and adrenal glands is also observed in depression. This HPA dysregulation affects neurotransmitter availability, oxidative stress, and inflammation, and it also contributes to neurodegeneration.

An interaction with the HPA axis provides a mechanism that mediates the protective effects of saffron and crocin against chronic stress-induced impairment of learning and memory. It claimed that crocin can decrease the corticosterone response to chronic restraint stress (Ghadrdoost et al., 2011). P95 p96 It has been reported that intraperitoneal administration of saffron water extract or safranal reduced stress-induced corticosterone plasma level elevation by interacting with some of the parts of HPA axis (Hooshmandi et al., 2011; Halataei et al., 2011; Adrian et al., 2014).

Amyloid-β

Aβ is formed by the processing of a transmembrane protein, amyloid precursor protein. Aβ buildup in the brain is projected to be an early toxic occasion in the pathogenesis of Alzheimer's disease, which is the most ordinary form of dementia linked with plaques and tangles. Aβ may make up a core path for the rising number of NDDs, including Huntington's diseases, AD, and PD, which may lead to the development of a novel treatment strategy against diverse degenerative diseases (Chen et al., 2017).

Crocetin is considered to be an important component in saffron which bears good beneficial values for AD. Crocetin inhibit Aβ fibrillization and stabilize Aβ oligomers. It was also reported that crocetin can lower the overall insoluble amyloid, insoluble Aβ42, and soluble Aβ40 in the hippocampus, cerebellum, and cerebral cortex, which enhanced the learning and memory (Zhang et al., 2018). Saffron and two of its constituents (crocin-1 and crocetin) known to slow down Aβ aggregation, and crocin-1 also inhibits tau aggregation (Inoue et al., 2018). Any pathological changes in blood brain barrier (BBB) in AD relates to the accumulation of Aβ peptides, and elevated levels of cerebral Aβ impair the BBB integrity and function. Results have been demonstrated that *C. sativus* extract has been documented to enhance the tightness of bEnd-3 cells–based BBB model as observed by reduced permeability of LY in a concentration dependent manner in the range of 0.22–2.2 µg/mL. Furthermore, *C. sativus* extract elevates the transport of 125I-Aβ40 from basolateral (B) to apical (A) compartment across the b End-3 cells by 15% ($P < .01$). This increase in Aβ transport is associated with concentration-dependent increase in P-gp expression by 17% ($P < .05$) and 42% ($P < .01$) at 1.1 and 2.2 µg/mL, respectively. Consumption of *C. sativus* extract has been found to reduce total Aβ by 53%, Aβo, which is a central player in causing neurotoxicity and initiating the pathological and cognitive disturbances, by 63%, Aβ40 by 73% and Aβ42 levels by 63%. On the other hand, crocin administration reduces total Aβ levels, Aβ40 by 25% and Aβ42 levels by 29% (Batarseh et al., 2017). Trans-crocin-4, saffron extract, and DMC affect the Aβ1-40-fibrillogenesis. Amyloid fibrils formation can be inhibited by the extraction of *C. sativus* stigmas, which depends on time and concentration. When the saffron extract was allowed to incubate with Aβ1-40, its effects decreased because of oxidation or any other chemical transformations that lessen the activeness of saffron constituents. Trans-Crocin-4, which is considered to be the principle crocin constituent of stigmas, inhibits Aβ fibrillogenesis. Crocin constituents also found to inhibit the in vitro amyloid aggregation (Mirmosayyeb et al., 2017). Papandreou et al. has found an inhibitory effect of saffron extract and crocin on fibrillogenesis of Aβ40 in vitro (Papandreou et al., 2006). It was further investigated the effect of crocin on fibrillogenesis of Aβ42 by thioflavin T-based fluorescence assay, DNA binding shift assay, CD spectroscopy, and transmission electron microscopy. Ghaghaei et al. found that crocin prevented Aβ42-mediated amyloid fibril formation in vitro, probably through the stabilization of helical structure, and resulted in the dissolution of previously formed aggregates (Ghahghaei et al., 2013). Furthermore, it has been demonstrated that crocin inhibited Aβ fibril formation and destabilized preformed Aβ fibrils (Ahn et al., 2011; Finley and Gao, 2017; Zhang et al., 2018). Transcrocetin at low molecular doses are shown to enhance the Aβ42 degradation in monocytes of AD by the upregulation of the lysosomal protease cathepsin B. CA074Me, a potent and selective cathepsin B inhibitor, counteracted such trans-crocetin—induced effect. Trans-crocetin, which is a carotenoid, improves the clearance of Aβ42 by the involving cathepsin B, and this could be a new antiamyloid strategy in AD. Trans-crocetin decreased the level of intracellular Aβ42 and also increased the levels of the Aβ42-degrading lysosomal protease CatB, which suggests a potential mechanism by which monocytic Aβ42 degradation ability can be restored (Tiribuzi et al., 2017).

CONCLUSION

In the aforementioned lines and data, it may be concluded saffron has neuroprotective action because of its chemical constituents such as crocin, picrocrocin, safranal, and many others. These chemical constituent act by different mechanisms of action such as nuclear factor-κB (NF-κB) pathway, B-cell lymphoma and B-cell lymphoma—associated X protein regulation, C-Fos protein regulation, p53 signaling pathway, Kelch-like ECH-associated protein 1—nuclear factor (erythroid-derived 2)-like two signaling, CCA AT-enhancer-binding protein homologous protein/Wnt/β-catenin pathway, MAPK pathway, PI3K pathway, Notch signaling pathway, GRK pathway, cAMP response element-binding protein, brain-derived neurotropic factor, VGF nerve growth factor inducible, glutamate signaling, GABAergic-benzodiazepine receptor regulation, serotonergic signaling, dopaminergic signaling, acetyl-cholinergic signaling, hypothalamic pituitary adrenal axis regulation, and Aβ. Evidently, majority of the mechanisms are not exactly known for saffron, so there is a huge scope for future research on therapeutic benefits along with pharmacological mechanisms of saffron and its actives in brain diseases.

REFERENCES

Adalier, N., Parker, H., 2016. Vitamin E, turmeric and saffron in treatment of Alzheimer's disease. Antioxidants 5 (4), E40.

Ahn, J.H., Hu, Y., Hernandez, M., Kim, J.R., 2011. Crocetin inhibits beta-amyloid fibrillization and stabilizes beta-amyloid oligomers. Biochem. Biophys. Res. Commun. 414 (1), 79–83. https://doi.org/10.1016/j.bbrc.2011.09.025.

Ahmad, A.S., Ansari, M.A., Ahmad, M., Saleem, S., Yousuf, S., Hoda, M.N., Islam, F., 2005. Neuroprotection by crocetin in a hemi-parkinsonian rat model. Pharmacol. Biochem. Behav. 81 (4), 805–813.

Andersson, J.D., Halldin, C., 2013. PET radioligands targeting the brain GABAA/benzodiazepine receptor complex. J. Label. Comp. Radiopharm. 56 (3–4), 196–206. https://doi.org/10.1002/jlcr.3008.

Asadi, F., Jamshidi, A.H., Khodagholi, F., Yans, A., Azimi, L., Faizi, M., Vali, L., Abdollahi, M., Ghahremani, M.H., Sharifzadeh, M., 2015. Reversal effects of crocin on amyloid β-induced memory deficit: modification of autophagyor apoptosis markers. Pharmacol. Biochem. Behav. 139 (Pt A), 47–58. https://doi.org/10.1016/j.pbb.2015.10.011.

Asrari, N., Yazdian-Robati, R., Abnous, K., Razavi, B.M., Rashednia, M., Hasani, F.V., Hosseinzadeh, H., 2018. Antidepressant effects of aqueous extract of saffron and its effects on CREB, P-CREB, BDNF, and VGF proteins in rat cerebellum. J. Pharmacopuncture 21 (1), 35–40. https://doi.org/10.3831/KPI.2018.21.005.

Batarseh, Y.S., Bharate, S.S., Kumar, V., Kumar, A., Vishwakarma, R.A., Bharate, S.B., Kaddoumi, A., 2017. Crocus sativus extract tightens the blood-brain barrier, reduces amyloid β load and related toxicity in 5XFAD mice. ACS Chem. Neurosci. 8 (8), 1756–1766. https://doi.org/10.1021/acschemneuro.7b00101.

Berger, F., Hensel, A., Nieber, K., 2011. Saffron extract and trans-crocetin inhibit glutamatergic synaptic transmission in rat cortical brain slices. Neuroscience 180, 238–247. https://doi.org/10.1016/j.neuroscience.2011.02.037.

Binder, D.K., Scharfman, H.E., 2004. Brain-derived neurotrophic factor. Growth Factors (3), 123–131.

Bolhasani, S.Z., Bathaie, Yavari, I., Moosavi-Movahedi, A.A., Ghaffari, M., 2005. Separation and purification of some components of Iranian saffron. Asian J. Chem. 17 (2), 725–729.

Chen, G.F., Xu, T.H., Yan, Y.1, Zhou, Y.R., Jiang, Y., Melcher, K., Xu, H.E., 2017. Amyloid beta: structure, biology and structure-based therapeutic development. Acta Pharmacol. Sin. 38 (9), 1205–1235. https://doi.org/10.1038/aps.2017.28.

Colovic, M.B., Krstic, D.Z., Lazarevic-Pasti, T.D., Bondzic, A.M., Vasic, V.M., 2013. Acetylcholinesterase inhibitors: Pharmacology and toxicology. Curr. Neuropharmacol. 11, 315–335.

Dar, R.A., Kumar, B., Tiwari, S., Pitre, S., 2012. Indirect Electrochemical Analysis of Crocin in Phytochemical Sample. E-J. Chem. 9 (2), 918–925.

Deshmukh, P., Unni, S., Krishnappa, G., Padmanabhan, B., 2017. The Keap1-Nrf2 pathway: promising therapeutic target to counteract ROS-mediated damage in cancers and neurodegenerative diseases. Biophys Rev 9 (1), 41–56. https://doi.org/10.1007/s12551-016-0244-4.

Dorri, S.A., Hosseinzadeh, H., Abnous, K., Hasani, F.V., Robati, R.Y., 2015. Razavi BM Involvement of brain-derived neurotrophic factor (BDNF) on malathion induced depressive-like behavior in subacute exposure and protective effects of crocin. Iran J Basic Med Sci 18 (10), 958–966.

Esalatmanesh, S., Biuseh, M., Noorbala, A.A., Mostafavi, S.A., Rezaei, F., Mesgarpour, B., Mohammadinejad, P., Akhondzadeh, S., 2017. Comparison of saffron and fluvoxamine in the treatment of mild to moderate obsessive-compulsive disorder: a double blind randomized clinical trial. Iran. J. Psychiatry 12 (3), 154–162.

Ettehadi, H., Seyedeh, M., Mina, R., Jamal, S., Hedayat, S., Mahdi, H., Farzad, A., 2013. Aqueous Extract of Saffron

(*Crocus sativus*) Increases Brain Dopamine and Glutamate Concentrations in Rats. J. Behav. Brain Sci. 3, 315–331.

Finley, J.W., Gao, S., 2017. A perspective on *Crocus sativus* L. (saffron) constituent crocin: a potent water-soluble antioxidant and potential therapy for Alzheimer's disease. J. Agric. Food Chem. 65 (5), 1005–1020. https://doi.org/10.1021/acs.jafc.6b04398.

Ghahghaei, A., Bathaie, S.Z., Kheirkhah, H., Bahraminejad, E., 2013. The protective effect of crocin on the amyloid fibril formation of Aβ42 peptide in vitro. Cell. Mol. Biol. Lett. 18 (3), 328–339. https://doi.org/10.2478/s11658-013-0092-1.

Ghadrdoost, B., Vafaei, A.A., Rashidy-Pour, A., Hajisoltani, R., Bandegi, A.R., Motamedi, F., Haghighi, S., Sameni, H.R., Pahlvan, S., 2011. Protective effects of saffron extract and its active constituent crocin against oxidative stress and spatial learning and memory deficits induced by chronic stress in rats. Eur. J. Pharmacol. 667 (1–3), 222–229. https://doi.org/10.1016/j.ejphar.2011.05.012.

Ghalandari-Shamami, M., Nourizade, S., Yousefi, B., Vafaei, A.A., Pakdel, R., Rashidy-Pour, A., 2019. Beneficial effects of physical activity and crocin against adolescent stress induced anxiety or depressive-like symptoms and dendritic morphology remodeling in prefrontal cortex in adult male rats. Neurochem. Res. https://doi.org/10.1007/s11064-019-02727-2.

Ghasemi, T., Abnous, K., Vahdati, F., Mehri, S., Razavi, B.M., Hosseinzadeh, H., 2015. Antidepressant effect of Crocus sativus aqueous extract and its effect on CREB, BDNF, and VGF transcript and protein levels in rat Hippocampus. Drug Res. 65 (7), 337–343. https://doi.org/10.1055/s-0034-1371876.

Gismondi, A., 2012. Biochemical, antioxidant and antineoplastic properties of Italian saffron (*Crocus sativus* L.). Am. J. Plant Sci. 3, 1573–1580.

Halataei, B.A., Khosravi, M., Arbabian, S., Sahraei, H., Golmanesh, L., Zardooz, H., Jalili, C., Ghoshooni, H., 2011. Saffron (*Crocus sativus*) aqueous extract and its constituent crocin reduces stress-induced anorexia in mice. Phytother Res. 25 (12), 1833–1838. https://doi.org/10.1002/ptr.3495.

Harris, S.L., Levine, A.J., 2005. The p53 pathway: positive and negative feedback loops. Oncogene 24 (17), 2899–2908.

Hashimoto, K., 2018. Essential role of Keap1-Nrf2 signaling in mood disorders: overview and future perspective. Front. Pharmacol. 9, 1182. https://doi.org/10.3389/fphar.2018.01182.

Hooshmandi, Z., Rohani, A.H., Eidi, A., Fatahi, Z., Golmanesh, L., Sahraei, H., 2011. Reduction of metabolic and behavioral signs of acute stress in male Wistar rats by saffron water extract and its constituent safranal. Pharm. Biol. 49, 947–954. https://doi.org/10.3109/13880209.2011.558103.

Hosseinali, E., Seyedeh, M., Mina, R., Jamal, S., Hedayat, S., Mahdi, H., Farzad, A., 2013. Aqueous extract of saffron (*Crocus sativus*) increases brain dopamine and glutamate concentrations in rats. J. Behav. Brain Sci. 3, 315–331.

Hosseinzadeh, H., Jahanian, Z., 2010. Effect of *Crocus sativus* L. (saffron) stigma and its constituents, crocin and safranal,

on morphine withdrawal syndrome in mice. Phytother Res. 24 (5), 726–730. https://doi.org/10.1002/ptr.3011.

Hosseinzadeh, H., Sadeghnia, H.R., 2007. Protective effect of safranal on pentylenetetrazol-induced seizures in the rat: involvement of GABAergic and opioids systems. Phytomedicine 14 (4), 256–262.

Hosseinzadeh, H., Sadeghnia, H.R., Rahimi, A., 2008. Effect of safranal on extracellular hippocampal levels of glutamate and aspartate during kainic acid treatment in anesthetized rats. Planta Med. 74 (12), 1441–1445. https://doi.org/10.1055/s-2008-1081335.

Inoue, E., Shimizu, Y., Masui, R., Hayakawa, T., Tsubonoya, T., Hori, S., Sudoh, K., 2018. Effects of saffron and its constituents, crocin-1, crocin-2, and crocetin on α-synuclein fibrils. J. Nat. Med. 72 (1), 274–279. https://doi.org/10.1007/s11418-017-1150-1.

James, H., Jessica, M., Sriparna, B., Aynara, W., Ryan, M., Jessie, S., Brent, M., 2016. Regulation of the hypothalamic-pituitary-adrenocortical stress response. Comp. Physiol. 6 (2), 603–621.

Javadi, B., Sahebkar, A., Emami, S.A., 2013. A survey on saffron in major islamic traditional medicine books. Iran J Basic Med Sci 16 (1), 1–11.

Ables, Jessica L., Breunig, Joshua J., Eisch, Amelia J., Rakic, Pasko, 2011. Not(ch) just development: Notch signalling in the adult brain. Nat Rev Neurosci 12 (5), 269–283.

Jiang, H., Zhang, X., Wang, Y., Zhang, H., Li, J., Yang, X., Zhao, B., Zhang, C., Yu, M., Xu, M., Yu, Q., Liang, X., Li, X., Shi, P., Bao, T., 2017. Mechanisms underlying the antidepressant response of acupuncture via PKA/CREB signaling pathway. Neural Plast. 2017, 4135164. https://doi.org/10.1155/2017/4135164.

Jiang, C., Lin, W.J., Sadahiro, M., Labonté, B., Menard, C., Pfau, M.L., Tamminga, C.A., Turecki, G., Nestler, E.J., Russo, S.J., Salton, S.R., 2018. VGF function in depression and antidepressant efficacy. Mol. Psychiatry 23 (7), 1632–1642. https://doi.org/10.1038/mp.2017.233.

Khazdair, M.R., Boskabady, M.H., Hosseini, M., Rezaee, R., M Tsatsakis, A., 2015. The effects of Crocus sativus (saffron) and its constituents on nervous system: a review Avicenna. J Phytomed 5 (5), 376–391.

Kim, E.K., Choi, E.J., 2010. Pathological roles of MAPK signaling pathways in human diseases. Biochim. Biophys. Acta 1802 (4), 396–405. https://doi.org/10.1016/j.bbadis.2009.12.009.

Koh, S.H., Lo, E.H., 2015. The role of the PI3K pathway in the regeneration of the damaged brain by neural stem cells after cerebral infarction. J. Clin. Neurol. 11 (4), 297–304. https://doi.org/10.3988/jcn.2015.11.4.297.

Lewis, J., John, M., Brameld, H., Preeti, H., Neuroendocrine Role for, V.G.F., 2015. Front. Endocrinol. 6, 3.

Linardaki, Z.I., Orkoula, M.G., Kokkosis, A.G., Lamari, F.N., Margarity, M., 2013. Investigation of the neuroprotective action of saffron (*Crocus sativus* L.) in aluminum-exposed adult mice through behavioural and neurobiochemical assessment. Food Chem. Toxicol. 52, 163–170. https://doi.org/10.1016/j.fct.2012.11.016.

Linardaki, Z.I., Lamari, F.N., Margarity, M., 2017. Saffron (*Crocus sativus* L.) tea intake prevents learning/memory defects and neurobiochemical alterations induced by aflatoxin B1 exposure in adult mice. Neurochem. Res. 42 (10), 2743–2754. https://doi.org/10.1007/s11064-017-2283-z.

Liu, Z., Xu, X.H., Liu, T.Y., Hong, Z.Y., Urade, Y., Huang, Z.L., Qu, W.M., 2012. Safranal enhances non-rapid eye movement sleep in pentobarbital-treated mice. CNS Neurosci. Ther. 18 (8), 623–630. https://doi.org/10.1111/j.1755-5949.2012.00334.x.

Lopresti, A.L., Drummond, P.D., 2014. Saffron (*Crocus sativus*) for depression: a systematic review of clinical studies and examination of underlying antidepressant mechanisms of action. Hum. Psychopharmacol. 29 (6), 517–527. https://doi.org/10.1002/hup.2434.

Luchicchi, A., Bloem, B., Viaña, J.N., Mansvelder, H.D., Role, L.W., 2014. Illuminating the role of cholinergic signaling in circuits of attention and emotionally salient behaviors. Front. Synaptic Neurosci. 6, 24. https://doi.org/10.3389/fnsyn.2014.00024. eCollection 2014.

Maguschak, K.A., Ressler, K.J., 2012. A role for WNT/β-Catenin signaling in the neural mechanisms of behavior. J. Neuroimmune Pharmacol. 7 (4), 763–773. https://doi.org/10.1007/s11481-012-9350-7. Epub 2012 Mar 15.

Mazumder, A.G.1, Sharma, P., Patial, V., Singh, D., 2017. Crocin attenuates kindling development and associated cognitive impairments in mice via inhibiting reactive oxygen species-mediated NF-κB activation. Basic Clin. Pharmacol. Toxicol. 120 (5), 426–433. https://doi.org/10.1111/bcpt.12694.

Masaki, M., Aritake, K., Tanaka, H., Shoyama, Y., Huang, Z.L., Urade, Y., 2012. Crocin promotes non-rapid eye movement sleep in mice. Mol. Nutr. Food Res. 56 (2), 304–308.

Mathieu, P., Adami, P.V., Morelli, L., 2013. Notch signaling in the pathologic adult brain. Biomol. Concepts 4 (5), 465–476. https://doi.org/10.1515/bmc-2013-0006.

Mehri, S., Abnous, K., Mousavi, S.H., Shariaty, V.M., Hosseinzadeh, H., 2012. Neuroprotective Effect of Crocin on Acrylamide-induced Cytotoxicity in PC12 cells. Cell Mol. Neurobiol 32, 227–235. https://doi.org/10.1007/s10571-011-9752-8.

Mizoguchi, T., Minakuchi, H., Ishisaka, M., Tsuruma, K., Shimazawa, M., Hara, H., 2017. Behavioral abnormalities with disruption of brain structure in mice overexpressing VGF. Sci. Rep. 7 (1), 4691. https://doi.org/10.1038/s41598-017-04132-7.

Mohamadpour, A.H., Ayati, Z., Parizadeh, M.R., Rajbai, O., Hosseinzadeh, H., 2013. Safety evaluation of crocin (a constituent of saffron) tablets in healthy volunteers. Iran J Basic Med Sci 16 (1), 39–46.

Mohammadi, E., Mehri, S., Badie Bostan, H., Hosseinzadeh, H., 2018 . Protective effect of crocin against d-galactose-induced aging in mice. Avicenna J. Phytomed. 8 (1), 14–23.

Mojaverrostami, S., Bojnordi, M.N., Ghasemi-Kasman, M., Ebrahimzadeh, M.A., Hamidabadi, H.G., 2018. A review of herbal therapy in multiple sclerosis. Adv. Pharmaceut. Bull. 8 (4), 575–590. https://doi.org/10.15171/apb.2018.066.

Mokhtari Hashtjini, M., Pirzad Jahromi, G., GH1, M., Esmaeili, D., Javidnazar, D., 2018. Aqueous extract of saffron administration along with amygdala deep brain stimulation promoted alleviation of symptoms in post-traumatic stress disorder (PTSD) in rats. Avicenna J Phytomed. 8 (4), 358–369.

Nam, K.N., Park, Y.M., Jung, H.J., Lee, J.Y., Min, B.D., Park, S.U., Jung, W.S., Cho, K.H., Park, J.H., Kang, I., Hong, J.W., Lee, E.H., 2010. Anti-inflammatory effects of crocin and crocetin in rat brain microglial cells. Eur. J. Pharmacol. 648 (1–3), 110–116. https://doi.org/10.1016/j.ejphar.2010.09.003. Epub 2010 Sep 18.

Neve, Kim A., Seamans, Jeremy K., Tranthamdavidson, Heather, 2004. Dopamine receptor signaling. J.Rec. Signal Trans. 24 (3), 165–205.

Nemat Shahi, M., Asadi, A., Behnam Talab, E., Nemat Shahi, M., 2017. The impact of saffron on symptoms of withdrawal syndrome in patients undergoing maintenance treatment for opioid addiction in sabzevar parish in 2017. Adv. Met. Med. 2017, 1079132. https://doi.org/10.1155/2017/1079132.

Nishitoh, H., 2012. CHOP is a multifunctional transcription factor in the ER stress response. J. Biochem. 151 (3), 217–219. https://doi.org/10.1093/jb/mvr143.

Pan, P.K., Qiao, L.Y., Wen, X.N., 2016. Safranal prevents rotenone-induced oxidative stress and apoptosis in an in vitro model of Parkinson's disease through regulating Keap1/Nrf2 signaling pathway. Cell. Mol. Biol. 62 (14), 11–17. https://doi.org/10.14715/cmb/2016.62.14.2.

Papandreou, M.A., Kanakis, C.D., Polissiou, M.G., Efthimiopoulos, S., Cordopatis, P., Margarity, M., Lamari, F.N., 2006. Inhibitory activity on amyloid-beta aggregation and antioxidant properties of Crocus sativus stigmas extract and its crocin constituents. J. Agric. Food Chem. 54 (23), 8762–8768.

Papandreou, M.A., Tsachaki, M., Efthimiopoulos, S., Cordopatis, P., Lamari, F.N., Margarity, M., 2011. Memory enhancing effects of saffron in aged mice are correlated with antioxidant protection. Behav. Brain Res. 219 (2), 197–204. https://doi.org/10.1016/j.bbr.2011.01.007.

Papaliagkas, V., Anogianaki, A., Anogianakis, G., Ilonidis, G., 2007. The proteins and the mechanisms of apoptosis: a mini-review of the fundamentals. Hippokratia 11 (3), 108–113.

Penela, P., Murga, C., Ribas, C., Lafarga, V., Mayor Jr., F., 2010. The complex G protein-coupled receptor kinase 2 (GRK2) interactome unveils new physiopathological targets. Br. J. Pharmacol. 160 (4), 821–832. https://doi.org/10.1111/j.1476-5381.2010.00727.x.

Picciotto, M.R., Higley, M.J., Mineur, Y.S., 2012. Acetylcholine as a neuromodulator: cholinergic signaling shapes nervous system function and behaviour. Neuron 76 (1), 116–129.

Prinston, J.E., Emlaw, J.R., Dextraze, M.F., Christian, J., Tessier, G., Javier Pérez Areales, F., McNulty, M.S., Corrie, J., daCosta, B., 2017. Ancestral reconstruction approach to acetylcholine receptor structure and function. Structure 25, 1–8.

Rai, S.N., Dilnashin, H., Birla, H., Singh, S.S., Zahra, W., Rathore, A.S., Singh, B.K., Singh, S.P., 2019. The role of PI3K/akt and ERK in neurodegenerative disorders. Neurotox. Res. 35 (3), 775–795. https://doi.org/10.1007/s12640-019-0003-y.

Rafieipour, F., Hadipour, E., Emami, S.A., Asili, J., Tayarani-Najaran, Z., 2019. Safranal protects against beta-amyloid peptide-induced cell toxicity in PC12 cells via MAPK and PI3 K pathways. Metab. Brain Dis. 34 (1), 165–172. https://doi.org/10.1007/s11011-018-0329-9.

Rao, S.V., Muralidhara, Yenisetti, S.C., Rajini, P.S., 2016. Evidence of neuroprotective effects of saffron and crocin in a Drosophila model of Parkinsonism. Neurotoxicology 52, 230–242. https://doi.org/10.1016/j.neuro.2015.12.010.

Ravindran, A.V., Balneaves, L.G., Faulkner, G., Ortiz, A., McIntosh, D., Morehouse, R.L., Ravindran, L., Yatham, L.N., Kennedy, S.H., Lam, R.W., MacQueen, G.M., Milev, R.V., Parikh, S.V., CANMAT depression work group, 2016. Canadian network for Mood and anxiety treatments (CANMAT) 2016 clinical guidelines for the management of adults with major depressive disorder: section 5. Complementary and alternative medicine treatments. Can. J. Psychiatr. 61 (9), 576–587. https://doi.org/10.1177/0706743716660290.

Razavi, B.M., Sadeghi, M., Abnous, K., Hasani, F.V., Hosseinzadeh, H., 2017. Study of the Role of CREB, BDNF, and VGF Neuropeptide in Long Term Antidepressant Activity of Crocin in the Rat Cerebellum. Iranian Journal of Pharmaceutical Research 16 (4), 1452–1462.

Sadeghnia, H.R., Shaterzadeh, H., Forouzanfar, F., Hosseinzadeh, H., 2017. Neuroprotective effect of safranal, an active ingredient of Crocus sativus, in a rat model of transient cerebral ischemia. Folia Neuropathol 55 (3), 206–213.

Sadeghnia, H.R., Cortez, M., Liu, D., Hosseinzadeh, H., Snead, O.C., 2008. Antiabsence effects of safranal in acute experimental seizure models: EEG and autoradiography. J Pharm Pharmaceut Sci 11 (3), 1–14. www.cspsCanada.org.

Sangiovanni, E., Brivio, P., Dell'Agli, M., Calabrese, F., 2017. Botanicals as modulators of neuroplasticity: focus on BDNF. Neural Plast. 2017, 5965371. https://doi.org/10.1155/2017/5965371.

Sarris, J., Panossian, A., Schweitzer, I., Stough, C., Scholey, A., 2011. Herbal medicine for depression, anxiety and insomnia: a review of psychopharmacology and clinical evidence. Eur. Neuropsychopharmacol. 21 (12), 841–860. https://doi.org/10.1016/j.euroneuro.2011.04.002.

Shafiee, M., Arekhi, S., Omranzadeh, A., Sahebkar, A., 2018. Saffron in the treatment of depression, anxiety and other mental disorders: current evidence and potential mechanisms of action. J. Affect. Disord. 227, 330–337. https://doi.org/10.1016/j.jad.2017.11.020.

Shih, R.H., Wang, C.Y., Yang, C.M., 2015. NF-kappaB signaling pathways in neurological inflammation: a mini review. Front. Mol. Neurosci. 8, 77. https://doi.org/10.3389/fnmol.2015.00077. eCollection 2015.

Skladnev, N.V., Johnstone, D.M., 2017. Neuroprotective properties of dietary saffron: more than just a chemical scavenger? Neural Regen. Res. 12 (2), 210–211.

Tiribuzi, R., Crispoltoni, L., Chiurchiù, V., Casella, A., Montecchiani, C., Del Pino, A.M., Maccarrone, M., Palmerini, C.A., Caltagirone, C., Kawarai, T., Orlacchio, A., Orlacchio, A., 2017. Trans-crocetin improves amyloid-β degradation in monocytes from Alzheimer's Disease patients. J. Neurol. Sci. 372, 408–412. https://doi.org/10.1016/j.jns.2016.11.004.

Vahdati Hassani, F., Naseri, V., Razavi, B.M., Mehri, S., Abnous, K., Hosseinzadeh, H.1, 2014. Antidepressant effects of crocin and its effects on transcript and protein levels of CREB, BDNF, and VGF in rat hippocampus. Daru 22 (1), 16. https://doi.org/10.1186/2008-2231-22-16.

Velazquez, F.N., Caputto, B.L., Boussin, F.D., 2015. c-Fos importance for brain development. Aging (N Y) 7 (12), 1028–1029.

Wang, K., Zhang, L., Rao, W., Su, N., Hui, H., Wang, L., Peng, C., Tu, Y., Zhang, S., Fei, Z., 2015. Neuroprotective effects of crocin against traumatic brain injury in mice: involvement of notch signaling pathway. Neurosci. Lett. 591, 53–58. https://doi.org/10.1016/j.neulet.2015.02.016.

Willard, S.S., Koochekpour, S., 2013. Glutamate, glutamate receptors, and downstream signaling pathways. Int. J. Biol. Sci. 9 (9), 948–959. https://doi.org/10.7150/ijbs.6426. eCollection 2013.

Wirth, A., Holst, K., Ponimaskin, E., 2017. How serotonin receptors regulate morphogenic signalling in neurons. Prog. Neurobiol. 151, 35–56. https://doi.org/10.1016/j.pneurobio.2016.03.007.

Yu, J.Z., Rasenick, M.M., 2012. Receptor signaling and the cell biology of synaptic transmission. Handb. Clin. Neurol. 106, 9–35. https://doi.org/10.1016/B978-0-444-52002-9.00002-4.

Zhang, G.F., Zhang, Y., Zhao, G., 2015. Crocin protects PC12 cells against MPP (+)-induced injury through inhibition of mitochondrial dysfunction and ER stress. Neurochem. Int. 89, 101–110. https://doi.org/10.1016/j.neuint.2015.07.011.

Zhang, J., Wang, Y., Dong, X., Liu, J., 2018. Crocetin attenuates inflammation and amyloid-β accumulation in APPsw transgenic mice. Immun. Ageing 15, 24.

Zheng, Y.Q., Liu, J.X., Li, X.Z., Xu, L., 2010. Effects and mechanism of Weinaokang on reperfusion-induced vascular injury to cerebral microvessels after global cerebral ischemia. Chin. J. Integr. Med. 16 (2), 145–150. https://doi.org/10.1007/s11655-010-0145-5.

CHAPTER 11

Assessment of Crocus sativus L., and Its Bioactive Constituents as Potential Anti-Anxiety Compounds. Basic and Clinical Evidence

NIKOLAOS PITSIKAS

INTRODUCTION

Anxiety

Anxiety is among the most serious and devastating mental disorders. It can be considered as an adaptive psychological, physiological, and behavioral situation which induces coping when compared with a probable menace (Steimer, 2002). The result of a conspicuous number of epidemiological studies indicates that anxiety-related disorders have the highest lifetime prevalence estimates (13.6%–28.8%) and the earliest age of onset (11 years) among the various psychiatric diseases (Kessler et al., 2005a, 2005b).

Several types of this psychiatric disease such as generalized anxiety disorder (GAD), specific phobias (agoraphobia, social phobia, etc.), posttraumatic stress disorder (PTSD), obsessive-compulsive disorder (OCD), and panic disorder have been described. Common symptoms of all these disorders are temporary worry and exaggerated fear. In particular, GAD comprises persistent and excessive anxiety and worry about ordinary, routine issues. Specific phobias are characterized by intense anxiety when a subject is exposed to a particular object or social situation and desires to avoid it. PTSD is manifested with different reexperiencing, avoidance/numbing, and hyperarousal symptoms after exposure to a life-threatening event that results in psychological trauma. OCD is an anxiety disorder involving the presence of excessive thoughts (obsessions) that are accompanied by repetitive actions (compulsions). Panic disorder includes recurrent episodes of sudden feelings of major anxiety, fear, or terror that can yield their higher expression within few minutes (panic attacks).

All the aforementioned pathologies represent a serious public health issue all around the world (Steimer, 2002).

Different pharmacological approaches are currently used to alleviate the symptoms of this psychiatric illness. Agents acting on the γ-aminobutyric acid (GABA), serotonergic, and noradrenergic neurotransmission, as are benzodiazepines, partial agonists of the serotonergic 5-HT$_{1A}$ receptor, selective serotonin reuptake inhibitors (SSRIs), and serotonin noradrenaline reuptake inhibitors (SNRIs), are widely used for this purpose (Hoffman and Mathew, 2008).

In spite of it, some types of anxiety do not respond satisfactorily to challenge with the aforementioned medications (Hammer et al., 2004; Van Ameringen et al., 2004). Moreover, benzodiazepines, SSRIs, and SNRIs can be linked with undesired effects, such as sedation, cognitive impairments, dependence and withdrawal, sexual malfunction, gastrointestinal effects, and increment of body weight. In addition, buspirone, a 5-HT$_{1A}$ receptor partial agonist is not largely used, although it is generally well tolerated with few side effects because its efficiency is weaker and onset of action, similarly to SSRIs and SNRIs, is slower with respect to the benzodiazepines (Cryan and Sweeney, 2011).

Based on the aforementioned evidence, there is an imperative requirement to unfold new compounds for the therapy of this serious psychiatric disease (Gorman, 2003). Among the various alternative approaches for the treatment of anxiety, the implication of the plant saffron (Crocus sativus L.) and its constituents as potential antianxiety agents has recently been proposed. In

Saffron. https://doi.org/10.1016/B978-0-12-818462-2.00011-5

the present review, I intend to evaluate with a critical spirit the therapeutic potential of *Crocus sativus* L. (*C. sativus*) and its active components for the treatment of anxiety. Current analysis indicates that these molecules might represent an interesting alternative for the pharmacotherapy of anxiety.

C. sativus

C. sativus is a perennial plant and a member of the Iridaceae family, the line of Liliaceae. This herb is cultivated in various nations all around the world with moderate and dry climates such as Azerbaijan, China, France, Greece, Egypt, India, Iran, Israel, Italy, Mexico, Morocco, Spain, and Turkey. The spice saffron is the final product of this plant. Saffron, in filaments, is the dried dark-red stigmas of *C. sativus* flower. The weight of each stigma of this herb is circa 2 mg, and each flower contain three stigmatas; 150,000 flowers, thoroughly collected, are required to obtain 1 kg of spice. Saffron has a characteristic color, aroma, and taste. It is used either as a food ingredient or as a perfume (Liakopoulou-Kyriakides and Kyriakidis, 2002). In traditional medicine, saffron is largely used as a therapeutic agent for the treatment of pathologies related to cardiovascular, respiratory, gastroenteric, and nervous system (for review see Rios et al., 1996). Moreover, saffron has broadly been used in the Persian folk medicine for attenuating cognitive disorders (Akhondzadeh, 2007).

The chemical profile of C. sativus

An assay of *C. sativus* stigmas has evidenced the presence of circa 150 volatile and nonvolatile components. Up to our days, less than 50 components, however, have been recognized. Terpenes, terpene alcohols, and the respective esters are the constituents of the volatile components of saffron (Winterhalter and Straubinger, 2000).

Crocin, crocetin, picrocrocin, safranal, and flavonoids such as quercetin and kaempferol are the prevailing nonvolatile compounds (Liakopoulou-Kyriakides and Kyriakidis, 2002). Crocins, glucosyl esters of crocetin, are water-soluble carotenoids and are accountable for saffron's typical color. The glycoside of safranal, picrocrocin, is responsible for the bitter taste of the spice. Safranal, the main component of the distilled essential oil, is a monoterpene aldehyde and confers the typical flavor (Tarantilis et al., 1995; Kanakis et al., 2004). The chemical structures of *C. sativus*, crocin, and safranal which seem to be implicated in anxiety are plotted in Fig. 11.1.

Pharmacological profile of C. sativus and its constituents

Based on a plethora of preclinical and clinical findings, an interesting pharmacological profile of saffron and its bioactive ingredients is emerging.

Effects of *C. sativus* and its constituents on nonneurological/neuropsychiatric pathologies. In a series of in vitro and in vivo studies, the anticancer action of *C. sativus* has been revealed. Furthermore, in a series of in vitro and in vivo studies, it has been demonstrated that this spice and its active components expressed antinociceptive and antiinflammatory properties and were able to diminish atherosclerosis and hepatic damage, attenuate hyperlipidemia, confer protection from myocardial injury, and consistently reduce blood pressure (for review, see Rios et al., 1996; Abdullaev and Espinosa-Aguirre, 2004; Bathaie and Mousavi, 2010; Alavizadeh and Hosseinzadeh, 2014).

What emerges from these findings is that *C. sativus* and its active ingredients seem to display a beneficial effect in various preclinical models of different diseases. Interestingly, up to now, there is lack of clinical data supporting the therapeutic efficiency of saffron in the aforementioned diseases. Therefore, clinical studies should be designed and performed to properly address this issue.

Effects of *C. sativus* and its constituents on pathologies of the central nervous system. Preclinical research has revealed that the aqueous and ethanolic extracts of *C. sativus* and safranal possess anticonvulsant properties. In addition, these molecules were found to be protective in animal models of Parkinson's disease (PD) and cerebral ischemia (for review, see Pitsikas, 2015).

Accumulating experimental evidence shows that both *C. sativus* and crocin were efficacious in counteracting disruption of memory in animal models related to Alzheimer's disease (AD), cerebral injuries, or schizophrenia. The outcome of human studies designed to assess the efficiency of saffron in alleviating memory problems, a common feature of AD, indicates that the effects exerted by *C. sativus* on cognition, although weak, were similar than those displayed by the reference drugs donepezil and memantine. It is important to underline that in all human studies, treatment performed with saffron did not produce noticeable undesired effects (for review, see Pitsikas, 2015, 2016).

In a series of preclinical studies, an antidepressant-like effect of *C. sativus*, crocin, and safranal was observed

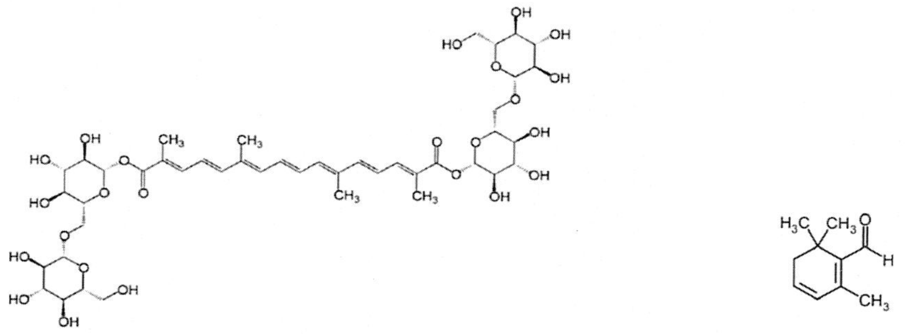

Crocin   **Safranal**

FIG. 11.1   Chemical structures of crocin and safranal.

(Hosseinzadeh et al., 2004). In agreement with the aforementioned facts, clinical research findings suggest that saffron is efficacious for the treatment of mild-to-moderate depression (Akhondzadeh et al., 2004; Noorbala et al., 2005). Moreover, it has been reported that saffron alleviated sexual malfunction in humans caused by treatment with the SSRI antidepressant agent fluoxetine (Kashani et al., 2012; Modabbernia et al., 2012).

Up to now, there is little information concerning a potential therapeutic action of saffron in schizophrenia. In this context, it has been reported that crocin attenuated psychotomimetic effects, including cognition deficits, in animal models of this devastating psychiatric disease, reflecting abnormal glutamatergic or dopaminergic activity (Georgiadou et al., 2014; Pitsikas and Tarantilis, 2017). Further studies are mandatory aiming to elucidate this important issue.

Safety studies. Toxicological investigations performed in rodents that received saffron extracts have shown that the hematological and the biochemical parameters of the rodents remained at physiological levels (Nair et al., 1991). Furthermore, it has been found that the oral LD_{50} of *C. sativus* was 20.7 g/kg when it was delivered as a decoction in mice (Abdullaev, 2002). In line with what is mentioned previously, mice treated acutely (up to 3 g, either orally [p.o.] or intraperitoneally [i.p.]) and repeatedly with crocin (15−180 mg/kg, i.p.) did not show alterations in a series of biochemical, hematological, and pathological markers recorded (Hosseinzadeh et al., 2010).

The safety of *C. sativus* extracts and crocin have been confirmed in investigations performed in humans. In particular, in a double-blind, placebo-controlled study carried out on healthy volunteers, a 7-day challenge with saffron (200−400 mg/day) did not induce significant abnormalities. It caused only some minor clinical

and laboratory parameter changes such as hypotension, reduced platelets, and bleeding time and increased creatinine and blood urea nitrogen levels (Modagheghi et al., 2008).

In agreement with the aforementioned points are the findings of another clinical trial conducted on healthy participants who received 20 mg/day of crocin for 30 consecutive days. Treatment with crocin did not produce any alteration of various hematological, biochemical, hormonal, and urinary parameters recorded (Mohamadpour et al., 2013).

Finally, administration of very high doses of saffron (1.2−2 g) in healthy volunteers induced nausea, diarrhea, vomiting, and bleeding (Schmidt et al., 2007). In summary, saffron and its main bioactive components can be considered as safe natural products displaying very low toxicity.

EFFECTS OF *C. SATIVUS* AND ITS CONSTITUENTS ON ANXIETY
Preclinical Evidence

Table 11.1 summarizes the preclinical studies performed, aiming to assess the efficiency of *C. sativus* and its bioactive components as potential antianxiety agents.

In a series of behavioral investigations performed in the rat, the anxiolytic-like effect of crocin was revealed (Pitsikas et al., 2008; Georgiadou et al., 2012). In particular, acute challenge with 50 mg/kg of crocin, similar to the reference drug diazepam (1.5 mg/kg), augmented the time to enter the dark chamber, did not influence the number of transitions between the different chambers of the apparatus, and increased the time spent in the illuminated chamber of the light/dark box (Pitsikas et al., 2008). Additionally, crocin (30 and 50 mg/kg, acutely) reduced compulsive episodes (excessive self-

TABLE 11.1
Effects of Crocus sativus L. and its Active Constituents on Animal Models of Anxiety

Species	Agent	Dose Range	Route	Behavioral Test	Effect	Reference
Rat	Crocin	15, 30, 50 mg/kg	i.p. acute	Light/dark box Motor activity	Anxiolytic-like (50 mg/kg) effect No effect	Pitsikas et al. (2008)
Mouse	CSAE Crocin Safranal	56, 80, 320, 560 mg/kg 50, 200, 600 mg/kg 0.05, 0.15, 0.35 mL/kg	i.p. acute i.p. acute i.p. acute	EPM Open field Rotarod	CSAE (56, 80 mg/kg), safranal (0.15, 0.35 mL/kg) anxiolytic effect. Crocin was ineffective. CSAE (dose-dependently), crocin (200–600 mg/kg), reduced motility, grooming, rearing, leaning. Safranal (0.05, 0.15 mL/kg) reduced motility; (0.15, 0.35 mL/kg) increased grooming, leaning, rearing. CSAE (dose-dependently) decreased motor coordination. Crocin and safranal were ineffective.	Hosseinzadeh and Noraei (2009)
Mouse	CSAE CSEE Crocin Safranal	1, 5, 10 mg/kg 1, 5, 10 mg/kg 1, 5, 10 mg/kg 1, 5, 10 mg/kg	i.p. acute i.p. acute i.p. acute i.p. acute	Food intake	CSAE and crocin decreased stress-induced anorexia. Plasma corticosterone levels were not increased in CSAE and crocin-treated mice. CSEE and safranal were ineffective.	Halatei et al. (2011)
Rat	Crocins m-CPP	15, 30 mg/kg 0.6 mg/kg	i.p. acute i.p. acute.	Measurement of grooming behavior Motor activity	Attenuated mCPP-induced excessive grooming (anxiolytic effect). No effect	Georgiadou et al. (2012)
Rat	CSAE DBS CSAE + DBS	5 mg/kg	i.p. sub- chronic	CFC EPM c-fos expression	CSAE alone reduced freezing behavior CSAE alone anxiolytic-like effect DBS alone ineffective CSAE + DBS anxiolytic-like effect CSAE alone decreased c-fos expression in amygdala CSAE + DBS decreased c-fos expression in amygdala CSAE, DBS and their combination increased serum corticosterone levels	Mokhtari-Hashtjini et al. (2018)

CSAE, Crocus sativus aqueous extracts; *CSEE*, Crocus sativus ethanolic extracts; *CFC*, contextual fear conditioning; *DBS*, deep brain stimulation; *EPM*, elevated plus maze; *i.p.*, intraperitoneally; *mCPP*, 1-(3-chlorophenyl)piperazine.

grooming) in rats caused by the serotonergic 5-HT$_{2c}$ receptor agonist m-CPP (0.6 mg/kg) (Georgiadou et al., 2012). Importantly, crocin did not affect the motor activity of the rats. The outcome of these experiments proposes that crocin displays an antianxiety action, which cannot be ascribed to alterations in motility (Pitsikas et al., 2008; Georgiadou et al., 2012).

Additionally, it has been reported that aqueous extracts of saffron (56 and 80 mg/kg) and safranal (0.15 and 0.35 mL/kg) as well diazepam (3 mg/kg) acutely injected in mice induced an anxiolytic-like effect since they augmented the time spent in the open arms of an elevated plus maze. At higher dose range (320 and 560 mg/kg), saffron did not express any anxiolytic effect. Of note, in this study, all doses of saffron tested caused sedation since they diminished the motor abilities of mice. Similarly, low doses of safranal (0.05 and 0.15 mL/kg) reduced rodents' motor activity and increased self-grooming activity and rearing episodes. Crocin (50−600 mg/kg) did not influence the performance of mice in the elevated plus maze test, but at 200 and 600 mg/kg, it induced hypomotility (Hosseinzadeh and Noraei, 2009).

The findings of this experimentation (Hosseinzadeh and Noraei, 2009) appear to be in disagreement with other reports (Pitsikas et al., 2008; Georgiadou et al., 2012) in which the anxiolytic effect of crocin observed was not confounded by sedation. These contrasting results may be ascribed to the different species of animals used and to diverse study protocols applied.

Furthermore, a single injection of aqueous extracts of saffron (1−10 mg/kg), crocin (1−10 mg/kg) but not of ethanolic extracts of C. sativus (1−10 mg/kg) and safranal (1−10 mg/kg) diminished anorexia caused by stress and did not affect serum corticosterone concentrations in mice. Overall, these findings propose that saffron and crocin might possess an antistress profile (Halatei et al., 2011).

Finally, subchronic treatment with aqueous extracts of saffron (5 mg/kg, once a day for seven consecutive days) alone or in combination with amygdala deep brain stimulation (DBS) reduced anxiety symptoms, evaluated in the elevated plus maze test, in a rat model of PTSD. The same group also reported that either saffron or the combination of it with DBS normalized plasmatic corticosterone concentrations and diminished c-fos expression in rat's amygdala (Mokhtari-Hashtjini et al., 2018).

As a whole, although few, the preclinical results here reported propose an antianxiety effect of C. sativus and crocin of a certain consistency. In spite of it, there are some limitations underlying these promising preclinical results. First, data were revealed in experiments carried out in male rodents using acute treatment schedule with the exception of the study by Mokhtari-Hashtjini et al. in which a subchronic treatment condition was applied. In addition, the effects of this spice and its bioactive ingredients were tested solely in animal models of anxiety which are based on the conflict between the desire to explore and avoidance of new spaces (Bouwknecht and Paylor, 2008). Finally, there is a lack of information concerning the effects of these molecules on preclinical models resembling phobias or panic attacks.

Clinical Evidence

Table 11.2 summarizes the results of the clinical studies conducted, in which the efficiency of saffron on anxiety was evaluated.

A first randomized double-blind trial was conducted in 102 patients for herniorrhaphy surgery. Administration of saffron (25 mg/day) for 32 weeks reduced anxiety symptoms in these preoperative patients (Basiri-Mohadam et al., 2016). Subsequently, a double-blind, randomized and placebo-controlled study was performed with 62 anxiety patients. Treatment with 50 mg of C. sativus capsule, twice per day, for 12 weeks, significantly affected Back Anxiety Inventory (BAI) questionnaire, eliciting thus an antianxiety action of saffron (Mazidi et al., 2016).

Furthermore, in a subsequent double-blind randomized study, an anti-OCD effect of saffron was observed. Specifically, 46 patients with mild-to-moderate OCD were treated with saffron (15 or 30 mg/day saffron for 10 weeks), and the efficacy of treatment was compared with that of the SSRI fluvoxamine (100 mg/day). Utilizing the Yale-Brown Obsessive Compulsive Scale (Y-BOCS), saffron was identified to be efficacious as fluvoxamine in alleviating OCD symptoms. A weak point of this study was the lack of a placebo group and the small number of participants (Esalatmanesh et al., 2017).

A subsequent double-blind randomized trial indicated that using the Depression, Anxiety and Stress Scale (DASS-21) affron, a standardized stigmas extract of saffron, administered for a shorter period (4 weeks) and at a lower dose range (22−28 mg/day), except to prior experimentations, reduced anxiety (28 mg/day) in 128 low-mood healthy participants. The authors, however, acknowledged that the subjective nature of self-reporting of low mood at screening might be a weak point of this study (Kell et al., 2017).

Another double-blinded randomized trial aiming to evaluate the antianxiety effects of saffron was conducted in 40 patients with mild-to-moderate GAD, under treatment with the SSRI sertraline. Using the Hamilton Anxiety Rating Scale (HAM-A), the combination of saffron

(450 mg/day for 6 weeks) with sertraline (50 mg/day) attenuated GAD symptoms. The limitation of this study resides to the small number of participants and to impossibility, for ethical concerns, to assess the effects of saffron alone (Jafarnia et al., 2017).

Lopresti et al. evaluated the efficacy of affron as an antianxiety agent in a small size of samples (80 adolescents) suffering from mild-to-moderate anxiety using the Revised Child Anxiety and Depression Scale (RCADS) as the outcome measure. In this double-blind, placebo-controlled trial, affron (14 mg/day, twice per day, for 8 weeks) lowered anxiety symptoms accordingly to the view of the adolescent patients (self-report). By contrast, these presumed beneficial effects were not supported by parents. This could represent a limit in the utilization of self-report questionnaires as the only parameter recorded of treatment efficiency. Validation through clinician-rated measures may, thus, be cautious in subsequent experiments. This inconsistency observed between adolescents and reports of first degree relatives may depend on parents' own status of mental health (Lopresti et al., 2018).

Finally, the therapeutic effect of administration of saffron in 54 type 2 diabetic patients suffering from mild to moderate comorbid depression-anxiety (CDA) was evaluated using the HAM-A scale. Saffron given at 30 mg/day for 8 weeks lowered anxiety symptoms in the diabetics. In spite of it, also the present clinical trial suffers from different limitations such as the small sample size and the lack of a dose-response effect (Milajerdi et al., 2018).

Collectively, the outcome of the clinical trials aiming to test the ability of saffron in alleviating anxiety symptoms propose an anxiolytic effect of it, which importantly was not confounded by adverse side effects. On the other hand, all these human studies, although promising, present some limitations, including the narrow dose range tested, the small number of participants, and the lack of information regarding the effects of other main components of saffron on anxiety disorders.

Potential mechanism(s) of Action of C. sativus and its Constituents in anxiety Disorders

The mechanism(s) through which *C. sativus* and its bioactive components exert their antianxiety effects is not yet clarified. It has been previously demonstrated that the effects of crocin on an animal model of anxiety were not different than those exerted by the benzodiazepine anxiolytic diazepam (Pitsikas et al., 2008). It is well documented that the antianxiety effects of benzodiazepines are mediated by their agonistic action on the $GABA_A$ receptor. In this context, it has been observed that some other flavonoids isolated from plants express an affinity for the benzodiazepine-binding site at the $GABA_A$ receptor (Ai et al., 1997;

TABLE 11.2
Summary of Clinical Trials on *Crocus sativus* L., as Treatment for Anxiety.

Design of Study	Duration of Study	Severity of Disease	Agent	Dose Range	Route	Effect	Reference
Double-blind	32 weeks	Presurgery patients	Cs	25 mg/day	p.o.	Anxiolytic and safe.	(Basiri-Mohadam et al., 2016)
Double-blind	12 weeks	Anxiety	Cs	50 mg/twice per day	p.o.	Anxiolytic and safe	(Mazidi et al., 2016)
Double-blind	10 weeks	Mild to moderate OCD	Cs	15 mg/twice per day	p.o.	Effective and safe	Esalatmanesh et al. (2017)
Double-blind		Low mood	affron		p.o.		(Kell et al., 2017)
Double-blind	4 weeks	healthy	Cs	22–28 mg/day	p.o.	Anxiolytic and safe (28 mg/day)	(Jafarnia et al., 2017)
Double-blind		volunteers	Sertraline	450 mg/day	p.o.		(Lopresti et al., 2018)
Double-blind	6 weeks	Mild to moderate GAD under treatment with sertraline	affron Cs	(50 mg/day) 14 mg/twice per day	p.o.	Anxiolytic and safe Anxiolytic and safe	(Milajerdi et al., 2018)
	8 weeks	Youth anxiety		30 mg/day		Anxiolytic and safe	
	8 weeks	Type-2 diabetic patients suffering from CDA					

CDA, comorbid depression anxiety; *Cs*, *Crocus sativus* L.; *GAD*, generalized anxiety disorder; *OCD*, obsessive compulsive disorder; *p.o.*, orally.

Marder et al., 2001). It cannot be excluded that the anxiolytic effects of saffron and its components are exerted by the aforementioned mechanism.

In addition, a consistent body of evidence suggests the involvement of inflammation and oxidative stress in the pathogenesis of anxiety. Specifically, it has been reported that different inflammatory markers including cytokines and C-reactive proteins are elevated in anxiety disorders (for review, see Michopoulos et al., 2017). The outcome of preclinical studies indicates a consistent increase in reactive oxygen species (ROS) accumulation in neurons and lipid and protein peroxidation in rodents' hippocampus and amygdala (Salim, 2014). In line with what is mentioned previously, clinical research has shown that different oxidative biomarkers were found elevated in patients with social phobia, PTSD, and OCD (for review, see Smaga et al., 2015).

The well-known potent antiinflammatory and antioxidant properties of saffron and its bioactive ingredients revealed in different preclinical studies may provide an explanation for the therapeutic action of these agents in anxiety disorders. In particular, saffron was found to significantly reduce different proinflammatory factors including cytokines, B cells, to inhibit interleukin (IL)-1β-induced activation of the nuclear factor kappa B (NF-κB) and decrease the mRNA expression of tumor necrosis factor α (TNFα) (for review, see Boskabady and Farkhondeh, 2016).

Moreover, in a broad number of preclinical reports, the antioxidant profile of C. sativus and its components has also been evidenced. These molecules decreased the high plasmatic concentrations of malondialdehyde (MDA), glutathione peroxidase enzyme activity (GSHPx), and inhibited ROS production. Additionally, saffron increased superoxide dismutase (SOD), total glutathione (GSH), and catalase (CAT) (Boskabady and Farkhondeh, 2016).

CONCLUSIONS AND FUTURE PLANS

In summary, although few, the preclinical results here presented propose an antianxiety effect of C. sativus and crocin of a certain consistency. Various important issues, however, have not yet been addressed. Future studies should evaluate the efficacy of these molecules as anxiolytics in all types of anxiety disorders (there is a lack of information concerning the effects of these agents on preclinical models resembling phobias or panic attacks), by using also female rodents and both acute and chronic treatment schedules. Regarding this issue, it is important to emphasize that anxiety disorders are occurring with higher frequency to women than men (Hu and Zhu, 2017). Finally, future research should examine the potential antianxiety action of saffron and its main constituents using a variety of behavioral procedures including the ultrasonic vocalization, the stress-induced hypothermia, and various conflict tests such as the Geller-Seifter and the Vogel conflict tests (Bouwknecht and Paylor, 2008).

Clinical research results, although promising, might be considered preliminary because the number of participants was inconsistent. Nevertheless, it is worth to underline the good safety profile of saffron which was observed in all human studies.

Future multicenter clinical trials, therefore, should be conducted, aiming to definitively establish the potential anxiolytic effects of saffron and its constituents. These future studies should evaluate the efficacy of saffron and its components in the entire spectrum of anxiety disorders, using a wide dose range and most importantly recruiting an appropriate number of participants. A summary of some further investigations aiming to examine the efficacy of saffron and its bioactive components as anxiolytics is illustrated in Table 11.3.

TABLE 11.3
Summary of Future Studies Designed to Evaluate the Role of C. sativus and its Constituents in Anxiety—Key Proposals

Preclinical research

Male versus female rodents

Unconditioned non—exploration-driven anxiety-related tests versus conditioned non—exploration-driven anxiety-related tests

Acute versus repeated drug treatment

Animal models of panic attacks and phobias

Clinical research

Studies of the effects of saffron alone in patients of all the different anxiety types

Use of broad dose range of C. sativus

Appropriate number of participants

REFERENCES

Abdullaev, F.I., 2002. Cancer chemoprotective and tumoricidal properties of saffron (*Crocus sativus* L.). Exp. Biol. Med. 227, 20—25.

Abdullaev, F.I., Espinosa-Aguirre, J.J., 2004. Biomedical properties of saffron and its potential use in cancer therapy and chemoprevention trials. Cancer Detect. Prev. 28, 426—432.

Ai, J., Dekermendjian, K., Wang, X., Nielsen, M., Witt, M.R., 1997. 6-methylflavone, a benzodiazepine receptor ligand with antagonistic properties on rat brain and human recombinant GABA(A) receptors in vitro. Drug Dev. Res. 41, 99—106.

Akhondzadeh, S., Fallah-Pour, H., Afkham, K., Jamshidi, A.H., Khalighi-Cigaroudi, F., 2004. Comparison of *Crocus sativus* L., and imipramine in the treatment of mild to moderate depression: a pilot double-blind, randomized trial. BMC Complement Altern. Med. 4, 12—16.

Akhondzadeh, S., 2007. Herbal medicine in the treatment of psychiatric and neurological disorders. In: Abate, L. (Ed.), Low-cost Approaches to Promote Physical and Mental Health: Theory, Research and Practice. Springer, New York, USA, pp. 119—138.

Alavizadeh, S.H., Hosseinzadeh, H., 2014. Bioactivity assessment and toxicity of crocin: a comprehensive review. Food Chem. Toxicol. 64, 65—80.

Basiri-Mohadam, M., Hamzei, A., Moslem, A.R., Pasban-Noghabi, S., Ghorbani, N., Ghenaati, J., 2016. Comparison of the anxiolytic effects of saffron (Crocus sativus L.) and diazepam before herniorrhaphy surgery: a double blind randomized clinical trial. Zahedan J. Res. Med. Sci. 18.

Bathaie, S.Z., Mousavi, S.Z., 2010. New applications and mechanisms of action of saffron and its important ingredients. Crit. Rev. Food Sci. Nutr. 50, 761—786.

Boskabady, M.H., Farkhondeh, T., 2016. Antiinflammatory, antioxidant and immunomodulatory effects of Crocus sativus L. and its main constituents. Phytother Res. 30, 1072—1094.

Bouwknecht, J.A., Paylor, R., 2008. Pitfalls in the interpretation of genetic and pharmacological effects of anxiety-like behaviour in rodents. Behav. Pharmacol. 19, 385—402.

Cryan, J.F., Sweeney, F.F., 2011. The age of anxiety: role of animal models of anxiolytic action in drug discovery. Br. J. Pharmacol. 164, 1129—1161.

Esalatmanesh, S., Biuseh, M., Noorbala, A.A., Mostafavi, S.A., Rezaei, F., Mesqarpour, B., Mohammadinejad, P., Akhondzadeh, S., 2017. Comparison of saffron and fluvoxamine in the treatment of mild to moderate obsessive-compulsive disorder: a double blind randomized clinical trial. Iran. J. Psychiatry 12, 154—162.

Georgiadou, G., Tarantilis, P.A., Pitsikas, N., 2012. Effects of the active constituents of Crocus Sativus L., crocins in an animal model of obsessive-compulsive disorder. Neurosci. Lett. 528, 27—30.

Georgiadou, G., Grivas, V., Tarantilis, P.A., Pitsikas, N., 2014. Crocins the active constituents of *Crocus Sativus* L., counteracted ketamine-induced behavioural deficits in rats. Psychopharmacology 231, 717—726.

Gorman, J.M., 2003. New molecule targets for antianxiety interventions. J. Clin. Psychiatry 64, 28—35.

Halatei, B.S., Khosravi, M., Sahrei, H., Golmanesch, L., Zardooz, H., Jalili, C., Ghoshoomi, H., 2011. Saffron (Crocus sativus) aqueous extract and its constituent crocin reduces stress-induced anorexia in mice. Phytother Res. 25, 1833—1838.

Hammer, M.B., Robert, S., Fruech, B.S., 2004. Treatment-resistant posttraumatic stress disorder: strategies for intervention. CNS Spectr. 9, 740—752.

Hoffman, E.J., Mathew, S.J., 2008. Anxiety disorders: a comprehensive review of pharmacotherapies. Mt. Sinai J. Med. 75, 248—262.

Hosseinzadeh, H., Karimi, G., Niapoor, M., 2004. Antidepressant effects of *crocus sativus* stigma extracts and its constituents, crocins and safranal in mice. J. Med. Plants 3, 48—58.

Hosseinzadeh, H., Noraei, N.B., 2009. Anxiolytic and hypnotic effect of *Crocus sativus* aqueous extract and its constituent, crocins and safranal in mice. Phytother Res. 23, 768—774.

Hosseinzadeh, H., Motamedshariaty, V.S., Sameni, A.K., Vahabzadeh, M., 2010. Acute and sub-acute toxicity of crocin, a constituent of *Crocus sativus* L., (saffron), in mice and rats. Pharmacologyonline 2, 943—951.

Hu, Y., Zhu, D.Y., 2017. Hippocampus and nitric oxide. Vitam. Horm. 96, 127—160.

Jafarnia, N., Ghorbani, Z., Nokhostin, M., Manayi, A., Nourimajad, S., Jahroni, S.R., 2017. Effect of saffron (*Crocus sativus* L.) as an add-on therapy to sertraline in mild to moderate generalized anxiety disorder: a double blind randomized controlled trial. Arch. Neurosci. 4, e14332.

Kanakis, C.D., Daferera, D.J., Tarantilis, P.A., Polissiou, M.G., 2004. Qualitative determination of volatile compounds and quantitative evaluation of safranal and 4-hydroxy-2,6,6-trimethyl-1-cyclohexene-1-carboxaldehyde. J. Agric. Food Chem. 52, 4515—4521.

Kashani, L., Raisi, F., Saroukhani, S., Sohrabi, H., Modabbemia, A., Nasehi, A.A., Jamshidi, A., Ashrafi, M., Mansouri, P., Gheli, P., Akhondzadeh, S., 2012. Saffron for treatment of fluoxetine-induced sexual dysfunction in women: randomized double-blind placebo-controlled study. Hum. Psychopharmacol. 28, 54—60.

Kell, G., Rao, A., Beccaria, G., Clayton, P., Inarejos-Garcia, A.M., Prodanov, M., 2017. Affron a novel saffron extract (*Crocus sativus* L.) improves mood in healthy adults over 4 weeks in a double-blind, parallel, randomized, placebo-controlled clinical trial. Complement. Ther. Med. 33, 58—64.

Kessler, R.C., Berglund, P., Demler, O., Jin, R., Merikangas, K.R., Walters, E.E., 2005a. Lifetime prevalence and age-of-onset distributions of DSM-IV disorders in the national comorbidity survey replication. Arch. Gen. Psychiatry 62, 593—602.

Kessler, R.C., Chiu, W.T., Demler, O., Merikangas, K.R., Walters, E.E., 2005b. Prevalence, severity, and comorbidity of 12-month DSM-IV disorders in the national comorbidity survey replication. Arch. Gen. Psychiatry 62, 617—627.

Liakopoulou-Kyriakides, M., Kyriakidis, D., 2002. *Crocus Sativus*-biological active constituents. Stud. Nat. Prod. Chem. 16, 293–312.

Lopresti, A.L., Drummond, P.D., Inarejos-Garcia, A.M., Prodanov, M., 2018. Affron, a standardised extract from saffron (*Crocus sativus* L.) for the treatment of youth anxiety and depressive symptoms> a randomised, double-blind, placebo-controlled study. J. Affect. Disord. 232, 349–357.

Marder, M., Estiu, G., Blanch, L.B., Viola, H., Wasowski, C., Medina, J.H., Paladini, A.C., 2001. Molecular modelling and QSAR analysis of the interaction of flavone derivatives with the benzodiazepine binding site of the GABA(A) receptor complex. Bioorg. Med. Chem. 9, 323–335.

Mazidi, M., Shemshian, M., Mousavi, S.H., Norouzi, A., Kermani, T., Moghiman, T., Sadeghi, A., Mokhber, N., Ghayour-Mobarhan, M., Ferns, G.A., 2016. A double-blind, randomized and placebo-controlled trial of Saffron (*Crocus sativus* L.) in the treatment of anxiety and depression. J. Complement. Integr. Med. 13, 195–199.

Michopoulos, V., Powers, A., Gillespie, C.F., Ressler, K.J., Jovanovic, T., 2017. Inflammation in fear- and anxiety-based disorders: PTSD, GAD and beyond. Neuropsychopharmacology 42, 254–270.

Milajerdi, A., Jazayeri, S., Shirzadi, E., Hashemzadeh, N., Azizqoi, A., Djazayery, A., Esmaillzadeh, A., Akhondzadeh, S., 2018. The effects of alcoholic extract of saffron (*Crocus sativus* L.) on mild to moderate comorbid depression-anxiety, sleep quality, and life satisfaction in type 2 diabetes mellitus: a double-blind, randomized and placebo-controlled clinical trial. Complement. Ther. Med. 41, 196–202.

Modabbernia, A., Sohrabi, H., Nasehi, A.A., Raisi, F., Saroukhani, S., Jamshidi, A., Tabrizi, M., Asshrafi, M., Akhondzadeh, S., 2012. Effect of saffron on fluoxetine-induced sexual impairment in men: randomized double-blind placebo-controlled trial. Psychopharmacology 223, 381–388.

Modagheghi, M.H., Shahabian, M., Esmaeli, H.A., Rajbai, O., Hosseinzadeh, H., 2008. Safety evaluation of saffron (*Crocus sativus*) tablets in healthy volunteers. Phytomedicine 15, 1032–1037.

Mohamadpour, A.H., Ayati, Z., Parizadeh, M.R., Rajbai, O., Hosseinzadeh, H., 2013. Safety evaluation of crocin (a constituent of saffron) tablets in healthy volunteers. Iran J. Basic Med. Sci. 16, 39–46.

Mokhtari-Hashtjini, M., Pirzad-Jahromi, G., Meftahi, G.H., Esmaeili, D., Javidnazar, D., 2018. Aqueous extract of saffron administration along with amygdala deep brain stimulation promoted alleviation of symptoms in post-traumatic stress disorder (PTSD) in rats. Avicenna J. Phytomed. 8, 358–369.

Nair, S.C., Panikkar, B., Panikkar, K.R., 1991. Antitumor activity of saffron. Cancer Lett. 57, 109–114.

Noorbala, A.A., Akhondzadeh, S., Tahmacebi-Pour, N., Jamshidi, A.H., 2005. Hydro-alcoholic extract of *Crocus sativus* L., versus fluoxetine in the treatment of mild to moderate depression: a double-blind, randomized trial. J. Ethnopharmacol. 97, 281–284.

Pitsikas, N., Boultadakis, A., Georgiadou, G., Tarantilis, P.A., Sakellaridis, N., 2008. Effects of the active constituents of *Crocus Sativus* L., crocins, in an animal model of anxiety. Phytomedicine 15, 1135–1139.

Pitsikas, N., 2015. The effects of Crocus sativus L. and its constituents on memory: basic studies and clinical applications. Evid. Based Complement. Altern. Med. 926284.

Pitsikas, N., 2016. Constituents of saffron (*Crocus sativus* L.) as potential candidates for the treatment of anxiety disorders and schizophrenia. Molecules 21, 303.

Pitsikas, N., Tarantilis, P.A., 2017. Crocins the active constituents of *Crocus sativus* L., counteracted apomorphine-induced performance deficits in the novel object recognition task, but not novel object location task, in rats. Neurosci. Lett. 644, 37–42.

Rios, J.L., Recio, M.C., Ginger, R.M., Manz, S., 1996. An update review of saffron and its active constituents. Phytother Res. 10, 189–193.

Salim, S., 2014. Oxidative stress and psychological disorders. Curr. Neuropharmacol. 12, 140–147.

Schmidt, M., Betti, G., Hensel, A., 2007. Saffron in phytotherapy: pharmacology and clinical uses. Wien. Med. Wochenschr. 157, 315–319.

Smaga, I., Niedzielska, E., Gawlik, M., Moniczewski, A., Krzek, I., Przegalinski, E., Pera, J., Filip, M., 2015. Oxidative stress as an etiological factor and a potential treatment target of psychiatric disorders. Part 2. Depression, anxiety, schizophrenia and autism. Pharmacol. Rep. 67, 569–580.

Steimer, T., 2002. The biology of fear-and anxiety-related behaviors. Dialogues Clin. Neurosci. 28, 123–137.

Tarantilis, P.A., Tsoupras, G., Polissiou, M., 1995. Determination of saffron (*Crocus sativus* L.) components in crude plant extract using high-performance liquid chromatography-UV/Visible photodiode-array detection-mass spectrometry. J. Chromatogr. 699, 107–118.

Van Ameringen, M., Mancini, C., Pipe, B., Bennett, M., 2004. Optimizing treatment in social phobia: a review of treatment resistance. CNS Spectr. 9, 753–762.

Winterhalter, P., Straubinger, M., 2000. Saffron-renewed interest in an ancient spice. Food Rev. Int. 16, 39–59.

CHAPTER 12

Protecting Mechanisms of Saffron Extract Against Doxorubicin Toxicity in Ischemic Heart

NATHALIE CHAHINE • RAMEZ CHAHINE

INTRODUCTION

Doxorubicin (DOX) is an effective chemotherapeutic drug. It is used in the treatment of many hematologic and solid tumor malignancies (example: lung cancers, breast cancers, sarcomas, leukemia, Hodgkin's disease, non-Hodgkin lymphoma). DOX belongs to the antitumor anthracycline antibiotic class of drugs; it is derived from Streptomyces bacteria. However, DOX induces a dose-dependent cardiotoxicity owing to free radical formation, membrane lipid peroxidation, and mitochondrial damage (Simunek et al., 2009; Mordente et al., 2012; Tacar et al., 2013). Drug cardiotoxicity is one of the main reasons for nonapproval, relabeling, warnings, and withdrawal of DOX. In this context, cardiac side effect is a major concern to the pharmacological manufacturing.

Many therapeutic modalities have been used to limit DOX toxicity. In this context, the use of DOX analogs such as epirubicin and idarubicin has spread. At the dose of 50 mg/m^2, DOX and epirubicin provided identical response rates and survivals. The cardiac toxicity was significantly lower in patients treated with epirubicin. On the other hand, for the most serious forms of tumors in a metastatic situation, the use of less cardiotoxic analogs can lead to an increase in doses, which no longer brings a benefit because the toxicity becomes equivalent to that of conventional dose of DOX (Kaklamani et al., 2003; Ryberg et al., 2008; Kaya et al., 2013).

It is also recommended to limit the total cumulative dose of anthracyclines to reduce cardiotoxicity. A maximum cumulative dose has been defined for each anthracycline. However, this strategy did not give satisfactory results because of the great variability of individual tolerance. This limitation may lead to stopping a treatment in a patient who could withstand larger doses without showing cardiotoxicity. In addition, the decrease in maximum peak concentration does not eliminate the risk of cardiotoxicity, as some patients have developed ischemic cardiomyopathy with cumulative doses below the dose limits (To et al., 2003; Van Dalen et al., 2009).

One of the approaches to try to reduce the myocardial toxicity of anthracyclines is to administer them as a continuous infusion. Numerous clinical trials have been performed using continuous infusion for several days in a row rather than a bolus injection every 3 weeks. The prolongation of the duration of infusion of DOX did not offer any advantages in terms of cardioprotection compared with the conventional administration scheme. In addition, the mucosal toxicity is much greater; adding to this, a considerable increase in the length of hospitalization poses economic problems. As a result, this approach has been abandoned in clinical practice (Lipshultz et al., 2002; Pun and Neilan, 2016).

A surrogate method involves the development of encapsulated anthracyclines within liposomal structures. By acting as a vehicle for cytotoxic agents, liposomes promote their distribution in the tumor by limiting their diffusion into healthy tissues. Their size prevents them from crossing the capillaries in the heart, which should significantly reduce the risk of cardiotoxicity (Theodoulou and Hudis, 2004). Phase II studies have been completed in adults demonstrating reduction of cardiac toxicity while maintaining antitumor activity; but, no phase III data exist with liposomal anthracyclines, so studies need to be completed. On the other hand, the cost of these drugs and their longer preparation times may be significant barriers to wider use (Lawrie et al., 2013).

Saffron. https://doi.org/10.1016/B978-0-12-818462-2.00012-7

The mechanisms of myocardial toxicity of anthracyclines rely on the formation of reactive oxygen species (ROS), thus several antioxidant therapies have been proposed to limit the production of $O_2^{\bullet-}$, H_2O_2, and $OH^{\bullet}$ radicals. In vitro research has focused on several compounds with antioxidant and cardioprotective properties. In contrast, in vivo approaches were sometimes disappointing. Several trials of cardioprotective drugs have been published, for instance, antioxidant substances such as coenzyme Q, N-acetylcysteine, vitamin E, and vitamin C. These compounds have useful effects on models of myocardial damage triggered by anthracyclines in animals; however, they do not avoid cardiotoxicity in humans. For that reason, we found a certain discrepancy between the importance of ROS formation, which induces the cardiotoxicity of anthracyclines, and the absence of results obtained clinically with regard to antioxidant defenses (Zamorano et al., 2016; Songbo et al., 2019).

In animals overexpressing enzymes with antioxidant activity such as catalase or MnSOD, it was shown that myocardial damage due to DOX was decreased. Results have shown that subsequent incubation of cells with catalase and DOX limits the degree of cardiac damage due to catalase (Cardinale et al., 2015). The impact of free radicals concerning the cardiotoxicity of anthracyclines has been established (Menna et al., 2012; Abdel-Qadir et al., 2017). Probucol is an antilipidemic agent that also acts as a powerful antioxidant; its chemical structure is close to that of vitamin E. It prevents the myocardial lesions induced by DOX in several animal models, by increasing the activity of SOD and myocardial glutathione-peroxidase, which are reduced by anthracyclines. No death was detected in the group of rats treated with probucol-DOX combination against 32% mortality in the group of rats treated with DOX alone, without affecting the antitumor activity. This protection is not obtained by the other hypolipidemic agents, devoid of antioxidant action (El-Demerdash et al., 2003; Smith et al., 2010; Avila et al., 2018).

It is important to note that cancers often occur in elderly along with other diseases. However, preexisting heart problem is generally considered as exclusion criteria in clinical investigation when analyzing the effectiveness and side effects of anticancer drugs (Vera-Badillo et al., 2013). Since the potential effects of DOX on the ischemic heart have not been studied in details, it is thus necessary to consider the off-target impact of anticancer treatments in pathological situations such as ischemia/reperfusion injury.

Myocardial ischemia/reperfusion (IR) is an insufficiency in blood perfusion. There is shifting of the myocardium from an aerobic to an anaerobic metabolism due to an imbalance between O_2 supply and demand (Rosano et al., 2008). It is crucial to restore the coronary flow to the ischemic heart because IR induces loss of contractile function and yields myocardial damage. However, reperfusion after ischemia can bring injury to the myocardium. Excessive amount of ROS production is an important mechanism of reperfusion injury. When the dioxygen is restored into an ischemic myocardium, O_2 will undertake serial reduction, leading to the establishment of ROS. Powerful ROS are formed during the first few minutes of reflow and play a critical role in reperfusion injury (Braunersreuther and Jaquet, 2012; Smart, 2017). In this context, oxidative stress is an imbalance between production and destruction of free radicals, which induces many harmful effects on cellular metabolism. It is important to note that ROS accumulation results from the overproduction of free radicals in addition to the decrease of free radicals scavenger systems (Su et al., 2013).

At the subcellular level (Fig. 12.1), signaling through phosphatidylinositol 3-kinase (PI3K)/protein kinase B (AKT)/mammalian target of rapamycin (mTOR) and the extracellular signal regulated kinases (ERK) pathways coordinate multiple cellular activities such as cell survival, proliferation, metabolism, motility, and cancer progression (Li et al., 2008). Mainly, it has a crucial role in heart development and diseases (Wang, 2007). In this context, the ` (RISK) pathways (phosphorylation cascades) facilitate cell survival during cardiac IR injuries (Hausenloy and Yellon, 2004). In fact, protection of mitochondrial integrity and downregulation of proapoptotic proteins come from the activation of RISK pathways. In addition, downregulation of the same signaling pathways, including AKT and ERK, has also been associated with DOX-induced damage and apoptosis of cardiomyocytes (Gabrielson et al., 2007).

PI3K and downstream AKT are signal-transduction enzymes. PI3K has the capacity to phosphorylate inositol ring in inositol phospholipids of the plasma membrane; it is a lipid kinase. AKT induces the phosphorylation of important downstream targets and regulates inflammatory responses, apoptosis, and cellular activation; it is the essential mediator of the PI3K/AKT signaling pathway (Cantley, 2002; Zhang et al., 2012).

IR-induced injuries might be cured by mediators that act on the PI3K/AKT signaling pathway (Han et al., 2012). In addition, a hypoxia-induced factor-1α (HIF-1α) is positively regulated by PI3K/AKT/mTOR pathway (Zhong et al., 2000). Activation of PI3K/AKT pathway by fibroblast growth factor-2 stops ROS-induced apoptosis and protects heart from IR injury. It can improve left ventricular function and decrease infarct size (Wang et al., 2012).

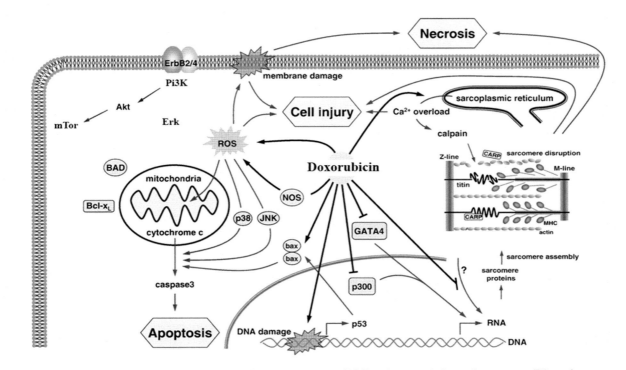

FIG. 12.1 Signaling pathways of reactive oxygen species (ROS) and apoptosis in cardiomyocytes: Effect of doxorubicin (DOX) and/or ischemia/reperfusion (IR) injury.

mTOR kinase is a main regulator of cardiac function, it is essential for homeostasis and normal regulation of cardiac structure and metabolism. It stimulates mitochondrial function and have an impact on cardiac energy deprivation, ischemia, pathogenesis, and progression of myocardial ischemia/reperfusion injury (Parra et al., 2014). Cardiac mTOR is a controller of oxidative stress by promoting oxidative metabolism and mitochondrial biogenesis (Cunningham et al., 2007). mTOR increases mitochondrial clearance, modulates autophagy, and protects cardiomyocytes from oxidative stress-induced toxicity via the activation of protein kinase B (Pal et al., 2014).

Mitogen-activated protein kinase (MAPK) family includes distinct isoforms of protein kinase subfamilies. These isoforms connect molecules with different affinity and can activate diverse signaling pathways. MAPKs transport extracellular signals to their intracellular targets in response to many stress stimuli, thus regulating cell differentiation, growth, and function (Gerits et al., 2007). MAPK are classified as (1) ERK 1/2 (44/42 kDa), activated by growth hormone receptors, via Ras/Raf pathway, and (2) JNK 1/2 (stress activated

kinases-Jun-NH2-terminal kinases 1/2) and p38 MAPK α/β activated by cellular stresses including ROS, heat shock, inflammatory cytokines and ischemia, via MKK4/MKK7 and MKK3/MKK6 pathways, respectively (Vassalli et al., 2012). p38 MAPK activation was increased by ischemia/reperfusion. p38 MAPK inhibition limits infarct size and polymorphonuclear accumulation in mouse hearts subjected to IR injury. This proposed a possible role for p38 MAPK as a mediator of myocardial IR injury (Gao et al., 2002; Kaiser et al., 2004). Studies have shown a protective role for ERK signaling pathway against IR injury (Das et al., 2009; Yang et al., 2011). Consequently, this pathway has been well-known as a principal constituent of the RISK pathway (Hausenloy and Yellon, 2004).

The exact mechanism of the DOX-induced cardiotoxicity and its progression to heart failure still remain unknown. However, evidence has shown that increased oxidative stress and cardiomyocyte apoptosis play important roles in the DOX-induced cardiotoxicity. Owing to its unique chemical structure, DOX is likely to generate ROS by redox cycling (Lou et al., 2006). In addition, DOX decreases the levels of the endogenous antioxidant enzymes that are responsible for scavenging the free radicals (Ludke et al., 2009). Under these conditions, free radicals are generated, and oxidative stress, which is characterized by an imbalance between prooxidants and antioxidants, is stimulated. Oxidative stress directly or indirectly activates several signaling pathways which leads to cardiomyocyte apoptosis and, ultimately, to heart failure (Zhang et al., 2009). Cellular oxidative stress activates an array of kinase pathways that modulate cardiomyocyte fate and response to anthracyclines. Signaling through RISK pathway is a cascade of carefully orchestrated series of events beginning from the cell surface and leading to controlled gene expression in the nucleus (Steelman et al., 2008). Regulation of these cascades is mediated by a sequence of kinases, phosphatases and exchange proteins. Some mutations could induce uncontrolled regulation (Lee et al., 2008). In cardiomyocytes with oxidative stress or DOX treatment, the ERK and PI3K/AKT pathways are changed. Studies have proved weakening cardiac contractile function, left ventricular remodeling, and cardiomyocyte loss during heart failure. AKT activation might protect heart function by inhibiting apoptosis. In addition, p38 MAPK inhibition might reduce cellular inflammatory reactions (Chaanine and Hajjar, 2011).

α-Actinin, troponin C, and myosin light chain are contractile proteins and markers of cardiac injury. Damage in these proteins is considered a main cause of the IR or DOX-induced reduction in myocardial contractile function (Wallace et al., 2004). Moreover, the mitochondria-dependent intrinsic apoptotic pathway plays a significant part in cardiac cell injury (Murphy and Steenbergen, 2008). mPTP opening results in free passage of cytochrome c, loss of the mitochondrial membrane potential, and caspase-3 activation (Listenberger et al., 2001). Therefore, antioxidative therapeutic agents could be a major way to counteract the cardiotoxicity induced by IR and DOX. Whether antioxidant could reverse chemotherapy-induced cardiotoxicity is not well understood. Thus, the relationship between oxidative stress, IR, and DOX-induced damage and the effect of SAF on cardioprotective signaling pathway is complicated and needs more data.

The protective system preventing radical-mediated organ failure, disease progression, and aging is known as the antioxidant defensive mechanism. The radicals should be converted to metabolically nondestructive molecules or scavenged immediately after formation, thereby preventing free radical damage. Attention has been paid to the natural sources of antioxidants, such as phenolic and flavonoid compounds (Zhao and Zhao, 2010; Akhlaghi and Bandy, 2009). In this context, saffron is a spice holding antioxidant activities attributed to crocin and safranal (bioactive compounds) (Karimi et al., 2010).

Saffron comes from dehydrated stigmata of *Crocus sativus* that belongs to Iridaceae family. *C. sativus* is an autumn flowering perennial plant mostly used in medicine and food as a fragrance and colorant spice (FAO, 2012). It is widely cultivated in Iran, India, and Greece. Commercial saffron is a spice consisting of dried red stigma; it is considered the most expensive spice in the world (SharafEldin et al., 2008, 2015). Saffron is rather adapted to hill sides and mountain valleys (altitude between 600 and 1700 m) (Agayev et al., 2007). It can be cultivated in a dry and infertile place where there is an extreme water shortage in summer. This is one of the valuable herbs in the world because it requires properly plucked stigma from the flowers. Variation and high quality of final products are due to the harvest process involved (Khazdair et al., 2015).

Saffron was used as both medicine and spice (Dwyer et al., 2011). The stigma of saffron has been used as a medicine for its expectorant, aphrodisiac, and antispasmodic effects (Wang et al., 2010); it was used in various opioid preparations for pain relief (Schmidt et al., 2007). Also, saffron has been used in coloring tunics in Spain and by the Babylonian culture in 2400 B.C. (Yasmin and Nehvi, 2013). Approximately 1 kg of this valuable spice is made using 150,000 flowers that must be carefully picked (Pitsikas, 2016). The price for 1 kg of saffron spice can reach 5000 US$. The growth of local saffron manufacture in Lebanon is therefore essential. Approximately 150 volatile and nonvolatile compounds were detected from the chemical analysis of *C. sativus*. However, about 50 constituents have been identified as the phytochemicals agents in saffron which are responsible for many pharmacological actions in the body. The major constituents of saffron are crocin, picrocrocin, and safranal (Winterhalter and Straubinger, 2000). Saffron is widely used in food processing industry as flavoring agents and colorant. It has an intense fragrance and is characterized by its bitter taste caused by the presence of picrocrocin (Himeno and Sano, 1987). The bright yellow-orange color is mainly due to the degraded carotenoid compounds, crocin, and crocetin (Gohari et al., 2013). The stigma was shown to contain carbohydrates, minerals, mucilage, vitamins B1 and B2, and pigments. Crocin, crocetin, carotene, lycopene, anthocyanin, alpha-carotene, beta-carotene, and zeaxanthin are oil-soluble pigments that can be found in the stigma (Bhat and Broker, 1953; Nørbæk and Kondo, 1998).

Safranal is the main constituent of total essential oil of *C. sativus* (Himeno and Sano, 1987). The secondary metabolites present in the petals of *C. sativus* are tannins, anthocyanins, and flavonoids (Galati et al., 1994; Fatehi et al., 2003). The main phytochemicals that may contribute to the biological activities of *C. sativus* are crocin, picrocrocin, and safranal. These active components have shown several pharmacological effects such as anticonvulsant, antidepressant, anti-inflammatory, antitumor, antioxidant, antidepression, and memory-improving effects (Moshiri et al., 2014; Akhondzadeh Basti et al., 2008). The therapeutic doses of saffron exhibited no significant toxicity in both clinical and experimental investigations (Bostan et al., 2017). In placebo-controlled and double-blinded study, the result showed that treatment for 1 week with saffron tablet (200 and 400 mg/day) has no adverse effect (Ayatollahi et al., 2014). Further research is needed regarding saffron mechanism of action, effectiveness, and safety. More data are recommended for a better understanding of publications bias.

Thus, the aim of the present study was to:

1) Extract the main components (safranal and crocin) from saffron stigma grown in Lebanon, HPLC analysis, and determination of the antioxidant activity.
2) Investigate in cardiomyocytes, the possible protective effect of saffron and DOX treatment combined to ischemia-reperfusion conditions on cell survival and cytotoxicity in vitro.
3) Test the potential chronic cardioprotective effects of saffron extracts given to rabbits in the presence or absence of DOX under normal or ischemic condition in vivo.

MATERIALS AND METHODS
Preparation of Saffron Extract
The Lebanese saffron used was grown in the Beqaa Valley. For each protocol, 2 g of dried stigmas of saffron were suspended in 400 mL of a methanol-water mixture (50:50, v/v) and then left for 24 h in the dark, on a magnetic stirrer at 4°C. The solution was then filtered, and the filtrate placed in a rotavapor at 40° C to evaporate the methanol; the resulting solution was refrigerated for 3 days and then lyophilized for 48 h. The yield of saffron extraction from dried stigmas is then calculated.

HPLC Analysis
For the quantitative analysis of saffron extracts, we used an Agilent HPLC (1100 series) with a multisolvent system equipped with a quaternary pump, a degasser, an injector, a UV detector with variable wavelength diode array (DAD), Spherisorb RP C18 column 20-cm long, 4.6-mm ID, particle size 10 μm with a pore diameter of 80 Å. The mobile phase is made up of a linear gradient of methanol (10%–100%) in water (15% acetonitrile) with a flow rate of 1.0 mL/min and an injection volume of 20 μL. The samples were analyzed in duplicate. Seven different concentrations (1, 0.5, 0.25, 0.125, 0.062, 0.03, and 0.015) of the internal standard (2-nitroaniline) were prepared and used to create the calibration curve. Picrocrocin was detected at 250 nm, safranal at 310 nm, and crocin at 440 nm.

Determination of Total Polyphenols
Polyphenols possess significant antioxidant activity; their content can be determined by measuring the Folin-Ciocalteu index. Thus, the determination of the phenolic compounds is based on the method using the Folin-Ciocalteu reagent. This reagent consists of a mixture of phosphotungstic acid and phosphomolybdic acid. Oxidation of phenols reduces this reagent in a mixture of blue oxides of tungsten and molybdenum. The intensity of the color produced has a maximum absorption at 725 nm. It is proportional to the level of oxidized phenolic compounds and therefore to the amount of polyphenols present in the extracts (Ortiz et al., 2013). The absorbance of saffron polyphenols (at 725 nm) was 0.2489, and its corresponding concentration was 16 mg GAE/L (GAE: gallic acid equivalent).

Experimental Protocol for Cultured Cardiomyocytes
H9c2 cardiomyocytes were cultured in modified Dulbecco's Modified Eagle's Medium containing 4.5 g/L of glucose + 10% of fetal calf serum + 1% of a mixture of penicillin (100 IU/mL)/streptomycin (100 μg/mL) antibiotics. They were cultured in 96-well or 6-well plates and subjected to the following protocol (Fig. 12.2): Group 1, control—cells were cultured in a complete media in normoxia and were not subjected to any treatment. Group 2, SAF: cells were incubated in 10 μg/mL of saffron for 16 h. Group 3, IR: cells were subjected to 8 h of hypoxia followed by 16 h of reoxygenation. Group 4, DOX: cells were incubated in 4 μmol/L of DOX for 3 h. Group 5, IR + DOX: cells were subjected to 8 h of hypoxia, followed by 16h of reoxygenation in the presence of 4 μmol/L of DOX for 3 h at reperfusion. Group 6, IR + SAF: cells were subjected to 8 h of hypoxia followed by 16 h reoxygenation in the presence of 10 μg/mL of SAF during 16 h at reperfusion. Group 7, DOX + SAF: cells were incubated in 10 μg/mL of SAF for 16 h and 4 μmol/L of DOX for

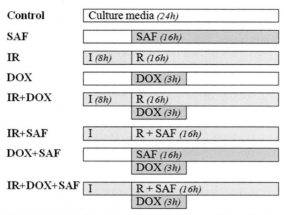

FIG. 12.2 Experimental protocol for doxorubicin effect on H9c2 cardiomyocytes subjected to ischemia/reperfusion in the absence or presence of saffron at reperfusion (n = 3). SAF, saffron; DOX, doxorubicin; I, ischemia; R, reperfusion.

3 h. Group 8, IR + DOX + SAF: cells were subjected to 8 h of hypoxia followed by 16 h of reoxygenation in the simultaneous presence of 10 µg/mL of SAF for 16 h and 4 µmol/L of DOX for 3 h at reperfusion. Cell viability, LDH cytotoxicity, and Western blot analysis were performed.

Experimental Protocol for Chronic Administration of DOX and Saffron in Rabbits

In this study, 50 male rabbits were randomly divided into five groups (n = 10–12/group) (Fig. 12.3). Group 1, control: without any treatment. Group 2, IR: no treatment on animals, then isolated hearts is subjected to IR. Group 3, SAF + IR: animals are treated orally with an optimal dose of SAF extracts (5 mg/kg weight/day) for 6 weeks, then isolated hearts are subjected to IR. Group 4, DOX + IR: animals are treated with a single dose (intraperitoneal) of DOX (2.5 mg/kg weight) per week for 4 weeks starting from the third week, and then isolated hearts are subjected to IR. Group 5, SAF + DOX + IR: treated with SAF as for group 3, then with DOX as for group 4, and then, the isolated hearts are subjected to IR. Heart isolation was performed 1 week after the end of treatment; the surviving rabbits were sacrificed and their hearts isolated and perfused according to the Langendorff model. Hearts are maintained for a period of 15 min of stabilization, then subjected to 30-min period of global ischemia (I) followed by 30 min of reperfusion (R). Pathological symptoms, left ventricular pressure (LVP), left ventricular end-diastolic ventricular pressure (LVEDP), heart rate (HR), coronary flow (CF), arrhythmias, and glutathione peroxidase were determined.

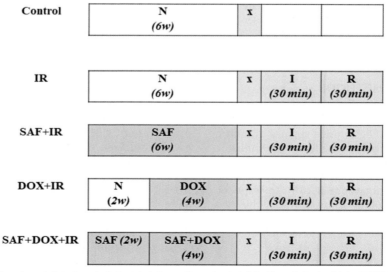

FIG. 12.3 Experimental protocol of chronic intraperitoneal administration of doxorubicin (DOX) to rabbits for 4 weeks (w) in the presence or absence of saffron extracts (SAF) administered per os, followed by heart isolation submitted to ischemia (I)/reperfusion (R) (n = 10–12). N, normal serum; x, heart isolation followed by 15 min of stabilization.

RESULTS

Effect of Saffron Extracts on DOX Toxicity in Hypoxic H9c2 Cells

The percentages of cytotoxicity and cell viability were measured to evaluate the effect of SAF on IR- and DOX-induced cardiomyocytes cell death. H9c2 were exposed to 8 h of hypoxia and 16 h of reoxygenation, with or without DOX (4 μmol/L for 3h) treatment during reoxygenation, (miming IR) in the presence or absence of SAF (10 μg/mL for 16h) at reoxygenation. MTT and LDH release assays were used. The results in Table 12.1 indicated that IR aggravates DOX-induced cell injury (IR + DOX) inducing decrease cell viability to 24% ($P < .05$) (vs. control) and increased LDH activity to 192% (vs. control). Treatment with 10 μg/mL SAF at reperfusion (IR + SAF and IR + DOX + SAF) or treatment with 10 μg/mL SAF and DOX (DOX + SAF) significantly ($P < .05$) reduced IR- and DOX-induced cytotoxicity by increasing cell viability and reducing LDH activity close to control values.

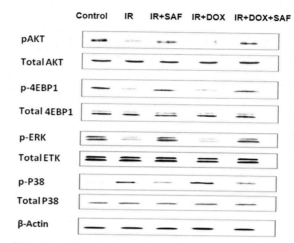

FIG. 12.4 Western blot analysis of protein kinases: p-AKT, p-4EBP1, p-ERK, and p-P38 in H9c2 cardiomyocytes. H9c2 were subjected to IR (8h/16h), with or without DOX (4 μmol/L for 3h) treatment at reperfusion, in the presence or absence of SAF (10 μg/mL for 16h) at reperfusion. Total-AKT, -4EBP1, -ERK, -P38, and β-Actin are the internal control for equal loading of proteins.

Saffron Extract Effects on Phosphorylation of AKT, 4EBP1, ERK, and P38 in H9c2 Cells

We estimated the level of phosphorylation of AKT, 4EBP1, ERK, and P38 using western blotting to clarify the signaling pathways involved in SAF protection against IR and DOX injury. H9c2 were subjected to IR (8h/16h), with or without DOX (4 μmol/L for 3h) treatment at reperfusion, in the presence or absence of SAF (10 μg/mL for 16 h) at reperfusion. Fig. 12.4 shows the levels of p-AKT, p-4EBP1, p-ERK, and p-P38 in response to SAF and DOX treatment at reperfusion. IR and IR + DOX treatment caused a significant ($P < .05$) reduction in the levels of p-AKT, p-4EBP1, and p-ERK and a rise in the level of p-P38 as compared with control. This effect was reversed in H9c2 cells exposed to SAF at reperfusion (IR + SAF and IR + DOX + SAF).

Animal Observation

Under our experimental conditions, treatment with DOX (a single IP dose of 2.5 mg/kg body weight per week) for 4 weeks resulted in premature mortality of 4 out of 12 rabbits as well as other pathological symptoms (Table 12.2). Oral pretreatment with an optimal dose of SAF extracts (5 mg/kg body weight per day) for 6 weeks in combination with DOX (a single IP dose of 2.5 mg/kg body weight per week) for 4 weeks

TABLE 12.1

Saffron (SAF), ischemia/reperfusion (IR), and doxorubicin (DOX) Effects on H9c2 cardiomyocytes. The percentage of cell viability (MTT assay) and LDH cytotoxicity (LDH assay) were determined. H9c2 cells were treated in normoxia (control); subjected to 8 h of ischemia followed by 16 h of reperfusion; treated with DOX (4 μmol/L for 3 h); treated with SAF (10 μg/mL for 16 h). Doxorubicin and saffron were added at reperfusion (post-treatment). The results are expressed as a percentage and represent the mean ± standard deviation of 3 experiments, * p <0.05 vs control, † p <0.05 vs IR, #p<0.05 vs DOX, #p <0.05 vs IR+DOX.

Parameters	Cell viability (%)	LDH cytotoxicity (%)
Control	100	100
SAF	130	105
IR	56*	151*
DOX	54*	145*
IR+DOX	24*	192*
IR+SAF	89†	106†
DOX+SAF	85#	107#
IR+DOX+SAF	70#	140#

TABLE 12.2
Effect of saffron (SAF) administration (5 mg/kg) on doxorubicin (DOX)-induced changes of body weight before and after treatment, pathological symptoms (ascites, diarrhea, lethargy, epistaxis), and premature mortality, in rabbits.

Parameters	n	Weight before (kg)	Weight after (kg)	Ascites	Diarrhea	Lethargy	Epistaxis	Premature mortality
Control	10	1.9±0.10	2.1±0.11	0/10	0/10	0/10	0/10	0
SAF	10	2.0±0.12	2.1±0.10	0/10	0/10	0/10	0/10	0
DOX	12	2.1±0.11	1.8±0.11	4/12	5/12	12/12	4/12	4
SAF+DOX	10	2.0±0.11	2.0±0.12	1/10	2/10	5/10	1/10	1

TABLE 12.3
Changes in cardiodynamic parameters (LVP, LVEDP, CF and HR) in response to different treatments with saffron and doxorubicin followed by ischemia-reperfusion on rabbits hearts. DOX: doxorubicin; SAF: saffron (5 mg/kg); IR: ischemia-reperfusion; LVP: left ventricular pressure; LVEDP: left ventricular end diastolic pressure; HR: heart rate; CF: coronary flow; B: before ischemia; A: 30 min after reperfusion. *p <0.05 vs IR; #p <0.05 vs IR+DOX (n = 6).

Parameters	LVP MMHG		LVEDP MMHG		HR BEAT/MIN		CF ML/MIN	
	B	A	B	A	B	A	B	A
Control	120±12	124±12.5	10±1	10±1.1	163±16.4	159±15.9	24±2.4	23.7±2.4
IR	124±12.4	98±9.8	10±1.2	15±1.5	164±16.3	141±14.2	23.5±2.5	18.7±1.9
SAF+IR	122±12.2	118±11.8*	10±1.1	12±1.2*	162±16.5	152±15.3*	23.7±2.4	21.9±2.2*
DOX+IR	122±12.3	80±8	10±1.2	17±1.8	163±16.3	135±13.3	23.7±2.5	16.5±1.7
SAF+DOX +IR	121±12.1	105±10.5#	10±1.3	13.5±1.4#	162±16.4	148±14.9	23.6±2.3	19.8±2#

resulted in a significant decrease in this mortality (1 out of 10) and a decrease in the severity of other pathological symptoms. No mortality or symptoms were observed in the control or SAF group.

Cardiodynamic Parameters

One week after the end of the treatment, the surviving rabbits were sacrificed, and their hearts were isolated and perfused according to the Langendorff model and subjected to 30 min of global ischemia, followed by 30 min of reperfusion. All hearts survived until the end of the protocol without mortality. Table 12.3 shows the changes in LVP, LVEDP, CF and HR, before ischemia (B) and 30 min after reperfusion (R). Hearts from rabbits treated with IR or DOX + IR are only able to partially recover their contractility. Hearts from rabbits pretreated with SAF (SAF + IR and SAF + DOX + IR)

are able to recover $(P < .05)$ and reach values near to preischemia.

Electrophysiological Parameters

Hearts from the control group showed no significant arrhythmias. A period of ventricular tachycardia (VT), ventricular fibrillation (VF), and frequent premature ventricular contractions (PVC) appear at reperfusion, following a global ischemia of 30 min. PVC, VT, and VF last a few seconds to a minute for IR group. PVC increases significantly, but VT and VF are still present with no noticeable changes for the DOX + IR group. VT, VF, and PVC are markedly reduced in hearts from rabbits given daily saffron for 6 weeks and subjected to ischemia-reperfusion (SAF + IR). However, hearts from rabbits treated with SAF + DOX + IR show a decrease in VT and VF, but less pronounced for PVC (Table 12.4).

TABLE 12.4

Number of PVCs (premature ventricular contractions) and percentages of ventricular tachycardia and ventricular fibrillation (VT/VF) of control hearts and hearts subjected to ischemia-reperfusion (IR) after administration of doxorubicin (DOX) with or without saffron extracts (SAF) 5 mg/kg in rabbits. *p <0.05 compared to Control; #p <0.05 compared to IR (n = 6).

Parameters	Control	IR	SAF+IR	DOX+IR	SAF+DOX+IR
PVC (n)	4±2	51±8*	18±4*#	89±14*#	47±10*
VT/VF (%)	0	100*	40*#	100*	60*#

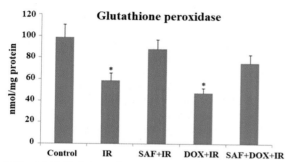

FIG. 12.5 Variation of glutathione peroxidase activity in control heart tissues and hearts subjected to ischemia-reperfusion (IR) after treatment with doxorubicin (DOX) with or without saffron extracts (SAF) 5 mg/kg in rabbits. *$P < .05$ compared to control (n = 6).

Biochemical Parameters

Fig. 12.5 shows that glutathione peroxidase, an antioxidant enzyme, decreases in the hearts of rabbits subjected to IR and DOX + IR relatively to the control. These values improve significantly in the hearts of rabbits treated with saffron, SAF + IR, and SAF + DOX + IR.

DISCUSSION

Primarily, it is important to note that the extracts of the stigmas of saffron flowers that have been used for all the protocols of our study are not adulterated; they come from the same saffron plant in the plain of Beqaa. Because drying of stigmas is a very delicate step, all measures have been taken to ensure good dehydration to prevent the development of molds which will affect its quality and therefore its biological properties. Saffron must lose about 4/5 of its weight, and the remaining moisture content must be at most 10% according to the international ISO standard. The stigmas after drying should be to the touch neither too dry nor too soft, and the color should be dark red

and uniform. Being very hygroscopic, saffron is preserved after drying in a dry place and protected from the air.

The methanol-water extractions were retained for all the protocols of our thesis, although several extractions were made from the dried stigmas. Indeed, through our literature search, we noticed that most studies on saffron are performed on methanolic extracts, which facilitates comparison with others. In addition, our yields are close to those found in the literature, namely between 40% and 42%. The lyophilization allowed us a good preservation of the extracts and to prepare each experimentation session a fresh solution and exact concentration.

It was important to quantify the active components of saffron, namely safranal and crocin; it is the latter that play the leading role in the antioxidant activity of saffron. Of the esterified carotenoid C20 family, there are six types of crocin, the major compound being crocin 4 or alpha crocin (Tarantilis et al., 1995). The HPLC analyzes we performed on our extracts supported what these authors found (Table 12.5). Moreover, the determination of the polyphenols in our samples also revealed values, not only in the average of the concentrations found in different rudders, but our extracts can be classified, according to the international standards ISO, among the high-end rudders of the world.

It is known that the toxicity caused by DOX affects heart function harmfully (Minotti et al., 2004), but its effect on cardiomyocyte viability and signaling after IR remains subtle. Actually, cancer patient's mortality on anthracycline treatment is due to cardiac problems (Mertens et al., 2008). Consequently, it is imperative to understand the effect of anthracyclines on cardiac dysfunction during IR injuries to develop beneficial strategies for patients with ischemic heart disease undergoing chemotherapy.

The increased production of free radical species is a main event involved in cardiovascular pathologies. However, the presence of effective cardioprotective

TABLE 12.5
Saffron active constituents: Lebanese saffron sample, compared to four other samples from different origins. Values are expressed in mg/g of total extract obtained by HPLC analysis.

	Lebanon (Bekaa)	Italy	India	Iran
Safranal	5.22	5.24	4.75	3.27
Picocrocin	18.76	11.64	5.22	31.57
Trans crocin4	36.75	37.54	40.77	38.41
Trans crocin3	29.33	22.16	30.36	23.58
Trans crocin2	2.45	2.61	2.84	1.33
Trans crocin2'	1.88	1.01	2.16	1.15
cis crocin4	6.75	9.10	10.14	4.73
cis crocin2	1.12	3.29	0.23	0.12
TOTAL	102.26	92.59	96.44	104.6

molecules against the toxic effects of anthracyclines is unclear (Li and Shah, 2004). Therefore, attention has been paid to the natural sources of antioxidants. Saffron is a natural plant having an antioxidant effect and is a rich source of flavonoids (Wattanapitayakul et al., 2005). Phenol and flavonoid neutralize free radical damage and significantly attenuate the risk of cardiovascular disease (Akhlaghi and Bandy, 2009).

We assessed the effect of SAF on H9c2 cytotoxicity comprising of DOX treatment under IR conditions. H9c2 cells have been used as a model to investigate the protective effect of many compounds against DOX-induced cardiotoxicity, these include carvedilol (Spallarossa et al., 2004), rosmarinic acid (Kim et al., 2005), and plantainoside D (Kim et al., 2007). SAF showed a protecting effect against DOX- and/or IR-induced injuries by reducing cytotoxicity, increasing cell viability, reducing the phosphorylation of P38 in DOX and/or IR cells, and restoring the decline in the phosphorylation of AKT, 4EBP1, and ERK.

We described an innovative cardioprotective role for SAF against IR- and DOX-induced toxicity. While high concentration of SAF 100 mg/mL presented anticancer effects (Abdullaev, 2002), low concentration (10 μg/mL) presented favorable effects on stressed cells. Treatment of control cells with 10 μg/mL SAF did not cause toxicity, proposing that SAF is used to avoid toxicity on H9c2 cells at low doses for 16 h. Hence, it may well be used without causing adverse effects to the heart.

Remarkably, our study revealed that treatment with SAF (10 μg/mL during 16h) at reperfusion protects the myocardium from both ischemia and DOX injuries (Chahine et al., 2016).

AKT/mTOR/4EBP1 and ERK are essential components of signaling pathways implicated in cardiomyocyte viability. Our results show that AKT, 4EBP1, and ERK phosphorylation were decreased in DOX-treated cells and at a higher range when H9c2 cells were exposed to IR and DOX. Our results are in agreement with previous work concerning DOX-induced cardiotoxicity (Taniyama and Walsh, 2002). Treatment with saffron extract during reperfusion conserved the phosphorylation of these pathway constituents. AKT and ERK are fundamental to the RISK pathway, concerning cell proliferation and survival (Yellon and Hausenloy, 2007). mTOR/4EBP1 pathway is a major signaling axis downstream of PI3K/AKT which is important for protein translation (Fingar and Blenis, 2004). Initiating these signaling pathways revealed a decrease in hypertrophic response and stimulate cardiomyocyte function and survival in vitro and in vivo (Matsui and Rosenzweig, 2006). These results indicate that saffron maintained the activation of ERK and PI3K/AKT/mTOR/4EBP1 pathway in IR- and DOX-treated cardiomyocytes.

Furthermore, P38 MAPK is an essential cell cycle regulator used by cardiomyocytes to control proliferation. Activated P38 MAPK phosphorylates downstream signaling molecules important for cardiomyocyte hypertrophy, and it induces cell cycle exit (Liang and Molkentin, 2003). Saffron inverted the rise in the level of p-P38 MAPK caused by IR and DOX, and this resulted in protection against cardiomyocyte apoptosis. Earlier study stated that SAF scavenge free radicals in vitro (Makhlouf et al., 2011). The antiapoptotic properties of SAF detected in the current study can be related with the antioxidant properties of SAF. This proposes that the cardioprotective effect of SAF at reperfusion against IR- and DOX-induced cardiotoxicity could be due to the free radical–scavenging capacity of SAF.

These findings demonstrate that saffron extract is likely to be a cardioprotective compound. SAF improved the cardiomyocyte survival, activated the AKT/mTOR/4EBP1, and inhibited the P38 MAPK pathway in IR- and DOX-treated cardiomyocytes.

Rabbit heart perfused according to the Langendorff method is one of the most studied models of cardiac physiology and pathophysiology. Many types of clinically observed arrhythmias could be reproduced in the rabbit heart model (Lou et al., 2011).

In our experimental conditions, treatment with DOX caused the mortality of 1/3 of the rabbits, whereas pretreatment with saffron decreases the mortality to 1/10. Moreover, during reperfusion, rabbit's hearts receiving SAF and DOX showed improved cardiodynamic parameters in comparison with hearts from rabbits treated with IR and DOX without saffron. Concerning glutathione peroxidase, which is the key enzyme in the transformation of radicals into less toxic products, its activity decreases in the myocardium subjected to ischemia-reperfusion after the treatment with DOX (DOX + IR), whereas pretreatment with saffron is capable of significantly counteracting this decrease (SAF + DOX + IR).

These findings demonstrate that saffron protects the heart from DOX and ischemia-reperfusion injury in a chronic protocol with isolated rabbit heart model. This cardioprotective effect is, at least in part, strongly linked to the antioxidant properties of saffron.

Finally, we first reported the evidence that Lebanese saffron extracts protect against DOX-induced myocardial toxicity in conditions of IR. SAF has potent antioxidant and antiapoptotic properties, resulting in prevention of cardiac injury and amelioration of cell survival in vitro and in vivo.

ACKNOWLEDGMENTS

Authors wish to thank Pr Hassane Makhlouf for providing saffron stigmas and Pr Laurent Martiny for the help in cardiomyocytes culture in his laboratory at the Faculty of Sciences, University of Reims. Funds were provided in part from Lebanese University.

REFERENCES

Abdel-Qadir, H., Ong, G., Fazelzad, R., Amir, E., Lee, D.S., 2017. Interventions for preventing cardiomyopathy due to anthracyclines: a Bayesian network meta-analysis. Ann. Oncol. 28, 628–633.

Abdullaev, F., 2002. Cancer chemopreventive and tumoricidal properties of saffron (*Crocus sativus* L.). Exp. Biol. Med. 227, 20–25.

Agayev, Y.M., Shakib, A.M., Soheilivand, S., Fathi, M., 2007. Breeding of saffron (*Crocus sativus*): possibilities and problems. Acta Hortic. 739, 203–207.

Akhlaghi, M., Bandy, B., 2009. Mechanisms of flavonoid protection against myocardial ischemia-reperfusion injury. J. Mol. Cell. Cardiol. 46, 309–317.

Akhondzadeh Basti, A., Ghoreishi, S.A., Noorbala, A.A., Akhondzadeh, S.H., Rezazadeh, S.H., 2008. Petal and stigma of *Crocus sativus* L. in the treatment of depression: a pilot double-blind randomized trial. J. Med. Plants 7 (4), 29–36.

Avila, M.S., Ayub-Ferreira, S.M., de Barros Wanderley Jr., M.R., das Dores Cruz, F., Gonçalves Brandão, S.M., Rigaud, V.O.C., et al., 2018. Carvedilol for prevention of chemotherapy-related cardiotoxicity: the CECCY trial. J. Am. Coll. Cardiol. 71, 2281–2290.

Ayatollahi, H., Javan, A.O., Khajedaluee, M., Shahroodian, M., Hosseinzadeh, H., 2014. Effect of *Crocus sativus* L. (saffron) on coagulation and anticoagulation systems in healthy volunteers. Phytother. Res. 28, 539–543.

Bhat, J.V., Broker, R., 1953. Riboflavine and thiamine contents of saffron, *Crocus sativus* Linn. Nature 172, 544.

Bostan, H.B., Mehri, S., Hosseinzadeh, H., 2017. Toxicology effects of saffron and its constituents: a review. Iran. J Basic Med. Sci. 20, 110–121.

Braunersreuther, V., Jaquet, V., 2012. Reactive oxygen species in myocardial reperfusion injury: from physiopathology to therapeutic approaches. Curr. Pharmaceut. Biotechnol. 13 (1), 97–114.

Cantley, L.C., 2002. The phosphoinositide 3-kinase pathway. Science 296 (5573), 1655–1657.

Cardinale, D., Colombo, A., Bacchiani, G., Tedeschi, I., Meroni, C.A., Veglia, F., et al., 2015. Early detection of anthracycline cardiotoxicity and improvement with heart failure therapy. Circulation 131, 1981–1988.

Chaanine, A.H., Hajjar, R.J., 2011. AKT signalling in the failing heart. Eur. J. Heart Fail. 13 (8), 825–829.

Chahine, N., Nader, M., Duca, L., Martiny, L., Chahine, R., 2016. Saffron extracts alleviate cardiomyocytes injury induced by doxorubicin and ischemia-reperfusion in vitro. Drug Chem. Toxicol. 39 (1), 87–96.

Cunningham, J.T., Rodgers, J.T., Arlow, D.H., Vazquez, F., Mootha, V.K., Puigserver, P., 2007. mTOR controls mitochondrial oxidative function through a YY1-PGC-1alpha transcriptional complex. Nature 450 (7170), 736–740.

Das, A., Salloum, F.N., Xi, L., Rao, Y.J., Kukreja, R.C., 2009. ERK phosphorylation mediates sildenafil-induced myocardial protection against ischemia-reperfusion injury in mice. Am. J. Physiol. 296 (5), H1236–H1243.

Dwyer, A.V., Whitten, D.L., Hawrelak, J.A., 2011. Herbal medicines, other than St.John's wort, in the treatment of depression: a systematic review. Altern. Med. Rev. 16, 40–49.

El-Demerdash, E., Ali, A.A., Sayed-Ahmed, M.M., Osman, A.M., 2003. New aspects in probucol cardioprotection against doxorubicin-induced cardiotoxicity. Cancer Chemother. Pharmacol. 52 (5), 411–416.

FAO, 2012. Country Compass: Killing Heroin with Saffron. Non Wood News, pp. 45–62.

Fatehi, M., Rashidabady, T., Fatehi-Hassanabad, Z., 2003. Effects of *Crocus sativus* petals' extract on rat blood pressure and on responses induced by electrical field stimulation in the rat isolated vas deferens and Guinea-pig ileum. J. Ethnopharmacol. 84, 199–203.

Fingar, D.C., Blenis, J., 2004. Target of rapamycin (TOR): an integrator of nutrient and growth factor signals and coordinator of cell growth and cell cycle progression. Oncogene 23, 3151–3171.

Gabrielson, K., Bedja, D., Pin, S., Tsao, A., Gama, L., Yuan, B., Muratore, N., 2007. Heat shock protein 90 and ErbB2 in the cardiac response to doxorubicin injury. Cancer Res. 67, 1436–1441.

Galati, E.M., Monforte, M.T., Kirjavainen, S., Forestieri, A.M., Trovato, A., Tripodo, M.M., 1994. Biological effects of hesperidin, a citrus flavonoid. (Note I): antiinflammatory and analgesic activity. Farmaco 40, 709–712.

Gao, F., Yue, T.L., Shi, D.W., Lopez, B.L., Ohlstein, E.H., Barone, F.C., Ma, X.L., 2002. p38 MAPK inhibition reduces myocardial reperfusion injury via inhibition of endothelial adhesion molecule expression and blockade of PMN accumulation. Cardiovasc. Res. 53 (2), 414–422.

Gerits, N., Kostenko, S., Moens, U., 2007. In vivo functions of mitogen-activated protein kinases: conclusions from knock-in and knock-out mice. Transgenic Res. 16 (3), 281–314.

Gohari, A.R., Saeidnia, S., Mahmoodabadi, M.K., 2013. An overview on saffron, phytochemicals, and medicinal properties. Pharmacogn. Rev. 7, 61–66.

Han, J.Q., Yu, K.Y., He, M., 2012. Effects of puerarin on the neurocyte apoptosis and p-Akt (Ser473) expressions in rats with cerebral ischemia/reperfusion injury. Zhongguo Zhong Xi Yi Jie He Za Zhi 32 (8), 1069–1072.

Hausenloy, D.J., Yellon, D.M., 2004. New directions for protecting the heart against ischaemia-reperfusion injury: targeting the reperfusion injury salvage kinase (RISK)-pathway. Cardiovasc. Res. 61, 448–460.

Himeno, H., Sano, K., 1987. Synthesis of crocin, picrocrocin and safranal by saffron stigma-like structures proliferated *in vitro*. Agric. Biol. Chem. 51, 2395–2400.

Kaiser, R.A., Bueno, O.F., Lips, D.J., Doevendans, P.A., Jones, F., Kimball, T.F., Molkentin, J.D., 2004. Targeted inhibition of p38 mitogen-activated protein kinase antagonizes cardiac injury and cell death following ischemia-reperfusion in vivo. J. Biol. Chem. 279 (15), 15524–15530.

Kaklamani, V.G., Gradishar, W.J., 2003. Epirubicin versus doxorubicin: which is the anthracycline of choice for the treatment of breast cancer? Clin Breast Cancer 4 (Suppl 1), S26–33.

Karimi, E., Oskoueian, E., Hendra, R., Jaafar, H.Z., 2010. Evaluation of *Crocus sativus* L. stigma phenolic and flavonoid compounds and its antioxidant activity. Molecules 15, 6244–6256.

Kaya, M.G., Ozkan, M., Gunebakmaz, O., Akkaya, H., Kaya, E.G., Akpek, M., et al., 2013. Protective effects of nebivolol against anthracycline-induced cardiomyopathy: a randomized control study. Int. J. Cardiol. 167, 2306–2310.

Khazdair, M.R., Boskabady, M.H., Hosseini, M., Rezaee, R., Tsatsakis, A.M., 2015. The effects of *Crocus sativus* (saffron) and its constituents on nervous system: a review. Avicenna J. Phytomed. 5, 376–391.

Kim, D.S., Kim, H.R., Woo, E.R., 2005. Inhibitory effects of rosmarinic acid on adriamycin-induced apoptosis in H9c2 cardiac muscle cells by inhibiting reactive oxygen species and the activations of c-Jun N-terminal kinase and extracellular signal-regulated kinase. Biochem. Pharmacol. 70, 1066–1078.

Kim, D.S., Woo, E.R., Chae, S.W., 2007. Plantainoside D protects adriamycin-induced apoptosis in H9c2 cardiac muscle cells via the inhibition of ROS generation and NF-kappaB activation. Life Sci. 80, 314–323.

Lawrie, T.A., Rabbie, R., Thoma, C., Morrison, J., 2013. Pegylated liposomal doxorubicin for first-line treatment of epithelial ovarian cancer. Syst. Rev. 10, CD010482.

Lee, J.T., Lehmann, B.D., Terrian, D.M., Chappell, W.H., Stivala, F., Libra, M., Martelli, A.M., Steelman, L.S., McCubrey, J.A., 2008. Targeting prostate cancer based on signal transduction and cell cycle pathways. Cell Cycle 7 (12), 1745–1762.

Li, J.M., Shah, A.M., 2004. Endothelial cell superoxide generation: regulation and relevance for cardiovascular pathophysiology. Am. J. Physiol. Regul. Integr. Comp. Physiol. 287, 1014–1030.

Liang, Q., Molkentin, J.D., 2003. Redefining the roles of p38 and JNK signaling in cardiac hypertrophy: dichotomy between cultured myocytes and animal models. J. Mol. Cell. Cardiol. 35, 1385–1394.

Li, L., Qu, Y., Mao, M., Xiong, Y., Mu, D., 2008. The involvement of phosphoinositid 3-kinase/Akt pathway in the activation of hypoxia-inducible factor-1alpha in the developing rat brain after hypoxia-ischemia. Brain Res. 1197, 152–158.

Lipshultz, S.E., Giantris, A.L., Lipsitz, S.R., Kimball Dalton, V., Asselin, B.L., Barr, R.D., 2002. Doxorubicin administration by continuous infusion is not cardioprotective: the Dana-Farber 9101 acute lymphoblastic leukemia protocol. J. Clin. Oncol. 20 (6), 1677–1682.

Listenberger, L.L., Ory, D.S., Schaffer, J.E., 2001. Palmitate-induced apoptosis can occur through a ceramide-independent pathway. J. Biol. Chem. 276, 14890–14895.

Lou, H., Kaur, K., Sharma, A.K., Singal, P.K., 2006. Adriamycin-induced oxidative stress, activation of MAP kinases and apoptosis in isolated cardiomyocytes. Pathophysiology 13 (2), 103–109.

Ludke, A.R., Al-Shudiefat, A.A., Dhingra, S., Jassal, D.S., Singal, P.K., 2009. A concise description of cardioprotective strategies in doxorubicin-induced cardiotoxicity. Can. J. Physiol. Pharmacol. 87 (10), 756–763.

Lou, Q., Li, W., Efimov, I.R., 2011. Multiparametric optical mapping of the Langendorff-perfused rabbit heart. J. Vis. Exp. 55, e3160.

Makhlouf, H., Saksouk, M., Habib, J., Chahine, R., 2011. Determination of antioxidant activity of saffron taken from the flower of *Crocus sativus* grown in Lebanon. Afr. J. Biotechnol. 10, 8093–8100.

Matsui, T., Rosenzweig, A., 2006. Convergent signal transduction pathways controlling cardiomyocyte survival and function: the role of PI 3-kinase and Akt. J. Mol. Cell. Cardiol. 38, 63–71.

Menna, P., Paz, O.G., Chello, M., Covino, E., Salvatorelli, E., Minotti, G., 2012. Anthracycline cardiotoxicity. Expert Opin. Drug Saf. 11 (Suppl. 1), S21–S36.

Mertens, A.C., Liu, Q., Neglia, J.P., Wasilewski, K., Leisenring, W., Armstrong, G.T., et al., 2008. Cause-specific late mortality among 5-year survivors of childhood cancer: the childhood cancer survivor study. J. Natl. Cancer Inst. 100, 1368–1379.

Minotti, G., Menna, P., Salvatorelli, E., Cairo, G., Gianni, L., 2004. Anthracyclines: molecular advances and pharmacologic developments in antitumor activity and cardiotoxicity. Pharmacol. Rev. 56, 185–229.

Mordente, A., Meucci, E., Silvestrini, A., Martorana, G.E., Giardina, B., 2012. Anthracyclines and mitochondria. Adv. Exp. Med. Biol. 942, 385–419.

Moshiri, M., Vahabzadeh, M., Hosseinzadeh, H., 2014. Clinical applications of saffron (Crocus sativus) and its constituents: a review. Drug Res. 64, 1–9.

Murphy, E., Steenbergen, C., 2008. Mechanisms underlying acute protection from cardiac ischemia-reperfusion injury. Physiol. Rev. 88, 581–609.

Nørbæk, R., Kondo, T., 1998. Anthocyanins from flowers of Crocus (Iridaceae). Phytochemistry 47, 1–4.

Ortiz, J., Marín-Arroyo, M.R., Noriega-Domínguez, M.J., Navarro, M., Arozarena, I., 2013. Color, phenolics, and antioxidant activity of blackberry (Rubus glaucus Benth.), blueberry (Vaccinium floribundum Kunth.), and apple wines from Ecuador. J. Food Sci. 78 (7), C985–C993.

Pal, R., Palmieri, M., Loehr, J.A., Li, S., Abo-Zahrah, R., Monroe, T.O., et al., 2014. Src-dependent impairment of autophagy by oxidative stress in a mouse model of Duchenne muscular dystrophy. Nat. Commun. 5, 4425.

Parra, V., Verdejo, H.E., Iglewski, M., Del Campo, A., Troncoso, R., Jones, D., et al., 2014. Insulin stimulates mitochondrial fusion and function in cardiomyocytes via the Akt-mTOR-NFκB-Opa-1 signaling pathway. Diabetes 63 (1), 75–88.

Pitsikas, N., 2016. Constituents of saffron (Crocus sativus L.) as potential candidates for the treatment of anxiety disorders and schizophrenia. Molecules 21 (3), 303.

Pun, S.C., Neilan, T.G., 2016. Cardiovascular side effects of small molecule therapies for cancer. Eur. Heart J. 37 (36), 2742–2745.

Rosano, G.M., Fini, M., Caminiti, G., Barbaro, G., 2008. Cardiac metabolism in myocardial ischemia. Curr. Pharmaceut. Des. 14, 2551–2562.

Ryberg, M., Nielsen, D., Cortese, G., Nielsen, G., Skovsgaard, T., Andersen, P.K., 2008. New insight into epirubicin cardiac toxicity: competing risks analysis of 1097 breast cancer patients. J. Natl. Cancer. Inst. 100 (15), 1058–1067.

Schmidt, M., Betti, G., Hensel, A., 2007. Saffron in phytotherapy: pharmacology and clinical uses. Wien. Med. Wochenschr. 157, 315–319.

SharafEldin, M., Elkholy, S., Fernández, J.A., Junge, H., Cheetham, R., Guardiola, J., Weathers, P., 2008. Bacillus subtilis FZB24 affects flower quantity and quality of saffron (Crocus sativus). Planta Med. 74, 1316–1320.

SharafEldin, M., Elkholy, S., Hosokawa, M., Yanagawa, K., Nawata, E., Takagi, K., Fernández, J.A., 2015. Saffron flowers with augmented number of stigmata. Zeitschrift für Arznei Gewürzpflanzen 20, 84–87.

Simunek, T., Stérba, M., Popelová, O., Adamcová, M., Hrdina, R., Gersl, V., 2009. Anthracycline-induced cardiotoxicity: overview of studies examining the roles of oxidative stress and free cellular iron. Pharmacol. Rep. 61, 154–171.

Smart, N., 2017. Prospects for improving neovascularization of the ischemic heart: lessons from development. Microcirculation 24 (1), 12335.

Smith, L.A., Cornelius, V.R., Plummer, C.J., et al., 2010. Cardiotoxicity of anthracycline agents for the treatment of cancer: systematic review and meta-analysis of randomised controlled trials. BMC Cancer 10, 337.

Songbo, M., Lang, H., Xinyong, C., Bin, X., Ping, Z., Liang, S., 2019. Oxidative stress injury in doxorubicin-induced cardiotoxicity. Toxicol. Lett. 307, 41–48.

Spallarossa, P., Garibaldi, S., Altieri, P., 2004. Carvedilol prevents doxorubicin-induced free radical release and apoptosis in cardiomyocytes in vitro. J. Mol. Cell. Cardiol. 37, 837–846.

Steelman, L.S., Abrams, S.L., Whelan, J., Bertrand, F.E., Ludwig, D.E., Bäsecke, J., et al., 2008. Contributions of the Raf/MEK/ERK, PI3K/PTEN/Akt/mTOR and Jak/STAT pathways to leukemia. Leukemia 22 (4), 686–707.

Su, H., Ji, L., Xing, W., Zhang, W., Zhou, H., Qian, X., et al., 2013. Acute hyperglycaemia enhances oxidative stress and aggravates myocardial ischaemia/reperfusion injury: role of thioredoxin-interacting protein. J. Cell Mol. Med. 17 (1), 181–191.

Tacar, O., Sriamornsak, P., Dass, C.R., 2013. Doxorubicin: an update on anticancer molecular action, toxicity and novel drug delivery systems. J. Pharm. Pharmacol. 65, 157–170.

Taniyama, Y., Walsh, K., 2002. Elevated myocardial Akt signaling ameliorates doxorubicin-induced congestive heart failure and promotes heart growth. J. Mol. Cell. Cardiol. 34, 1241–1247.

Tarantilis, P.A., Tsoupras, G., Polissiou, M., 1995. Determination of saffron (Crocus sativus L.) components in crude plant extract using high-performance liquid chromatography-UV-visible photodiode-array detection-mass spectrometry. J. Chromatogr. A. 699 (1–2), 107–118.

Theodoulou, M., Hudis, C., 2004. Cardiac profiles of liposomal anthracyclines: greater cardiac safety versus conventional doxorubicin? Cancer 100, 2052–2063.

To, H., Ohdo, S., Shin, M., Uchimaru, H., Yukawa, E., Higuchi, S., et al., 2003. Dosing time dependency of doxorubicin-induced cardiotoxicity and bone marrow toxicity in rats. J. Pharm. Pharmacol. 55 (6), 803–810.

Van Dalen, E.C., Van der Pal, H.J., Caron, H.N., Kremer, L.C., 2009. Different dosage schedules for reducing cardiotoxicity in cancer patients receiving anthracycline chemotherapy. Cochrane Database Syst. Rev. (4), CD005008.

Vassalli, G., Milano, G., Moccetti, T., 2012. Role of mitogen-activated protein kinases in myocardial ischemia-reperfusion injury during heart transplantation. J. Transplant. 2012, 928954.

Vera-Badillo, F.E., Al-Mubarak, M., Templeton, A.J., Amir, E., 2013. Benefit and harms of new anti-cancer drugs. Curr. Oncol. Rep. 15, 270–275.

Wallace, K.B., Hausner, E., Herman, E., et al., 2004. Serum troponins as biomarkers of drug-induced cardiac toxicity. Toxicol. Pathol. 32, 106–121.

Wang, Y., 2007. Mitogen-activated protein kinases in heart development and diseases. Circulation 116, 1413–1423.

Wang, Y., Han, T., Zhu, Y., Zheng, C.J., Ming, Q.L., Rahman, K., et al., 2010. Antidepressant properties of bioactive fractions from the extract of *Crocus sativus* L. J. Nat. Med. 64, 24–30.

Wang, Z., Zhang, H., Xu, X., Shi, H., Yu, X., Wang, X., et al., 2012. bFGF inhibits ER stress induced by ischemic oxidative injury via activation of the PI3K/Akt and ERK1/2 pathways. Toxicol. Lett. 212 (2), 137–146.

Wattanapitayakul, S.K., Chularojmontri, L., Herunsalee, A., 2005. Screening of antioxidants from medicinal plants for cardioprotective effect against doxorubicin toxicity. Basic Clin. Pharmacol. Toxicol. 96, 80–87.

Winterhalter, P., Straubinger, M., 2000. Saffron—renewed interest in an ancient spice. Food Rev. Int. 16, 39–59.

Yang, X., Liu, Y., Yang, X.M., Hu, F., Cui, L., Swingle, M.R., et al., 2011. Cardioprotection by mild hypothermia during ischemia involves preservation of ERK activity. Basic Res. Cardiol. 106 (3), 421–430.

Yasmin, S., Nehvi, F.A., 2013. Saffron as a valuable spice: a comprehensive review. Afr. J. Agric. Res. 8, 234–242.

Yellon, D.M., Hausenloy, D.J., 2007. Myocardial reperfusion injury. N. Engl. J. Med. 357, 1121–1135.

Zamorano, J.L., Lancellotti, P., Rodriguez Muñoz, D., Aboyans, V., Asteggiano, R., Galderisi, M., et al., 2016. ESC position paper on cancer treatments and cardiovascular toxicity developed under the auspices of the ESC committee for practice guidelines: the task force for cancer treatments and cardiovascular toxicity of the European society of cardiology (ESC). Eur. Heart J. 37, 2768–2801.

Zhang, F., Ding, T., Yu, L., Zhong, Y., Dai, H., Yan, M.J., 2012. Dexmedetomidine protects against oxygen-glucose deprivation-induced injury through the I2 imidazoline receptor-PI3K/AKT pathway in rat C6 glioma cells. J. Pharm. Pharmacol. 64 (1), 120–127.

Zhang, Y.W., Shi, J., Li, Y.J., Wei, L., 2009. Cardiomyocyte death in doxorubicin-induced cardiotoxicity. Arch. Immunol. Ther. Exp. 57 (6), 435–445.

Zhao, Y., Zhao, B., 2010. Protective effect of natural antioxidants on heart against ischemia-reperfusion damage. Curr. Pharmaceut. Biotechnol. 11, 868–874.

Zhong, H., Chiles, K., Feldser, D., Laughner, E., Hanrahan, C., Georgescu, M.M., et al., 2000. Modulation of hypoxia-inducible factor 1alpha expression by the epidermal growth factor/phosphatidylinositol 3-kinase/PTEN/AKT/FRAP pathway in human prostate cancer cells: implications for tumor angiogenesis and therapeutics. Cancer Res. 60 (6), 1541–1545.

FURTHER READING

Calixto, J.B., Beirith, A., Ferreira, J., Santos, A.R., Filho, V.C., Yunes, R.A., 2000. Naturally occurring antinociceptive substances from plants. Phytother Res. 14, 401–418.

Negbi, M., 1999. Saffron: *Crocus Sativus L.* Harwood Academic, Amsterdam, The Netherlands.

Rothermel, B.A., Abel, E.D., Zorzano, A., Lavandero, S., 2014. Insulin stimulates mitochondrial fusion and function in cardiomyocytes via the Akt-mTOR-NFκB-Opa-1 signaling pathway. Diabetes 63 (1), 75–88.

CHAPTER 13

Beneficial Effects of Saffron (*Crocus sativus* L.) in Ocular Diseases

MÜBERRA KOŞAR • K. HÜSNÜ CAN BAŞER

INTRODUCTION

Crocus sativus L. (saffron) belongs to the Crocoideae, the subfamily of the family of Iridaceae (rich in endemic species) and has the highest economic value. Saffron, the most expensive spice in the world, is obtained by manual collection, drying, and then powdering of 2.5- to 3.2-cm-long dark orange stigmas of flowers (Fig. 13.1). Approximately, 160 kg of saffron flowers are required to obtain 1 kg of dry stigma, and the difficulty of cultivation is the main reason for its expensiveness. Today, saffron is cultivated in European countries as well as Turkey, Greece, Israel, Pakistan, India, Iran, Egypt, Azerbaijan, China, Japan, and Australia (Rios et al., 1996; Shahi et al., 2016).

The name saffron comes from Arabic language and means yellow due to the color carotenoid constituents. It is stated that Anatolia and the Eastern Mediterranean region is the homeland of saffron, and some reports state that saffron was brought to Anatolia by the Turks during their migration from Central Asia. Homeros and Hippocrates noted that saffron had been cultivated in the Kashmir region of Iran and India throughout the ages (Javadi et al., 2013). The Mongols introduced saffron to China, the Arabs to Spain, and the Crusaders to Western Europe. It has been used in ancient Greek, Roman, and Egyptian civilizations for painting, perfume, medicine, and cooking purposes. There are records indicating Cleopatra's use of a saffron perfume. In the Middle East, saffron has been cultivated for at least 4000 years for use as an aromatic sweetener, perfume, dye, medicine, and even as an aphrodisiac. Saffron has, at times, been valued same as gold (Giaccio, 2004).

Saffron, a valuable drug, is also of great importance in medicine. Many scientific data on the use of saffron in various diseases are recorded in the scientific literature. Traditional use of saffron has been confirmed by modern studies and has taken its place in modern medicine. According to these scientific studies, saffron, which has been used in the treatment of depression, nervous system diseases, heart diseases, endocrine system diseases, and immunological diseases, has also been used safely in the treatment of ocular diseases in recent years (Mousavi et al., 2011). Ocular disorders, especially mild-to-moderate glaucoma and retinal maculopathy disorders, are treated in a short time with saffron. For this purpose, many preparations, including saffron extract, containing crocin and crocetin as active ingredients are used in treatment (Rios et al., 1996; Broadhead et al., 2016).

In this review, details on the use of saffron in ocular diseases, its effective compounds, and in vivo and clinical studies will be given. Especially, glaucoma and age-related retinal maculopathy diseases will be covered.

CHEMICAL PROFILE OF SAFFRON

Saffron contains more than 150 volatile, flavoring, and phenolic compounds. These compounds are generally in the form of glycosides with different sugar molecules. Apart from them, fatty acids (palmitic, oleic, linoleic acids, *etc.*), vitamins (riboflavin and thiamine), and flavonoids (kaempferol, delphinidin, quercetin, derivatives, etc.) were also detected in the saffron (Rios et al., 1996; Shahi et al., 2016).

Among the secondary metabolites of saffron, the most important are the colored compound crocin ($C_{44}H_{64}O_{24}$), bitter-tasting compound picrocrocin ($C_{16}H_{26}O_7$), and fragrant compound safranal ($C_{10}H_{14}O$) (Fig. 13.2) (Bagur et al., 2018).

Saffron. https://doi.org/10.1016/B978-0-12-818462-2.00013-9

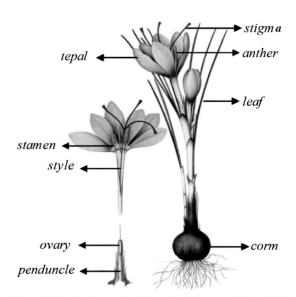

FIG. 13.1 Structure of different parts of saffron plant. (Adapted from Shahi, T., Assadpour, E., Jafari, S.M., 2016. Main chemical compounds and pharmacological activities of stigmas and tepals of 'red gold'; saffron. Trends Food Sci. Technol. 58, 69–78.)

Crocin, which constitutes more than 10% of the dry saffron mass, has been used as a chemotherapeutic agent according to the recent studies due to its water solubility and inhibitory effect on the growth of cells. Crocin significantly inhibited breast cancer cells, pancreatic cancer cells, and human rhabdomyosarcoma cells. Picrocrocin, derived from zeaxanthin, which is carotenoid by oxidative degradation. Picrocrocin ratio is approximately 4% within the stigmas of dry saffron. Safranal which is the volatile ingredient of saffron, found in 70% in dry mass, is derived from picrocrocin during drying and storage periods by hydrolysis (Fig. 13.2) (Shahi et al., 2016; Bagur et al., 2018).

The stability of saffron is very low and sensitive to pH changes, degraded by light and many oxidants. Therefore, the storage conditions of saffron are very important and should be checked (Bagur et al., 2018).

Carotenoids of Saffron

The carotenoids within the plants are synthesized by chloroplasts and chromoplasts. Saffron contains hydrophilic and lipophilic carotenoids that are most active compounds for many diseases and ocular diseases as well. C-40 containing zeaxanthin, α-carotene, and β-carotene; lycopene; and other carotenoids are known as lipophilic carotenoids of saffron. Hydrophilic

carotenoids are crocins (C-20) which are found in saffron in 6%–16% ratio. The solubility of crocins within saffron depends on their sugars. Generally, ester forms of crocetin as monoglycosyl or diglycosyl polyene series were isolated from aqueous fraction of saffron (Shahi et al., 2016; Bagur et al., 2018).

Crocins have deep red color and give their color to the water easily and quickly, and this property is used for identification and quality control of saffron. Because of these color properties, the saffron is used in food industries as a natural dye. After oxidative degradation of zeaxanthine, which is C-40 carotenoid, C-10-containing picrocrocin, hydroxysafranal, safranal, and C-20 containing crocetin, crocin are obtained (Fig. 13.2). Owing to changing of pH values within the media, dry saffron is easily oxidized and chemically breaks down by lights and other oxidants (Shahi et al., 2016; Bagur et al., 2018).

Many of the biological effects of saffron are due to the carotenoid compounds it contains. These effects are due to the strong antioxidant activity of carotenoids. Radicals that occur during metabolic reactions are responsible for the oxidation events in our body. Oxidative damage to cells also causes many diseases to occur in organs. The effects of saffron's carotenoid extract against oxidation are due to (1) interaction with enzymes and (2) ROS direct suppression. In both mechanisms, crocetin was effective and the effect of safranal was shown to be weaker (Bolhassani et al., 2014; Bagur et al. (2018).

The group of active compounds that are effective in the treatment of ophthalmological diseases especially for glaucoma and age-related macular degeneration (AMD) are crocins which are water-soluble carotenoids. The activities of crocins for glaucoma and AMD treatment were evaluated in in vitro, in vivo, and clinical studies (Falsini et al., 2010; Bisti et al., 2014; Bagur et al., 2018).

OCULAR DISEASES
Glaucoma

Glaucoma, also known as eye pressure, is an eye disease that results from increased intraocular pressure, resulting in blindness when untreated. Inside the eye, there is a fluid circulating in the front to feed the tissues. This liquid is produced in the eye. In some eyes, this fluid cannot be ejected because of obstruction in the canals and elevated intraocular pressure. This causes damage in the optic nerve (Fig. 13.3) (Weinreb and Khaw, 2004).

Glaucoma, at the beginning, may go unnoticed. It progresses slowly over the years and wreaks havoc. The vision decreases gradually, and when the complaints begin, permanent damage to the visual field is located. In case of acute glaucoma crisis, the eye pressure increases suddenly. The eye also has symptoms

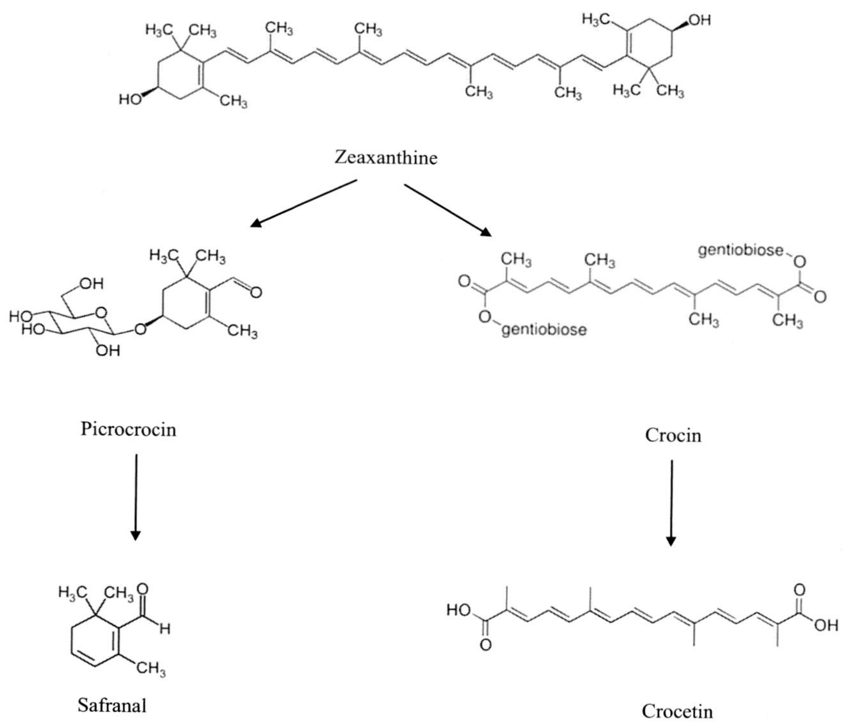

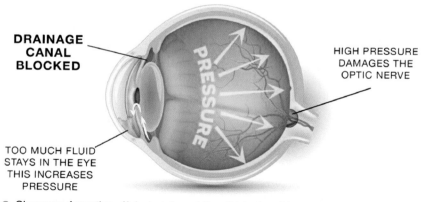

Zeaxanthine

Picrocrocin

Crocin

Safranal

Crocetin

FIG. 13.2 Main active components of saffron stigma.

DRAINAGE CANAL BLOCKED

PRESSURE

HIGH PRESSURE DAMAGES THE OPTIC NERVE

TOO MUCH FLUID STAYS IN THE EYE THIS INCREASES PRESSURE

FIG. 13.3 Glaucoma formation. (Adapted from https://iristech.co/glaucoma-signs-and-symptoms/, April 2019.)

such as redness, pain, blurred vision, and seeing colored rings around lights, in addition to nausea and vomiting. Diagnosis can be made earlier in such patients (Foster et al., 2002; Weinreb and Khaw, 2004).

The purpose of glaucoma treatment is to improve the visual quality of patients. Glaucoma treatment may be implemented by drugs, laser treatment, and surgical treatment. Treatment usually starts with medication; laser or surgical treatment is applied if the damage persists. Appropriate treatment is applied depending on the patient's condition. Early or late diagnosis, the patient's age, and whether or not to use drugs properly are important factors. Treatment cannot bring back the old vision but only prevents more vision loss. Selective laser trabeculoplasty (SLT) is an alternative treatment option for glaucoma. It provides a supportive solution when the treatment is not enough in patients receiving medication. It can only be applied to open-angle glaucoma. SLT, which is very effective in correctly selected patients, is a simple treatment method of 3–4 min with no side effects and no harm. It can reduce eye pressure by 20% –30%. The effectiveness of the treatment, which can be administered every 6 months, continues between 6 months and 2 years (Dietlein et al., 2009).

Age-Related Macular Degeneration

AMD is a macula (*Macula lutea*, center of the retina) disease. *Macula lutea* contains the lutein and zeaxanthin as photoreceptors that are responsible for yellow colorization. These xanthophyll isomers and their action mechanisms were discovered in 1980s. In 1866, the absorption of blue light within the same receptors was described, and then the similar absorption spectra with carotenoids were shown within the macula in 1945 (Beatty et al., 1999; Gehrs et al., 2006).

Generally, increasing of oxidation in the macula AMD occurs, and antioxidant pigments found in the macula are known as protective agents. Decreasing the level of macular pigments causes macular degeneration. In the treatment of macular degeneration, carotenoid-containing supplements are used (Beatty et al., 1999). AMD is the main reason for blindness in over 65 elderly patients. The scientific literature contains various results according to the countries, age groups, and etc (Bird et al., 1995; Gehrs et al., 2006).

Two different types of AMD diseases are known: dry AMD (atrophic type) and wet AMD (neovascular type). Dry type of AMD is the main reason for more than 20% of the blindness in patients (Gehrs et al., 2006)

1. Dry-type AMD: It is a common form of the disease, which results in slow but progressive visual impairment. This disease, which can progress without notice, constitutes approximately 85%–90% of AMD. Dry type is known as chronic AMD and generally some visual impairment and progresses to severe blind develops (Fig. 13.4) (Ambati and Fowler, 2012).

2. Wet-type AMD: A more serious form of disease which progresses rapidly. This disease is the leading cause of vision loss in older ages and occurs in approximately 10%–15% of AMD patients. Age-type AMD is caused by abnormal development of blood vessels at the back of the eye. These blood vessels can cause blood and fluid leakage, causing loss of your central vision. Age type intensive care

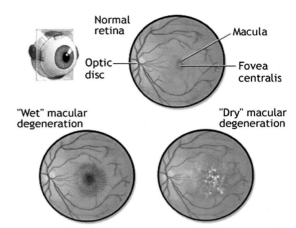

FIG. 13.4 Dry and wet macular degeneration. (Adapted from https://www.medicalmarijuana.com/, April 2019.)

unit can affect your ability to see both near and far as you look at a photo or reading the number of the bus (Fig. 13.4) (Ambati and Fowler, 2012).

The macula covers a very small area called the yellow spot in the middle of the retina layer and responsible for sharp vision (Fig. 13.4). Our vision is weaker in the center of the macula toward sharper edges. Macular degeneration is the result of damage to this yellow point (Beatty et al., 1999; Gehrs et al., 2006).

Retinal areas outside the macula are protected from environmental lights. Therefore, macular degeneration does not lead to complete blindness, but as in Fig. 13.1, it may make the close study and reading impossible without various optical auxiliary devices. The main risk factor for the development of degeneration within the macula is age. It is a retinal disease that causes serious vision loss, especially in the 50-year-old population in developed countries. It is the known cause of visual loss in western countries in people older than 65 years. Severe vision loss increases with age (Gehrs et al., 2006).

What are the risk factors for macular degeneration?

- Age: Age is the most important risk factor for macular degeneration. AMD is observed in one in three adults older than 75 years.
- Smoking: Cigarette smoking is one of the factors that increase the risk of developing the AMD. The retina produces high levels of oxygen consumption. Each factor that affects the access of the oxygen to the retina has a negative effect on vision.
- Genetic factors: People with a family of yellow dot diseases have a higher risk of developing this disease.
- Gender: Women are more likely to have yellow spot disease. However, since the life span of women is

longer, this can be explained by the fact that women have more time to develop the disease.

- Long lifetime sun exposure: Ultraviolet rays directly damage the retinal tissue and lead to the accumulation of harmful products in the retina.
- Dietary and/or low nutritional value, antioxidant-free diet: It is determined that the rate of macular degeneration is higher in individuals with high nutritional value, low nutritional value, and low antioxidant diet.
- Inactivity: People who do not exercise regularly are more likely to be affected by AMD. Owing to inactivity in dry macular degeneration, failure of the retina to obtain adequate oxygen causes cell death in the macula. Exercises to improve cardiovascular health have a positive effect on the development of macular degeneration (Ambati and Fowler, 2012).

Treatment of AMD

Dry-type AMD cannot be treated with conventional therapies, and only neovascularization therapy, which is an emerging type of treatment is possible (Nowak, 2006) In addition, antioxidant supplement treatment plays a role in delaying of progression in 20%–25% ratio (Friedman et al., 2004; Beatty et al., 1999; Nowak, 2006).

General treatment methods applied for treatment of wet-type AMD are as follows (Nowak, 2006):

1. Photodynamic therapy
2. Thermal laser photocoagulation
3. Transpupillary thermotherapy
4. Antiangiogenic agents
   a. Pegaptanib sodium (Macugen)
   b. Bevacizumab (Avastin)
   c. Ranibizumab (rhuFab V2; Lucentis)
   d. Anecortave acetate (Retaane)
   e. Triamcinolone acetonide
   f. Squalamine lactate (Evizon)
   g. Sirna-027 (small interfering RNA, siRNA)
   h. VEGF-Trap (VEGF-Trap$_{R1R2}$; soluble decoy receptor)
   i. Angiostatin, endostatin, and PEDF (Pigment epithelium-derived factor)

In addition, stem cell transplantation has been tried for the treatment of AMD in recent years. Phase I and II studies of some pharmaceutical industries with the stem cells are ongoing. These studies aim to treat especially dry-type macular degeneration using human embryogenic stem cells.

In addition, antioxidant supplementation is also applied for the treatment of AMD as an additional therapy. The use of ascorbic acid, α-tocopherol, glutathione, zinc, and macular carotenoids (lutein and zeaxanthin) plays a both preventive and treatment role against the AMD. Especially, macular carotenoids are well-known and important agents for macular degeneration (Nowak, 2006).

SAFFRON CAROTENOIDS FOR THE TREATMENT OF GLAUCOMA AND AMD

Saffron has strong antioxidant properties because of its polar carotenoids. These polar carotenoids are known as crocin and crocetin and are particularly effective in the treatment of ocular diseases. They protect retinal cells from oxidation and help them to perform their functions when used in the treatment of age-related maculopathy (Broadhead et al., 2015; Heitmar et al., 2019).

Many plant products produced for this purpose contain extracts carrying these polar carotenoids. In the scientific studies conducted in this field, extracts containing carotenoids were used. In vitro, in vivo, and clinical trials have been confirmed to be particularly effective in the treatment of AMD and glaucoma of saffron carotenoids. As a result of the treatment with extracts administered at daily doses of 20–50 mg for 3 months, clinical studies showed statistically significant improvement compared with the control group (Heitmar et al., 2019).

An in vitro assay with pure crocin inhibited damage to the photoreceptors because of concentration in the primary retina cell culture (EC$_{50}$: 30 mM). In an in vivo study with crocin derivatives isolated from saffron, it was noted that the blood flow in the eye was accelerated and crocin derivatives caused increased vascular enlargement and increased oxygenation (Alavizadeh and Hosseinzadeh, 2014; Xuan et al., 1999).

Clinical Trials for Ocular Diseases with Saffron

Clinical studies with saffron or its extracts were published on three different ocular diseases such as diabetic maculopathy, age-related maculopathy, and glaucoma. Saffron and its active compound crocin have shown significant activities in the clinical trials using the antidiabetic, antiapoptotic, antioxidant, antiinflammatory, antihypertensive, antiatherogenic, and neuroprotective mechanisms in the ocular diseases (Heitmar et al., 2019).

Diabetic macular edema is a main problem especially for patients with type 2 diabetes. These patients were treated with carotenoid fraction of saffron which contains crocin. Crocin is used for preventive or therapeutic purposes for patients with diabetic macular edema. Because of these properties of crocin, many pharmaceutical products contain crocin as an active constituent for maculopathy in the market. Some clinical studies were performed with ready-to-use pharmaceutical preparation to reduce the inflammation in the retinal tissue (Heitmar et al., 2019).

Sepahi et al. (2018) tried 5-mg or 15-mg crocin supplements per day for 3 months in the test group with diabetic macular edema. During the study, HbA1c, fasting blood sugar levels, central macular thickness, and best-corrected visual acuity were measured in every month. After 3 months of application, differences between 15 mg of crocin and placebo for fasting blood sugar level were 18, and for HbA1c, it was 0.76. In the same study, ophthalmic examinations such as central macular thickness and best-corrected visual acuity were also measured, and statistically significant results were found for the 15-mg crocin group. It was concluded that the 15-mg crocin administration per day for patients with diabetic maculopathy improved all symptoms.

In another clinical study, mild and moderate retinal maculopathy was treated with saffron supplement orally. Up to 50-year-old patients with mild and moderate retinal maculopathy were administered orally 20 mg of saffron supplement per day for 3 months. Statistically significant differences were obtained for best-corrected visual acuity and multifocal electroretinogram response density and latency between test and placebo groups after 3 months. In this study, some other safety properties were also measured, and no adverse and side effects were found at the end (Broadhead et al., 2019).

P2X7 receptors that are responsible for the health of retina occur in our nervous system and retinal inner and outer cells as well. According to literature information, the age-related retinal maculopathy which is the neurodegenerative ocular disease is related to P2X7 receptors. In an in vitro study (Corso, 2016), saffron was tested on mouse primary retinal cells and mouse retinal photoreceptor-derived 661W cells, which were high-concentration ATP-stressed. Saffron increased the viability of both cells and reduced the intracellular calcium level. Owing to the in vitro results, the treatment effects of saffron in the neurodegenerative disease were shown using mouse retinal cell cultures and corrected the relation between P2X7 receptors and age-related maculopathy (Corso, 2016).

Saffron extract was evaluated for dry-type age-related retinal maculopathy clinically, and the patients took saffron as 50 mg of extract in a gelatin capsule with 250 mg of starch for a period of 3 months. After the treatment period, different ophthalmological parameters such as contrast sensitivity, retinal thickness, and visual acuity were evaluated. Contrast sensitivity and visual acuity were improved significantly, whereas retinal thickness did not change (Riazi et al., 2017).

The oxidative damage plays a role in glaucoma, which is characterized by intraocular hypertension. In a clinical study, the patients with glaucoma were administered 30 mg/day of aqueous saffron extract orally during 1-month period. The intraocular pressures of both test and control groups were measured, and statistically significant results showing a decrease were obtained from test group. The pressure of control group was changed from 12.9 ± 3.7 to 10.6 ± 3.0 by water extract of saffron in 3 weeks (Bonyadi et al., 2014).

Saffron was evaluated in another clinical trial against AMD in 20-mg/day dose during 3 months. In this study, 25 patients were used in both groups as test and placebo, and their focal electroretinograms and other clinical scores were recorded as baseline and end point. The focal electroretinograms of test group were significantly increased by saffron in 3 months. They indicated that the responsible compounds were carotenoids in the treatment of AMD because of their antioxidant properties (Falsini et al., 2010).

CONCLUSION

As a result of clinical studies performed with the extracts of carotenoids of saffron, it has been shown that statistically significant results are obtained in both glaucoma and AMD. In these studies, patients older than 50 years were selected, and 20–50 mg of daily dose was administered orally for 3 months. As a result of the studies, different data were evaluated, and statistically significant results were obtained. According to these studies, significant results were obtained especially in the treatment of diabetes and glaucoma and maculopathy diseases that are related to diabetes and age. In addition, the levels of various biochemical substances related to diabetes in patients with diabetes also reached normal limits.

The activity of saffron depends on the crocin and crocetin, which are saffron carotenoids formed from zeaxanthin. Saffron carotenoids are the responsible components because of their antioxidant properties for the ocular diseases such as glaucoma and AMD.

At the end, saffron can be recommended for both preventive and therapeutic purposes, especially in the treatment of diabetic glaucoma and AMD.

REFERENCES

Alavizadeh, S.H., Hosseinzadeh, H., 2014. Bioactivity assessment and toxicity of crocin: a comprehensive review. Food Chem. Toxicol. 64, 65–80.

Ambati, J., Fowler, B.J., 2012. Mechanisms of age-related macular degeneration. Neuron 75, 26–39.

Bagur, M.J., Salinas, G.L.A., Jiménez-Monreal, A.M., Chaouqi, S., Llorens, S., Martínez-Tomé, M., Alonso, G.L., 2018. Saffron: an old medicinal plant and a potential novel functional food. Molecules 23, 30.

Beatty, S., Boulton, M., Henson, D., Koh, H.-H., Murray, I.J., 1999. Macular pigment and age related macular degeneration. Br. J. Ophthalmol. 83, 867–877.

Bird, A.C., Bressler, N.M., Bressler, S.B., Chisholm, I.H., Coscas, G., Davis, M.D., de Jong, P.T., Klaver, C.C., Klein, B.E., Klein, R., et al., 1995. An international classification and grading system for age-related maculopathy and age-related macular degeneration. Surv. Ophthalmol. 39, 367–374.

Bisti, S., Maccarone, R., Falsini, B., 2014. Saffron and retina: neuroprotection and pharmacokinetics. Vis. Neurosci. 31, 355–361.

Bolhassani, A., Khavari, A., Bathaie, S.Z., 2014. Saffron and natural carotenoids: biochemical activities and anti-tumor effects. Biochim. Biophys. Acta 1845, 20–30.

Bonyadi, M.H.J., Yazdani, S., Saadat, S., 2014. The ocular hypotensive effect of saffron extract in primary open angle glaucoma: a pilot study. BMC Complement. Altern. Med. 14, 399.

Broadhead, G.K., Grigg, J.R., Chang, A.A., McCluskey, P., 2015. Dietary modification and supplementation for the treatment. Nutr. Rev. 73, 448–462.

Broadhead, G.K., Chang, A., Grigg, J.R., Mccluskey, P., 2016. Efficacy and safety of saffron supplementation: current clinical findings. Crit. Rev. Food Sci. Nutr. 56, 2767–2776.

Broadhead, G.K., Grigg, J.R., McCluskey, P., Hong, T., Schlub, T.E., Chang, A.A., 2019. Saffron therapy for the treatment of mild/moderate age-related macular degeneration: a randomised clinical trial. Graefes Arch. Clin. Exp. Ophthalmol. 257, 31–40.

Corso, L., Cavallero, A., Baroni, D., Garbati, P., Prestipino, G., Bisti, S., Nobile, M., Picco, C., 2016. Saffron reduces ATP-induced retinal cytotoxicity by targeting P2X7 receptors. Purinergic Signalling 12, 161–174.

Dietlein, T.S., Hermann, M.M., Jordan, J.F., 2009. The medical and surgical treatment of glaucoma. Dtsch. Arztebl. Int. 106, 597–605.

Falsini, B., Piccardi, M., Minnella, A., Savastano, C., Capoluongo, E., Fadda, A., Balestrazzi, E., Maccarone, R., Bisti, S., 2010. Influence of saffron supplementation on retinal flicker sensitivity in early age-related macular degeneration. Investig. Ophthalmol. Vis. Sci. 51, 6118–6124.

Foster, P.J., Buhrmann, R., Quigley, H.A., Johnson, G.J., 2002. The definition and classification of glaucoma in prevalence surveys. Br. J. Ophthalmol. 86, 238–242.

Friedman, D.S., O'Colmain, B.J., Muñoz, B., Tomany, S.C., McCarty, C., de Jong, P.T., Nemesure, B., Mitchell, P., Kempen, J., 2004. Prevalence of age-related macular degeneration in the United States. Arch. Ophthalmol. 122, 564–572.

Gehrs, K.M., Anderson, D.H., Johnson, L.V., Hageman, G.S., 2006. Age-related macular degeneration—emerging pathogenetic and therapeutic concepts. Ann. Med. 38, 450–471.

Giaccio, M., 2004. Crocetin from saffron: an active component of an ancient spice. Crit. Rev. Food Sci. Nutr. 44, 155–172.

Heitmar, R., Brown, J., Kyrou, I., 2019. Saffron (Crocus sativus L.) in ocular diseases: a narrative review of the existing evidence from clinical studies of age-related macular degeneration. Nutrients 11, 649.

Javadi, B., Sahebkar, A., Emami, S.A., 2013. A survey on saffron in major islamic traditional medicine books. Iran. J. Basic Med. Sci. 16, 1–11.

Mousavi, S.Z., Bathaie, S.Z., 2011. Historical uses of saffron: identifying potential new avenues for modern research. Avicenna J. Phytomed. 1, 57–66.

Nowak, J.Z., 2006. Age-related macular degeneration (AMD): pathogenesis and therapy. Pharmacol. Rep. 58, 353–363.

Riazi, A., Panahi, Y., Alishiri, A.A., Hosseini, M.A., Zarchi, A.A.K., Sahebkar, A., 2017. The impact of saffron (Crocus sativus) supplementation on visual function in patients with dry age-related macular degeneration. Ital. J Med. 11, 196–201.

Rios, J.L., Recio, M.C., Giner, R.M., Manez, S., 1996. An update review of saffron and its active constituents. Phytother Res. 10, 189–193.

Sepahi, S., Mohajeri, S.A., Hosseini, S.M., Khodaverdi, E., Shoeibi, N., Namdari, M., Tabassi, S.A.S., 2018. Effects of crocin on diabetic maculopathy: a placebo-controlled randomized clinical trial. Am. J. Ophthalmol. 190, 89–98.

Shahi, T., Assadpour, E., Jafari, S.M., 2016. Main chemical compounds and pharmacological activities of stigmas and tepals of 'red gold'; saffron. Trends Food Sci. Technol. 58, 69–78.

Weinreb, R.N., Khaw, P.T., 2004. Primary open-angle glaucoma. Lancet 363, 1711–1720.

Xuan, B., Zhou, Y.-H., Li, N., Min, Z.-D., Chiou, G.C.Y., 1999. Effects of crocin analogs on ocular blood flow and retinal function. J. Ocul. Pharmacol. Ther. 15, 143–152.

CHAPTER 14

Saffron Shifts the Degenerative and Inflammatory Phenotype in Photoreceptor Degeneration

SILVIA BISTI* • STEFANO DI MARCO* • MARIA ANNA MAGGI • MATTIA DI PAOLO • MARCO PICCARDI • BENEDETTO FALSINI

SAFFRON CHEMISTRY

Crocus sativus L. belongs to the Iridaceae family, and commonly it is known as saffron. The flowers of *Crocus sativus* L. are composed of six violet petals, three yellow stamens, and a white filiform stem that culminates in three red stigmas, representing only 7.4% of the total weight of the fresh flower. From about 170,000 saffron flowers, together weighing more than 68 kg, 1 kg of spice can be obtained (Serrano-Díaz et al., 2014).

The different cultures together with the geoclimatic characteristics of the territory determine a different chemical composition that characterizes the final product. Saffron is one of the most expensive spices in the world, but high cost leads to a high rate of counterfeiting. The scientific community's interest in this product, however, is not only the intent of guaranteeing its authenticity to the consumer. Advanced pharmacological studies have in fact highlighted its numerous beneficial effects including the neuroprotective and antioxidant activity (see Stone et al., 2018 for ref.).

This is why a complete knowledge of this product is fundamental, from which more than 150 chemical compounds have been extracted, but only about a third of them have been identified (Bathaie et al., 2014). Saffron has primary metabolites, ubiquitous species in nature, such as carbohydrates, minerals, fats, vitamins, amino acids, and proteins as well as a large number of compounds belonging to different classes of secondary metabolites. These are nonubiquitous metabolism products but are still important for the development or reproduction of the organism, such as carotenoids, monoterpenes, and flavonoids, including mainly anthocyanins.

Among the secondary metabolites of saffron, the derivatives of crocetin (crocins) and the safranal are the most studied.

Carotenoids are the most important constituents of the spice, from which it derives its color. They include fat-soluble ones, such as α- and β-carotene, lycopene, zeaxanthin, and the apocarotenoid crocetin ($C_{20}H_{24}O_4$), and water-soluble ones, such as the polyene esters of the mono- and diglycoside crocetin, the crocins.

Crocetin is derived from the carotenoid zeaxanthin of the xanthophyll class and constitutes approximately 0.3% of the total weight of the plant's stigmas. It is a polyether dicarboxylic acid present mostly in its "*all-trans*" form, the *13-cis* form and its derivatives are minor components (Fig. 14.1).

Crocins are a family of carotenoids very soluble in water as mono- and diglycosylated esters of the dicarboxylic acid crocetin (Lozano et al., 1999). They make up 3.5% of the weight of the stigmas in the plant. The glycosidic carotenoids of saffron, like all glycosides, are usually thermally labile and photochemically sensitive, especially if in solution. As well as their precursor, the crocins exist in the two isomeric form: *13-cis* and "*all-trans*" (Fig. 14.2).

Furthermore, esterification of crocetins occurs in either of its end groups or only on one and with different saccharide residues on their anomeric carbon. The most common carbohydrates found in these molecules are D-glucose, β-D-gentiobiose (disaccharide made up of two D-glucose units with a 1β-6'-glycosidic bond), tri-β-D-glucose and the β-D-neapolitanose. *All-trans* glycosylated carotenoids show two absorption bands in the visible region. The first, at 256 nm, is due to the ester bond with the saccharide component, and the second is

---

*Equally contributing.

Saffron. https://doi.org/10.1016/B978-0-12-818462-2.00014-0

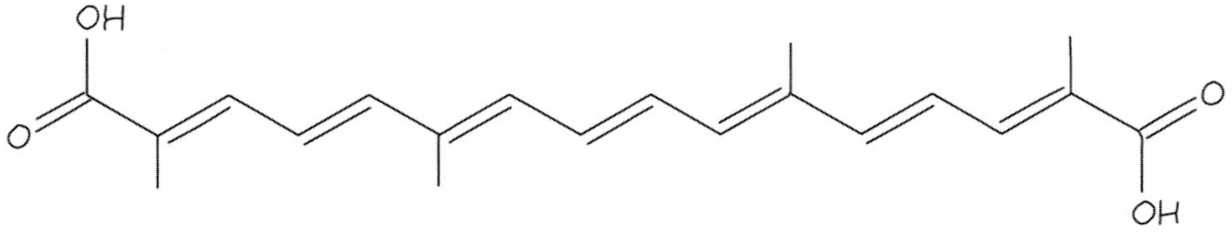

FIG. 14.1 Structure of the *all-trans* crocetin.

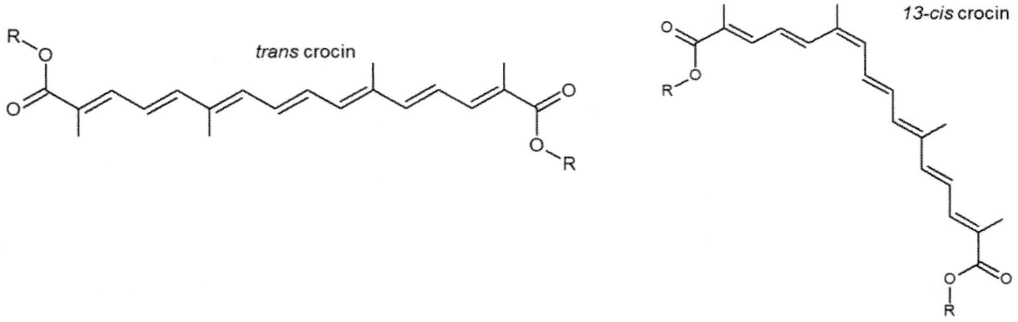

FIG. 14.2 Structure of *trans* and *cis* crocins.

located between 400 and 500 nm, with a maximum at 441 nm. The *cis* isomers have three bands in the same region because there is also an absorption at about 325 nm. This is due to the presence of a double bond with a *cis* configuration in a conjugated polyene (Fig. 14.3).

There is a great variety of crocins because there are different combinations of carbohydrates that can go to esterify one or both carboxyl groups and both isomeric forms. Although these crocins differ in the substituents and in the configuration, they have very similar chemical–physical properties, in particular the polarity. These similarities make their separation and subsequent identification extremely difficult.

Among the oxidation products of carotenoids, we find two compounds: picocrocin and safranal that give the spice bitterness strength and aroma strength, respectively. They are, respectively, the monoterpene glycoside (picocrocin) and the cyclic monoterpene aldehyde (safranal). According to the most accredited hypothesis, the precursor is considered to be zeaxanthin, which is broken at both ends by the enzyme CsZCD (*Crocus sativus* zeaxanthin cleavage dioxygenase) to generate the crocetin dialdehyde (Bouvier et al., 2003), which can be oxidized and esterified by different glucosyltransferases to give the crocins (Moraga et al., 2004), and the picocrocin. The picocrocin ($C_{16}H_{26}O_7$), which constitutes

3.7% of the weight of the stigma, has been identified only in the genus *Crocus* of which the only edible spice is the *Crocus sativus* L.; therefore, it constitutes the molecular marker of the saffron. During the drying process, the β-glucosidase enzyme acts on the picocrocin to release the 4-hydroxy-2,6,6-trimethyl-1-cyclohexene-1-carboxyaldehyde (HTCC, $C_{10}H_{16}O_2$) (Himeno and Sano, 1987), which by dehydration is transformed into safranal ($C_{10}H_{14}O$), with a characteristic absorption band at 310 nm. This is present with a percentage of 0.02% in the stigma and is the major component of the volatile fraction of saffron (Fig. 14.4).

The chemical composition of saffron is the digital fingerprint of this spice and is fundamental for its geographical traceability. Saffron traceability is important because this spice is among foods more subject to adulteration (Moore et al., 2012).

A chemo metric treatment of experimental data was used for geographical classification studies of saffron. These data were collected using different analytical methods, such as high performance liquid chromatography (D'Archivio et al., 2016), gas chromatography (D'Archivio et al., 2018), elemental analysis of bioelements (Maggi et al., 2011), or trace inorganic elements (D'Archivio et al., 2014).

Among the saffron metabolites identified with the different analysis methods that play an important role

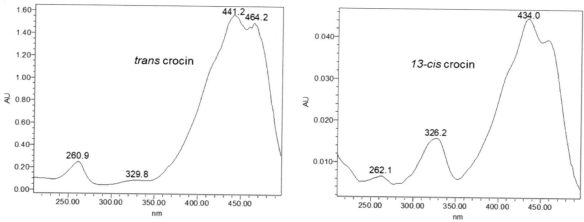

FIG. 14.3 Adsorption spectrum *trans* and *cis* crocins.

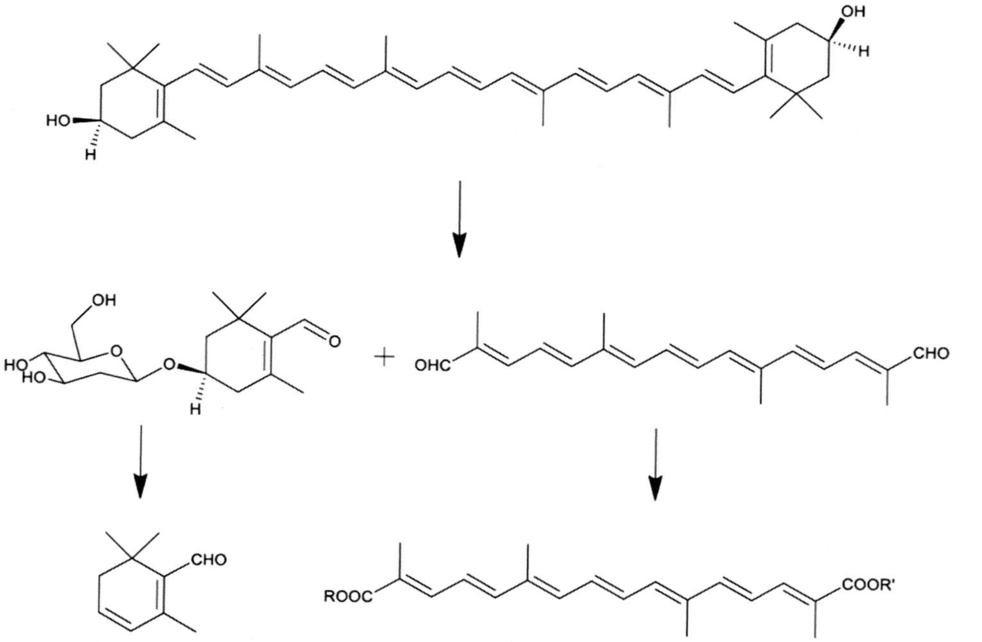

FIG. 14.4 Main hypothesis on the biosynthesis of the esters of crocetin, picrocrocin, and safranal *in Crocus sativus L.*

in the geographical classification, there are crocins, flavonoids, free amino acids, and the components of the volatile fraction (ketones and terpenic aldehydes, safranal).

Another technique also used for traceability studies is the analysis by UV–visible spectrophotometry (D'Archivio and Maggi, 2017) used with other physicochemical analysis, to determine the quality of saffron according to ISO Normative (ISO, 2010, 2011). From absorbance values at 440, 257, and 330 nm of aqueous extract, associated with coloring strength, flavor or bitterness strength, and aroma strength, respectively, to the three quality categories of saffron. Recently, it became clear that the chemical composition of saffron is not only relevant for its quality and traceability but is an essential requirement to define saffron efficacy in treating neurodegenerative processes.

PHOTORECEPTORS

Visual perception initiates in the retina by the activation of photoreceptors by quanta of light. Light photoisomerizes the 11-*cis*-retinal (11-*cis*-RAL) chromophore of photoreceptor visual pigments to an all-*trans* configuration. This gives rise to a complex series of events (see for ref. Kiser and Palczewski, 2016) that analyze the visual scene in terms of time, space, and color components to be transferred to higher visual centers. Photoreceptors are neurons highly specialized to accomplish the sophisticated task of transforming energy into electric signals; the only language recognized by the peripheral and central nervous system. They have a very high metabolism and a unique way to maintain their function (Léveillard et al., 2019; Narayan et al., 2017; Stone et al., 2008) so much so that both the choroid plexus and retinal pigment epithelium (RPE) are fundamental to support their requirements (Léveillard et al., 2019; Yu et al., 2019). On this basis, it is easy to understand that the extremely high specialization of photoreceptors makes them fragile to cope with internal and external stresses including aging. One of the main challenges for photoreceptor function and survival is oxidative stress.

Oxidative Damage in Acquired and Inherited Photoreceptor Degenerations

Photoreceptors absorb light, and this process leads to oxidation of their membrane lipids when both intensity and time exposure are increased (Organisciak et al., 1992; Tanito et al., 2006; Wiegand et al., 1983). It is possible to induce morphological and functional damage associated to the increased oxidative stress, as it is suggested by increased production of endogenous antioxidants (Gosbell et al., 2006; Organisciak et al., 1992; Penn et al., 1987) and that exogenous antioxidants are protective (Costa et al., 2008; Gosbell et al., 2006; Logvinov et al., 2005; Ranchon et al., 1999; Stahl and Sies, 2005; Tomita et al., 2005; Xie et al., 2007; Yılmaz et al., 2007) for cones (Komeima et al., 2006; Shen et al., 2005) as well as rods (Chrysostomou et al., 2008; Jozwick et al., 2006; Valter et al., 2009). The stress-induced death of photoreceptors is accompanied by damage to the survivors (Chrysostomou et al., 2008; Jozwick et al., 2006). It is interesting to note that in degenerative events starting with a genetic mutation of

rods the progression is often associated to the increased oxygen level and consequently accumulation of superoxide radicals induced by death of high oxygen consumer photoreceptor and the activation of nicotinamide adenine dinucleotide (Yu et al., 2000; Usui et al., 2009).

Superoxide radicals attack macromolecules, causing oxidative damage and the production of other molecules such as nitric oxide that generates peroxynitrite, a particularly damaging free radical that amplifies the damage (Komeima et al., 2008). Progressively antioxidant defense and repairing mechanism lose their efficiency and cell damage and apoptosis progress. Looking at cone density and distribution, it is possible to hypothesize that they start to die in periphery and then apoptosis moves posteriorly as it is observed in many retinal dystrophies. During this process, free radicals are continuously produced; thus, any treatment able to preserve cones has to be provided the entire life. An antioxidant treatment is efficient whether is able to reduce oxidative damage below a threshold to maintain active self-protective mechanisms in an effort to reduce dysfunction and apoptosis. Both long-term and short-term experiments are important to evaluate the efficacy of drugs and the possibility to rescue damaged but still viable cells.

Saffron (*Crocus sativus* Extract) Neuroprotection

Maccarone et al. (2008) tested whether the ancient spice "saffron" had good potentiality in protecting retina against the damage induced by light and results were very promising (see also Bisti et al., 2014 for ref.). Albino rats (Sprague–Dawley) were fed with saffron (1 mg/kg/day) for 21 days before exposing them to bright continuous light 1000 lux per 24 h. Animals were sacrificed either immediately at the end of the exposure or after a week treatment was continued until experimental session was completed. Photoreceptors death was defined with two techniques: direct measure of dying neurons and count of survivors. In addition, function was determined by recording flash ERG. Photoreceptor layer (ONL) resulted largely protected, as it was retinal function. Interestingly, the fibroblast growth factor (FGF2) was not upregulated as it happened in β-carotene-treated animals (Maccarone et al., 2008) where only morphology was maintained but not function. FGF2 upregulation was proved to abolish ERG response (Gargini et al., 2004). These results confirmed the hypothesis that saffron treatment might protect retina from stress probably acting as a regulator of a variety of functions including cell death

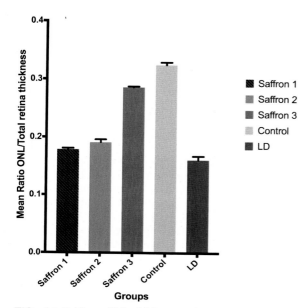

FIG. 14.9 Mean ONL thickness of dorsal retina as a function of animal treatment. At each point, the thickness of the ONL was calculated as the ratio between the thickness of the ONL and the thickness of the total retina. Relative statistics is reported in Table 14.2. Data are expressed as mean ± standard error.

A longitudinal open-label study in an outpatient ophthalmology setting was conducted to evaluate whether the observed functional benefits from saffron supplementation may extend over a longer follow-up duration. Twenty-nine early AMD patients (age range: 55–85 years) with a baseline visual acuity >0.3 were enrolled. They had dietary saffron supplementation (20 mg/day) over an average period of treatment of 14 (±2) months. Clinical examination and FERG (Falsini et al., 2010) were recorded every 3 months over a follow-up of 14 (±2) months. Retinal sensitivity, 1/over the threshold, was the main outcome measure. After 3 months of supplementation, mean FERG sensitivity improved by 0.3 log units compared to baseline values ($P < .01$), and mean visual acuity improved by two Snellen lines compared to baseline values (0.75–0.9, $P < .01$). These changes remained stable over the follow-up period 14 (±2) months (Piccardi et al., 2012). A second follow-up was performed to determine whether the functional effects of dietary supplementation with saffron are influenced by major risk genotypes such as complement factor H (CFH) and age-related maculopathy susceptibility 2 (ARMS2). Marangoni et al. (2013) longitudinally evaluated 33 early AMD patients, screened for CFH (rs1061170) and ARMS2 (rs10490924) polymorphisms and receiving saffron oral supplementation (20 mg/day) over an average period of treatment of 11 months (range, 6–12). FERG amplitude and macular sensitivity, the reciprocal value of the estimated FERG amplitude threshold, were the main outcome measures. After 3 months of supplementation, mean FERG amplitude and FERG sensitivity improved significantly when compared to baseline values ($P < .01$). These changes were stable throughout the follow-up period. No significant differences in clinical and FERG improvements were observed across different CFH or ARMS 2 genotypes (Marangoni et al., 2013). These results indicate that the functional effect of saffron

but not after placebo supplementation compared to baseline (mean change after saffron: 0.26 log units; mean change after placebo: 0.0003 log units). The results indicate that short-term dietary saffron supplementation improves retinal flicker sensitivity in early AMD. Although such results need to be further replicated, and the clinical significance is yet to be evaluated, they provided important clues that nutritional saffron carotenoids may impact AMD in novel and unexpected ways, possibly beyond their antioxidant properties (clinicaltrials.gov: NCT00951288).

TABLE 14.2
Statistical analysis of data reported in Fig. 14.9

	Saffron 1	Saffron 2	Saffron 3	Control	Light Damage
Saffron 1		Not significant	$P < .0001$	$P < .0001$	Not significant
Saffron 2	Not significant		$P < .0001$	$P < .0001$	$P < .005$
Saffron 3	$P < .0001$	$P < .0001$		$P < .005$	$P < .0001$
Control	$P < .0001$	$P < .0001$	$P < .005$		$P < .0001$
Light Damage	Not significant	$P < .005$	$P < .0001$	$P < .0001$	

supplementation in individual AMD patients is not related to the major risk genotypes of disease. Recently, the efficacy of saffron treatment in AMD patients has been confirmed by different groups (Broadhead et al., 2019; Riazi et al., 2016). Although there are some differences in dosage and efficacy, we might suppose that this is due to the chemical composition of the saffron used as evidence has been provided that an appropriate ratio among crocins increases the neuroprotective efficacy.

Stargardt

Stargardt disease 1 (STGD1 # 248,200) is a severe hereditary recessive macular dystrophy (Blacharski, 1988) characterized by the progressive retinal degeneration of rod and cone photoreceptors, with central retina (macula) involvement and the appearance of orange/yellow flecks distributed around the macula and/or the midretinal periphery (Noble and Carr, 1979) Mutations in the gene encoding an ATP-binding cassette (ABC) transporter (ABCA4 have been demonstrated to be responsible for STGD1 (Allikmets, 1997). Deficiency in ABCA4 function eventually leads to exaggerated production of bis-retinoids, the main components of lipofuscin, which may cause photooxidative damage and RPE degeneration (reviewed by Tanna et al., 2017 and Kim et al., 2006). Oxidative damage is a major mechanism involved in ABCA4-related retinopathy. Damaging retinal mechanisms of mutant "Abca4/-" retinas have been extensively investigated in the past, and much evidence (Sparrow et al., 2003; Weng et al., 1999) leads to the hypothesis that photoreceptors die because of RPE 'poisoning' by lipofuscin accumulation and the loss of the RPE support role. A2E arises from the condensation of phosphatidyl-ethanolamine and all-*trans*-retinal released from photoactivated rhodopsin (Sparrow et al., 2000), likely leading to the increased absorption of blue lights and phototoxic RPE cell damage in vivo. These compounds cannot readily be metabolized in RPE cells and trigger RPE cell degeneration through prevalent oxidative damage, which, in turn, might lead to photoreceptor dysfunction and death (Chen et al., 2012). The mutation-induced disease may affect both rod and cone photoreceptors at relatively early stages. In vitro studies (Sun and Nathans, 2001) also demonstrated that "Abca4" itself is an efficient target of all-*trans*-retinal-mediated photooxidative damage. However, several other mechanisms, occurring in parallel or in a cascade of events, might contribute to the disease development and progression. A second important aspect of the degenerative process is the activation of the inflammation cascade and

downregulation of antiinflammatory defenses. Both aspects have been recently discussed. Radu and collaborators reported that A2E accumulation causes oxidative stress, complement activation, and downregulation of protective complement-related proteins in the "Abca4 −/−" mouse model (Radu et al., 2011), while in Kohno et al. (2013) it has been shown that microglial activation increases retinal degeneration. Recently, a clinical trial was performed in patients with Stargardt disease (Falsini et al., 2014). The aim of this study was to investigate the effect of saffron (S) supplementation on central retinal function in STG/FF patients carrying ABCA4 mutations. In a randomized, double-blind, placebo-controlled, cross-over study (clinicaltrials.gov: NCT01278277), 31 patients with ABCA4-related STD/FF and a visual acuity ≥0.25 were randomly assigned to assume oral S (20 mg/day) or placebo (P) over a 6-month period, and then reverted to P or S supplementation for a further 6-month period. Full ophthalmic examination and FERG recordings were performed at baseline and after 6 months of either S or P. FERGs were recorded in response to a 41 Hz, sinusoidally modulated (93.5%) uniform field presented to the macular region (18 degrees) on a light-adapting background. For each FERG response, the Fourier-isolated fundamental harmonic component was measured, and the noise level at this component was estimated. Main outcome measures were FERG amplitude (in microV), signal-to-noise amplitude ratio (S/N in dB), and phase (in degrees). In all patients, either S or P was well tolerated, and no side effects were observed. After P, FERG amplitude decreased from baseline (mean change: 0.18 log μV, $P < .05$). After S, FERG amplitude was unchanged. Throughout the follow-up, mean S/N was above the cut-off threshold of 3.5 dB. FERG phase and visual acuity were unchanged. The results indicate that dietary saffron is well tolerated and free of side effects. The FERG outcomes of this study support the potential of antioxidant therapeutic strategies to prevent the progression of ABCA4-related central retinal degeneration/dysfunction, Fig. 14.10 shows an example of results obtained in one patient. The FERG results shown are recorded before and after 6 months of saffron supplementation in an STDG patient with 0.7 visual acuity. It can be noted that amplitude showed a slight increase (about 20%) from baseline, whereas phase was unchanged.

The results indicate that dietary saffron is well tolerated and free of side effects. The FERG outcomes of this study support the potential of this therapeutic strategy to prevent the progression of ABCA4-related central retinal degeneration/dysfunction.

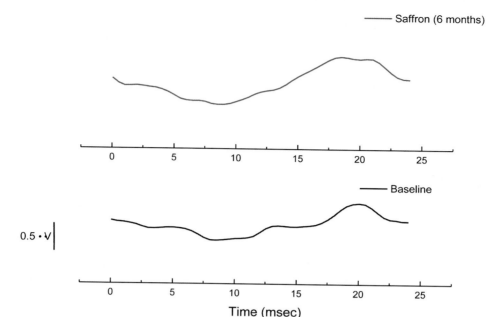

FIG. 14.10 Representative examples of FERG responses obtained from a Stargardt disease patient before and after 6 months of saffron supplementation. FERGs were recorded in response to sinusoidally flickering stimuli presented to the macular region (18°) and modulated at 41 Hz. Visual acuity was 0.7 at baseline and 0.8 after saffron.

CONCLUSIONS

We reviewed and presented original data on saffron treatment in retinal neurodegeneration, both in animal models and patients with AMD and Stargardt. Several conclusions can be drawn looking at the experimental data. Saffron does not have a unique way of action. Although the chemistry of its components suggests a strong antioxidant activity, it was proved that it is able to modulate the activity of many genes and eventually slowing down the progression of neurodegenerative diseases by modulating the activation of negative events including neuroinflammation. In addition, although saffron presents a quite stable genetic content, its reproduction is by cloning of corms, its neuroprotective efficacy strongly depends on the ratio among crocins (see Fig. 14.9), and why it happens is under investigation. This information has to be taken into account when saffron is used for treatment, and it can explain some discrepancies among results. Interestingly, this optimal ratio cannot be predicted by belonging to one of the three quality categories (I, II, and III). Saffron could be category I and not having the right ratio. An additional observation comes from the fractions experiment. Although crocins (fraction 100%) present a high neuroprotective activity, the entire saffron seems to introduce an added value even if not highly statistically significant. Altogether all these evidences point in the direction of a recently put forward idea that saffron treatment might induce "acquired resilience" and counteract dismetabolic negative events (Stone et al., 2018).

ACKNOWLEDGMENTS

We thank Lucia Corso and James Ashely for helping with cell cultures, Alessio Cavalli for its contribution with the "fractions experiments" and Giuseppe Cinquegrana for its contribution in the "Behavioral Experiments."

BF is supported by a grant of Fondi di Ateneo, Linea D3 "Nutrition and Aging" of Universita' Cattolica del S. Cuore, Rome, Italy.

SDM position is supported by Essse Caffè srl.

The grant providers (Hortus Novus srl, Universita' Cattolica del S. Cuore, Essse Caffè srl) had no role in study design, data collection and analysis, decision to publish, or preparation of the manuscript.

Disclosure Statements:

A patent "Compositions based on saffron for the prevention and/or treatment of degenerative eye disorders" covering the topic of this manuscript has been filed on March 20, 2015 (W02015/145316) and is owned by Hortus Novus srl.

S.B. and M.A.M. are inventors of the patent.

S.B. holds a nonremunerative relationship with Hortus Novus srl.

REFERENCES

Allikmets, R., 1997. A photoreceptor cell-specific ATP-binding transporter gene (ABCR) is mutated in recessive Stargardt macular dystrophy. Nat. Genet. 17, 122. https://doi.org/10.1038/ng0997-122a.

Bathaie, S., Farajzade, A., Hoshyar, R., 2014. A review of the chemistry and uses of crocins and crocetin, the carotenoid natural dyes in saffron, with particular emphasis on applications as colorants including their use as biological stains. Biotech. Histochem. 89, 401–411. https://doi.org/10.3109/10520295.2014.890741.

Bisti, S., Maccarone, R., Falsini, B., 2014. Saffron and retina: neuroprotection and pharmacokinetics. Vis. Neurosci. 31, 355–361. https://doi.org/10.1017/S0952523814000108.

Blacharski, P.A., 1988. Fundus flavimaculatus. Retin. Dystrophies Degener. 135–159.

Bouvier, F., Suire, C., Mutterer, J., Camara, B., 2003. Oxidative remodeling of chromoplast carotenoids: identification of the carotenoid dioxygenase CsCCD and CsZCD genes involved in Crocus secondary metabolite biogenesis. Plant Cell 15, 47–62.

Bringmann, A., Pannicke, T., Grosche, J., Francke, M., Wiedemann, P., Skatchkov, S.N., Osborne, N.N., Reichenbach, A., 2006. Müller cells in the healthy and diseased retina. Prog. Retin. Eye Res. 25, 397–424. https://doi.org/10.1016/j.preteyeres.2006.05.003.

Broadhead, G.K., Grigg, J.R., McCluskey, P., Hong, T., Schlub, T.E., Chang, A.A., 2019. Saffron therapy for the treatment of mild/moderate age-related macular degeneration: a randomised clinical trial. Graefes Arch. Clin. Exp. Ophthalmol. 257, 31–40. https://doi.org/10.1007/s00417-018-4163-x.

Chen, Y., Okano, K., Maeda, T., Chauhan, V., Golczak, M., Maeda, A., Palczewski, K., 2012. Mechanism of all-trans-retinal toxicity with implications for stargardt disease and age-related macular degeneration. J. Biol. Chem. 287, 5059–5069. https://doi.org/10.1074/jbc.M111.315432.

Chrysostomou, V., Stone, J., Stowe, S., Barnett, N.L., Valter, K., 2008. The status of cones in the rhodopsin mutant P23H-3 retina: light-regulated damage and repair in parallel with rods. Invest. Ophthalmol. Vis. Sci. 49, 1116–1125. https://doi.org/10.1167/iovs.07-1158.

Corso, L., Cavallero, A., Baroni, D., Garbati, P., Prestipino, G., Bisti, S., Nobile, M., Picco, C., 2016. Saffron reduces ATP-induced retinal cytotoxicity by targeting P2X7 receptors. Purinergic Signal. 12, 161–174. https://doi.org/10.1007/s11302-015-9490-3.

Costa, B.L., Fawcett, R., Li, G.-Y., Safa, R., Osborne, N.N., 2008. Orally administered epigallocatechin gallate attenuates light-induced photoreceptor damage. Brain Res. Bull. 76, 412–423. https://doi.org/10.1016/j.brainresbull.2008.01.022.

D'Archivio, A.A., Giannitto, A., Maggi, M.A., Ruggieri, F., 2016. Geographical classification of Italian saffron (Crocus sativus L.) based on chemical constituents determined by high-performance liquid-chromatography and by using linear discriminant analysis. Food Chem 212, 110–116. https://doi.org/10.1016/j.foodchem.2016.05.149.

D'Archivio, A.A., Di Pietro, L., Maggi, M.A., Rossi, L., 2018. Optimization using chemometrics of HS-SPME/GC—MS profiling of saffron aroma and identification of geographical volatile markers. Eur. Food Res. Technol 244, 1605–1613. https://doi.org/10.1007/s00217-018-3073-9.

D'Archivio, A.A., Giannitto, A., Incani, A., Nisi, S., 2014. Analysis of the mineral composition of Italian saffron by ICP-MS and classification of geographical origin. Food Chem 157, 485–489. https://doi.org/10.1016/j.foodchem.2014.02.068.

D'Archivio, A.A., Maggi, M.A., 2017. Geographical identification of saffron (Crocus sativus L.) by linear discriminant analysis applied to the UV-visible spectra of aqueous extracts. Food Chem 219, 408–413. https://doi.org/10.1016/j.foodchem.2016.09.169.

Di Marco, F., Di Paolo, M., Romeo, S., Colecchi, L., Fiorani, L., Spana, S., Stone, J., Bisti, S., 2014. Combining neuroprotectants in a model of retinal degeneration: no additive benefit. PLoS One 9, e100389. https://doi.org/10.1371/journal.pone.0100389.

Dunn, K.C., Aotaki-Keen, A.E., Putkey, F.R., Hjelmeland, L.M., 1996. ARPE-19, a human retinal pigment epithelial cell line with differentiated properties. Exp. Eye Res. 62, 155–169. https://doi.org/10.1006/exer.1996.0020.

Falsini, B., Piccardi, M., Minnella, A., Savastano, C., Capoluongo, E., Fadda, A., Balestrazzi, E., Maccarone, R., Bisti, S., 2010. Influence of saffron supplementation on retinal flicker sensitivity in early age-related macular degeneration. Invest. Opthalmol. Vis. Sci. 51, 6118. https://doi.org/10.1167/iovs.09-4995.

Falsini, B., Piccardi, M., Fadda, A., Martelli, F., Gentili, E., Minnella, A., Bertelli, M., Maccarone, R., Bisti, S., 2014. Targeting oxidative damage in ABCA4-related retinal degeneration: a phase I/II clinical trial with a dietary saffron extract. In: Investigative Ophthalmology & Visual Science. ARVO Abstract. p. Control ID: 1892203.

Gargini, C., Bisti, S., Demontis, G.C., Valter, K., Stone, J., Cervetto, L., 2004. Electroretinogram changes associated with retinal upregulation of trophic factors: observations following optic nerve section. Neuroscience 126, 775–783. https://doi.org/10.1016/j.neuroscience.2004.04.028.

Gosbell, A.D., Stefanovic, N., Scurr, L.L., Pete, J., Kola, I., Favilla, I., de Haan, J.B., 2006. Retinal light damage: structural and functional effects of the antioxidant glutathione peroxidase-1. Invest. Opthalmol. Vis. Sci. 47, 2613–2622. https://doi.org/10.1167/iovs.05-0962.

Himeno, H., Sano, K., 1987. Synthesis of crocin, picrocrocin and safranal by saffron stigma-like structures proliferated *in vitro*. Agric. Biol. Chem. 51, 2395−2400. https://doi.org/10.1080/00021369.1987.10868396.

ISO 3632-1, 2011. Saffron (*Crocus sativus* L.) Part 1 (Specification). International Organization for Standardization Genève, Switzerland.

ISO 3632-2, 2010. Saffron (*Crocus sativus* L.) Part 2 (Test Methods). International Organization for Standardization Genève, Switzerland.

Jozwick, C., Valter, K., Stone, J., 2006. Reversal of functional loss in the P23H-3 rat retina by management of ambient light. Exp. Eye Res. 83, 1074−1080. https://doi.org/10.1016/j.exer.2006.05.012.

Kim, S.R., Nakanishi, K., Itagaki, Y., Sparrow, J.R., 2006. Photo-oxidation of A2-PE, a photoreceptor outer segment fluorophore, and protection by lutein and zeaxanthin. Exp. Eye Res. 82, 828−839. https://doi.org/10.1016/j.exer.2005.10.004.

Kiser, P.D., Palczewski, K., 2016. Retinoids and retinal diseases. Annu. Rev. Vis. Sci. 2, 197−234. https://doi.org/10.1146/annurev-vision-111815-114407.

Kohno, H., Chen, Y., Kevany, B.M., Pearlman, E., Miyagi, M., Maeda, T., Palczewski, K., Maeda, A., 2013. Photoreceptor proteins initiate microglial activation via Toll-like receptor 4 in retinal degeneration mediated by all-trans-retinal. J. Biol. Chem. 288, 15326−15341. https://doi.org/10.1074/jbc.M112.448712.

Komeima, K., Rogers, B.S., Lu, L., Campochiaro, P.A., 2006. Antioxidants reduce cone cell death in a model of retinitis pigmentosa. Proc. Natl. Acad. Sci. USA 103, 11300−11305. https://doi.org/10.1073/pnas.0604056103.

Komeima, K., Usui, S., Shen, J., Rogers, B.S., Campochiaro, P.A., 2008. Blockade of neuronal nitric oxide synthase reduces cone cell death in a model of retinitis pigmentosa. Free Radic. Biol. Med. 45, 905−912. https://doi.org/10.1016/j.freeradbiomed.2008.06.020.

Léveillard, T., Philp, N.J., Sennlaub, F., 2019. Is retinal metabolic dysfunction at the center of the pathogenesis of age-related macular degeneration? Int. J. Mol. Sci. 20, 762. https://doi.org/10.3390/ijms20030762.

Logvinov, S.V., Plotnikov, M.B., Varakuta, E.Y., Zhdankina, A.A., Potapov, A.V., Mikhulya, E.P., 2005. Effect of ascovertin on morphological changes in rat retina exposed to high-intensity light. Bull. Exp. Biol. Med. 140, 578−581. https://doi.org/10.1007/s10517-006-0029-z.

Lozano, P., Castellar, M., Simancas, M., Iborra, J., 1999. A quantitative high-performance liquid chromatographic method to analyse commercial saffron (*Crocus sativus* L.) products. J. Chromatogr. A 830, 477−483. https://doi.org/10.1016/S0021-9673(98)00938-8.

Maccarone, R., Di Marco, S., Bisti, S., 2008. Saffron Supplement Maintains Morphology and Function after Exposure to Damaging Light in Mammalian Retina. Investig. Opthalmology Vis. Sci. 49, 1254. https://doi.org/10.1167/iovs.07-0438.

Maccarone, R., Rapino, C., Zerti, D., di Tommaso, M., Battista, N., Di Marco, S., Bisti, S., Maccarrone, M., 2016. Modulation of type-1 and type-2 cannabinoid receptors by saffron in a rat model of retinal neurodegeneration. PLoS One 11, e0166827. https://doi.org/10.1371/journal.pone.0166827.

Marangoni, D., Falsini, B., Piccardi, M., Ambrosio, L., Minnella, A.M., Savastano, M.C., Bisti, S., Maccarone, R., Fadda, A., Mello, E., Concolino, P., Capoluongo, E., 2013. Functional effect of Saffron supplementation and risk genotypes in early age-related macular degeneration: a preliminary report. J. Transl. Med. 11, 228. https://doi.org/10.1186/1479-5876-11-228.

Marco, F.D., Romeo, S., Nandasena, C., Purushothuman, S., Adams, C., Bisti, S., Stone, J., 2013. The time course of action of two neuroprotectants, dietary saffron and photobiomodulation, assessed in the rat retina. Am. J. Neurodegener. Dis. 2, 208−220.

Maggi, L., Carmona, M., Kelly, S.D., Marigheto, N., Alonso, G.L., 2011. Geographical origin differentiation of saffron spice (Crocus sativus L. stigmas) - Preliminary investigation using chemical and multi-element (H, C, N) stable isotope analysis. Food Chem 128, 543−548. https://doi.org/10.1016/j.foodchem.2011.03.063.

Moraga, A.R., Nohales, P.F.F., Gómez-Gómez, L., Pérez, J.A., 2004. Glucosylation of the saffron apocarotenoid crocetin by a glucosyltransferase isolated from *Crocus sativus* stigmas. Planta 219, 955−966. https://doi.org/10.1007/s00425-004-1299-1.

Moore, J.C., Spink, J., Lipp, M., 2012. Development and application of a database of food ingredient fraud and economically motivated adulteration from 1980 to 2010. J. Food Sci. 77, R118−R126. https://doi.org/10.1111/j.1750-3841.2012.02657.x.

Narayan, D.S., Chidlow, G., Wood, J.P., Casson, R.J., 2017. Glucose metabolism in mammalian photoreceptor inner and outer segments. Clin. Exp. Ophthalmol. 45, 730−741. https://doi.org/10.1111/ceo.12952.

Natoli, R., Zhu, Y., Valter, K., Bisti, S., Eells, J., Stone, J., 2010. Gene and noncoding RNA regulation underlying photoreceptor protection: microarray study of dietary antioxidant saffron and photobiomodulation in rat retina. Mol. Vis. 16, 1801−22.

Noble, K.G., Carr, R.E., 1979. Stargardt's disease and fundus flavimaculatus. Arch. Ophthalmol. 97, 1281−1285. https://doi.org/10.1001/archopht.1979.01020020023005.

Organisciak, D.T., Darrow, R.M., Jiang, Y.I., Marak, G.E., Blanks, J.C., 1992. Protection by dimethylthiourea against retinal light damage in rats. Invest. Ophthalmol. Vis. Sci. 33, 1599−1609.

Penn, J.S., Naash, M.I., Anderson, R.E., 1987. Effect of light history on retinal antioxidants and light damage susceptibility in the rat. Exp. Eye Res. 44, 779−788. https://doi.org/10.1016/S0014-4835(87)80041-6.

Piccardi, M., Marangoni, D., Minnella, A.M., Savastano, M.C., Valentini, P., Ambrosio, L., Capoluongo, E., Maccarone, R., Bisti, S., Falsini, B., 2012. A longitudinal follow-up study of saffron supplementation in early age-related macular degeneration: sustained benefits to central retinal function. Evidence-based complement. Altern. Med. 2012, 1−9. https://doi.org/10.1155/2012/429124.

Radu, R.A., Hu, J., Yuan, Q., Welch, D.L., Makshanoff, J., Lloyd, M., McMullen, S., Travis, G.H., Bok, D., 2011. Complement system dysregulation and inflammation in the retinal pigment epithelium of a mouse model for stargardt macular degeneration. J. Biol. Chem. 286, 18593–18601. https://doi.org/10.1074/jbc.M110.191866.

Ranchon, I., Gorrand, J.M., Cluzel, J., Droy-Lefaix, M.T., Doly, M., 1999. Functional protection of photoreceptors from light-induced damage by dimethylthiourea and Ginkgo biloba extract. Invest. Ophthalmol. Vis. Sci. 40, 1191–1199.

Riazi, A., Panahi, Y., Alishiri, A.A., Hosseini, M.A., Karimi Zarchi, A.A., Sahebkar, A., 2016. The impact of saffron (*Crocus sativus*) supplementation on visual function in patients with dry age-related macular degeneration. Ital. J Med. 10, 196–201. https://doi.org/10.4081/itjm.2016.758.

Serrano-Díaz, J., Sánchez, A.M., Martínez-Tomé, M., Winterhalter, P., Alonso, G.L., 2014. Flavonoid determination in the quality control of floral bioresidues from *Crocus sativus* L. J. Agric. Food Chem. 62, 3125–3133. https://doi.org/10.1021/jf4057023.

Shen, J., Yang, X., Dong, A., Petters, R.M., Peng, Y.W., Wong, F., Campochiaro, P.A., 2005. Oxidative damage is a potential cause of cone cell death in retinitis pigmentosa. J. Cell. Physiol. 203, 457–464. https://doi.org/10.1002/jcp.20346.

Sparrow, J.R., Nakanishi, K., Parish, C.A., 2000. The lipofuscin fluorophore A2E mediates blue light-induced damage to retinal pigmented epithelial cells. Invest. Ophthalmol. Vis. Sci. 41, 1981–1989.

Sparrow, J.R., Fishkin, N., Zhou, J., Cai, B., Jang, Y.P., Krane, S., Itagaki, Y., Nakanishi, K., 2003. A2E, a byproduct of the visual cycle. Vis. Res. 43, 2983–2990.

Stahl, W., Sies, H., 2005. Bioactivity and protective effects of natural carotenoids. Biochim. Biophys. Acta 1740, 101–107. https://doi.org/10.1016/j.bbadis.2004.12.006.

Stone, J., van Driel, D., Valter, K., Rees, S., Provis, J., 2008. The locations of mitochondria in mammalian photoreceptors: relation to retinal vasculature. Brain Res. 1189, 58–69. https://doi.org/10.1016/j.brainres.2007.10.083.

Stone, J., Mitrofanis, J., Johnstone, D.M., Falsini, B., Bisti, S., Adam, P., Nuevo, A.B., George-Weinstein, M., Mason, R., Eells, J., 2018. Acquired resilience: an evolved system of tissue protection in mammals. Dose Response 16, 155932581880342. https://doi.org/10.1177/1559325818803428.

Sun, H., Nathans, J., 2001. ABCR, the ATP-binding cassette transporter responsible for Stargardt macular dystrophy, is an efficient target of all-trans-retinal-mediated photooxidative damage in vitro. Implications for retinal disease. J. Biol. Chem. 276, 11766–11774. https://doi.org/10.1074/jbc.M010152200.

Tanito, M., Yoshida, Y., Kaidzu, S., Ohira, A., Niki, E., 2006. Detection of lipid peroxidation in light-exposed mouse retina assessed by oxidative stress markers, total hydroxyoctadecadienoic acid and 8-iso-prostaglandin F2alpha. Neurosci. Lett. 398, 63–68. https://doi.org/10.1016/j.neulet.2005.12.070.

Tanna, P., Strauss, R.W., Fujinami, K., Michaelides, M., 2017. Stargardt disease: clinical features, molecular genetics, animal models and therapeutic options. Br. J. Ophthalmol. 101, 25–30. https://doi.org/10.1136/bjophthalmol-2016-308823.

Tomita, H., Kotake, Y., Anderson, R.E., 2005. Mechanism of protection from light-induced retinal degeneration by the synthetic antioxidant phenyl- N-tert -butylnitrone. Invest. Opthalmol. Vis. Sci. 46, 427. https://doi.org/10.1167/iovs.04-0946.

Usui, S., Oveson, B.C., Lee, S.Y., Jo, Y.-J., Yoshida, T., Miki, A., Miki, K., Iwase, T., Lu, L., Campochiaro, P.A., 2009. NADPH oxidase plays a central role in cone cell death in retinitis pigmentosa. J. Neurochem 110, 1028–1037. https://doi.org/10.1111/j.1471-4159.2009.06195.x.

Valter, K., Kirk, D.K., Stone, J., 2009. Optimising the structure and function of the adult P23H-3 retina by light management in the juvenile and adult. Exp. Eye Res. 89, 1003–1011. https://doi.org/10.1016/j.exer.2009.08.009.

Weng, W., Li, L., van Bennekum, A.M., Potter, S.H., Harrison, E.H., Blaner, W.S., Breslow, J.L., Fisher, E.A., 1999. Intestinal absorption of dietary cholesteryl ester is decreased but retinyl ester absorption is normal in carboxyl ester lipase knockout mice. Biochemistry 38, 4143–4149. https://doi.org/10.1021/bi981679a.

Wiegand, R.D., Giusto, N.M., Rapp, L.M., Anderson, R.E., 1983. Evidence for rod outer segment lipid peroxidation following constant illumination of the rat retina. Invest. Ophthalmol. Vis. Sci. 24, 1433–1435.

Xie, Z., Wu, X., Gong, Y., Song, Y., Qiu, Q., Li, C., 2007. Intraperitoneal injection of ginkgo biloba extract enhances antioxidation ability of retina and protects photoreceptors after light-induced retinal damage in rats. Curr. Eye Res. 32, 471–479. https://doi.org/10.1080/02713680701257621.

Yu, D.Y., Cringle, S.J., Su, E.N., Yu, P.K., 2000. Intraretinal oxygen levels before and after photoreceptor loss in the RCS rat. Invest. Ophthalmol. Vis. Sci 41, 3999–4006.

Yu, D.-Y., Cringle, S.J., Yu, P.K., Balaratnasingam, C., Mehnert, A., Sarunic, M.V., An, D., Su, E.-N., 2019. Retinal capillary perfusion: spatial and temporal heterogeneity. Prog. Retin. Eye Res. 70, 23–54. https://doi.org/10.1016/j.preteyeres.2019.01.001.

Yılmaz, T., Aydemir, O., Özercan, İ.H., Üstündağ, B., 2007. Effects of vitamin E, pentoxifylline and aprotinin on light-induced retinal injury. Ophthalmologica 221, 159–166. https://doi.org/10.1159/000099295.

CHAPTER 15

Saffron—Immunity System

SHAISTA QADIR • SABEEHA BASHIR • RIFFAT JOHN

INTRODUCTION

Living organisms, especially animals are at a constant threat of infection from microorganisms because of the ideal environment that they provide for their survival. Most microorganisms thrive in warm temperatures, especially those close to body temperature. Besides, moisture content of the cells along with their rich supply of nutrients is also an ideal habitat for their growth. To survive and function properly, animals defend themselves effectively against these invasions. The body's inbuilt system that defends it against the constant attack by microorganisms is called the immune system. It is the immune system that keeps one healthy as one can stimulate this system to protect itself whenever they are exposed to an attack from bacteria, fungi, virus, parasites, and other toxic/foreign substances that invade their body. It is also involved in the body's response to injury and trauma. It is essential for one's survival as it controls and influences all aspects of the health. The healthier the immune system is, the better a body can cope with the many toxic substances it may encounter. A weakened or underactive immune system because of different conditions such as cancer, diabetes, major trauma, travel, heavy exercises, burns, UV lights (Moodycliffe et al., 2000), or everyday physical or emotional stress (Segerstrom and Miller, 2004) makes it susceptible to a number of diseases and finally results in death, if proper immune response is not stimulated.

Immune response is strictly regulated for the protection of a body. It can lead to severe damage if allowed to act in an uncontrolled manner. Because of its importance in an individual's health and survival, it is necessary that the immune system should remain in a balanced condition. Even a small and temporary gap should be closed immediately. When out of balance, it not only fails to protect the body but can even attack it, mistake "self"

cells for invading pathogens, resulting in enfeebling the immune system and autoimmune diseases such as lupus and rheumatoid arthritis. Many natural products/plant products and their derivatives have a chance of maintaining healthy status of an individual (Lee et al., 2005; Teixeira et al., 2005; Tripathi et al., 2005) with the advantages of low cost and total safety (Rahal et al., 2009). Functioning of the immune system is interrelated with the central nervous system and the endocrine system (Cotman, 1987). Its protective role, starting with the recognition of self and nonself entities and substances, puts the immune system in a vital position between a healthy and a diseased state of an individual.

The basic forms of immune response are of two types, the antibody and the cell-mediated response. Immunological tolerance is regarded as a special form of these two basic forms. The antibody-mediated responses provide protection against noncell-associated invaders, like bacteria or parasites. The production of the antibodies is stimulated by the foreign invaders (antigens), which then quicken their destruction. This response is responsible for the development of resistance against many infectious agents. However, it does not work alone against all invaders. Some organisms can enter the body (*Mycobacterium tuberculosis*) and hide themselves from the attack of antibody molecules. Same is the case of viruses that grows and proliferates within the living cells without elimination by the antibodies. These infected cells are destroyed by special killer cells called cytotoxic cells, which is a cell-mediated immune response.

The major function of the immune system is to not only protect an individual against the infectious diseases but also to prevent the development of abnormal cells within the body. It does not usually react against normal body components and is therefore said to be tolerant of self-components. The ability to differentiate between "self" and "not self" and to respond to microbial attack is found in both invertebrates and vertebrates. However, it is remarkably sophisticated and advanced among vertebrates (Sharma et al., 2017), where the complex immune system is capable to generate a limitless variety of cells and molecules to arrest enormous array of infections and undesirable substances by the collective activities of the myeloid system, lymphocytes, thymus, and spleen. The system works throughout the whole body because of the close regulation of humoral and cellular factors. Besides a vast range of specialized cells of immune system, many small soluble extracellular proteins or glycoproteins (usually smaller than 30 kDa) are secreted by its cells through inducible response to some injury (Mogensen, 2009). These protein molecules secreted are called cytokines/messenger proteins. Cytokines communicate with lymphocytes, inflammatory cells, and hematopoietic cells to regulate immune and inflammatory response (Mogensen, 2009), in an antigen-nonspecific manner. The most important and diverse of these cytokines are the lymphokines secreted by lymphocytes (The helper T cells—Th cells)) and macrophages, they are also called the interleukins. At least 90 lymphokine-mediated activities have been recognized. Among the interleukins (ILs), interleukins-2, secreted by Th1 cells and interleukins-1 secreted by macrophages are very crucial. In addition, interferons—the antiviral or regulatory proteins, chemokines that play an important role in inflammatory reactions, tumor necrosis factor family, and transforming growth factor family are also equally important to both innate and acquired types of immunity modulations. Components of innate immunity involved in immunomodulation are array of cells including natural killer (NK) cells, NKT-cells, T-cells, macrophages, granulocytes (neutrophils, eosinophils, and basophils), and dendritic cells, while B-cells naïve CD4+ T-cells, differentiated CD4+ T-cells including helper T-cells (TH1, TH2, and TH17 cells), induced regulatory T-cells, and natural regulatory T-cells (Kaiko et al., 2008). Components of both innate and adaptive immunity along with the complement system, which modulates both innate and adaptive immunity response (Dunkelberger and Song, 2010; Iwasaki and Medzhitov, Iwasaki and Medzhitov, 2010), interact and work together to protect the body from infection and disease.

Ancient medical literature suggests that many disease conditions are interrelated with all the components of immune system. For example, in diseases of the central nervous system, the cytokines (chemokine) have a predominant role as in a variety of psychiatric disorders abnormal secretions of these chemicals have been demonstrated. Various neurochemicals, neuroendocrine, and neuroimmune substances have appeared at the command of cytokines. The role of chemokine has been well established in depression Alzheimer's disease (Rubio-Perez and Morillas-Ruiz, 2012), and schizophrenia. Many behavioral changes such as emotions, stress, and physiological processes like infection, etc., have all been demonstrated to trigger cytokine secretion. Thus, even cytokine network is an important and complicated web of interactions between all the cell types of the immune system mediated by different proteins.

Different parts of a plant or a plant whole have been used in different systems of well-known traditional medicine—Unani medicine, Chinese medicine, Yoga, Siddha, Homeopathy, and Indian Ayurveda (Gurib-Fakim, 2006) from ancient times as a remedy for a number of diseases (Fabricant ad Farnsworth, 2001), because of their promotive, preventive, corrective, and curative approach. They were mostly taken in their crude form (unprocessed) as teas or decoction or tinctures (alcoholic extracts), decoctions (boiled extracts), and syrups (extracts of herbs made with syrup or honey) or applied externally as poultices, balms, and essential oils (Gurib-Fakim, 2006). Advances in biological research such as cell biology, genetics, biochemistry and other fields, made at an amazing rate, continuously support the evidences of the use of plants in curing a vast range of diseases and disorders among humans as they used to be the modulators of the complex immune system. Through a number of investigations conducted in the area, it is being explored that due to the presence of pharmacologically active compounds such as alkaloids, flavonoids, terpenoids, polysaccharides, lactones, and glycosides, natural products are responsible to cause alterations in the immunomodulatory properties (Sharma et al., 2017). Immunomodulators refer to those substances capable of inducing, amplifying, and inhibiting any component or phase of the immune system. These compounds have been reported to have multiple immunomodulatory actions including modulating cytokine secretion, histamine release, immunoglobulin secretion, class switching, cellular coreceptor expression, lymphocyte expression, phagocytosis, and so on (Spelman et al., 2006). The enhancement of immune response is known as immunostimulation while inhibition of immune responsiveness is termed as immunosuppression (Chauhan, 2010). From a therapeutic point of view, immunomodulation refers to a process and a course of action in which an immune response is altered to a desired level (Archana et al., 2011).

Modulation of immune response with the help of plant products to promote health and eliminate diseases is still a topic of interest and is gaining popularity in both consumer and scientific world day by day (Hashemi and Davoodi, 2012; Upadhayay et al., 2011). According to the World Health Organization, even today, at least 80% of people in developing countries depend largely on traditional systems of medicine for the control and treatment of various diseases. Disadvantages of synthetic drugs and chemicals in their adverse side effects and high cost are becoming known to the people (Mahima et al., 2012). A number of plants/herbal products have been worked out with various animal model systems such as mice, rats, chicken, and guinea pigs, as well as human cell lines during last few decades in different parts of the world for their possible immunomodulatory properties (Mahima et al., 2012). Some of these are *Azadirachta indica* bark, *Woodfordia fruticosa* flowers, *Picrorhiza kurroa* roots, and *Jatropha multifida* latex (Labadi et al., 1989), *Terminalis arjuna* stem bark, *Piper longum*, and *Crocus sativus* L. stigmas and petals (Boskabady and Farkhodeh, 2016). Here, the potent role of *crocus sativus* as an immunomodulator and as a biomedicine has been discussed.

Saffron is considered to be the native of south Europe. It is widely cultivated in many countries (Rios et al., 1996) such as Italy, Persia, Australia, China, Turkey, France Germany, Switzerland, Iran and some parts of Jammu and Kashmir. It has been growing here since ages and is cultivated on a commercial scale in the vast field in the Karewa lands of Pampore (5300 ft above sea level). It tolerates an enormous variety of ecological edaphic, as well as environmental conditions but is well adapted to areas with cold winters and warm, dry summers (−15°C or −20°C in winter and 35−45°C) in summer. It needs a rich, sandy, or loamy, well-drained soil free from decaying humus and clay (Srivastava et al., 1985). The plant is propagated by corms that last upto 10−15 years, new corms being produced yearly and the old ones rotting away. A new corm is produced by every growing bud and about 10 buds are grown on a flowering-size corm, factors affecting sprouting should be highly considered. The size of the daughter corms is important equally, and usually corms of flowering size are taken for planting. The relationships between flower number, corm size, and weight of stigmatic lobes have been described by De Mastro and Ruta (1993). The plants bloom from October to December; during this period, heavy rains are harmful. Stigmas and styles are parted and dehydrated in the sun or over low heat on sieves in earthen pots. The tripartite stigmas taken from freshly collected flowers along with about 50 mm portion of style, dried in the sun constitute pure saffron. As its small filaments are picked up by hand, it is of no surprise that it is world's most expensive spice (Muzaffar et al., 2015; Sánchez-Vioque et al., 2012)

Saffron is a noteworthy medicinal and spicy plant due to its powerful odor and intensive natural yellow color. Saffron is composed of sugars, water, soluble extracts, fibers, nitrogenous matter, and volatile oil. It is rich in vitamins like thiamine ($0.7−4\ \mu g.g^{-1}$) and riboflavin ($56−138\ \mu g.g^{-1}$). The active components crocin, picrocrocin, and safranal have been unraveled for large number of probable medicinal uses. The pharmacological properties of active components of saffron are due to their unique chemical structure, although, for determination of accurate dosage for human consumption, clinical trials are required to remove any chances of adverse effects thereby (Razak et al., 2017) (Table 15.1).

PHYTOCHEMISTRY

Saffron contains a number of metabolites that gives it a distinct and unique color, flavor, and smell. Carotenoids are colored compounds such as ester of crocin (color glycoside) that are responsible for its principal color, and picrocrocin, which is the glycoside precursor of safranal (2,6,6-trimethyl-1,3-cyclohexadiene-1-carbox aldehyde), the most abundant of all the volatile compounds is responsible for the aroma of saffron (Maggi et al., 2011) and bitter taste. Besides, saffron contains more than 150 volatile and aroma-yielding compounds. It also has many nonvolatile active components, many of which are carotenoids and flavonoids including zeaxanthin, various α- and β-carotenes, lycopene, rutin, quercetin, luteolin, and hesperidin. The

TABLE 15.1 Chemical Composition of Saffron (Srivastava et al., 2010).	
Chemicals	**Amount (%)**
Non-nitrogenous	Traces
Miscellaneous	40.5
Minerals	1.0−1.5
Lipids	3.0−8.0
Cellulose	4.0−7.0
Polypeptides	11.0−14.0
Carbohydrates	12.0−15.0
Water	14.0−19.0

volatiles present with a very strong odor are mainly terpenes, terpene alcohols, and their esters with glucose, gentiobiose, neapolitanose, or triglucose sugar moieties (Carmona et al., 2007; Lozano et al., 2000; Tarantilis et al., 1995) (Table 15.2).

PHARMACOLOGY

In traditional medicine, as well as in modern pharmacology, saffron has been widely used throughout the world in the treatment of numerous diseases due to its innumerable effect on the respiratory system, nervous system (insomnia, paralysis), the digestive system (flatulence, stomach disorders, colic (Khorasany and Hosseinzadeh, 2016) the cardiovascular system (heart disease), and disorders such as smallpox, scarlet fever, gout, and eye disease. From different studies, it has been seen that saffron also acts as an appetizer. It has been reported that saffron and its constituents have antitumor (Patel et al., 2017; Samarghandian et al., 2014) antiinflammatory, antinociceptive (Hosseinzadeh and Younesi, 2002), antioxidant (Farahmand et al., 2013), antidepressant (Ghasemi et al., 2015; Samarghandian et al., 2013; Charle, 2012) hypolipidemic and could improve memory as well learning abilities in rats (Sheng et al., 2006; Hosseinzadeh and Ziaei,

2006). Its active compounds show sedative, aphrodisiac, chemopreventive, diaphoretic, immunomodulatory, antioxidant (Chen et al., 2008; Kanaris et al., 2007), insulin-resistance reducing (Xi et al., 2005), and hypoglycemic (Mohajeri et al., 2009) effects. Progress has been seen in those suffering from allergies, flu, rheumatoid arthritis, hepatitis, heart disease, bacterial/viral infections, colds, asthma, aging, chemical intoxication, skin infections, etc. and is also found helpful in treating cancers (Hoshyar and Mollaei, 2017; Umashanker and Shruti, 2011; Mathew et al., 2010).

Evidence also showed that saffron and its constituents reduce lipid peroxidation in various tissues (Farahmand et al., 2013; Hosseinzadeh et al., 2012; Samarghandian et al., 2011, 2014) following oxidative damages in rats. One of the most important factors responsible for these activities is the modulation of immune responses. It had been shown that saffron reduced the IgM level and improved the IgG level; it increases the percentage of monocytes, and thus is a potential immunomodulator. Other study concluded that saffron petal extract causes an increase in antibody response without any alteration in hematological parameters or histology of spleen (Rahmani et al., 2017) (Fig. 15.1.)

ANTIINFLAMMATORY AND ANTIOXIDATIVE PROPERTIES

Inflammation is a response of body tissues to physical injury and irritation. Although inflammation is a part of the healing process sometimes, reducing inflammation by taking nonsteroidal (naproxen, ibuprofen, and aspirin) and steroidal drugs is helpful, though not always necessary. Many natural items such as olive oil, tomatoes, walnuts, leafy greens, fatty fish, blueberries, and oranges are known to reduce the risk of inflammation. However, these dietary solutions do not alone hold the key to controlling inflammation; they can help to boost the immune system to react in a measured way. There are many plants such as *Harpagophytum procumbens*, ginger, turmeric, cannabis, and saffron from which active compounds are isolated with the same properties.

Many studies were performed on mice models to evaluate antiinflammatory activity of saffron, and the results revealed that extracts of stigma as well as petals have antiinflammatory activity, suppressed inflammatory pain response, and decreased number of neutrophils (Hosseini et al., 2018; Tamaddonfard et al., 2013; Hosseinzadeh and Younesi, 2002).

In one of the experiments, the effect of various extracts on severe inflammation in mice using xylene-

TABLE 15.2 Various Metabolites Present in Saffron (Srivastava et al., 2010).	
Metabolites	**Amount (%)**
Water-soluble components	53.0
Water	10.0
Pentosans	8.0
Gums	10.0
Starch	6.0
Carotenoids	1.0
Nonvolatile oils	6.0
Volatile oils	1.0
Protein	12.0
Inorganic matter ("ash")	6.0
Fiber (crude)	5.0
α-crocin	2.0
Lipids	12.0
HCl-soluble ash	0.5
Pectins	6.0

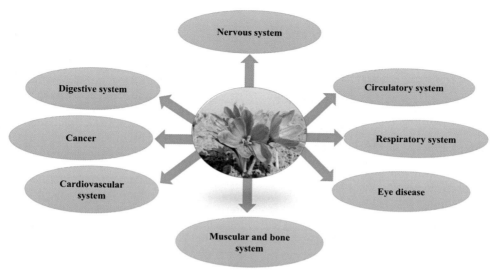

FIG. 15.1 Saffron folkloric uses (Abdullaev FI, 2002).

induced ear edema was studied. The stigma extracts showed weak-to-moderate effect against acute inflammation. In chronic inflammation, induced by formalin, both aqueous and ethanolic stigma extracts, as well as ethanolic petal extract, exerted antiinflammatory effects as induced paw edema in rats is significantly reduced in a dose-dependent manner. The aqueous petal extract did not exhibit significant antiinflammatory activity. In higher doses, the aqueous and ethanolic extracts of stigma showed significant activity against the acute inflammation. Crocus extract also inhibits xylene-induced swelling of the mouse ear (Ma et al., 1998). The antiinflammatory role of stigma extract of saffron has also been elucidated during rheumatoid arthritis (RA) in female Swiss albino mice of 12−14 weeks old. RA is a systemic autoimmune disorder characterized by inflammation of the synovial joints and concomitant destruction of cartilage and bone (Turco, 1963).

Antiinflammatory properties of saffron are due to the occurrence of various active ingredients such as crocus glycosides crocetin, safranal, crocine, flavonoids (Bolhassani et al., 2014; Poma et al., 2012; Ma et al., 1998) tannins, anthocyanins, alkaloids, and saponin and by the synergistic action of these active ingredients in the maintenance of immune homeostasis.

Samarghandian et al., 2017 investigated the immunomodulatory role of the aqueous saffron extract on streptozotocin (STZ)-induced diabetic rats. They determined the role of saffron extract in the regulation and expression of inflammatory cytokines (tumor necrosis factor TNF-α and IL-6) in diabetic rats, by using the RT-PCR analysis, in the presence or absence of different saffron extract concentrations. Due to the absence of this condition, control rats did not show expression of inflammatory cytokines; by contrast, both inflammatory cytokines (TNF-α and IL-6) were expressed by diabetic rats. Regarding groups treated with saffron extracts, the low concentration of saffron extract (10 mg/kg/day) inhibited the expression of inflammatory cytokine only to some extent and, the treatment of diabetic rats with the highest saffron extract concentration (40 mg/kg/day) significantly reduced the levels of proinflammatory cytokine, so that it was found to be similar with the control animals. Saffron treatment severely reduced the expression of TNF-α and IL-6 mRNA in dose-dependent manner. They concluded that, compared to untreated diabetic rats, diabetic rats inhibited the expression of inflammatory cytokines in the abdominal aorta.

Other experimental data suggest that saffron helps to reduce inflammation by inhibiting the cyclooxygenase (COX)/prostaglandin-endoperoxide synthase, enzyme activity (Zeinali et al., 2019) both in vitro and in vivo. COX is responsible for prostanoid formation, including thromboxane and prostaglandins such as prostacyclin. In this study, antiinflammatory activity in vivo was observed using two animal edema model tests, and it was concluded that crocin exhibits obvious antiinflammatory effects and may be one of the active ingredients in *Crocus sativus* that can modulate inflammatory processes (Litalien ad Beaulieu, 2011).

ANTIOXIDATIVE PROPERTIES

Aerobic life is constantly exposed to a number of endogenous oxidants that invariably cause marked alteration in the electron transport in mitochondrial respiration, enzymatic activities such as lipoxygenase and xanthine oxidase, and the NADPH oxidase/myeloperoxidase system of phagocytes. This results in the production of toxic oxygen species such as hydroxyl radicals ($^\bullet$OH), hydrogen peroxide (H_2O_2), superoxide radicals ($O_2^{\bullet-}$), singlet oxygen ($^1O_2$), and hydroxyl radicals ($^\bullet$OH) commonly called reactive oxygen species (ROS) (Foyer et al., 1997). The production of endogenous ROS is highly regulated under normal conditions, and endogenous antioxidants neutralize the effect of free radicals (Kattappagari et al., 2015). There are also many exogenous sources of oxidants such as natural dietary constituents, UV radiation, natural radioactive gases, and environmental pollutants like heavy metals that generate ROS (Van Wijk et al., 2008). It has been observed that low levels of ROS play a pivotal role in complex signaling cascades as they act as signals for the activation of various stress-responsive and defense pathways, transcription factor activation, apoptosis, protein phosphorylation cell differentiation, cell immunity, and as secondary messengers in the regulation of cardiac and vascular cell functioning. As far as the role of ROS is considered, the balance between their production and scavenging is a most crucial step for proper growth and development. Due to the variety of the processes that produce ROS during metabolism, an uncontrolled oxidation of various biomolecules occurs (Wu et al., 2013), which is associated with changes in their structure and functions (Lobo et al., 2010; Halliwel, 1994). Imbalance between oxidant/antioxidant in favor of oxidants results in oxidative stress that causes biological modification. This makes the biological system susceptible to injury caused by oxidative stress. Amid of this, enzymatic antioxidants play a crucial role in maintaining ROS homeostasis, for example, catalase (CAT), superoxide dismutase (SOD), and the two enzymes of glutathione redox cycle, that is, glutathione reductase (GR) and glutathione peroxidase.

Given the previously mentioned mechanisms used by living organisms to detoxify ROS, it is clearly important to establish how the administration of various natural products causes the enzymes involved in these detoxification processes to have a detrimental or stimulating effect. The experiments conducted on the subject have produced results that demonstrate that antioxidant responses are probably related both to levels of damage and to the concentration of these enzymes already present or induced by them. The mechanism involved by some of the important antioxidants is discussed briefly as follows:

Superoxide Dismutase

SOD is a group of metalloenzymes virtually present in all living organisms. It is a highly efficient catalyst, involved as a first line of defense among the enzymatic mechanisms against the removal of superoxide, with rates being almost diffusion inhibited. Superoxide can be formed by flavoprotein dehydrogenases enzymatically. Moreover, the autoxidation of ferredoxins, hydroquinones, thiols, and reduced hemoproteins in electron transport systems (chloroplast and mitochondria) can form superoxide nonenzymatically under normal conditions. Superoxide is not as toxic as other oxygen species but is possibly involved in membrane damage, lipid peroxidation, cellular toxicity, and single strand breaks in DNA (Fridovich, 1986). It results in production of hydroxyl radical by reacting with hydrogen peroxide in the metal catalyzed Haber—Weiss reaction. It also causes the inactivation of glutathione and peroxidase catalase as well as NAD(P)H and epinephrine oxidation (Fridovich, 1986). It is implicated in sunscald damage during high light and heat. Using a dismutation reaction catalyzed by the enzyme family, superoxide dismutase, superoxide is converted to hydrogen peroxide. SOD plays a pivotal role in the antioxidant pathway (Foyer et al., 1994; Salin, 1988). SOD catalyzes a reaction in which two identical substrates have different metabolic fates; in this case, one molecule of superoxide is oxidized and the other is reduced.

$$O^{\bullet-}_2 + O^{\bullet-}_2 + 2H^+ \rightarrow H_2O_2 + O_2$$

SODs are classified according to their metal factors present at their active sites, as FeSOD, MnSOD, or Cu—Zn SOD (Weisiger and Fridovich, 1973; Liou et al., 1993). They are mainly seen within cell, especially cytoplasm and other organelles (mitochondria); another type of SOD called extracellular SOD (EC SOD), which was first described by Marklund in the year 1982 (Marklund, 1982), also contains copper and zinc.

Catalase

The catalases are present in both prokaryotes and eukaryotes. They catalyze the dismutation of H_2O_2 to water and oxygen:

$$2H_2O_2 \rightarrow 2H_2O + O_2$$

The sources of H_2O_2 generation are P450 oxidases of the endoplasmic reticulum, electron transport chain of mitochondria, intercellular sources of H_2O_2 generation include peroxisome and reactions catalyzed by their associated dehydrogenases and oxidases, and H_2O_2 can easily permeate cell membranes and put DNA to a major threat by generation of highly reactive hydroxyl radicals (OH⁻) through the interaction of H_2O_2 with transitional metal ions such as Fe^{2+} in Fenton-type reactions. Catalases are chiefly in peroxisomes and reduce H_2O_2 without consuming cellular reducing equivalents, that is, it is a very effective means of eliminating H_2O_2 from cells. Modulation in CAT activity as an attribute of saffron extracts has been reported depending upon the duration, dose of the treatment, and the test organism under study. Alteration in CAT activity is reported by a number of workers with administration of varied saffron extract concentrations. These alterations were attributed to its additive function for oxidative stress.

Glutathione Levels

Glutathione (γ-glutamyl-cysteinyl-glycine) is the most abundant form of organic sulfur in living organisms, forming a major source of nonprotein thiol, apart from that incorporated into proteins (Dixon et al., 1998; May et al., 1998; Bergmann and Rennenberg, 1993). The chemical reactivity of the glutathione thiol group makes it particularly suitable for all organisms to serve a wide range of biochemical functions. It has an oxidative reduction potential of −0.23 V, which enables it to act for numerous biological reactions as an effective electron acceptor and donor. It has multiple functions in living systems as well as functioning as a translocatable store of organic sulfur (Hell, 1997). It appears to function as an intracellular signaling agent, responsive to changes in the extracellular environment (Sanchez- Fernandez et al., 1997). GSH has been also implicated in the regulation of enzyme activities, in DNA synthesis, in maintaining the viability of mitochondria, and in the regulation of gene expression possibly via thiol sensitive transcription factors (Wingsle and Karpinski, 1996; Kulik and Storz, 1994).

Reduced glutathione is one of the most efficient scavengers of peroxides arising as a by-product of cellular metabolism or during oxidative stress (Noctor and Foyer, 1998). As an antioxidant, glutathione together with ascorbate and other enzymes, SOD and *Ascorbate peroxidase-(APX)* controls the cellular concentration of H_2O_2 and $O^\cdot{}^-_2$. Here, it protects cell against damage from free radicals. The reactivation of these antioxidants requires adequate amounts of reduced glutathione. The efficiency with which the oxidized dithiol (GSSG) can be converted back to GSH during the reductive inactivation of peroxides contributes to the centrality of glutathione (May et al., 1998).

Under normal conditions, glutathione is predominantly present in its reduced form (GSH), with only a small portion present in its fully oxidized state (GSSG). The size of reduced glutathione pool shows marked alteration in response to a number of biotic and abiotic environmental conditions. Under some stress conditions, oxidation of GSH is accompanied by net glutathione degradation (Foyer et al., 1997). However, most of the studies have shown that glutathione accumulates in response to increased Reactive oxygen species (ROS) generation or is constitutively higher in organisms adapted to exacting conditions (Arora et al., 2002; Willekens et al., 1997; May and Leaver, 1993). Differences in GSH content may be wholly or partly due to modulated rates of GSH biosynthesis.

Ascorbate

Ascorbate (As) is the most effective hydrophilic physiological antioxidant found in living organisms. It is one of the major antioxidant for protection against diseases and degenerative processes caused by oxidant stress. Its ability to show antioxidant properties is related to the fact that dehydrogenase radical is far less reactive than many radicals are (Rose and Bode, 1993). To reduce this radical to ascorbate, enzymatic systems exist in vivo using NADH or GSH as a source of power reduction. Of the many functions ascribed to As, relatively few are well characterized. It is clear however, that As is a major primary antioxidant (Nijs and Kelley, 1991), reacting directly with hydroxyl radicals, superoxide, and singlet oxygen (Buettner and Jurkiewiez, 1996). Ascorbate plays an important role in preserving the activities of enzymes that contain prosthetic transition metal ion (Padh, 1990). Ascorbate is also a powerful secondary antioxidant, reducing the oxidized form of α-tocopherol an important antioxidant in aqueous phase (Padh, 1990).

Recent years have seen a large number of reports that correlate with an increase in one or more antioxidant systems while combating against different pathological conditions.

Glutathione Reductase

GR is an important antioxidant enzyme that plays a critical role in the metabolism of GSH, reducing GSSG to GSH using reducing equivalents derived from glucose through the pentose phosphate pathway and NADPH-dependent mechanism. The enzyme's function is to keep the reduced GSH cell concentration high and its oxidized form, GSSG, low (Wu et al., 2013; Ballatorie et al., 2009). GSH is significantly advantageous over GSSG under healthy physiological conditions (Ballatori et al., 2009; Wu et al., 2004)

$$GSSG + NADPH + H^+ \rightarrow 2GSH + NADP^+$$

GR isoforms are mainly found in cytoplasm and mitochondrial matrix and chloroplast (Yan et al., 2013). They range in size from about 90 to 140 KDa and usually contain two protein subunits, each with a flavin dinucleotide at their active site. NADPH appears to reduce the flavin nucleotide, which then transfers its electrons to a disulfide bridge (-S-S-) in the enzyme. The formed groups of two-sulfydryls (-SH) interact with GSSG and reduce it to GSH. GR's activity suggests that the normal cell's GSH/GSSG ratio is kept high. The use of NADPH acts as an energy sink that can have an indirect impact on the electron transport system's efficiency. GR is also known to play an important role in the protecting organism against oxidative damage by maintaining a high GSH/GSSG ratio.

Glutathione Peroxidase

Glutathione peroxidase (GPx) catalyzes the oxidation of glutathione at the cost of a hydroperoxidase, which might be hydrogen peroxide.

$$ROOH + 2\,GSH \rightarrow GSSG + H_2O + ROH$$

Lipid hydroperoxides play an important role in repairing damage cell resulting from lipid peroxidation. Selenium is required for activation of glutathione peroxidase. The activity of this particular enzyme is reduction of glutathione (Holben and Smith, 1999).

MODULATION OF ANTIOXIDANT SYSTEMS BY SAFFRON EXTRACTS

Saffron is a rich source for antioxidants that are known to prevent/delay different pathogenic conditions. Its antioxidant activity has been observed to be more as compared to tomatoes and carrots (Papandreou et al., 2006). Although, the exact mechanism by which saffron and its constituents influence the therapeutic role in diseases prevention is yet to be fully elucidated. However, the recent research has revealed that saffron extracts from stamens, petals, and entire flowers, which were considered waste products in the production of saffron, modulates/enhances the activity of various enzymes involved in oxidative stress including SOD, GPx, CAT, and malondialdehyde (MDA) in various test organisms. These medicinal properties of saffron can be attributed to a number of its compounds such as crocetin, crocins, phenolics, and flavonoids (Samarghandian et al., 2014; Gohari et al., 2013) and other substances that enhance the antioxidant capacity and proinflammatory cytokines (Uliana et al., 2015; Karimi et al., 2010; Poma et al., 2012), as have been shown in different in vivo and in vitro models (Hosseinzadeh et al., 2010; Hosseinzadeh and Sadeghnia, 2005). Thus, saffron shows remarkable antioxidant and radical scavenging (Khajuria et al., 2010) properties that can act by a protective mechanism similar to the carotenoid supplementation mechanism (Kanakis et al., 2007; Giaccio, 2004).

Saffron extract has also been shown to have protective effects on genotoxin-induced oxidative stress in Swiss albino mice (Hariri et al., 2011). Saffron administration in diabetic rats enhanced the activity of antioxidant enzymes such as CAT and GPx significantly compared to the diabetic control group (Hasanpour et al., 2018). Moreover, these components have been found to reduce the lipid peroxidation and enhance the antioxidant status. The activity of SOD is altered under the administration of different extracts of saffron as reported by various workers (Goli et al., 2012; Makhlouf et al., 2011; Karimi et al., 2010; Papandreou et al., 2006). Saffron extract controls the reduction of antioxidant enzymes such as GR and SOD in mice induced with RA (Rathore et al., 2015) and thereby help in quenching free radicals and exert protective effect against oxidative damage (Bilal et al., 2014). In addition, DPPH (1,1-diphenyl-2-picryl-hydrazyl) radical scavenging test has shown radical scavenging effect of saffron extract and its bioactive constituents crocin and safranal.

In one research on male albino rats, whole body exposure to gamma radiation (6.5 Gy) produced an imbalance in the brain and eye of rats between oxidant and antioxidant species (El-Azime et al., 2014). A significant rise in the levels of MDA, AOPP (advanced oxidation protein products), and PC (protein carbonyl) followed by substantial reductions in the total activity of CAT, SOD, and GPx and GSH was recorded. However, experimental animals supplemented with aqueous saffron extract before exposure to gamma radiation exhibits a significant reduction in the severity of oxidative stress caused by radiation and modification of catecholamines in the organs under investigation. The decrease in antioxidants could result from their increased use to neutralize the excess of free radicals generated in the body following exposure to ionizing radiation, where SOD catalyzes the reduction of $O_2^{\bullet-}$ to H_2O_2, most of which are broken down by CAT into oxygen and water. According to them, due to the existence of related bioactive compounds with antioxidant properties, saffron exerts its modulating impact in the organs under investigation. The important increase in SOD, CAT, and GPx activities and the content of GSH suggests its potential impact in improving antioxidant protection.

The changes in activities of antioxidant enzymes MDA, CAT, SOD, and GSH in liver and serum nitric oxide (NO) of rats 2, 10, and 20 months old were studied in the presence and absence of saffron extracted to determine the effect of saffron on the status of selected oxidative stress parameters. The results of this study showed that the saffron extract was found to be effective in enhancing the activity of the GST and decreasing the MDA level in the liver homogenates as well as decreasing the level of serum NO. Thus, saffron extract can be effective to protect susceptible aged liver from oxidative damage by balancing the oxidative system (Samarghandian et al., 2016). The antioxidant properties of the aqueous saffron extract on STZ-induced diabetic rats were also investigated by Samarghandian et al., 2017. They reported that extract of saffron reduced MDA, blood triglycerides, glucose total lipids, and cholesterol levels significantly and increased GSH, CAT, and SOD activities in diabetic groups as compared with the untreated groups, in a dose-dependent manner.

Among the responses of animals to oxidative stress under the administration of saffron extract, the increases in the pool of GSH have been measured in many test animals. Concerted efforts in recent years have given indications of physiological significance of saffron-induced changes in the pool size of GSH and mechanisms of GSH functions, which serve to maintain redox poise during stress. A number of workers have noted a stimulating impact of saffron extract on the formation of GSH (Samarghandian et al., 2017). The GSH reacts with free radicals and is a key substratum for glutathione peroxidase and glutathione-S-transferase that participates in the ROS defense mechanisms. Saffron extract caused an increase in plasma GSH content, which could boost the GSH/GSSG ratio and reduce lipid peroxidation; hence, aldehydic concentration, thus improving the regulation of serum glucose that saffron, safranal, and crocin can efficiently regulate glycemia in the alloxane-induced rat model.

ANTIMICROBIAL ACTIVITY

Antibiotics are powerful medicines that are being used for the treatment of certain infectious diseases when our immune system cannot fight the causal organisms. However, people are overusing antibiotics, and this overuse contributes toward the increasing number of bacterial infections that become resistant to drugs used in human infection treatment. This scenario has resulted researchers to search for new antimicrobials from different plant sources (Karaman et al., 2003), particularly those using traditional medicine systems (Manoj et al., 2010; Sumitra and Yogesh, 2010).

Different parts of saffron, such as stamen, are also known to have antimicrobial activity like many other spices (garlic, mustard, red chilli, turmeric, clove, cinnamon, fenugreek, black pepper, and ginger) and is often considered as immune enhancing (Babaei et al., 2014; Tilak and Devasagayam, 2006; Rajendhran et al., 1998). Its antimicrobial activity from different extracts has been worked out by various workers ad confirmed against many bacterial strains and fungi used as test organisms (Sovrlić et al., 2015; Jalal et al., 2015; Kamble and Patil (2007); Sekine et al. (2007); Nakhaei et al. (2008). For example, ethyl acetate extract of various parts of saffron including stamen, stigma, and corolla showed strong antimicrobial activity (Vahidi et al., 2002) when tested against different bacteria (*Staphylococcus epidermidis, Micrococcus luteus, Staphylococcus aureus* and *E. coli*) and fungi (*Cladosporium* sp., *Candida albicans*, and *Aspergillus niger*). Muzaffar et al. (2016) also recorded powerful antimicrobial activity of methanol extracts and petroleum ether of saffron stigmas against different bacterial strains (*Klebsiella pneumonia, Proteus vulgaris, Pseudomonas aeruginosa, Escherichia coli*, and *Staphylococcus aureus*) and fungi (*Aspergillus niger, Candida albicans*, and *Aspergillus fumigatus*). According to them, both petroleum ether of methanolic extracts and petroleum ether of *C. sativus* stigmas have great potential as antimicrobial compounds against fungi and bacteria. However, the findings showed that the extracts had powerful bactericidal impacts than fungicidal ones. They can therefore be used in the therapy of infectious diseases induced by resistant microbes and can be widely used in pharmaceutical, food, and medical applications. In addition, antimicrobial effects of mixtures of aqueous, ethanolic, and methanolic extracts of petal were observed against the foodborne pathogens, and the results have confirmed that such extracts show antimicrobial activity against most of the pathogenic bacteria (Gandomi et al., 2012). An in vitro antimicrobial activity of the total flavonoid from petal and stamen of *Crocus sativus* against 25 different microorganism strains was investigated and confirmed by Chen et al. (2017). The antimicrobial activities of saffron extracts are due to the presence of volatile and/or water-soluble safranal and crocin compounds (Soureshjan and Heidari, 2014; Pintado et al., 2011; Carmona et al., 2007).

ANTINOCICEPTIVE ACTIVITY

Antinociception also known as nocioception/nociperception is the body's response to potentially toxic stimuli, like harmful chemicals (e.g., capsaicin, formalin), mechanical injury (e.g., cutting, crushing), or adverse temperatures (heat and cold) by the sensory nervous system.

Many analgesic drugs produced by chemical synthesis have potential side effects (Zendehdel et al., 2011). Furthermore, available analgesics relieve only pain as a symptom without affecting its cause (Tripathi, 1999). Moreover, some drugs like morphine and nonsteroidal antiinflammatory drugs (NSAIDs), which are the drugs of choice for the treatment of pain, have been known to cause dependence and tolerance upon its prolonged usage (Rang et al., 2011). Therefore, natural products obtained from different parts of medicinal plants that have been used as analgesic drugs in folk medicine, together with the new plants are being investigated for their role as a source of new drugs with potential therapeutic effects in pain management. The phenomenon is known as antinociceptive activity. A number of plants (*Clinacanthus nutans, Muntingia calabura, Bauhinia purpurea, Piper solmsianum* C. DC. var. solmsianum, *Orbignya speciosa* Mart. (Babassu) *Sabicea grisea* var., *Teucrium polium,Crocus sativus* L. etc.) have been screened out for antinociceptive properties. A harmful stimulus in various animal model systems is deliberately applied followed by administration of plant extracts to study pain, efficacy, dose, and duration of these extracts to manage pain and promote health (Zendehdel et al., 2011; Abdul Rahim et al., 2016; Zakaria et al., 2011, 2014; Pinheiro et al., 2012; de Oliveira et al., 2012). These systems use particularly formalin, acetic acid or carrageenan in models of inflammatory pain (Tamaddonfard et al., 2013) and chronic constriction injury, nerve crush injury, in models of neuropathic pain (Tamaddonfard et al., 2014; Amin and Hosseinzadeh, 2012). Attempts are also being made to understand the mechanism of pain modulation with the help of these plant-based medications having fewer or, possibly, no side effects. This will also provide alternatives to conventional analgesics like opiates and NSAIDs.

The antinociceptive effects of extract of saffron petal aqueous, stigma, and ethanolic maceration have been reported by a number of scientists against chemical and thermal pain test (Hosseinzadeh and Shariaty, 2007; Hosseinzadeh and Younesi, 2002). These studies had reported that antinociceptive activity of saffron is due to flavonoids, tannins, and anthocyanins, particularly safranal which is one of the chief components of saffron. The analgesic role of safranal has been credited to its ability to suppress nonneural cell (glial) activation and proinflammatory cytokines production in the central nervous system (Zhu and Yang, 2014). Other studies have demonstrated that various flavonoids

such as quercetin, rutin, biflavonoids, hesperidin, and luteolin produced significant antinociceptive activity in the test organisms (Bittar et al., 2000; Calixto et al., 2000; Ramesh et al., 1998; Galati et al., 1994; Starec et al., 1988; Ma et al., 1988). Thus, antinociceptive property could be related to the presence of several bioactive compounds based on flavonoids and their synergistic action with nonvolatile bioactive compounds, which in turn activate signaling cascades responsible for regulating pain perception. In one of the experiments carried on male albino mice of 20–25 g, the antinociceptive activity of saffron was determined using hot-plate and chemical tests (writhing and formalin) (Hosseinzadeh and Shariaty, 2007). The formalin tests in mice is the most acceptable model of nociception, as it encompasses inflammatory, neurogenic, and central mechanisms of nociception (Hunskaar and Hole, 1987) and is sensitive to opioid agents, NSAIDs and other mild analgesics. Safranal was found to slow the abdominal constrictions induced by acetic acid at doses 0.1, 0.3, and 0.5 mL/kg/ip and also to increase the pain threshold of mice against the thermal source at 30 min after treatment. Safranal at doses of 0.05 mL/kg/ip significantly reduced pain-related responses at lower doses (0.05 and 0.025 mL/kg/ip) in the formalin test. According to them, Safranal decreased the number of abdominal constrictions induced by dose-dependent injection of acetic acid and naloxone did not inhibit safranal's antinociceptive activity. Therefore, it is possible that safranal analgesic effects are likely mediated by inhibiting prostaglandin synthesis or action and this effect is not mediated through opioid receptors that exert their analgesic effects through supraspinal and spinal receptors. Their results clearly showed that in chemical (formalin and acid acetic tests) methods safranal has antinociceptive activity and this effect can be more peripherally medicated. According to Li Puma et al. (2019) by partial agonism and selective desensitization of the transient receptor potential ankyrin 1 (TRPA1) channel, which mediates pain signals in nociceptors, saffron may exert analgesic properties. They assessed acute nociception in C57BL/6, $Trpv1^{+/+}$ and $Trpv1^{-/-}$, $Trpa1^{+/+}$ and $Trpa1^{-/-}$, or $Trpv4^{+/+}$ and $Trpv4^{-/-}$ mice, after intraplantar (i.pl.) injection (20 μL/paw) of safranal (0.2–20 nmol), capsaicin (0.2 nmol), AITC (10 nmol), GSK1016790A (2 nmol), or their vehicle (7% and 0.5% DMSO). Immediately after injection, mice were individually placed in plexiglass chambers and the amount of time (seconds) spent shaking and licking the injected paw was recorded for a period of 5 min, Nociception induced by safranal (20 nmol) was also assessed

TABLE 15.3
Role of Different Components of Saffaron.

Component	Antiinflammatory	Antioxidant	Antimicrobial	Antinoceptive
Crocin	+	+	+	−
Crocetin	+	+	−	−
Flavonoid	+	+	−	+
Phenols	+	−	−	−
Safranal	+	+	+	+
Saponin	+	−	−	−
Tannin	+	−	−	+

'+' indicates presence of activity '−' indicates absence of activity.

60 min after intraperitoneal (i.p.) treatment with HC-030031 (100 mg/kg) or 30 min after capsazepine (4 mg/kg) or HC-067047 (10 mg/kg) or their vehicle (all, 4% tween 80 plus 4% DMSO in isotonic saline, 0.9% NaCl). Safranal (0.5−1 mg/kg, i.g.) was administered every day for five consecutive days in another experimental setting. Every day, 60 min after administration of safranal, that is, AITC (10 nmol), capsaicin (0.2 nmol), or GSK1016790A (2 nmol) or their vehicles (0.5% DMSO) were administered (20 μL, i.pl.) and acute nociceptive response was recorded. They evaluated the role of three main saffron constituents in the function of TRP channels expressed in nociceptors, and in the function of TRP channels especially that of TRPA1, expressed in nociceptors, is affected by the three main saffron constituents. They evaluated the role of three main constituents of saffron in the function of TRP channels especially that of TRPA1. Finally, safranal induces selective desensitization of the TRPA1 channel, thereby attenuating neuronal excitation resulting in nociception and release of Calcitonin Gene-Related Peptide (CGRP). This surprising TRPA1-desensitization mechanism could possibly explain the analgesic effects attributed to saffron (Table 15.3.)

CONCLUSION AND FUTURE ASPECTS

Saffron has an important role in the cure and prevention of many diseases through the modulation of antioxidant, antiinflammatory, antitumor, antimicrobial, and antidiabetic activity as have been well documented. More research is needed to explain its role along with the mechanisms of managing health through alterations of various physiological and biochemical pathways. These days the popularity of herbal treatment among the masses is gaining much interest, so more research based on animal models and clinical trials is needed to expand the understanding of saffron and its active constituent's role in diseases prevention.

REFERENCES

Abdullaev, F.I., 2002. Cancer chemopreventive and tumoricidal properties of saffron (Crocus sativus L.). Exp. Biomed. 227 (1), 20−25.

Amin, B., Hosseinzadeh, H., 2012. Evaluation of aqueous and ethanolic extracts of saffron, Crocus sativus L., and its constituents, safranal and crocin in allodynia and hyperalgesia induced by chronic constriction injury model of neuropathic pain in rats. Fitoterapia 83, 888-895.

Archana, S.J., Paul, R., Tiwari, A., 2011. Indian medicinal plants: a rich source of natural immuno-modulator. Int. J. Pharmacol. 7, 198−205.

Arora, A., Sairmam, R.K., Srivastava, G.C., 2002. Oxidative stress and antioxidant system in plants. Curr. Sci. 82 (10), 10−25.

Babaei, A., Arshami, J., Haghparast, A., Mesgaran, M.D., 2014. Effects of saffron (Crocus sativus) petal ethanolic extract on hematology, antibody response, and spleen histology in rats. Avicenna J. Phytomed. 4, 103−109.

Ballatori, N., Krance, S.M., Notenboom, S., Shi, S., Tieu, K., Hammond, C.H.L., 2009. Glutathione dysregulation and the etiology and progression of human diseases. Biol. Chem. 390, 191−214.

Bergmann, L., Rennenberg, H., 1993. Glutathione Metabolism in Plants: Sulphur Nutrition and Assimilation in Higher Plants. SPB Academic Publishing, The Hauge, The Neatherlands, pp. 61−75.

Bilal, I., Chowdhury, A., Davidson, J., Whitehead, S., 2014. Phytoestrogens and prevention of breast cancer: the contentious debate. World J. Clin. Oncol. 5 (4), 705−712.

Bittar, M., de Souza, M.M., Yunes, R.A., Lento, R., Delle Monache, F., Cechinel Filho, V., 2000. Antinociceptive activity of I3, II8-binaringenin, a biflavonoid present in plants of the guttiferae. Planta Med. 66, 84−86.

Bolhassani, A., Khavari, A., Bathaie, S.Z., 2014. Saffron and natural carotenoids: biochemical activities and anti-tumor effects. Biochim. Biophys. Acta 1845 (1), 20—30.

Boskabady, M.H., Farkhodeh, T., 2016. Antiinflammatory, antioxidant, and immunomodulatory effects of *Crocus sativus* L. And its main constituents. Phytother Res. 30 (7), 1072—1094.

Buettner, G.R., Jurkiewicz, B.A., 1996. Catalytic metals, ascorbate and free radicals: combinations to avoid. J. Radiat. Res. 145 (5), 532—541.

Calixto, J.B., Beirith, A., Ferreira, J., Santos, A.R., Cechinel Filho, V., Yunes, R.A., 2000. Naturally occurring antinociceptive substances from plants. Phytother Res. 14, 401—418.

Carmona, M., Zalacain, A., Salinas, M.R., Alonso, G.L., 2007. A new approach to saffron aroma. Crit. Rev. Food Sci. Nutr. 47, 145—159.

Charles, D.J., 2012. Saffron. In: Antioxidant Properties of Spices, Herbs and Other Sources. Springer, NY.

Chauhan, R.S., 2010. Nutrition, immunity and livestock health. Indian Cow 7, 2—13.

Chen, Y., Zhang, H., Tian, X., 2008. Antioxidant potential of crocins and ethanol extracts of Gardenia jasminoides ELLIS and *Crocus sativus* L.: a relationship investigation between antioxidant activity and crocin contents. Food Chem. 109 (3), 484—492.

Chen, K., Wang, X.M., Chen, F., Bai, J., 2017. In vitro antimicrobial and free radical scavenging activities of the total flavonoid in petal and stamen of crocus sativus. Indian J. Pharm. Sci. 79 (3), 482—487.

Cotman, C.W., 1987. The Neuro-Immune Endocrine Connection. Raven Pr.

De Mastro, G., Ruta, C., 1993. Relation between corm size ad saffron flowering. Acta Hortic. 344, 512—517.

De Oliveira, A.M., Conserva, L.M., de Souza, J.N., de Ferro, F., Almeida Brito, R.P., Lemos, L., 2012. Barreto E Antinociceptive and anti-inflammatory effects of octacosanol from the leaves of Sabicea griseavar. grisea in mice. Int. J. Mol. Sci. 1598—1611.

Dixon, D.P., Cummins, I., Cole, D.J., Edwards, R., 1998. Glutathione mediated detoxification systems in plants. Curr. Opin. Plant Biol. 1, 258—266.

Dunkelberger, J.R., Song, W.C., 2010. Complement and its role in innate and adaptive immune responses. Cell Res. 20 (1), 34—50.

El-Azime Abd, S.A., Sherif, N.H., Eltahawy, N.A., 2014. Efficacy of aqueous extract of saffron (*Crocus sativus* L.) in modulating radiation-induced brain and eye retina damage in rats. Egypt. J. Hosp. Med. 54, 101—108.

Fabricant, D.S., Farnsworth, N.R., 2001. The value of plants used in traditional medicine for drug discovery. Environ. Health Perspect. 109 (1), 69—75.

Farahmand, S.K., Samini, F., Samini, M., Samarghandian, S., 2013. Safranal ameliorates antioxidant enzymes and suppresses lipid peroxidation and nitric oxide formation in aged male rat liver. Biogerontology 14, 63—71.

Foyer, C.H., Harbinson, J., 1994. Oxygen metabolism and the regulation of photosynthetic electron transport. In: Foyer, C.H., Mullineaux, P.M. (Eds.), Causes of Photo-Oxidative Stress and Amelioration of Defense Systems in Plants. CRC Press, pp. 2—42.

Foyer, C.H., Lopez Delgado, H., Dat, J.F., Scott, I.M., 1997. Hydrogen peroxide and glutathione associated mechanism of acclamatory stress tolerance and signaling. Physiol. Plant. 100, 241—254.

Fridovich, 1986. Biological effect of superoxide radical. Arch. *Biochem. Biophys.* 247, 1—11.

Galati, E.M., Monforte, M.T., Kirjavainen, S., Forestieri, A.M., Trovato, A., Tripodo, M.M., 1994. Biological effects of hesperidin, a citrus flavonoid. (Note I): anti-inflammatory and analgesic activity. Farmaco 40, 709—712.

Gandomi Nasrabadi, H., Azami Sarokelaei, L., Misaghi, A., Abbaszadeh, S., Shariatifar, N., Tayyar Hashtjin, N., 2012. Antibacterial effect of aqueous and alcoholic extracts from petal of saffron (*Crocus sativus* L.) on some foodborne bacterial pathogens. J. Med. Plants Res. 12 (42), 189—196.

Ghasemi, T., Abnous, K., Vahdati, F., Mehri, S., Razavi, B.M., Hosseinzadeh, H., 2015. Antidepressant effect of *Crocus sativus* aqueous extract and its effect on CREB, BDNF, and VGF transcript and protein levels in rat hippocampus. Drug Res. 65, 337—343.

Giaccio, M., 2004. Crocetin from saffron: an active component of an ancient spice. Crit. Rev. Food Sci. Nutr. 44 (3), 155—172.

Gohari, A.R., Saeidnia, S., Mahmoodabadi, M.K., 2013. An overview on saffron, phytochemicals, and medicinal properties. Pharmacogn. Rev. 7 (13), 61.

Goli, S.A., Mokhtari, F., Rahimmalek, M., 2012. Phenolic compounds and antioxidant activity from Saffron (*Crocus sativus* L.). Petal J. Agric. Sci. 4 (10), 175—181.

Gurib-Fakim, A., 2006. Medicinal plants: traditions of yesterday and drugs of tomorrow. Mol. Asp. Med. 27 (1), 1—93.

Halliwell, B., 1994. Free radicals, antioxidants, and human disease: curiosity, cause, or consequence? Lancet 344, 721—724.

Hariri, A.T., Moallem, S.A., Mahmoudi, M., Hosseinzadeh, H., 2011. The effect of crocin and safranal, constituents of saffron, against subacute effect of diazinon on hematological and genotoxicity indices in rats. Phytomedicine 18 (6), 499—504.

Hasanpour, M., Ashrafi, M., Erjaee, H., Nazifi, S., 2018. The effect of saffron aqueous extract on oxidative stress parameters and important biochemical enzymes in the testis of streptozotocin-induced diabetic rats. Physiol. Pharmacol. 22, 28—37.

Hashemi, S.R., Davoodi, H., 2012. Herbal plants as new immuno-stimulator in poultry industry. Asian J. Anim. Vet. Adv. 7, 105—116.

Hell, R., 1997. Molecular physiology of plant surface metabolism. Planta 202, 138—148.

Holben, D.H., Smith, A.M., 1999. The diverse role of selenium within selenoproteins. J. Am. Diet. Assoc. 99, 836—843.

Hoshyar, R., Mollaei, H., 2017. A comprehensive review on anticancer mechanisms of the main carotenoid of saffron, crocin. J. Pharm. Pharmacol. 69, 1419—1427.

Hosseini, A., Razavi, B.M., Hosseinzadeh, H., 2018. Saffron (*Crocus sativus*) petal as a new pharmacological target. J. Basic Med. Sci. 21, 1091−1099.

Hosseinzadeh, H., Shariaty, V.M., 2007. Anti-nociceptive effect of safranal, a constituent of *Crocus sativus* (saffron), in mice. Pharmacologyonline 2, 498−503.

Hosseinzadeh, H., Younesi, H.M., 2002. Antinociceptive and anti-inflammatory effects of *Crocus sativus* L. stigma and petal extracts in mice. BMC Pharmacol. 2, 7−15.

Hosseinzadeh, H., Sadeghnia, H.R., 2005. Safranal, a constituent of *Crocus sativus* (saffron), attenuated cerebral ischemia induced oxidative damage in rat hippocampus. J. Pharm. Pharm. Sci. 8, 394−399.

Hosseinzadeh, H., Ziaei, T., 2006. Effects of *Crocus sativus* stigma extract and its constituents, crocin and safranal, on intact memory and scopolamine-induced learning deficits in rats performing the Morris water maze task. J. Med. Plants 5, 40−50.

Hosseinzadeh, H., Shamsaie, F., Mehri, S., 2010. Antioxidant activity of aqueous and ethanolic extracts of *Crocus sativus* L. stigma and its bioactive constituents cracin and Safranal. Pharmacog. Mag. 5, 419−424.

Hosseinzadeh, H., Sadeghnia, H.R., Ghaeni, F.A., Motamed Shariaty, V.S., Mohajeri, S.A., 2012. Effects of saffron (*Crocus sativus* L.) and its active constituent, crocin, on recognition and spatial memory after chronic cerebral hypo perfusion in rats. Phytother Res. 26, 381−386.

Hunskaar, S., Hole, K., 1987. The formalin test in mice: dissociation between inflammatory and non-inflammatory pain. Pain 30, 103−114.

Iwasaki, A., Medzhitov, R., 2010. Regulation of adaptive immunity by the innate immune system. Science 327 (5963), 291−295.

Jalal, T.K., Ahmed, I.A., Mikail, M., Momand, L., Draman, S., Isa, M.L.M., 2015. Evaluation of antioxidant, total phenol and flavonoid content and antimicrobial activities of *Artocarpus altilis* (breadfruit) of underutilized tropical fruit extracts. Appl. Biochem. Biotechnol. 175, 3231−3243.

Kaiko, G.E., Horvat, J.C., Beagley, K.W., Hansbro, P.M., 2008. Immunological decision-making: how does the immune system decide to mount a helper T-cell response? Immunology 123 (3), 326−338.

Kamble, V.A., Patil, S.D., 2007. Antimicrobial effects of certain spices and condiments used in an Indian indigenous system of medicine. Zeitschrift fur Arznei Gewurzpflanzen 12, 188−193.

Kanakis, C.D., Tarantilis, P.A., Polissiou, M.G., Diamantoglou, S., Tajmir-Riahi, H.A., 2007. An overview of DNA and RNA bindings to antioxidant flavonoids. Cell Biochem. Biophys. 49 (1), 29−36.

Kanaris, C.D., Tarantilis, P.A., Tajmir-Riahi, H.A., Polissiou, M.G., 2007. Crocetin, dimethylcrocetin, and safranal bind human serum albumin: stability and antioxidative properties. J. Agric. Food Chem. 55 (3), 970−977.

Karaman, I., Sahin, F., Güllüce, M., Ögütçü, H., Sengül, M., Adıgüzel, A., 2003. Antimicrobial activity of aqueous and methanol extracts of *Juniperus oxycedrus* L. J. Ethnopharmacol. 85, 213−235.

Karimi, E., Oskoueian, E., Hendra, R., Hawk, Z.E., 2010. Evaluation of *Crocus sativus* L. stigma phenolic and flavonoid compounds and its antioxidant activity. Molecules 15, 6244−6256.

Kattappagari, K.K., Ravi Teja, C.S., Kommalpati, R.K., Poosarla, C., Gontu, S.R., Reddy, V., 2015. Role of atioxidants in facilitatig the body functions. J. Orofac. Sci. 5 (7), 71−75.

Khajuria, D.K., Asad, M., Asdaq, S., Kumar, P., 2010. The potency of crocus sativus (saffron) and its constituent crocin as an immunomodulator in animals. Lat. Am. J. Pharm. 29.

Khorasany, A.R., Hosseinzadeh, H., 2016. Therapeutic effects of saffron (*Crocus sativus* L.) in digestive disorders: *Iran. J. Basic Med. Sci. 19, 455−469.

Kulik, I., Storz, G., 1994. Transcriptional regulators of the oxidative stress response in prokaryotes and eukaryotes. Redox Res. 1, 23−29.

Labadie, R., Van der Nat, J.M., Simons, J.M., Kroes, B.H., Kosasi, S., van den Berg, T.A., Van der Sluis, W.G., Abeysekera, A., Bamunuarachchi, A., De Silva, K.T., 1989. An ethnopharmacognostic approach to the search for immunomodulators of plant origin. Planta Med. 55 (04), 339−348.

Lee, J.D., Park, H.J., Chae, Y., Lim, S., 2005. An overview of bee venom acupuncture in the treatment of arthritis. Evid. Based Complement. Alternat. Med. 2 (1), 79−84.

Li Puma, S., Landini, L., Macedo Jr., S.J., Seravalli, V., Marone, I.M., Coppi, E., Patacchini, R., Geppetti, P., Materazzi, S., Nassini, R., De Logu, F., 2019. TRPA 1 mediates the antinociceptive properties of the constituent of *Crocus sativus* L., safranal. J. Cell Mol. Med. 23 (3), 1976−1986.

Liou, W., Chang, L.Y., Geuze, H.J., Strous, G.J., Crapo, J.D., Slot, J.W., 1993. Distribution of CuZn superoxide dismutase in rat liver. Free Radic. Biol. Med. 14, 201−207.

Litalien, C., Beaulieu, P., 2011. Chapter 117 − molecular mechanisms of drug actions: from receptors to effectors. Pediatr. Crit. Care 1553−1568.

Lobo, V., Patil, A., Phatak, A., Chandra, N., 2010. Free radicals, antioxidants and functional foods: impact on human health. Pharmacogn. Rev. 4, 118−126.

Lozano, P., Delgado, D., Gomez, D., Rubio, M., Iborra, J.L., 2000. A non-destructive method to determine the Safranal content of saffron (*Crocus sativus* L.) by supercritical carbon dioxide extraction combined with high-performance liquid chromatography and gas chromatography. J. Biochem. Biophys. Methods 43, 367−378.

Ma, S., Zhou, S., Shu, B., Zhou, J., 1998. Pharmacological studies on Crocus glycosides I. Effects on antiinflammatory and immune function. Zhong Cao Yao 29, 536−539.

Maggi, L., Sánchez, A.M., Carmona, M., Kanakis, C.D., Anastasaki, E., Tarantilis, P.A., Alonso, G.L., 2011. Rapid determination of safranal in the quality control of saffron spice (Crocus sativus L.). Food Chem. 127, 369−373.

Mahima, R.A., Deb, R., Shyma, K., Hari, L., Samad, A., Tiwari, R., Verma, A.K., Amit Kumar, A., Dhama, K., 2012. Immunomodulatory and therapeutic potentials of herbal, traditional/indigenous and ethnoveterinary medicines. Pak. J. Biol. Sci. 15, 754−774.

Makhlouf, H., Saksouk, M., Habib, J., Chahine, R., 2011. Determination of antioxidant activity of saffron \sstaken from the flower of Crocus sativus grown in Lebanon. Afr. J. Biotechnol. 10 (41), 8093–8100.

Manoj, M., Kailas, C., Balaji, V., Sajid, N., 2010. Effect of plants extracts. Int. J. Pharm Tech Res. 2, 899–901.

Marklund, S.L., 1982. Human copper-containing superoxide dismutase of high molecular weight. Proc. Natl. Acad. Sci. USA 79, 7634–7638.

Mathew, T., Mathew, Z., Dhama, K., 2010. Plants and herbs for the treatment of cancer in human and animals. In: Proceedings of the National Seminar on Advances in Animal Cancer Research in India: Diagnosis, Treatment and Clinical Management, Indian Veterinary Research Institute. *India Souvenir*, Izatnagar (U.P.), pp. 85–86.

May, M.J., Leaver, C.J., 1993. Oxidative stimulation of glutathione synthesis in *Arabidopsis thaliana* suspension culture. Plant Physiol. 103, 621–627.

May, M.J., Vernoux, T., Leaver, C., Montagu, M.V., Inze, D., 1998. Glutathione homeostasis in plants: implication for environmental sensing and plant development. J. Exp. Bot. 49 (321), 649–667.

Mogensen, T.H., 2009. Pathogen recognition and inflammatory signaling in innate immune defenses. Clin. Microbiol. Rev. 22 (2), 240–273.

Mohajeri, D., Mousavi, G., Doustar, Y., 2009. Antihyperglycemic and pancreas-protective effects of *Crocus sativus* L. (Saffron) stigma-ethanolic extract on rats with alloxan-induced diabetes. J. Biol. Sci. 9 (4), 302–310.

Moodycliffe, A.M., Nghiem, D., Clydesdale, G., Ullrich, S.E., 2000. Immune suppression and skin cancer development: regulation by NKT cells. Nat. Immunol. 1 (6), 521.

Muzaffar, S., Rather, S.A., Khan, K.H., Akhter, R., 2015. Nutritional composition and in vitro antioxidant properties of two cultivars of Indian saffron. J. Food Meas. Charact. 10 (1), 185–192.

Muzaffar, S., Rather, S.A., Khan, K.Z., 2016. In vitro bactericidal and fungicidal activities of various extracts of saffron (*Crocus sativus* L.) stigmas from Jammu and Kashmir, India. Cogent Food Agric. 2 (1), 1–7.

Nakhaei, M., Khaje-Karamoddin, M., Ramezani, M., 2008. Inhibition of *Helicobacter pylori* growth in vitro by saffron (*Crocus sativus* L.). Iran. J. Basic Med. Sci. 11, 91–99.

Nijs, D., Kelley, P.M., 1991. Vitamins C and E donate single hydrogen atoms *in vivo*. FEBS Lett. 284, 147–151.

Noctor, G., Foyer, C.H., 1998. Ascorbate and glutathione: keeping active oxygen under control. Plant Physiol. Plant Mol. Biol. 49, 249–279.

Padh, H., 1990. Cellular functions of ascorbic acid Biochem. Cell Biol 68, 1166–1173.

Papandreou, M.A., Kanakis, C.D., Polissiou, M.G., Efthimiopoulos, S., Cordopatis, P., Margarity, M., Lamari, F.N., 2006. Inhibitory activity on amyloid-beta aggregation and antioxida nt properties of Crocus sativus stigmas extract and its crocin constituents. J. Agric. Food Chem. 54 (23), 8762–8768.

Patel, S., Sarwat, M., Khan, T.H., 2017. Mechanism behind the anti-tumour potential of saffron (*Crocus sativus* L.): the molecular perspective. Crit. Rev. Oncol. Hematol. 115, 27–35.

Pinheiro, M.M., Boylan, F., Fernandes, P.D., 2012. Antinociceptive effect of the Orbignya speciosa Mart. (Babassu) leaves: evidence for the involvement of apigenin. Life Sci. 91 (9–10), 293–300.

Pintado, C., de Miguel, A., Acevedo, O., Nozal, L., Novella, J.L., Rotger, R., 2011. Bactericidal effect of saffron (*Crocus sativus* L.) on *Salmonella enterica* during storage. Food Control 22, 638–642.

Poma, A., Fontecchio, G., Carlucci, G., Chichiriccò, G., 2012. Anti-inflammatory properties of drugs from saffron crocus. Antiinflamm. Antiallergy Agents Med. Chem. 11 (1), 37–51.

Rahal, A., Kumar, A., Tulsi, 2009. A miracle herb in the hands of traditional house lady. In: Proceedings of the 10th Annual Convention of Indian Association of Lady Veterinarians and National Symposium on Contribution of Women Veterinarians in Upliftment of Livestock Production Through New Technologies, (CIALV'09), College of Veterinary Sciences and Animal Husbandry. Jawaharlal Nehru Krishi Vishwa Vidyalaya, Jabalpur.

Rahim, M.H.A, Zakaria, Z.A., Sani, M., Hijaz, M., Omar, M.H., Yakob, Y., Cheema, M.S., Ching, S.M., Ahmad, Z., Abdul Kadir, A., 2016. Methanolic extract of Clinacanthus nutans exerts antinociceptive activity via the opioid/nitric oxide-mediated, but cGMP-independent, pathways. Evid. Based Complement. Alternat. Med. https://doi.org/10.1155/2016/1494981.

Rahmani, A.H., Khan, A.A., Aldebasi, Y.H., 2017. Saffron (*Crocus sativus*) and its active ingredients: role in the prevention and treatment of disease. Pharmacogn. J. 9 (6), 873–879.

Rajendhran, J., Mani, M.A., Navaneethakannan, K., 1998. Antimicrobial activity of some selected medicinal plants. Geobios 25, 208–282.

Ramesh, M., Rao, Y.N., Rao, A.V., Prabhakar, M.C., Rao, C.S., Muralidhar, N., Reddy, B.M., 1998. Antinociceptive and anti-inflammatory activity of a flavonoid isolated from *Caralluma attenuata*. J. Ethnopharmacol. 62, 63–66.

Rang, H.P., Dale, M.M., Ritter, J.M., Flower, R.J., Henderson, G., 2011. Rang and Dales Phramacology Elsevier Churchill Livingstone, seventh ed. Edinburgh, UK.

Rathore, B., Jaggi, K., Thakur, S.K., Mathur, A., Mahdi, F., 2015. Anti-inflammatory activity of *Crocus sativus* extract in experimental arthritis. Int. J. Pharm. Sci. Res. 6 (4), 1473–1478.

Razak, S.I., Anwar Hamzah, M.S., Yee, F.C., Kadir, M.R., Nayan, 2017. A review on medicinal properties of saffron toward major diseases. J. Herbs, Spices, Med. Plants 23 (2), 98–116.

Rios, J.L., Recio, M.C., Giner, R.M., Manez, S., 1996. An update review of saffron and its active constituents. Phytother Res. 10, 189–193.

Rose, R.C., Bode, A.M., 1993. Biology of free radical scavengers: an evaluation of ascorbate. FASEB J. 7, 1135–1142.

Rubio-Pere, J.M., Morillas-Ruiz, J.M., 2012. A review: inflammatory process in Alzheimer's disease, role of cytokines. Sci. World J. https://doi.org/10.1100/2012/756357.

Salin, M.L., 1988. Toxic oxygen species and protective systems of the chloroplast. Physiol. Plant. 72, 681–689.

Samarghandian, S., Afshari, J.T., Davoodi, S., 2011. Suppression of pulmonary tumor promotion and induction of apoptosis by *Crocus sativus* L. extraction. Appl. Biochem. Biotechnol. 164, 238–247.

Samarghandian, S., Borji, S., Farahmand, S.K., Afshari, R., Davoodi, S., 2013. *Crocus sativus* L. (Saffron) stigma aqueous extract induces apoptosis in alveolar human lung cancer cells through caspase-dependent activation. BioMed Res. Int. 417928.

Samarghandian, S., Afshari, R., Sadati, A., 2014. Evaluation of lung and bronchoalveolar lavage fluid oxidative stress indices for assessing the preventing effects of safranal on respiratory distress in diabetic rats. Sci. World J 69 (2), 151–159, 2–6. Indian Heart J.

Samarghandian, S., Azimi- Nezhad, M.C., Farahmand, S.K., 2017. Immunomodulatory and antioxidant effects of saffron aqueous extract (*Crocus sativus* L.) on streptozotocin-induced diabetes in rats. Indian Heart J. 69 (2), 151–159.

Samarghandian Samani, A.S., Farkhondeh, T., Bahmani, M., 2016. Assessment the effect of saffron ethanolic extract (*Crocus sativus* L.) on oxidative damages in aged male rat liver, 8, 283–290.

Sanchez-Fernandez, R., Fricker, M., Corben, L.B., White, N.S., Sheard, N., Leaver, C.J., Van Montagu, M., Inzé, D., May, M.J., 1997. Cell proliferation and hair tip growth in the Arabidopsis root are under mechanistically different forms of redox control. Proc. Natl. Acad. Sci. 94 (6), 2745–2750.

Sánchez-Vioque, R., Rodríguez-Conde, M.F., Reina-Ureña, J.V., Escolano-Tercero, M.A., Herraiz-Peñalvera, D., Santana-Méridas, O., 2012. In vitro antioxidant and metal chelating properties of corm, tepal and leaf from saffron (*Crocus sativus* L.). Ind. Crops Prod. 39, 149–153.

Segerstrom, S.C., Miller, G.E., 2004. Psychological stress and the human immune system: a meta-analytic study of 30 years of inquiry. Psychol. Bull. 130 (4), 601–630.

Sekine, T., Sugano, M., Majid, A., Fujii, Y., 2007. Antifungal effects of volatile compounds from black zira (Bunium persicum) and other spices and herbs. J. Chem. Ecol. 33, 2123–2132.

Sharma, P., Kumar, P., Sharma, R., Gupta, G., Chaudrary, A., 2017. Immunomodulators: role of medicinal plants in immune system. Natl. J. Physiol. Pharm. Pharmacol. 7 (6), 552–556.

Sheng, L., Qian, Z., Zheng, S., Xi, L., 2006. Mechanism of hypolipidemic effect of crocin in rats: crocin inhibits pancreatic lipase. Eur. J. Pharmacol. 543, 116–122.

Soureshjan, E.H., Heidari, M., 2014. In vitro Variation in antibacterial activity plant extracts on *Glaucium elegans* and Saffron (*Crocus sativus* L.). Onios Electron. J. Biol. 10, 64–67.

Sovrlić, M., Vasiljević, P., Jušković, M., Mašković, P., Manojlović, N., 2015. Phytochemical, antioxidant and antimicrobial profiles of extracts of *Daphne alpina* (Thymelaeaceae) L leaf and twig from Mt Kopaonik (Serbia). Trop. J. Pharm. Res. 14, 1239–1248.

Spelman, K., Burns, J., Nichols, D., Winters, N., Ottersberg, S., Tenborg, M., 2006. Modulation of cytokine expression by traditional medicines. Altern. Med. Rev. 11, 128–150.

Srivastava, T.N., Rajasekharan, S., Badola, D.P., Shah, D.C., 1985. Important medicinal plants of Jammu and Kashmir i. kesar (saffron). Ancient Sci. Life 1, 68–73.

Srivastava, R., Ahmed, H., Dixit, R.K., 2010. *Crocus sativus* L.: a comprehensive review. Pharmacogn. Rev. 4 (8), 200.

Starec, M., Waitzov'a, D., Elis, J., 1998. Evaluation of the analgesic effect of RG-tannin using the "hot plate" and "tail flick" method in mice. Ceskoslovenska Farm. 37, 319–321.

Sumitra, C., Yogesh, B., 2010. Extraction of active compounds of some medical plants. Afr. J. Biotechnol. 9, 3210–3217.

Tamaddonfard, E., Farshid, A.A., Eghdami, K., Samadi, F., Erfanparast, 2013. A Comparison of the effects of crocin, safranal and diclofenac on local inflammation and inflammatory pain responses induced by carrageenan in rats. Pharmacol. Rep. 65 (5), 1272–1280.

Tamaddonfard, E., Farshid, A.A., Maroufi, S., 2014. Effects of safranal, a constituent of saffron, and vitamin E on nerve functions and histopathology following crush injury of sciatic nerve in rats. Phytomedicine 21, 717–723.

Tarantilis, P.A., Tsoupras, G., Polissiou, M., 1995. Determination of saffron (*Crocus sativus* L.) components in crude plant extracts using high- performance liquid chromatography-UV-visible photodiode-array detection-mass spectrometry. J. Chromatogr. 699, 107–118.

Teixeira, E.W., Negri, G., Meira, R.M.S.A., Message, D., Salatino, A., 2005. Plant origin of green propolis: bee behavior, plant anatomy and chemistry. Evid. Based Complement. Alternat. Med. 2 (1), 85–92.

Tilak, J.C., Devasagayam, T.P.A., 2006. Indian medicinal plants: a potential reservoir in health and disease. In: Kohli, K., Gupta, M., Tejwani, S. (Eds.), Contemporary Perspectives on Clinical Pharmacotherapeutics. Elsevier, New Delhi, pp. 29–43.

Tripathi, K.D., 1999. Essentials of Medical Pharmacology, fourth ed. Jaypee Brothers Medical Publishers (P) Ltd., New Delhi, India.

Tripathi, Y.B., Singh, K., Pandey, R.S., Kumar, M., 2005. BHUx: a patent polyherbal formulation to prevent atherosclerosis. Evid. Based Complement. Alternat. Med. 2 (2), 217–221.

Turco, G.L., 1963. Rheumatoid arthritis. Aggiorn. Clin. Ter. 4, 1–56.

Uliana, M.P., Silva, A.G.D., Fronza, M., Scherer, R., 2015. In vitro antioxidant and antimicrobial activities of *Costus spicatus*Swartz used in folk medicine for urinary tract infection in Brazil. Lat. Am. J. Pharm. 34, 766–772.

Umashanker, M., Shruti, S., 2011. Traditional Indian herbal medicine used as antipyretic, antiulcer, anti-diabetic and anticancer. Int. J. Res. Pharm. Chem. 1, 1152–1159.

Upadhayay, H.A., Kuma, A.K., Verma, A., Rahal, Mahajan, S., 2011. Medicinal values of hot aqueous extracts (HAE) of

Sonchus Asper (Prickly Sow Thistle) leaves against bacterial and mycotic pathogens. In: Proceedings of the World Congress for Man and Nature Global Climate Change and Biodiversity Conservation. Haridwar, India, Uttarakhand, India, p. 407.

Vahidi, H., Kamalineja, M., Sedaghati, N., 2002. Antimicrobial properties of Croccus sativus L. Iran. J. Pharm. Res. 1, 33–35.

Van Wijk, R., Van Wijk, E., Wiegant, F.A., Ives, J., 2008. Free radicals and low-level photon emission in human pathogenesis: state of the art. Indian J. Exp. Biol. 46, 273–309.

Weisiger, R.A., Fridovich, I., 1973. Mitochondrial superoxide simutase. Site of synthesis and intramitochondrial localization. J. Biol. Chem. 248, 4793–4796.

Willekens, H., Chamnongpol, S., Davey, M., Schraudner, M., Langebartels, C., Van Montagu, M., Inzé, D., Van Camp, W., 1997. Catalase is a sink for H_2O_2 and is indispensable for stress defence in C3 plants. EMBO J. 16 (16), 4806–4816.

Winglse, G., Karpinski, S., 1996. Differential redox regulation by glutathione and glutathione reductase and Cu-Zn SOD gene expression in Pinus sylvesties L. needles. Planta 198, 151–157.

Wu, G., Fang, Y.Z., Yang, S., Luoton, J.R., Turner, N.D., 2004. Glutathione metabolism and its implications for health. J. Nutr. 34, 489–49.

Wu, J.Q., Kosten, T.R., Zhang, X.Y., 2013. Free radicals, antioxidant defense system, and schizophrenia. Prog. Neuropsychopharmacol. Biol. Psychiatry 46, 200–206.

Xi, L., Qian, Z., Shen, X., N Wen, Y., 2005. Zhang: crocetin prevents dexamethasone-induced insulin resistance in rats. Planta Med. 71 (10), 917–922.

Yan, J., Ralston, M.M., Meng, X., Bongiovanni, K.D., Jones, A.L., Benndorf, R., 2013. Glutathione reductase is essential for host defense against bacterial infection. Free Radic. Biol. Med. 61, 320–332.

Zakaria, Z.A., Abdul Hisam, E.E., Rofiee, M.S., 2011. In vivo antiulcer activity of the aqueous extract of Bauhinia purpurea leaf. J. Ethnopharmacol. 137 (2), 1047–1054.

Zakaria, Z.A., Sani, M.H., Cheema, M.S., Kader, A.A., Kek, T.L., Salleh, M.Z., 2014. Antinociceptive activity of methanolic extract of Muntingia calabura leaves: further elucidation of the possible mechanisms. BMC Complement Altern. Med. 14 (1), 63.

Zeinali, M., Zirak, M., Rezaee, S., Karimi, G., Hosseinzadeh, H., 2019. Immunoregulatory and anti-inflammatory properties of Crocus sativus (Saffron) and its main active constituents: a review. Iran. J. Basic Med. Sci. 22 (4), 334–344.

Zendehdel, M., Taati, M., Jadidoleslami, M., Bashiri, A., 2011. Evaluation of pharmacological mechanisms of antinociceptive effect of Teucrium polium on visceral pain in mice. Iran. J. Vet. Res. 12 (4), 292–297.

Zhu, K.J., Yang, J.S., 2014. Anti-allodynia effect of safranal on neuropathic pain induced by spinal nerve transection in rat. Int. J. Clin. Exp. Med. 7, 4990–4996.

CHAPTER 16

The Effects of Saffron (*Crocus sativus*) and its Constituents on Immune System: Experimental and Clinical Evidence

AMIN MOKHTARI-ZAER • SAEIDEH SAADAT • VAHIDEH GHORANI •
ARGHAVAN MEMARZIA • MOHAMMAD HOSSEIN BOSKABADY

INTRODUCTION

Saffron, with a scientific name of *Crocus sativus (C. sativus)*, is widely used with a long history in traditional medicine according to the reports of Razi and Avicenna (Hosseinzadeh and Nassiri-Asl, 2013; Mollazadeh et al., 2015). In addition, saffron is used as a food additive, spice, and also for various medicinal purposes. Chemical studies of *C. sativus* have shown the presence of carotenoid components, mainly crocin, crocetin, picrocrocin, and safranal, which are the main constituents of the plant and are responsible for most of the pharmacological effects of the plant (Caballero-Ortega et al., 2007).

Crocus sativus belongs to the large family of Iridaceae, which consists of about 60 genera and 1500 species, and is mainly produced and grown in Iran, Spain, Greece, Turkey, India, and Morocco. The growth cycle of saffron lasts for at least 220 days, of which summer and autumn are the best seasons for its growth, and the flowering of saffron occurs in autumn (Dhar et al., 2017). The main part saffron responsible for therapeutic and pharmacologic effects of the plant is its stigma which has been focused by biomedical researchers in recent years (Caballero-Ortega et al., 2007). Saffron has been used as antispasmodic, aphrodisiac, sedative, carminative, appetizer, flatulence, expectorant, diaphoretic, tranquilizer, and eupeptic (Abdullaev and Espinosa-Aguirre, 2004; Rios et al., 1996). *C. sativus* showed several pharmacological activities including antidiabetic (Kianbakht and Mozaffari, 2009), immunomodulatory (Boskabady et al., 2011a,b), anticancer (Tseng et al., 1995), analgesic (Hosseinzadeh and Younesi, 2002), antimicrobial (Yousefi et al., 2014), antiatherogenic (Xu et al., 2005), cardioprotective (Zhang et al., 2009), and antioxidant (El-Beshbishy et al., 2012). The relaxant effect of saffron and its constituents on tracheal smooth muscle (Boskabady and Aslani, 2006), inhibitory effect on the calcium channel of heart (Boskabady et al., 2008), and its effect on Thh1/Th2 balance (Boskabady et al., 2011a,b) were also indicated. The other pharmacological effect of the plants include antigenotoxic (Premkumar et al., 2006), antimutagenic (Bhandari, 2015), antithrombotic (Yang et al., 2008), gastroprotective (El-Maraghy et al., 2015), renal protective (Hazman and Bozkurt, 2015), and hepatoprotective properties (Sun et al., 2014).

The components of this plant via modulating proinflammatory cytokines and immune factors can reduce inflammation and immunomodulatory effects (El-Beshbishy et al., 2012; Hassan et al., 2015). In addition, in several disorders such as asthma, cardiovascular disease, and allergic disorders, the role of saffron and its constituents were demonstrated (Aggarwal and Harikumar, 2009). Saffron-based compounds have been extensively investigated for pharmacological, clinical, and toxicological aspects (Bostan et al., 2017). The protective effects of saffron against chemical toxine (Razavi and Hosseinzadeh, 2015), including its protective effect on diazinon (Lari et al., 2015; Razavi et al., 2013), malathion (Mohammadzadeh et al., 2018), acrylamide (Mehri et al., 2015), and cumene hydroperoxide (Yousefsani et al., 2018a), have been reported.

Recent findings showed the positive effects of saffron and saffron petal extracts in the treatment of mild to moderate depression (Christodoulou et al., 2015). The medicinal properties of saffron may be related to a number of its components, such as crocetin, crocin, and safranal due to their antioxidant properties against reactive oxygen species (ROS) (Hosseinzadeh and Jahanian, 2010; Rezaee and Hosseinzadeh, 2013). Therefore, in this chapter, the effects of saffron (*Crocus*

Saffron. https://doi.org/10.1016/B978-0-12-818462-2.00016-4

sativous) and its constituents on immune system based on experimental and clinical evidence, will be reviewed.

THE EFFECT OF SAFFRON (*CROCUS SATIVUS*) AND ITS CONSTITUENTS ON HUMORAL AND CELL-MEDIATED IMMUNITY

The immune system is a complex biological system consisting of innate and adaptive immunity. The innate immune system provides an efficient first line of host defense, and it is essential for triggering the adaptive immune response. The adaptive immune system can be classified into cellular and humoral immunity. T cells and B cells are the main components of the adaptive, cellular immune system. T lymphocytes have two subtypes, including T helper cells (Th, CD4$^+$) and cytotoxic T cells (CTL, CD8$^+$). According to the local cytokine environment, naïve CD4$^+$ T cells differentiate into distinct subsets, including Th1, Th2, Treg, and Th-17 cells. Cellular immunity is stimulated by the presentation of antigens on human leukocyte antigen (HLA) receptors and the identification of these antigens by T cells. However, humoral immunity is mediated by the recognition of antigens by antibodies produced by B cells. Both innate and acquired immunity are influenced by *C. sativus* and its components. A brief overview of the currently available information is summarized below.

Humoral Immunity (Immunoglobulins/Antibody Titer)
Experimental studies
Bani et al. examined the effect of alcoholic extract of saffron on humoral immunity on sheep erythrocyte-specific haemagglutination antibody titer in mice. Cyclosporin at a dose of 5 mg/kg significantly inhibited antibody titer response, however, administration of *C. sativus* at a dose of 6.25 mg/kg significantly increased agglutinating antibody titer in mice. Saffron also increased the levels of IgG-1 and IgM antibodies of the primary and secondary immune response (Bani et al., 2011). Vijayabhargava and Asad, investigated the power of humoral mediated immunity induced by saffron and demonstrated that saffron as a suspension at doses of 50 and 100 mg/kg increased the level of serum immunoglobulins and circulating antibody titer. At 50 mg/kg, saffron, effectively stimulated humoral and cell-mediated immunity (Vijayabhargava and Asad, 2011).

In a toxicological study, the immunotoxic effect of safranal was investigated, and the results showed that the subacute exposure to safranal (0.1, 0.5, and 1 mL/kg) for 3 weeks did not exhibit significant changes in

mice antibody response (Riahi-Zanjani et al., 2015). In another work by Babaei et al., the effects of 0, 75, 150, 225, and 450 mg/kg saffron petal extract on the immune response was studied. Saffron petal extract pretreatment at the dose of 75 mg/kg resulted in a significant elevation in the level of IgG. The authors suggested that these effects might have resulted from the secretion of IFN-γ involved in the stimulation of B lymphocytes for IgG production (Babaei et al., 2014).

The effect of saffron on immunoglobulin production by B cells in allergic asthma condition has been investigated in one study. Xiong et al. investigated the effect of crocin on the ovalbumin (OVA)-induced allergic airway inflammation in mice. They demonstrated that crocin significantly inhibited the proliferation of IgE (Xiong et al., 2015).

Clinical studies
The immunological effects of saffron in a randomized, double-blind, placebo-controlled clinical trial of healthy volunteers were enrolled for daily oral administration of 100 mg saffron tablet for 6 weeks. After 3 weeks, a significant decrease in the level of IgG and a decrease in IgM level compared to the baseline and placebo were reported. However, after 6 weeks, these alterations returned to the baseline levels with no observable adverse effects (Kianbakht and Ghazavi, 2011).

Taken together, published data demonstrated that saffron and its constituent, crocin, augment the production of humoral immune responses.

Cell-Mediated Immunity (Phagocytic Activity)
Cell-mediated immunity which depends on T cells mediates the immune response and plays a central role in defense against pathogens, antitumor immunity, rejection of organ transplants, and development of autoimmune diseases. Cell-mediated immunity was assessed by evaluating T-cell proliferation, differentiation, and production of cytokines by T cells. Several studies suggested that saffron is capable of modulating many of these T-cell—mediated immune functions. Cytokines are molecules secreted by monocytes, lymphocytes, and a variety of other cells. They are usually produced in response to antigens, microbes, or physiological stress. Activated monocytes/macrophages produce proinflammatory cytokines including IL-1, TNF-α, and IL-6 that play a major role in inflammatory responses. Th1 cells release gamma interferon (IFN-γ) and IL-2, which predominantly promote cell-mediated immunity. Th2 cells produce cytokine, such as IL-4, IL-5, IL-6, and transforming growth factor (TGF-β) that

negatively regulate cell-mediated immunity. A brief review of the effects of saffron on each of these T-cell activities is presented below.

Saffron extracts

Saffron and its constituents have also been investigated for its effect on cytokine production in disease-specific conditions. Byrami et al. showed that saffron extract increased the level of serum IL-4 but decreased IFN-γ and IFN-γ/IL-4 ratio in the experimental asthma model (Byrami et al., 2013).

Crocin and crocetin

The regulation of cytokine production by saffron has been addressed in a number of studies. Nam et al. showed that the inhibition of LPS-induced production of TNF-α and IL-1β in rat brain microglia by crocin or crocetin (Nam et al., 2010). In another study, Li et al., it was shown that crocin inhibited proinflammatory IL-1β, IL-6, and TNF-α in rat intervertebral discs stimulated with LPS and demonstrated that suppression of the phosphorylation of JNK by crocin was responsible for the impairment of cytokine production (Li et al., 2015).

Yang et al. examined the effect of the crocetin on acute lung injury induced by lipopolysaccharide (LPS). Significant inhibition of IL-6, macrophage chemoattractant protein-1 (MCP-1), and TNF-α expression by crocetin was observed in lung tissue. The authors of the study concluded that the crocetin might be effective as a therapeutic agent in the attenuation of acute lung injury (Yang et al., 2012). Kawabata et al. studied the effect of the crocin on the expression of NF-κB, COX-2, iNOS, TNF-α, IL-1β, and IL-6 in DSS-induced colitis in mice. They showed that treatment with the crocin inhibited the mRNA NF-κB, COX-2, iNOS, TNF-α, IL-1β, and IL-6, suggesting that crocin might be beneficial in protecting against colorectal carcinogenesis (Kawabata et al., 2012). The effect of saffron (*Crocus sativus*) and its constituents on humoral and cell-mediated immunity was summarized in Table 16.1.

THE EFFECT OF SAFFRON (*CROCUS SATIVUS*) AND ITS CONSTITUENTS ON WBC AND PLATELETS

The innate immune system is the first line of defense against various pathogens and their products. The innate immune system includes several types of white blood cells (neutrophils, eosinophils, basophils, lymphocytes, monocytes, total white blood cells, and platelets). The immunomodulatory activity of saffron and its

main bioactive compounds might be related to its alteration of several types of white blood cells, which plays a role in several inflammatory diseases.

Saffron Extracts

Concerning the effects of saffron on WBC, Bayrami and coworkers showed that if the extract of saffron (0.1, 0.2, and 0.4 mg/mL) and safranal (4, 8, and 16 µg/mL in drinking water) were administered to asthmatic animals, the total and differential count of WBC were significantly reduced (Byrami et al., 2013). Administration of hydroethanolic extract of *C. sativus* (50, 100, and 200 mg/kg) on sensitized rats reduced WBC number and decreased the percentage of eosinophils and neutrophils in the lung lavage as compared with the untreated sensitized animals (Mahmoudabady et al., 2013). In a similar work, saffron hydroethanolic extract also significantly decreased WBC count, eosinophil and neutrophil percentages, and platelet count in the blood of sensitized rats. However, lymphocyte percentage was increased in the animals receiving 100 mg/kg of saffron hydroethanolic extract which was due to the reduction of total WBC count (Vosooghi et al., 2013).

Crocin

In another study, it was observed that the crocin decreased the numbers of total and differential leukocyte counts in BALF of a murine model of allergic airway inflammation (Xiong et al., 2015). In a similar study, the treatment of sensitized mice with crocin (25 mg/kg, orally) once daily for 16 days, reduced the differential cell counts (monocytes, 59%; neutrophils, 63%; and eosinophils, 58%) compared with untreated asthmatic mice (Yosri et al., 2017).

Collectively, published data indicate that saffron and its main bioactive compounds modulate total and differential leukocyte counts, which demonstrated immunomodulatory effects of saffron.

THE EFFECT OF SAFFRON (*CROCUS SATIVUS*) AND ITS CONSTITUENTS ON TH1, TH2, AND TH17 RESPONSES

The Immunomodulatory effects of saffron and its constituents were shown in several in vitro and in vivo studies, which will be reviewed in this section.

Saffron Extracts
In vivo *studies*

Immunomodulatory impact of saffron alcoholic extract had been studied in sensitized mice with fresh sheep red

TABLE 16.1
The Effect of saffron (Crocus sativus) and its Constituents on Humoral and Cell-mediated Immunity.

Extract/constituent	Dose	Model	Outcomes	Ref.
EE	1.56, 3.12, 6.25, 12.5, 25, 50 mg/kg, orally, 5 days	Sensitized mice	Increased agglutinating antibody, IgG-1 and IgM antibodies levels	Bani et al. (2011)
Saffron as a suspension	50 and 100 mg/kg	Indirect hemagglutination test	Increased serum immunoglobulins and circulating antibody levels	Vijayabhargava and Asad (2011)
Saffron tablet	100 mg/day for 6 weeks	Healthy men	Decrease IgG and IgM level in 3 weeks, but returning to the baseline in 6 weeks	Kianbakht and Ghazavi (2011)
Safranal	0.1, 0.5, and 1 mL/kg for 3 weeks	Mice model of immunotoxicity	Unchanged antibody, IL-4, and INF-γ levels	Riahi-Zanjani et al. (2015)
Saffron petal extract	0, 75, 150, 225, and 450 mg/kg	Immunization by SRBC	Elevation of IgG level due to 75 mg/kg	Babaei et al. (2014)
Crocin	100 mg/kg/day for 5 days	Ovalbumin-sensitized mice	Reduced IgE	Xiong et al. (2015)
Crocetin	20 and 40 μM	LPS-induced microglial activation	Reduced TNF-α and IL-1β	Nam et al. (2010)
Crocin	10, 50, and 100 μM	LPS-induced inflammation	Inhibited expression of IL-1β, IL-6, and TNF-α	Li et al. (2015)
EE	20, 40, and 80 mg/kg in drinking water, 31 days	Ovalbumin sensitized guinea pigs	Increased the level of serum IL-4 but decreased IFN-γ and IFN-γ/IL-4 ratio	Byrami et al. (2013)
Crocetin	50, 100 mg/kg, i.g., before and after LPS instillation	LPS-induced acute lung injury in mice	Decreased expressions of TNF-α and IL-6	Yang et al. (2012)
Crocin	50, 100, and 200 ppm, 4 weeks	Colitis-associated colon carcinogenesis in mice	Decreased expression of TNF-α, IL-1β, IL-6, IFN-γ	Kawabata et al. (2012)
EE	20, 40, and 80 mg/kg in drinking water for 31 days	Ovalbumin sensitized guinea pigs	Reduced total and differential count of WBC	Byrami et al. (2013)
Crocin	100 mg/kg/day for 5 days	Ovalbumin-sensitized mice	Decreased total and differential leukocyte counts	Xiong et al. (2015)
Crocin	25 mg/kg, orally once daily for 16 days	Ovalbumin sensitized mice	Reduced the differential cell counts (monocytes, neutrophils, and eosinophils)	Yosri et al. (2017)
HEE	50, 100, and 200 mg/kg	Ovalbumin sensitized rats	Reduced WBC count	Mahmoudabady et al. (2013)
HEE	100 mg/kg	Ovalbumin sensitized rats	Decreased WBC count	Vosooghi et al. (2013)

Abbreviations: EE, ethanolic extract; HEE, hydroethanolic extract; WBC, white blood cell.

blood cells (SRBC) injection. Oral administration of alcoholic extract of saffron at graded dose levels from 1.56 to 50 mg/kg (1.56, 3.12, 6.25, 12.5, 25, and 50 mg/kg orally daily once a day for 5 days) potentiated the Th2 response of humoral immunity causing the significant increases in agglutinating antibody titer in mice at a dose of 6.25 mg/kg and an elevation of CD19 + B cells and IL-4 cytokine. However, the plant showed no appreciable expression of the Th1 cytokines, IL-2, and IFN-γ (Bani et al., 2011).

The stimulatory effect of saffron on Th1 and a suppressive effect on Th2 cells in sensitized animals had been demonstrated. Treatment of ovalbumin sensitized guinea pigs with hydroethanolic extract of the plant (20, 40, and 80 mg/kg/day in drinking water for 31 days) decreased serum IL-4 concentration while increasing the IFN-γ levels and IFN-γ/IL-4 ratio. Therefore, saffron extract treatment of asthmatic guinea pigs may be effective in balancing Th1 and Th2 in the immune system (Byrami et al., 2013).

The effect of hydroalcoholic extract of saffron was evaluated on the clinical and immunological profile of experimental autoimmune diabetes in C57BL/6 mice. Treatment with extract of saffron (500 mg/kg orally for 3 weeks) markedly decreased the production of proinflammatory IL-17 and increased antiinflammatory IL-10 and TGF-β in the pancreatic cell population of diabetic mice compared with the vehicle-treated diabetic mice. The level of IFN-γ was downregulated in the lymphocyte population of the pancreatic cell isolated from diabetic mice after extract therapy (Faridi et al., 2018).

Antiinflammatory, antioxidant, and antiapoptotic effects of aqueous and ethanolic extracts of saffron (200 mg/kg, intraperitoneally for 7 days) were explored in the chronic constriction injury (CCI) model of neuropathic pain in rats. The lumbar spinal cord levels of proinflammatory cytokines including TNF-α, IL-1β, and IL-6 increased in CCI animals on days 3 and 7, which were suppressed by both extracts (Amin et al., 2014).

In vitro *studies*
The effects of three concentrations (50, 250, and 500 μg/mL) of macerated extract of saffron on IL-4, IL-10, and IFN-γ release of stimulated human peripheral blood mononuclear cells by phytohemagglutinin (PHA) and nonstimulated cells were evaluated. High concentrations of the extract (500 μg/mL) inhibited secretion of IFN-γ in stimulated cells and IL-10 secretion in both stimulated and nonstimulated cells. The extract showed a stimulatory effect on IFN-γ and IL-4

secretion in nonstimulated cells. The ratios of IFN-γ to IL-4 in the presence of all concentrations of saffron on stimulated cells were significantly higher than those in the control group (M.-H. Boskabady et al., 2011a,b).

These results suggested that treatment with various extract of saffron decreased the production of proinflammatory cytokines and increased antiinflammatory cytokines as well as caused a shift in Th1/Th2 balance toward Th2-dominant immunity by increased IL-4 cytokine expression levels rather than Th1 response in various disorders such as asthma, diabetes, constriction injury, and PHA-stimulated human peripheral blood mononuclear cells.

Safranal
In vivo *studies*
The antiinflammatory effects of safranal were investigated on high-fat diet and multiple low-dose streptozotocin induced type 2 diabetes rat model. Safranal treatment for 4 weeks decreased the levels of TNF-α and IL-1β in the plasma and pancreas tissue (Hazman and Ovalı, 2015).

In ovalbumin sensitized guinea pigs, safranal (4, 8, and 16 μg/mL in drinking water) decreased the serum level of IL-4 and increased IFN-γ and IFN-γ/IL-4 ratio. These results showed an increased Th1/Th2 balance in ovalbumin sensitized guinea pigs (Boskabady et al., 2014). Therefore, safranal may have preventive therapeutic values in asthma treatment by immunoregulatory effect.

In the diazinon immunotoxicity rat model, the protective effect of safranal has been indicated. Intraperitoneal (i.p.) injection of safranal (0.025, 0.05, and 0.1 mL/kg three times per week) decreased the diazinon induced TNF-α elevation (Hariri et al., 2010).

The effect of safranal on immune system function and cellularity has been evaluated in mice model of immunotoxicity. i.p. injection of three doses of safranal (0.1, 0.5 and 1 mL/kg) for 3 weeks, did not significantly changed theproductionIL-4 and INF-γ in isolated mice splenocytes and did not induce any marked effects in immune system parameters of mice (Riahi-Zanjani et al., 2015).

The neuroprotective effect of safranal was investigated in a rat model of traumatic injury to the spinal cord. Safranal (25, 50, 100 and 200 mg/kg, three times per day for 3 days after spinal cord injury) suppressed immunoreactivity and expression of the inflammatory cytokines IL-1β and TNF-α and increased expression of IL-10 after spinal cord injury. The most effective dose of safranal for spinal cord injury was 100 mg/kg (Zhang et al., 2015).

The antiallodynia effect of safranal was investigated in a model of neuropathic pain induced by spinal nerve transection in rats. Safranal (0.1 mg/kg, i.p. for 21 consecutive days) attenuated the pain sensitivity and inhibited the expression of TNF-α and IL-1β in ipsilateral dorsal horn of lumbar enlargement after surgery (Zhu and Yang, 2014).

In vitro *studies*

It has been indicated that safranal may affect cell viability and cytokine release of PHA stimulated and nonstimulated peripheral blood mononuclear cells (PBMCs). Safranal (0.5 and 1 mM) showed a stimulatory effect on IFN-γ secretion and increased IFN-γ/IL-4 ratio in PBMC supernatants of both nonstimulated and stimulated cells (Feyzi et al., 2016).

The aforementioned findings indicate that safranal treatment decreased the levels of TNF-α, IL-1β, and IL-4 but increased the levels of IL-10 and IFN-γ in the plasma, serum, and tissue in various conditions such as asthma, diabetes, immunotoxicity, neuronal traumatic injury, and PHA-stimulated human peripheral blood mononuclear cells. These results indicated potential therapeutic effect of safranal on the aforementioned disorders by shifting Th1/Th2 ratio toward Th1 activity.

Crocin

In vivo *studies*

The antiasthmatic effect of crocin in sensitized mice has been shown. Crocin treatment (100 mg/kg/day dissolved in 0.5% sodium carboxymethyl cellulose solution (CMC-Na; intragastric) for 5 days significantly decreased BALF levels of IL-4, IL-5, and IL-13 in ovalbumin-sensitized mice (Xiong et al., 2015).

The antiinflammatory and antiarthritic effects of crocin were investigated on type II collagen-induced arthritis (CIA) in rats. Crocin treatment (10, 20 or 40 mg/kg for 36 days) inhibited the mRNA expression levels of TNF-α, IL-17, IL-6 in the serum and ankle tissues of CIA rats (Liu et al., 2018). The antiarthritic potentiality of crocin was investigated on Freund's complete adjuvant-induced arthritis in rats. Crocin (10 and 20 mg/kg for 15 days) effectively neutralized the augmented serum levels of enzymatic and nonenzymatic (TNF-α, IL-1β, and IL-6) inflammatory mediators (Hemshekhar et al., 2012).

The gastroprotective effect of crocin was investigated in ethanol-induced gastric injury in rats. Prophylactic administration of crocin (50 mg/kg/day, i.p.) for three consecutive days increased ethanol-lowered levels of IL-6 and decreased ethanol-elevated TNF-α level (El-Maraghy et al., 2015). The possible inhibitory effects of crocin were investigated against colitis-associated colon carcinogenesis using an AOM/DSS mouse model. Dietary feeding with crocin (50, 100, and 200 ppm) for 4 weeks was able to decrease the mRNA expression of TNF-α, IL-1β, IL-6, and IFN-γ in the colorectal mucosa (Kawabata et al., 2012). Crocin (50 and 100 mg/kg, i.p. three times per week) reduced the TNF-α increment induced by diazinon in the colorectal mucosa and improved colitis and colitis-related colon carcinogenesis induced chemically in rats (Hariri et al., 2010).

In vitro *studies*

The antiophidian property of α-crocin against viper venom-induced oxidative stress was evaluated. Preincubation with α-crocin (1:10; venom: crocin, w/w for 10 min) inhibited venom-induced elevation of serum IL-1b, IL-6, and TNF-α levels (Santhosh et al., 2013). It is indicated that pretreatment with crocin considerably reduced LPS-induced production of TNF-α and IL-1β in culture media of primary microglia (Nam et al., 2010).

The reviewed articles indicated that crocin leads to decreased IL-1β, IL-4, IL-5, IL-6, IL-13, IL-17, and TNF-α, but increased IFN-γ/IL-4 ratio in the serum, BALF, and tissues in asthma, arthritis and gastrointestinal disorders associated with oxidative stress.

Crocetin

In vivo *studies*

It was shown that crocetin has a protective effect against LPS-induced acute lung injury in mice. Crocetin treatment (50 and 100 mg/kg, intragastric, 1, 12, 24, 36, and 48 h before LPS instillation, and 12 and 24 h after LPS instillation) significantly decreased LPS-induced elevation in TNF-α and IL-6 protein and mRNA expressions (Yang et al., 2012).

The protective effect of crocetin ester was investigated on isoproterenol-induced acute myocardial ischemia. Administration of crocetin ester (25 and 50 mg/kg, intragastric for 14 days) reduced the serum contents of proinflammatory cytokines including TNF-α, IL-1β, and IL-6 in isoproterenol-induced myocardial injury in rats (Huang et al., 2016). In an ischemia/reperfusion rat model, crocetin (50 mg/kg/day, intragastric for 1 week) reduced TNF-α concentration and the increased plasma level of IL-10 (Wang et al., 2014).

It was demonstrated that a bolus of 2 mg/kg (1 mL/kg) crocetin inhibited liver mRNA expression of TNF-α and IL-1β in hemorrhagic shock induced by withdrawing blood in rats (Yang et al., 2006). In a rat model of burn-induced intestinal injury, crocetin (100 and 200 mg/kg, i.p. immediately after burn injury) ameliorated TNF-α and IL-6 levels (Zhou et al., 2015).

The effect of crocetin (10, 20, and 40 mg/kg, intragastric, twice daily for 35 days) on methylcholanthrene (MCA)-induced uterine cervical cancer in mice showed that crocetin supplementation decreased the plasma level of IL-1β and TNF-α which were elevated in MCA mice (Chen et al., 2015).

In vivo *studies*

It is indicated that pretreatment with crocetin considerably reduced LPS-induced production of TNF-α and IL-1β in culture media of primary microglia (Nam et al., 2010).

The aforementioned studies reported the reduction effect of crocetin on the levels and expressions levels of proinflammatory cytokines including IL-1β, IL-6, and TNF-α, but it increased plasma level of IL-10 in myocardial, lung and intestinal injuries, and cancer.

THE EFFECT OF SAFFRON (*CROCUS SATIVUS*) AND ITS CONSTITUENTS ON IMMUNOREGULATORY PROTEINS

Saffron Extracts

In vivo *studies*

Antiinflammatory, antioxidant, and antiapoptotic effects of aqueous and ethanolic extracts of saffron were explored in the chronic constriction injury (CCI) model of neuropathic pain in rats. The ratio of Bax/Bcl2 proteins was elevated on day 3 but not on day 7, in CCI animals, as compared with sham-operated animals and decreased after treatment with both extracts (200 mg/kg administered at a dose of 1 mL/kg, i.p. for 7 days) (Amin et al., 2014).

Safranal

In vivo *studies*

The antiallodynia effect of safranal was investigated in spinal nerve transection model of rats. Safranal (0.1 mg/kg, i.p. for 21 consecutive days) attenuated the increase of mRNA levels of GFAP and OX-42 expression (glial activation markers) in dorsal horn after spinal nerve transection (Zhu and Yang, 2014). In a rat model of traumatic injury to the spinal cord, safranal treatment (25, 50, 100, and 200 mg/kg three times per day) for 3 days after spinal cord injury suppressed immunoreactivity and expression of p38 MAPK (Zhang et al., 2015).

Crocin

In vivo *studies*

The antiinflammatory and antiarthritic effects of crocin were investigated on type II collagen-induced arthritis (CIA) in rats. Crocin treatment (10, 20, or 40 mg/kg

for 36 days) inhibited the expression of CXCL8 in the serum of CIA rats. MMP-1, MMP-3, and MMP-13 protein expression levels of CIA rats with 40 mg/kg crocin treatment were decreased to the levels similar to normal rats (Liu et al., 2018). The antiarthritic potentiality of crocin was also investigated on Freund's complete adjuvant-induced arthritis in rats. Crocin (10 and 20 mg/kg for 15 days) effectively neutralized the augmented serum levels of nonenzymatic (NF-κB) and enzymatic (MMP-13, MMP-3, MMP-9, and HAases) inflammatory mediators (Hemshekhar et al., 2012).

In the ovalbumin-sensitized mice, crocin (100 mg/kg dissolved in 0.5% sodium carboxymethyl cellulose solution (CMC-Na) intragastric daily for 5 days) significantly decreased the levels of ovalbumin-specific IgE in serum, tryptase in BALF, and lung erythropoietin (EPO) activity and inhibited the expressions of eotaxin, p-ERK, p-JNK, and p-p38 protein (Xiong et al., 2015).

The gastroprotective effect of crocin was investigated against ethanol-induced gastric injury in rats. Prophylactic administration of crocin (50 mg/kg/day, i.p.) for three consecutive days decreased ethanol-elevated myeloperoxidase (MPO) activity and heat shock protein 70 (Hsp70) mRNA and protein levels (El-Maraghy et al., 2015).

The potential inhibitory effects of crocin were reported against inflammation-associated mouse colon carcinogenesis and chemically induced colitis in male ICR mice. Crocin feeding (50, 100, and 200 ppm, for 15 weeks) suppressed the proliferation and immunohistochemical expression of NF-κB but increased the NF-E2-related factor 2 (Nrf2) expression, in adenocarcinoma cells. Dietary feeding with crocin for 4 weeks was able to decrease the mRNA expression of NF-κB in the colorectal mucosa and increased the Nrf2 mRNA expression (Kawabata et al., 2012).

In vitro *studies*

Crocin also suppressed the effect of TNF-α on neuronally differentiated PC-12 cells and blocked the TNF-α–induced expression of Bcl-XS and LICE mRNAs. In addition, it could improve the cytokine-induced reduction of Bcl-XL mRNA expression (Soeda et al., 2001).

It is demonstrated that pretreatment with crocin effectively reduced LPS-elicited NF-κB activation in mouse microglial cell (Nam et al., 2010).

Therefore, saffron extract, safranal, and specially crocin treatment inhibited the expression of CXCL8, eotaxin, p-ERK, p-JNK, and p-p38 protein and decreased protein expression levels of MMP-1, MMP-3, MMP-9 MMP-13, HAases, tryptase, Hsp70 mRNA and protein levels, EPO and MPO activities as well as suppressed the proliferation and expression of NF-κB but increased Nrf2 expression in various inflammatory conditions such as neuronal injury, arthritis, asthma, gastro-intestinal disorders and cancer.

Crocetin

In vivo *studies*

Crocetin has a protective effect against LPS-induced acute lung injury in mice. Crocetin treatment (50 and 100 mg/kg intragastric, 1, 12, 24, 36, and 48 h before LPS instillation, and 12 and 24 h after LPS instillation) significantly decreased LPS-induced elevation of macrophage chemoattractant protein-1 (MCP-1) in the lung tissue. Also, crocetin decreased phospho-IκB expression and NF-κB activity in the lung tissue which had been induced by LPS (Yang et al., 2012).

The therapeutic effect of crocetin on an experimental model of endotoxin-induced disseminated intravascular coagulation has been investigated. Crocetin (3 mg/kg dissolved in DMSO, i.p., 30 min before the beginning of intravenous infusion of endotoxin) treatment in rabbits restored hemostatic indices changes such as plasma fibrinogen, protein C concentration, and fibrin deposition in the glomeruli (Tsantarliotou et al., 2013).

Administration of crocetin (100 μM/L intranasal, daily for 10 weeks) increased the levels of immunoregulatory proteins Foxp3 and TNF-α protein 8-like 2 (TIPE2) in regulatory T (Treg) cells in ovalbumin-sensitized mice (Ding et al., 2015). Crocetin may activate Foxp3through TIPE2 in asthma-associated Treg cells to mitigate the severity of asthma.

The protective effect of crocetin ester was investigated on isoproterenol-induced acute myocardial ischemia. Administration of crocetin ester (25 and 50 mg/kg intragastric) for 14 days could ameliorate the cardiac expressions of Rho, ROCK, p-IκB, and p−NF−κBp65 in isoproterenol-induced rats (Huang et al., 2016).

The effects of saffron and its constituents on Th1, Th2, and Th17 responses were shown in Table 16.2, and their effects on immunoregulatory proteins were summarized in Table 16.3.

The aforementioned studies showed that crocetin could decrease MCP-1, phospho-IκB expression, and NF-κB activity in the lung, restore plasma fibrinogen, protein C concentration, and fibrin deposition in the glomeruli, and increase the levels of immunoregulatory proteins Foxp3 and TIPE2 in Treg cells as well as ameliorate the cardiac expressions of Rho, ROCK, p-IκB, and p−NF−κBp65. These results showed that crocetin might modulate immune response pathways.

THE EFFECT OF SAFFRON (*CROCUS SATIVUS*) AND ITS CONSTITUENTS ON OXIDATIVE STRESS

Oxidative stress is a disturbance in the balance between free radicals (reactive oxygen species [ROS] and reactive nitrogen species [RNS]) production and antioxidant level that lead to damage in variety of tissues (Betteridge, 2000; Karimian et al., 2012). Thus, oxidative stress is important in pathogenesis of various diseases (Kim et al., 2012). The decrease of free radicals or increase of antioxidant level which occur via antioxidant properties of plants or their derivatives can delay or inhibit oxidative reactions (Hasani-Ranjbar et al., 2009; Rahmani et al., 2017). Medicinal plants with antioxidant activities contain phenolic acids, polyphenols, and flavonoids which scavenge free radicals and therefore prevent from the oxidative mechanisms (Del Bano et al., 2006). Saffron is classified as a potent plant antioxidant, which is related to its constituents mainly crocin with a strong antioxidant capacity (Mashmoul et al., 2013). The antioxidant activity of saffron has been reported in several studies based on in vivo and in vitro models. In these studies, the oxidant/antioxidant parameters including lipid peroxidation (LPO), glutathione (GSH), glutathione peroxidase (GPx), glutathione reductase (GR), superoxide dismutase (SOD), catalase (CAT), and malondialdehyde (MDA) are considered for investigating antioxidant effects of this plant (Dadkhah et al., 2014).

Saffron Extracts

In vivo *studies*

Daily administration of 25 mg/kg powdered stigmas of saffron administered by the drinking water for 20 weeks had a protective role against retinal damage induced by oxidative stress in high-fat diet mice. Total oxidative capacity (PerOX) was significantly higher in mice treated with saffron than that in the control group (Doumouchtsis et al., 2018). Similarly, treatment of hamsters under a high-fat diet with 100 mg/kg/day aqueous saffron extract through gavage for 10 days reduced MDA level, cholesterol, and some hepatic enzymes. Therefore, saffron could be effective in treatment of cardiovascular disease (Vakili et al., 2017).

Free access of aflatoxin B1 exposed−mice to saffron infusion (90 mg pure red styles of saffron/200 mL of hot water for 2 weeks) prevented learning/memory defects and reduction of MDA level in whole brain and cerebellum (Linardaki et al., 2017).

In a rat model of chronic stress induced oxidative stress in the hippocampus leading to learning and memory loss, the effect of saffron extract was assessed.

TABLE 16.2
The Effect of Saffron (*Crocus sativus*) and its Constituents on Th1, Th2, and Th17 Responses.

Extract/ Constituent	Method	Dose	Model	Outcomes	Ref.
EE	In vivo	1.56, 3.12, 6.25, 12.5, 25, 50 mg/kg, orally, 5 days	Sensitized mice with fresh sheep RBC	Increased IL-4, unchanged IL-2, and IFN-γ	Bani et al. (2011)
		20, 40, and 80 mg/kg in drinking water for 31 days	Ovalbumin sensitized guinea pigs	Decreased IL-4, Increased IFN-γ	Byrami et al. (2013)
HEE		500 mg/kg, orally for 3 weeks	Ovalbumin sensitized guinea pigs	Decreased IL-17, increased IL-10, and TGF-β	Faridi et al. (2018)
AE and EE		200 mg/kg, i.p., for 7 days	Chronic neuropathic pain in rats	Decreased TNF-α, IL-1β, and IL-6	Amin et al. (2014)
ME	In vitro	50, 250, and 500 μg/mL	Nonstimulated and PHA-stimulated human PBMC	Reduced IFN-γ in stimulated and IL-10 in stimulated and nonstimulated, increased IFN-γ, and IL-4 in nonstimulated cells	Boskabady et al. (2011a),b
Safranal	In vivo	0.2 mL/kg for 4 weeks	Streptozotocin-induced type 2 diabetes in rat	Decreased TNF-α and IL-1β	Hazman and Ovalı (2015)
		4, 8, and 16 μg/mL in drinking water	Ovalbumin sensitized guinea pigs	Decreased level of IL-4 Increased level of IFN-γ	Boskabady et al. (2014)
		0.025, 0.05 and 0.1 mL/kg, i.p. three times per week	Diazinon immunotoxicityin rat	DecreasedTNF-α	Hariri et al. (2010)
		0.1, 0.5 and 1 mL/kg, i.p., 3 weeks	Mice model of immunotoxicity	UnchangedIL-4 and INF-γ	Riahi-Zanjani et al. (2015)
		25, 50, 100, 200 mg/kg, 3 times/day, 3 days	Rat model of traumatic injury to the spinal cord	Decreased IL-1β and TNF-α Increased IL-10	Zhang et al. (2015)
		0.1 mg/kg, i.p., for 21 days	Spinal nerve induced neuropathic pain	Inhibited expression of TNF-α and IL-1β	Zhu and Yang (2014)
	In vitro	0.5 and 1 mM	PHA stimulated and nonstimulated PBMC	Increased IFN-γ/IL-4 ratio in stimulated and nonstimulated cells	Feyzi et al. (2016)
Crocin	In vivo	100 mg/kg/day i.g, 5 days	Ovalbumin-sensitized mice	Decreased IL-4, IL-5, and IL-13	Xiong et al. (2015)
		10, 20, or 40 mg/kg, 36 days	Type II collagen-induced arthritis in rats	Inhibited expression of TNF-α, IL-17, and IL-6	Liu et al. (2018)
		10 and 20 mg/kg, 15 days	Adjuvant-induced arthritis in rats	Inhibited TNF-α, IL-1β, and IL-6 levels	Hemshekhar et al. (2012)
		50 mg/kg/day, i.p., 3 days	Ethanol-induced gastric injury in rats	Increased IL-6, decreased TNF-α	El-Maraghy et al. (2015)
		50, 100, and 200 ppm, 4 weeks	Colitis-associated colon carcinogenesis in mice	Decreased expression of TNF-α, IL-1β, IL-6, IFN-γ	Kawabata et al. (2012)
		50 and 100 mg/kg, i.p., three times per week	Colon carcinogenesis induced chemically	Reduced TNF-α	Timcheh Hariri et al. (2010)

Continued

TABLE 16.2
The Effect of Saffron (Crocus sativus) and its Constituents on Th1, Th2, and Th17 Responses.—cont'd

Extract/ Constituent	Method	Dose	Model	Outcomes	Ref.
	In vitro	1:10; venom: crocin, w/w for 10 min	Viper venom-induced oxidative stress	Inhibited levels of IL-1b, IL-6, and TNF-α	Santhosh et al. (2013)
			Culture media of primary microglia	Reduced TNF-α and IL-1β	Nam et al. (2010)
Crocetin	In vivo	50, 100 mg/kg, i.g. before and after LPS instillation	LPS-induced acute lung injury in mice	Decreased expressions of TNF-α and IL-6	Yang et al. (2012)
		25 and 50 mg/kg, i.g., 14 days	Isoproterenol-induced acute MI	Reduced TNF-α, IL-1β, and IL-6	Huang et al. (2016)
		50 mg/kg/day, i.g., 1 week	Ischemia/reperfusion rat model	Reduced TNF-α, increased IL-10	Wang et al. (2014)
		A bolus of 2 mg/kg (1 mL/kg)	Hemorrhagic shock by blood withdrawal	Inhibited expression of TNF-α and IL-1β	Yang et al. (2006)
		100 and 200 mg/kg, i.p. after burn injury	Burn-induced intestinal injury in rat	Decreased TNF-α and IL-6	Zhou et al. (2015)
		10, 20, and 40 mg/kg, i.g., twice daily, 35 days	MCA-induced uterine cervical cancer in mice	Decreased IL-1β and TNF-α	Chen et al. (2015)
	In vitro		Culture media of primary microglia	Reduced TNF-α and IL-1β	Nam et al. (2010)

Abbreviations: AE, aqueous extract; EE, ethanolic extract; HEE, hydroethanolic extract; ME, macerated extract; RBC, red blood cell; i.p., intraperitoneal; i.g., intragastric; PBMC, peripheral blood mononuclear cells; PHA, phytohemagglutinin; MCA, methylcholanthrene; MI, myocardial ischemia.

Systemic administration of saffron extract (30 mg/kg/day) for 21 days improved oxidative stress markers (SOD, GPx, and GR levels) in the hippocampus (Ghadrdoost et al., 2011).

The oxidative stress in age-related diseases reduces activities of antioxidant markers. The effect of saffron in improving age-related oxidative damage in rat hippocampus was examined. The results showed that treatment of rats with the ethanolic extract of saffron for 28 days decreased NO and MDA levels while increasing antioxidant status in hippocampus tissue of rats (Samarghandian et al., 2017b). Treatment of old rats with saffron hydroethanolic extract (5, 10, 20 mg/kg/day; i.p) for 4 weeks also reduced the oxidative stress by reduction of MDA and increase of GSH levels in kidney tissue as well as decline of nitric oxide (NO) and MDA but enhancing GST level in liver tissue of aged rats (Samarghandian et al., 2016a,b).

A study reported the antioxidant effect of aqueous extract saffron on diabetic rats induced by streptozotocin. Injection (i.p.) of the extract (10, 20, and 40 mg/kg/day) for 4 weeks in diabetic rats reduced serum MDA level and increased SOD, CAT, and GSH levels compared with the untreated groups (Samarghandian

et al., 2017a). In addition, treatment of diabetic encephalopathy rats with 20, 40, and 80 mg/kg/day of aqueous extract of saffron as i.p. for 4 weeks ameliorated oxidative stress by reduction of SOD, CAT, and GSH contents (Samarghandian et al., 2014). The effect of saffron aqueous extract (200 mg/kg, i.p, for 5 weeks) on oxidative stress in the testis of streptozotocin-induced diabetic rats was also evaluated. The extract significantly enhanced CAT and GPx levels in testis of diabetic rats (Hasanpour et al., 2018).

The impact of freeze-dried aqueous extract of saffron on γ-radiation (RAD) induced oxidative stress in the liver and brain showed that the gavage of 40 mg/kg extract to RAD-exposed mice for 6 days reduced LPO while it enhanced GSH, GPx, and CAT contents (Koul and Abraham, 2017).

In an ischemia-reperfusion model of rabbit hearts, oral administration of saffron (at a concentration of 2 g/400 mL in a mixture of methanol and water) for 6 weeks increased GPx activity and thus showed a cardioprotective effect against ischemia-reperfusion injuries (Nader et al., 2016). Similarly, pretreatment of rats with hydroethanolic extract of saffron (5 mg/kg, 10 mg/kg, or 20 mg/kg; i.p) in a model of acute kidney

TABLE 16.3
The Effect of Saffron (*Crocus sativus*) and its Constituents on Immunoregulatory Proteins

Extract/ Constituent	Method	Dose	Model	Outcomes	Ref.
AE and EE	In vivo	200 mg/kg administered at a dose of 1 mL/kg, i.p. for 7 days	Chronic constriction injury of neuropathic pain in rats.	Decreased ratio of Bax/Bcl2 proteins	Amin et al. (2014)
Safranal	In vivo	0.1 mg/kg, i.p., for 21 days	Spinal nerve transection model of rats	Decreased expression of GFAP and OX-42	Zhu and Yang (2014)
		25, 50, 100, and 200 mg/kg three times per day for 3 days	Rat model of traumatic injury to the spinal cord	Decreased expression of p38 MAPK	Zhang et al. (2015)
Crocin	In vivo	10, 20, and 40 mg/kg for 36 days	Type II collagen-induced arthritis in rats.	Inhibited CXCL8 expression Decreased MMP-1, MMP-3, and MMP-13 expression	Liu et al. (2018)
		10 and 20 mg/kg for 15 days	Adjuvant-induced arthritis in rats	Decreased MMP-13, MMP-3, MMP-9, and HAases expression	Hemshekhar et al. (2012)
		100 mg/kg/day, i.g., for 5 days	Ovalbumin-sensitized mice	Decreased EPO, OVA-specific IgE, tryptase, inhibited eotaxin, p-ERK, p-JNK, and p-p38 protein expression	Xiong et al. (2015)
		50 mg/kg, i.p., for 3 days	Ethanol-induced gastric injury in rats	Decreased MPO and heat shock protein 70	El-Maraghy et al. (2015)
		50, 100, and 200 ppm, for 4 or 15 weeks	Mouse colon carcinogenesis and chemically induced colitis in ICR mice	Suppressed NF-κB expression	Kawabata et al. (2012)
	In vitro	100 μM/L/day	Neuronally differentiated PC-12 cells	Increased Nrf2 expression Inhibited Bcl-XS and LICE mRNAs expression	Soeda et al. (2001)
			Mouse microglial cell	Improved Bcl-XL expression Reduced activation of LPS-elicited NF-κB	Nam et al. (2010)
Crocetin	In vivo	50 and 100 mg/kg, i.g., before and after LPS instillation	LPS-induced acute lung injury in mice	Decreased MCP-1 and phospho-IκB expression Decreased NF-κB activity	Yang et al. (2012)
		3 mg/kg, i.p., 30 min before the beginning of endotoxin infusion	Endotoxin-induced disseminated intravascular coagulation in rabbits	Restored plasma fibrinogen, protein-C, and fibrin deposition	Tsantarliotou et al. (2013)
		100 μM/L/day, i.n., for 10 weeks	Ovalbumin-sensitized mice	Increased Foxp3 and TIPE2 in Treg cells	Ding et al. (2015)
		25 and 50 mg/kg, i.g., for 14 days	Isoproterenol-induced acute myocardial ischemia	Decreased Rho, ROCK, p-IκB and p–NF-κBp65 expression	Huang et al. (2016)

Abbreviations: OVA, ovalbumin; AE, aqueous extract; EE, ethanolic extract; i.p., intraperitoneal; i.g., intragastric; i.n., intranasal; EPO, erythropoietin; MPO, myeloperoxidase; MCP-1, macrophage chemoattractant protein-1; Nrf2, NF-E2-related factor 2; TIPE2, protein 8-like 2; Treg, regulatory T cells.

injury induced by ischemia-reperfusion showed reduction of the tissue MDA level in comparison to the untreated group (Mahmoudzadeh et al., 2017). The model of hepatic ischemia-reperfusion injury in rats was also used for revealing protective effects of saffron ethanolic extract. Oral administration of 20 mg/kg saffron extract for 2 h before ischemia insult restored SOD and CAT levels while inhibited intracellular ROS concentration in liver tissue (Pan et al., 2013).

Antioxidant effect of aqueous and ethanolic extracts of saffron in chronic constriction injury (CCI) model was evaluated. In this study, i.p. injection of both extract (200 mg/kg) in CCI rats for 7 days led to attenuation of MDA and increasing GSH levels (Amin et al., 2014).

Das et al. (2010) induced skin carcinoma by 7, 12 dimethyl ben-z[a]anthracene (DMBA) in mice and then treated animals with 200 mg/kg/day (orally) of saffron infusions for 12 weeks. The results illustrated that saffron extract suppresses oxidative stress by decline of LPO and increasing antioxidant enzymes activity (SOD, CAT, GPx, and glutathione S-transferase [GST]) in this model (Das et al., 2010).

In vitro studies

The effect of saffron ethanolic extract (2, 10, 20, and 40 µg/mL) against oxidative injury in endothelial cells showed a reduction in ROS production in treated cells with saffron extract (Rahiman et al., 2018).

The protective effect of hydroethanolic extract of saffron showed via an in vitro model of cardiomyocytes injury induced by doxorubicin and ischemia-reperfusion. Cardiomyocytes were subjected to simulated ischemia-reperfusion, with doxorubicin treatment at reperfusion, in the presence of the extract (10 µg/mL for 16) before ischemia or at reperfusion. Saffron extract protected cells against doxorubicin and ischemia-reperfusion toxicity through attenuating oxidative stress (Chahine et al., 2016).

The reviewed studies indicated the effect of various extracts of saffron on oxidative stress of cardiovascular and nervous systems. In age-related and also diabetics-induced reduction of antioxidant activities also, the protective effect of saffron was reported. In addition, saffron treatment also showed an antioxidant effect on liver, kidney and skin disorders associated with oxidative stress. Therefore, saffron could be effective in reducing various oxidative stress-related disorders.

Safranal
In vivo studies

To investigate the neuroprotective effect of safranal, a rat model of transient cerebral ischemia was used. In this model, 72.5 and 145 mg/kg of safranal was injected, i.p., at 0, 3, and 6 h after ischemic reperfusion injury. Increasing antioxidant capacity and improvement of oxidative stress markers such as decreasing MDA level and increasing total thiol content suggest protective effects of safranal (Sadeghnia et al., 2017). In a study conducted by Hosseinzadeh and Sadeghnia (2005), i.p. injection of safranal (727.5, 363.75, 145.5, and 72.75 mg/kg/day) prior to reperfusion and in the then every day for 3 days after induction of ischemia led to attenuation of oxidative damage induced by cerebral ischemia via reduction of MDA and increases of total thiol contents in rat model (Hosseinzadeh and Sadeghnia, 2005). In a rat model of cerebral ischemia induced by middle cerebral artery occlusion (MCAO), nasal route administration of 10 mg/kg of safranal mucoadhesive nanoemulsion (SMNE) led to a significant improvement in antioxidants activity including GPx, GR, SOD, and CAT (Ahmad et al., 2017).

Administration (i.p.) of 0.75 mg/kg/day of safranal for 21 days in immobilization-induced oxidative damage of rat brain resulted in enhancement of antioxidant enzymes including SOD, CAT, GPx, and GR, as well as reduction of MDA level (Samarghandian et al., 2017c). The evaluation of safranal effect on sciatic nerve function following crush injury indicated that i.p. injection of 0.05, 0.2, and 0.8 mg/kg safranal for 10 days restored blood MDA level (Tamaddonfard et al., 2014).

In a rat model, safranal effect on nephrotoxicity and oxidative stress induced by cisplatin was tested. Use of 200 mg/kg/day safranal by gavage for 5 days before (pretreatment) and after (posttreatment) administration of cisplatin showed enhanced levels of GSH and total antioxidant status (TAS) as well as reduction of MDA and total oxidant status (TOS) contents mainly pretreatment with safranal (Karafakıoğlu et al., 2017). In another study, the effect of safranal on the diabetic nephropathy-induced damage in rat renal tissue was investigated. Safranal administration for 4 weeks led to restoration of renal tissue oxidative stress parameters including TAS, TOS, GSH, and NO (Hazman and Bozkurt, 2015).

The evaluation of safranal effect against oxidative damage in aged rat brain (10 and 20 months) showed that injections of safranal (0.5 mg/kg/day, i.p.) for 30 caused reduction of MDA and increasing GSH, SOD, and GST contents (Samarghandian et al., 2015). Administration of safranal according to the aforementioned study also improved NO, MDA, and CAT in aged rat liver (Farahmand et al., 2013).

In vitro *studies*

In a study, protective effects of safranal (2−40 μM) against oxidative stress and apoptosis in endothelial cells were reported. Viability of cells in response to H_2O_2-induced toxicity and the amount of ROS in cells were measured. Improved viability and reduced ROS production were observed in the presence of safranal (Rahiman et al., 2018).

The reviewed articles demonstrated that safranal could be helpful in behavioral changes by control of brain oxidative response antioxidant. The antioxidant effects of safranal on liver, kidney, and skin disorders associated with oxidative stress were also shown. These results indicated the effect of safranal on oxidant and antioxidant imbalance through reduction oxidant agents and increase of antioxidant enzyme activities.

Crocin

In vivo *studies*

A study showed that gavage of rats with 100 mg/kg/day crocin for 15 days led to elimination of carbon tetrachloride (CCl4) induced brain damage through preventing oxidative stress, including increased GSH and TAS levels and CAT activities and decreased MDA and TOS levels and SOD activity (Altinoz et al., 2018). Malathion-induced Parkinson-like behaviors and neurochemical changes in rat after treatment with crocin showed that i.p. injection of 10, 20, or 40 mg/kg/day crocin for 28 days elevated serum GSH level while reduced MDA content relative to the Malathion group (Mohammadzadeh et al., 2018). In a model of spatial memory deficits and cortical oxidative damage in diabetic rats, i.p. administration of crocin at doses of 15, 30, and 60 mg/kg/day for 6 weeks reduced oxidative stress in diabetic rats by reduction of thiobarbituric acid reactive substance (TBARS), an index of lipid peroxidation, in cortex. It suggests that crocin could be useful in streptozotocin-induced memory dysfunction (Ahmadi et al., 2017). Similarly, the effect of crocin on brain oxidative damage and memory deficits in a rat model of Parkinson's disease was determined. Treatment of animals with 30 and 60 mg/kg/day of i.p. crocin for 6 weeks decreased TBARS and nitrite levels in the hippocampus and improved memory (Rajaei et al., 2016). In addition, neuroprotective effects of crocin on acrolein-induced toxicity in the rat brain were determined by Rashedinia et al. (2015). Administration (i.p.) of 12.5, 25, and 50 mg/kg/day for 2 weeks significantly reduced MDA level and increased GSH value in cerebral cortex tissue compared with the untreated group (Rashedinia et al., 2015).

In a rat model of cerebral ischemia reperfusion (IR) injury, pretreatment of animal with 40 mg/kg/day of crocin orally for 10 days significantly declined the TOS level compared with the IR group. Therefore, crocin could be effective in improving IR-mediated brain injury due to antioxidant property (Oruc et al., 2016). In another model of IR injury in retina, rats were pretreated with 50 mg/kg of crocin (i.p. injection) 30 min before and once daily after retinal IR injury. Crocin significantly enhanced GSH and SOD activities while also decreased the ROS and MDA levels after IR injury (Chen et al., 2015).

A study also demonstrated that beryllium chloride (BeCl2) -induced oxidative stress in the brain and liver of rats declined after i.p. injection of crocin (200 mg/kg) for 7 days. Restoration of SOD and CAT contents near to normal levels was results from crocin treatment (El-Beshbishy et al., 2012).

Diabetes-induced oxidative stress in rats attenuated antioxidant defense system of hepatic tissue. Treatment of diabetic rats with 40 mg/kg/day crocin for 8 weeks i.p. also improved antioxidant system via decrease of MDA and nitrate contents as well as increase in SOD and CAT levels in hepatic tissue (Yaribeygi et al., 2018). Another study also indicated hepatoprotective effects of crocin on acrylamide-induced liver injury in rats. Gavage of 50 mg/kg/day of crocin for 21 days led to biochemical changes in liver tissue such as decrease in MDA and TOS as well as elevation in GSH and TAS levels. Thus, crocin suppressed acrylamide-induced liver damage due to the strong antioxidant properties (Gedik et al., 2017). The protective effect of crocin on Bisphenol A-induced liver toxicity in rats via inhibition of oxidative stress was also reported. Injection (i.p.) of 5, 10, or 20 mg/kg/day of crocin for 30 days significantly improved GSH level in liver tissue (Hassani et al., 2017).

Patulin-induced oxidative stress was suppressed by injection of crocin (50, 100, and 250 mg/kg; i.p.) 3 h before patulin treatment in both liver and kidney tissues of mice. Therefore, crocin showed a preventive effect on patulin-induced nephrotoxicity and hepatotoxicity through reduction of LPO and improvement of antioxidant enzymes (Boussabbeh et al., 2016). In a model of zearalenone-induced oxidative stress, treatment of mice with 50, 100, and 250 mg/kg (i.p.) of crocin significantly restored oxidative stress markers including MDA, CAT, and SOD levels in the liver and kidney (Salem et al., 2015).

Pretreatment of rats with 20 mg/kg/day of crocin, orally for 7 days before induction of renal ischemia reperfusion, improved kidney functions via attenuation of oxidative stress markers including reduction of NO and MDA contents and increase of SOD and GSH levels (Abou-Hany et al., 2018).

The changes in oxidative stress parameters in rat kidney tissue after tartrazine induced nephrotoxicity and administration of crocin by gavage (50 mg/kg/day for 21 days) were investigated. The protective effect of crocin on nephrotoxicity was observed via reduction of MDA and TOS levels as well as increase in SOD, CAT, and TAS values compared with untreated rats (Erdemli et al., 2017). Cisplatin-induced renal oxidative stress rat model treated by crocin (100, 200, and 400 mg/kg, i.p. for 4 days) showed an increase in thiol and GPx concentrations as well as reduction of MDA level (Naghizadeh et al., 2010).

Salem et al. (2016) also examined a protective impact of crocin on zearalenone-induced oxidative stress in cardiac tissue of mice. Treatment of mice with 50, 100, and 250 mg/kg (i.p.) of crocin led to a significant decrease of zearalenone-induced toxicity via improvement of oxidative stress markers (Salem et al., 2016).

Oxidative stress has an important role in infarction-induced injury. In a study, the protective effect of crocin (20, 40, 60 mg/kg/day for 7 days) on myocardial infarction (MI)-induced injury in rats was examined. Injection of crocin as i.p. in rats exerted antioxidant effect in 40 and 60 mg/kg concentrations through increase of SOD and reduction of MDA and NO production (Wang et al., 2018).

The protective effect of crocin against heart oxidative stress in high-fat diet–induced diabetic rats was demonstrated. Oral administration of crocin (50 mg/kg/day) for 8 weeks significantly increased SOD, GPx, and CAT activities while reduced MDA level compared with diabetic animals (Ghorbanzadeh et al., 2016).

To explore the role of crocin in improvement of hemorrhagic shock (HS)-induced organ damages, HS rats were treated with 60 mg/kg of crocin as intravenously at the beginning of resuscitation. Evaluation of oxidative stress markers showed an increase of GSH and reduction of MDA levels in both serum and lung tissue in crocin-treated animals. Thus, crocin can protect organs from HS-induced damages during resuscitation due to its antioxidative property (Yang and Dong, 2017).

In a model of ovalbumin-induced asthma, an increase of antioxidant strength and reduction of oxidative stress by restoring MDA, SOD, and GSH levels in lung tissue were observed after treatment of mice with 25 mg/kg/day crocin, orally for 16 days (Yosri et al., 2017).

The protective effect of crocin against cigarette smoke exposure-mediated oxidative stress in rats was investigated. The results indicated that i.p. injection of 50 mg/kg/day crocin, three times per week for 2 months, restored GSH, SOD, CAT, and GPx in tissue of the lung to normal levels (Dianat et al., 2018).

Therapeutic effect of crocin on osteoarthritis symptoms was exhibited by relieving oxidative stress parameters. Rats were ingested crocin (30 mg/kg/day) for 10 days after induction of osteoarthritis by meniscectomy (MNX) surgery. The results showed reduction of LPO and increase in GSH and GPx activities after crocin treatment (Lei et al., 2017).

Oxidative stress and tissue injury induced by acute swimming exercise in rats were prevented by gavage of crocin at a dose of 20 mg/kg/day for 21 days. Crocin treatment led to a significant increase in GSH level and on the other hand decreased MDA level in several tissues such as liver and skeletal muscle compared with untreated exercise groups (Altinoz et al., 2016).

In a metabolic syndrome (MS) rat model, oral administration of 50 mg/kg/day crocin for 10 weeks has reduced increased levels of MDA and advanced glycation end products (AGEs) in MS rats. Therefore, metabolic syndrome was ameliorated by inhibiting oxidative stress (El-Fawal et al., 2018).

In vitro studies

Pretreatment of mitochondria extracted from rat liver with crocin (5, 10, and 25 µg/mL for 15 min) before induction of toxicity by Arsenic III significantly reduced mitochondrial ROS formation and LPO. Therefore, crocin ameliorates oxidative stress induced by Arsenic III through mitochondrial targeting (Yousefsani et al., 2018b).

In another study, antioxidant and antiapoptotic activities of crocin in endothelial cells were evaluated. The improvement in viability and oxidative injury in cells treated with 2–40 µM crocin suggest the protective effect of crocin on endothelial cells (Rahiman et al., 2018).

Yang et al. (2017) indicated that crocin can inhibit oxidative stress in microglial cells via activation of PI3K/Akt signaling pathway in a model of diabetic retinopathy. Pretreatment of cells with 0.1 or 1 µM of crocin for 24 h prior to induction of diabetes led to prevention of the oxidative stress through decline of ROS and NO levels (Yang et al., 2017).

The described studies showed antioxidant activity of crocin in various disorders of the brain and other parts of nervous system associated with oxidative stress. The effects of crocin in oxidative stress conditions of other organs such as cardiovascular, liver, kidney, and the lung were also shown. Therefore, crocin can contribute in antioxidant property of saffron via restoring oxidant/antioxidant agents such as LPO, MDA, SOD, CAT, thiol, GSH, etc. in animal and cellular models of oxidative stress injury.

Crocetin

In vivo *studies*

The protective effect of crocetin against ovary injury induced by cyclophosphamide (CPM) in mice was assessed. The mice gavaged by 100 mg/kg crocetin extract for 15 days and on the 15th day received a single dose (100 mg/kg i.p.) of CPM. The crocetin protected the ovary against CPM by modulating mitochondrial markers such as SOD level (Di Emidio et al., 2017).

A mouse model with neuropathic pain induced by spared nerve injury was used for investigating the role of crocetin in attenuation of oxidative stress as an important determinant of neuropathic pain. Crocetin (5–50 mg/kg) was infused into the subarachnoid space intrathecally for up to 12 days. The results indicated that crocetin attenuated the neuropathic pain and significantly inhibited oxidative stress through restoration of mitochondrial MnSOD activity (Wang et al., 2017).

Cardioprotective effect of crocetin was also observed in myocardial infracted (MI) rats. The oral administration of 50, 100, and 200 mg/kg/day crocetin for 15 days improved oxidative stress by increasing GSH and CAT levels as well as decreased MDA and SOD, which suggests the protective effect of crocetin on myocardial cells (Zhang et al., 2017). Similarly, protective effects of crocetin on myocardial injury in an ischemia/reperfusion rat model were observed. In this model, pretreatment of rats with 50 mg/kg/day as intragastric for 7 days caused decline of MDA and increasing SOD levels in serum. Therefore, crocetin can protect myocardial injury by inhibiting ROS production (Wang et al., 2014). Ishizuka and colleagues (2013) showed the effects of crocetin (20 mg/kg, orally) in retinal ischemia mice model. The administration of crocetin 1 h before the ischemia and at 6 and12 h after the start of reperfusion, then twice a day for the next 4 days, led to inhibition of 8-hydroxy-2-deoxyguanosine (an index of oxidative stress) and thus prevented ischemia-induced retinal damage (Ishizuka et al., 2013).

In a burn-induced intestinal injury rat model, i.p. injection of 100 and 200 mg/kg immediately after burn injury reduced oxidative stress through restoring MDA, CAT, SOD, and GPx in serum and small intestine tissue (Zhou et al., 2015).

The use of crocetin under in vivo condition protected skin damage induced by ultraviolet A (UV-A). Induction of oxidative stress in skin mice by UV-A irradiation for 8 h improved after oral administration of 100 mg/kg of crocetin. In addition, lipid peroxidation was reduced in the skin of mice (Ohba et al., 2016).

In vitro *studies*

Treatment of human skin-derived fibroblasts, followed by UV-A irradiation, with 0.1, 0.3, and 1 μM of crocetin resulted in a decrease of ROS production and cell death in these cells, especially with treatment of 1 μM (Ohba et al., 2016).

In another study, incubation of bovine spermatozoa with 1, 2.5, and 5 μM of crocetin for 120 or 240 min illustrated that 2.5-μM concentration of crocetin improved sperm quality and its fertilizing ability via regulating ROS and reduction of LPO under in vitro condition (Sapanidou et al., 2016).

The articles relating the effect antioxidant of crocetin indicated its preventive effect on oxidative stress in several organs including nervous, cardiovascular, digestive, and urogenital systems. Therefore, antioxidant properties of crocetin on several damages where free radicals have an effective role were reported by regulating ROS production and antioxidant levels under in vivo and in vitro conditions.

The effects of saffron and its constituents on oxidative stress were shown in Table 16.4.

CLINICAL APPLICATIONS OF THE EFFECT OF SAFFRON (*CROCUS SATIVUS*) AND ITS CONSTITUENTS ON IMMUNE SYSTEM

The effects of saffron and its constituents on the immune system have been demonstrated in various cellular and animal models (Zeinali et al., 2019). Therefore, saffron due to immunomodulatory properties can act as an immune modulator and protect the human body from infections, oxidant-induced stress, and cancers. Fighting infections, enhancing mood, inducing sleep, and modulating hormonal activity are ways to boost immune system of individuals by saffron.

Only a clinical trial reported the role of saffron in improving the immune system. In this randomized double-blind placebo-controlled clinical trial, immunomodulatory effects of saffron were assessed. The male subjects were administrated one tablet saffron (100 mg) every day for 6 weeks. The levels of the serum immunoglobulins including IgG, IgM, and IgAC3 and C4 complements were evaluated. The results indicated that administration of saffron for 3 weeks increased only the IgG level and decreased the IgM level compared with the baseline values, but levels of these

TABLE 16.4
The Effect of Saffron (Crocus sativus) and its Constituents on Oxidative Stress.

Extract/Constituent	Method	Dose	Model	Outcomes	Ref.
Powdered stigmas	In vivo	25 mg/kg/day in drinking water, 20 weeks	Retinal damage induced by oxidative stress in high-fat diet mice	Increased total oxidative capacity	Doumouchtsis et al. (2018)
AE		100 mg/kg/day, gavage,10 days	High-fat diet in hamster model	Reduced MDA	Vakili et al. (2017)
Saffron infusion		90 mg pure red styles/ 200 mL of hot water, 2 weeks	Aflatoxin B1 exposed-mice model	Reduced MDA	Linardaki et al. (2017)
Saffron extract		30 mg/kg/day, systemic administration, 21 days	Chronic stress-induced oxidative stress in a rat	Improved SOD, GPx, and GR	Ghaddoost et al. (2011)
EE		For 28 days	Age-related oxidative damage in rat hippocampus	Reduced NO and MDA Increased antioxidant	Samarghandian et al. (2017b)
HEE		5, 10, 20 mg/kg/day; i.p, 4 weeks	Old rat model	Reduced kidney tissue MDA. increased GSH Declined liver tissue NO and MDA but enhanced GST	Samarghandian et al. (2016a,b)
AE		10, 20, and 40 mg/kg/day, i.p, 4 weeks	STZ-induced diabetic rats	Reduced serum MDA Increased SOD, CAT, and GSH	Samarghandian et al. (2017a)
AE		20, 40, and 80 mg/kg/day, i.p, for 4 weeks	Diabetic encephalopathy in rats	Reduced SOD, CAT, and GSH	Samarghandian et al. (2014)
AE		200 mg/kg, i.p., 5 weeks	STZ-induced diabetic rats	Enhanced CAT and GPx levels in testis	Hasanpour et al. (2018)
AE		40 mg/kg, gavage, 6 days	RAD-induced oxidative stress	Enhanced GSH, GPx, and CAT contents	Koul and Abraham (2017)
Methanol and water mixture		2 g/400 mL in a mixture of methanol and water (50:50, v/v), 6 weeks	Ischemia-reperfusion model of rabbit hearts	Increased GPx activity	Nader et al. (2016)
HEE		5 mg/kg, 10 mg/kg, or 20 mg/kg; i.p.	Ischemia-reperfusion model of rat kidney	Reduced tissue MDA	Mahmoudzadeh et al. (2017)
EE		20 mg/kg, orally, for 2 h before ischemia insult	Hepatic ischemia-reperfusion injury in rats	Restored SOD and CAT; inhibited intracellular ROS	Pan et al. (2013)
AE and EE		200 mg/kg, i.p., 7 days	Chronic constriction injury model in rats	Attenuated MDA and increased GSH	Amin et al. (2014)
HEE		10 µg/mL for 16	Doxorubicin and ischemia-reperfusion induced cardiomyocytes injury	Attenuated oxidative stress	Chahine et al. (2016)
Saffron infusion		200 mg/kg/day, orally, 12 weeks	DMBA-induced skin carcinoma in mice	Declined LPO, increased SOD, CAT, GPx, and GST	Das et al. (2010)

Continued

		Model	Dose	Effect	Reference
EE	In vitro	Oxidative injury in endothelial cells	2, 10, 20, and 40 μg/mL	Reduced ROS production	Rahiman et al. (2018)
HEE		Doxorubicin and ischemia-reperfusion induced cardiomyocytes injury	10 μg/mL, 16 days	Attenuated oxidative stress	Chahine et al. (2016)
Safranal	In vivo	Transient cerebral ischemia in rat model	72.5 and 145 mg/kg, i.p., after induction of injury	Decreased MDA	Sadeghnia et al. (2017)
		Cerebral ischemia in rat model	727.5, 363.75, 145.5, and 72.75 mg/kg/day, i.p., 3 days	Increased total thiol	Hosseinzadeh and Sadeghnia (2005)
		Cerebral ischemia in rat model	10 mg/kg, nasal route	Reduced MDA; increased total thiol	Ahmad et al. (2017)
		Immobilization-induced oxidative damage in rat brain	0.75 mg/kg/day, i.p., 21 days	Improved GPx, GR, SOD, and CAT	Samarghandian et al. (2017a,b)
		Crush injury of sciatic nerve in rat model	0.05, 0.2, and 0.8 mg/kg, i.p., 10 days	Enhanced SOD, CAT, GPx, and GR, reduced MDA	Tamaddonfard et al. (2014)
		Cisplatin induced nephrotoxicity and oxidative stress in rat model	200 mg/kg/day, gavage, 5 days	Restored blood MDA	Karafakioglu et al. (2017)
		Diabetic nephropathy in rat model	No dose has been reported, 4 weeks	Enhanced GSH and TAS, Reduced MDA and TOS	Hazman and Bozkurt (2015)
		Oxidative damage model in aged rat brain	0.5 mg/kg day, i.p., 30 days	Restored TAS, TOS, GSH, and NO	Samarghandian et al. (2015)
		Oxidative damage model in aged rat liver	0.5 mg/kg day, i.p., 30 days	Reduced MDA, increased GSH, SOD, and GST	Farahmand et al. (2013)
	In vitro	H2O2-induced toxicity in endothelial cells	2–40 μM	Reduced ROS production	Rahiman et al. (2018)
Crocin	In vivo	Carbon tetrachloride-induced brain damage, rats	100 mg/kg/day, gavage, 15 days	Increased GSH and TAS and CAT Decreased MDA and TOS and SOD	Altinoz et al. (2018)
		Malathion-induced Parkinson and neurochemical changes, rats	10, 20, or 40 mg/kg/day, i.p., 28 days	Elevated serum GSH levels; reduced MDA	Mohammadzadeh et al. (2018)
		Cortical oxidative damage in diabetic rats	15, 30, and 60 mg/kg/day, i.p., 6 weeks	Reduced TBARS	Ahmadi et al. (2017)
		Rat model of Parkinson's disease	30 and 60 mg/kg/day, i.p., 6 weeks	Decreased TBARS and nitrite in hippocampus	Rajaei et al. (2016)
		Acrolein-induced toxicity in the rat brain	12.5, 25, and 50 mg/kg/day, i.p., for 2 weeks	Reduced MDA Increased GSH in cerebral cortex	Rashedinia et al. (2015)
		Rat model of cerebral ischemia reperfusion injury	40 mg/kg/day, orally, 10 days	Declined TOS level	Oruc et al. (2016)
		Rat model of ischemia reperfusion injury in retina	50 mg/kg, i.p., 30 min before and once daily after injury	Enhanced GSH and SOD; decreased ROS and MDA	Chen et al. (2015)
		BeCl2-induced oxidative stress in the liver and brain of rats	200 mg/kg, i.p., 7 days	Restored SOD and CAT	El-Beshbishy et al. (2012)

TABLE 16.4
The Effect of Saffron (Crocus sativus) and its Constituents on oxidative Stress—cont'd

Extract/Constituent	Method	Dose	Model	Outcomes	Ref.
		40 mg/kg/day, i.p., 8 weeks	Diabetes-induced oxidative stress in rats	Decreased MDA and nitrate; increased hepatic tissue SOD and CAT	Yaribeygi et al. (2018)
		50 mg/kg/day, gavage, 21 days	Acrylamide-induced liver injury in rats	Decreased MDA and TOS, Elevated GSH and TAS	Gedik et al. (2017)
		5, 10, or 20 mg/kg/day, i.p, for 30 days	Bisphenol A-induced liver toxicity in rats	Improved GSH level in liver tissue	Vahdati Hassani et al. (2017)
		50, 100 and 250 mg/kg, i.p., 3 h before patulin treatment	Patulin-induced nephrotoxicity and hepatotoxicity in mice	Reduced LPO Improved antioxidant enzymes	Boussabbeh et al. (2016)
		50, 100, and 250 mg/kg, i.p.	Zearalenone-induced oxidative stress in the liver and kidney of mice	Restored MDA, CAT, and SOD levels in the liver and kidney	Ben Salem et al. (2015)
		20 mg/kg/day, orally, 7 days	Renal ischemia reperfusion in rat model	Reduced NO and MDA; increased SOD and GSH	Abou-Hany et al. (2018)
		50 mg/kg/day, gavage, 21 days	Tartrazine- induced nephrotoxicity in rat model	Reduced MDA and TOS, Increased SOD, CAT and TAS	Erdemli et al. (2017)
		100, 200, and 400 mg/kg, i.p., 4 days	Cisplatin-induced renal oxidative stress in rat model	Increased thiol and GPx; reduced MDA	Naghizadeh et al. (2010)
		50, 100, and 250 mg/kg, i.p.	Zearalenone-induced oxidative stress in cardiac tissue of mice	Improved oxidative stress markers	Salem et al. (2016)
		20, 40, 60 mg/kg/day, i.p, 7 days	Myocardial infarction-induced injury in rats	Increased SOD Reduced MDA and NO	Wang et al. (2018)
		50 mg/kg/day, orally, 8 weeks	Heart oxidative stress in high-fat diet-induced diabetic rats	Increased SOD, GPx, and CAT Reduced MDA	Ghorbanzadeh et al. (2016)
		60 mg/kg, i.v, at beginning of resuscitation	Hemorrhagic shock-induced organ damages in rats	Increased GSH Reduced MDA	Yang and Dong (2017)
		25 mg/kg/day, orally, for 16 days	Ovalbumin- induced asthma in mice model	Restored MDA, SOD and GSH in lung tissue	Yosri et al. (2017)
		50 mg/kg/day, i.p, three times/week, 2 months	Cigarette smoke exposure-mediated oxidative stress, rats	Restored GSH, SOD, CAT, GPx in lung tissue	Dianat et al. (2018)
		30 mg/kg/day, orally, 10 days	Rat model of osteoarthritis	Reduced LPO Increased GSH and GPx	Lei et al. (2017)

		Dose/treatment	Model	Effect	Reference
		20 mg/kg/day, gavage, 21 days	Acute swimming exercise-induced oxidative stress and tissue injury in rats	Increase GSH and decreased MDA in liver and skeletal muscle	Altinoz et al. (2016)
		50 mg/kg/day, orally, 10 weeks	In a metabolic syndrome rat model	Reduced MDA Advanced glycation end products	El-Fawal et al. (2018)
	In vitro	5, 10 and 25 µg/mL for 15 min	Arsenic III-induced toxicity in mitochondria, rat liver	Reduced mitochondrial ROS and LPO	Yousefsani et al. (2018a,b)
		2–40 µM	Oxidative injury in endothelial cells	Improved viability and oxidative injury in cells	Rahiman et al. (2018)
		0.1 or 1 µM, 24 h prior to induction of diabetes	Diabetic retinopathy in microglial cells	Declined ROS and NO Inhibited oxidative stress	Yang et al. (2017)
Crocetin	In vivo	100 mg/kg, gavage, 15 days	Cyclophosphamide induced-ovary injury, mice	Modulated markers (SOD) in mitochondrial	Di Emidio et al. (2017)
		5–50 mg/kg, i.t,12 days	Neuropathic pain induced by spared nerve injury, mice	Restored mitochondrial SOD activity	Wang et al. (2017)
		50, 100 and 200 mg/kg/day, orally, f15 days	Myocardial infracted in rat model	Increased GSH and CAT Decreased MDA, SOD	Zhang et al. (2017)
		50 mg/kg/day, i.g, 7 days	Myocardial injury in ischemia/reperfusion, rat	Declined MDA Increased SOD	Wang et al. (2014)
		20 mg/kg, orally, before and after the ischemia reperfusion, 4 days	Retinal ischemia mice model	Inhibited 8-hydroxy-2-deoxyguanosine	Ishizuka et al. (2013)
		100 and 200 mg/kg, i.p.	Burn-induced intestinal injury rat model	Restored MDA, CAT, SOD and GPx in serum and small intestine tissue	Zhou et al. (2015)
	In vitro	100 mg/kg, orally	Skin damage induced by ultraviolet A in mice	Reduced LPO in skin	Ohba et al. (2016)
		0.1, 0.3, and 1 µM	Skin damage induced by ultraviolet A in mice	Decreased ROS production and cell death	Ohba et al. (2016)
		1, 2.5, and 5 µM, for 120 or 240 min	Bovine spermatozoa	Regulated ROS Reduced LPO	Sapanidou et al. (2016)

Abbreviations: AE, aqueous extract; EE, ethanolic extract; HEE, hydroethanolic extract; i.p. intraperitoneal; i.t., intrathecally; i.g., intragastrical; i.v., intravenously; BeCl2, beryllium chloride; STZ, streptozotocin; RAD, γ-radiation; DMBA, 7,12dimethylben-z[a]anthracene; ROS, reactive oxygen species; LPO, lipid peroxidation; GSH, glutathione; GPx, glutathione peroxidase; GR, glutathione reductase; SOD, superoxide dismutase; CAT, catalase; MDA, malondialdehyde; GST, glutathione S-transferase; NO, nitric oxide; TAS, total antioxidant status; TOS, total oxidant status.

parameters returned to the baseline after 6 weeks. Therefore, saffron has temporary immunomodulatory effects without any adverse effects (Kianbakht and Ghazavi, 2011).

CONCLUSION

This review article indicated various immunological effects of saffron and its constituents including in vivo and in vitro as well as a few clinical studies.

The published data demonstrated that saffron and its constituent, crocin, augment the production of humoral immune responses and modulate total and differential leukocyte counts, which demonstrated immunomodulatory effects of saffron.

These results of reviewed article showed decreased production of proinflammatory cytokines and increased antiinflammatory cytokines as well as caused a shift in Th1/Th2 balance toward Th2-dominant immunity by increased IL-4 cytokine expression levels rather than Th1 response in various disorders such as asthma, diabetes, constriction injury, and PHA-stimulated human peripheral blood mononuclear cells due to treatment with various extracts of saffron. Treatment with the saffron constituent such as safranal, crocin, and crocetin also decreased the levels of TNF-α, IL-1β, and IL-4 but increased the levels of IL-10 and IFN-γ in the plasma, serum, and tissue in various inflammatory conditions, which indicated the potential therapeutic effect of the plant constituents on inflammatory disorders by shifting the Th1/Th2 ratio toward Th1 activity.

Saffron extracts safranal, crocetin, and specially crocin treatment inhibited the expression of CXCL8, eotaxin, p-ERK, p-JNK, and p-p38 protein and decreased protein expression levels of MMP-1, MMP-3, MMP-9 MMP-13, HAases, tryptase, and Hsp70 mRNA and protein levels of EPO and MPO activities, as well as suppressed the proliferation and expression of NF-κB but increased Nrf2 expression in neuronal injury, arthritis, asthma, gastrointestinal disorders, and cancer.

Based on obtained results from reviewed studies, various extracts of saffron and its main constituents including safranal, crocin, and crocetin possessed a potent antioxidant effect on various disorders associated with oxidative stress imbalance in animal and cellular models. Therefore, the saffron extract and its main compounds could be useful for the treatment of diseases where free radicals have an effective role, by restoring oxidant/antioxidant agents such as LPO, MDA, SOD, CAT, thiol, GSH, etc.

Therefore, various extracts as well as different constituents of saffron could be of therapeutic values in inflammatory disorders because of their immunomodulatory effects. However, more clinical studies should be carried out on the effect of saffron and its constituents before they can be used in clinical practice.

REFERENCES

Abdullaev, F.I., Espinosa-Aguirre, J.J., 2004. Biomedical properties of saffron and its potential use in cancer therapy and chemoprevention trials. Cancer Detect. Prev. 28, 426−432.

Abou-Hany, H.O., Atef, H., Said, E., Elkashef, H.A., Salem, H.A., 2018. Crocin reverses unilateral renal ischemia reperfusion injury-induced augmentation of oxidative stress and toll like receptor-4 activity. Environ. Toxicol. Pharmacol. 59, 182−189.

Aggarwal, B.B., Harikumar, K.B., 2009. Potential therapeutic effects of curcumin, the anti-inflammatory agent, against neurodegenerative, cardiovascular, pulmonary, metabolic, autoimmune and neoplastic diseases. Int. J. Biochem. Cell Biol. 41, 40−59.

Ahmad, N., Ahmad, R., Abbas Naqvi, A., Ashafaq, M., Alam, M.A., Ahmad, F.J., Al-Ghamdi, M.S., 2017. The effect of safranal loaded mucoadhesive nanoemulsion on oxidative stress markers in cerebral ischemia. Artif. Cells Nanomed Biotechnol. 45, 775−787.

Ahmadi, M., Rajaei, Z., Hadjzadeh, M.A., Nemati, H., Hosseini, M., 2017. Crocin improves spatial learning and memory deficits in the Morris water maze via attenuating cortical oxidative damage in diabetic rats. Neurosci. Lett. 642, 1−6.

Altinoz, E., Erdemli, M.E., Gul, M., Aksungur, Z., Gul, S., Bag, H.G., Kaya, G.B., Turkoz, Y., 2018. Neuroprotection against CCl4 induced brain damage with crocin in Wistar rats. Biotech. Histochem. 93, 623−631.

Altinoz, E., Ozmen, T., Oner, Z., Elbe, H., Erdemli, M.E., Bag, H.G., 2016. Saffron (its active constituent, crocin) supplementation attenuates lipid peroxidation and protects against tissue injury. Bratisl. Lek. Listy 117, 381−387.

Amin, B., Abnous, K., Motamedshariaty, V., Hosseinzadeh, H., 2014. Attenuation of oxidative stress, inflammation and apoptosis by ethanolic and aqueous extracts of Crocus sativus L. stigma after chronic constriction injury of rats. An. Acad. Bras. Cienc. 86, 1821−1832.

Babaei, A., Arshami, J., Haghparast, A., Mesgaran, M.D., 2014. Effects of saffron (Crocus sativus) petal ethanolic extract on hematology, antibody response, and spleen histology in rats. Avicenna J. Phytomed. 4, 103.

Bani, S., Pandey, A., Agnihotri, V.K., Pathania, V., Singh, B., 2011. Selective Th2 upregulation by Crocus sativus: a neutraceutical spice. Evid Based Complement. Alternat. Med. 2011.

Betteridge, D.J., 2000. What is oxidative stress? Metabolism 49, 3−8.

Bhandari, P.R., 2015. *Crocus sativus* L.(saffron) for cancer chemoprevention: a mini review. J. Tradit. Complement. Med. 5, 81—87.

Boskabady, M.-H., Keyhanmanesh, R., Khameneh, S., Doostdar, Y., Khakzad, M.-R., 2011a. Potential immunomodulation effect of the extract of Nigella sativa on ovalbumin sensitized Guinea pigs. J. Zhejiang Univ. Sci. B 12, 201—209.

Boskabady, M.H., Aslani, M.R., 2006. Relaxant effect of *Crocus sativus* (saffron) on Guinea-pig tracheal chains and its possible mechanisms. J. Pharm. Pharmacol. 58, 1385—1390.

Boskabady, M.H., Byrami, G., Feizpour, A., 2014. The effect of safranal, a constituent of Crocus sativus (saffron), on tracheal responsiveness, serum levels of cytokines, total NO and nitrite in sensitized Guinea pigs. Pharmacol. Rep. 66, 56—61.

Boskabady, M.H., Seyedhosseini Tamijani, S.M., Rafatpanah, H., Rezaei, A., Alavinejad, A., 2011b. The effect of Crocus sativus extract on human lymphocytes' cytokines and T helper 2/T helper 1 balance. J. Med. Food 14, 1538—1545.

Boskabady, M.H., Shafei, M.N., Shakiba, A., Sefidi, H.S., 2008. Effect of aqueous-ethanol extract from *Crocus sativus* (saffron) on Guinea-pig isolated heart. Phyther. Res. 22, 330—334.

Bostan, H.B., Mehri, S., Hosseinzadeh, H., 2017. Toxicology effects of saffron and its constituents: a review. Iran. J. Basic Med. Sci. 20, 110.

Boussabbeh, M., Ben Salem, I., Belguesmi, F., Bacha, H., Abid-Essefi, S., 2016. Tissue oxidative stress induced by patulin and protective effect of crocin. Neurotoxicology 53, 343—349.

Byrami, G., Boskabady, M.H., Jalali, S., Farkhondeh, T., 2013. The effect of the extract of *Crocus sativus* on tracheal responsiveness and plasma levels of IL-4, IFN-gamma, total NO and nitrite in ovalbumin sensitized Guinea-pigs. J. Ethnopharmacol. 147, 530—535.

Caballero-Ortega, H., Pereda-Miranda, R., Abdullaev, F.I., 2007. HPLC quantification of major active components from 11 different saffron (*Crocus sativus* L.) sources. Food Chem. 100, 1126—1131.

Chahine, N., Nader, M., Duca, L., Martiny, L., Chahine, R., 2016. Saffron extracts alleviate cardiomyocytes injury induced by doxorubicin and ischemia-reperfusion in vitro. Drug Chem. Toxicol. 39, 87—96.

Chen, L., Qi, Y., Yang, X., 2015. Neuroprotective effects of crocin against oxidative stress induced by ischemia/reperfusion injury in rat retina. Ophthalmic Res. 54, 157—168.

Christodoulou, E., Kadoglou, N.P.E., Kostomitsopoulos, N., Valsami, G., 2015. Saffron: a natural product with potential pharmaceutical applications. J. Pharm. Pharmacol. 67, 1634—1649.

Dadkhah, A., Fatemi, F., Malayeri, M.R.M., Rasooli, A., 2014. Cancer chemopreventive effect of dietary Zataria multiflora essential oils. Turkish J. Biol. 38, 930—939.

Das, I., Das, S., Saha, T., 2010. Saffron suppresses oxidative stress in DMBA-induced skin carcinoma: a histopathological study. Acta Histochem. 112, 317—327.

Del Bano, M.J., Castillo, J., Benavente-García, O., Lorente, J., Martín-Gil, R., Acevedo, C., Alcaraz, M., 2006. Radioprotective— antimutagenic effects of rosemary phenolics against chromosomal damage induced in human lymphocytes by γ-rays. J. Agric. Food Chem. 54, 2064—2068.

Dhar, M.K., Sharma, M., Bhat, A., Chrungoo, N.K., Kaul, S., 2017. Functional genomics of apocarotenoids in saffron: insights from chemistry, molecular biology and therapeutic applications. Brief. Funct. Genomics 16, 336—347.

Di Emidio, G., Rossi, G., Bonomo, I., Alonso, G.L., Sferra, R., Vetuschi, A., Artini, P.G., Provenzani, A., Falone, S., Carta, G., 2017. The natural carotenoid crocetin and the synthetic tellurium compound AS101 protect the ovary against cyclophosphamide by modulating SIRT1 and mitochondrial markers. Oxid. Med. Cell. Longev. 2017.

Dianat, M., Radan, M., Badavi, M., Mard, S.A., Bayati, V., Ahmadizadeh, M., 2018. Crocin attenuates cigarette smoke-induced lung injury and cardiac dysfunction by anti-oxidative effects: the role of Nrf2 antioxidant system in preventing oxidative stress. Respir. Res. 19, 58.

Ding, J., Su, J., Zhang, L., Ma, J., 2015. Crocetin activates Foxp3 through TIPE2 in asthma-associated treg cells. Cell. Physiol. Biochem. 37, 2425—2433.

Doumouchtsis, E.K., Tzani, A., Doulamis, I.P., Konstantopoulos, P., Laskarina-Maria, K., Agrogiannis, G., Agapitos, E., Moschos, M.M., Kostakis, A., Perrea, D.N., 2018. Effect of saffron on metabolic profile and retina in apolipoprotein E—knockout mice fed a high-fat diet. J. Diet. Suppl. 15, 471—481.

El-Beshbishy, H.A., Hassan, M.H., Aly, H.A.A., Doghish, A.S., Alghaithy, A.A.A., 2012. Crocin "saffron" protects against beryllium chloride toxicity in rats through diminution of oxidative stress and enhancing gene expression of antioxidant enzymes. Ecotoxicol. Environ. Saf. 83, 47—54.

El-Fawal, R., El Fayoumi, H.M., Mahmoud, M.F., 2018. Diosmin and crocin alleviate nephropathy in metabolic syndrome rat model: effect on oxidative stress and low grade inflammation. Biomed. Pharmacother. 102, 930—937.

El-Maraghy, S.A., Rizk, S.M., Shahin, N.N., 2015. Gastroprotective effect of crocin in ethanol-induced gastric injury in rats. Chem. Biol. Interact. 229, 26—35.

Erdemli, M.E., Gul, M., Altinoz, E., Zayman, E., Aksungur, Z., Bag, H.G., 2017. The protective role of crocin in tartrazine induced nephrotoxicity in Wistar rats. Biomed. Pharmacother. 96, 930—935.

Farahmand, S.K., Samini, F., Samini, M., Samarghandian, S., 2013. Safranal ameliorates antioxidant enzymes and suppresses lipid peroxidation and nitric oxide formation in aged male rat liver. Biogerontology 14, 63—71.

Faridi, S., Delirezh, N., Froushani, S.M.A., 2018. Beneficial effects of hydroalcoholic extract of saffron in alleviating experimental autoimmune diabetes in C57bl/6 mice. Iran. J. Allergy, Asthma Immunol. 1—10.

Feyzi, R., Boskabady, M.H., Seyedhosseini Tamijani, S.M., Rafatpanah, H., Rezaei, S.A., 2016. The effect of safranal on Th1/Th2 cytokine balance. Iran. J. Immunol. 13, 263—273.

Gedik, S., Erdemli, M.E., Gul, M., Yigitcan, B., Bag, H.G., Aksungur, Z., Altinoz, E., 2017. Hepatoprotective effects of crocin on biochemical and histopathological alterations following acrylamide-induced liver injury in Wistar rats. Biomed. Pharmacother. 95, 764–770.

Ghadrdoost, B., Vafaei, A.A., Rashidy-Pour, A., Hajisoltani, R., Bandegi, A.R., Motamedi, F., Haghighi, S., Sameni, H.R., Pahlvan, S., 2011. Protective effects of saffron extract and its active constituent crocin against oxidative stress and spatial learning and memory deficits induced by chronic stress in rats. Eur. J. Pharmacol. 667, 222–229.

Ghorbanzadeh, V., Mohammadi, M., Mohaddes, G., Dariushnejad, H., Chodari, L., Mohammadi, S., 2016. Protective effect of crocin and voluntary exercise against oxidative stress in the heart of high-fat diet-induced type 2 diabetic rats. Physiol. Int. 103, 459–468.

Hariri, A.T., Moallem, S.A., Mahmoudi, M., Memar, B., Hosseinzadeh, H., 2010. Sub-acute effects of diazinon on biochemical indices and specific biomarkers in rats: protective effects of crocin and safranal. Food Chem. Toxicol. 48, 2803–2808.

Hasani-Ranjbar, S., Larijani, B., Abdollahi, M., 2009. A systematic review of the potential herbal sources of future drugs effective in oxidant-related diseases. Inflamm. Allergy – Drug Targets 8, 2–10.

Hasanpour, M., Ashrafi, M., Erjaee, H., Nazifi, S., 2018. The effect of saffron aqueous extract on oxidative stress parameters and important biochemical enzymes in the testis of streptozotocin-induced diabetic rats. Physiol. Pharmacol. 22, 28–37.

Hassan, M.H., Bahashawan, S.A., Abdelghany, T.M., Abd-Allah, G.M., Ghobara, M.M., 2015. Crocin abrogates carbon tetrachloride-induced renal toxicity in rats via modulation of metabolizing enzymes and diminution of oxidative stress, apoptosis, and inflammatory cytokines. J. Biochem. Mol. Toxicol. 29, 330–339.

Hassani, F.V., Mehri, S., Abnous, K., Birner-Gruenberger, R., Hosseinzadeh, H., 2017. Protective effect of crocin on BPA-induced liver toxicity in rats through inhibition of oxidative stress and downregulation of MAPK and MAPKAP signaling pathway and miRNA-122 expression. Food Chem. Toxicol. 107, 395–405.

Hazman, Ö., Bozkurt, M.F., 2015. Anti-inflammatory and antioxidative activities of safranal in the reduction of renal dysfunction and damage that occur in diabetic nephropathy. Inflammation 38, 1537–1545.

Hazman, Ö., Ovalı, S., 2015. Investigation of the anti-inflammatory effects of safranal on high-fat diet and multiple low-dose streptozotocin induced type 2 diabetes rat model. Inflammation 38, 1012–1019.

Hemshekhar, M., Santhosh, M.S., Sunitha, K., Thushara, R.M., Kemparaju, K., Rangappa, K.S., Girish, K.S., 2012. A dietary colorant crocin mitigates arthritis and associated secondary complications by modulating cartilage deteriorating enzymes, inflammatory mediators and antioxidant status. Biochimie 94, 2723–2733.

Hosseinzadeh, H., Jahanian, Z., 2010. Effect of Crocus sativus L.(saffron) stigma and its constituents, crocin and safranal, on morphine withdrawal syndrome in mice. Phyther. Res. 24, 726–730.

Hosseinzadeh, H., Nassiri-Asl, M., 2013. Avicenna's (Ibn Sina) the canon of medicine and saffron (Crocus sativus): a review. Phyther. Res. 27, 475–483.

Hosseinzadeh, H., Sadeghnia, H.R., 2005. Safranal, a constituent of Crocus sativus (saffron), attenuated cerebral ischemia induced oxidative damage in rat hippocampus. J. Pharm. Pharm. Sci. 8, 394–399.

Hosseinzadeh, H., Younesi, H.M., 2002. Antinociceptive and anti-inflammatory effects of Crocus sativus L. stigma and petal extracts in mice. BMC Pharmacol. 2, 7.

Huang, Z., Nan, C., Wang, H., Su, Q., Xue, W., Chen, Y., Shan, X., Duan, J., Chen, G., Tao, W., 2016. Crocetin ester improves myocardial ischemia via Rho/ROCK/NF-κB pathway. Int. Immunopharmacol. 38, 186–193.

Ishizuka, F., Shimazawa, M., Umigai, N., Ogishima, H., Nakamura, S., Tsuruma, K., Hara, H., 2013. Crocetin, a carotenoid derivative, inhibits retinal ischemic damage in mice. Eur. J. Pharmacol. 703, 1–10.

Karafakıoğlu, Y.S., Bozkurt, M.F., Hazman, Ö., Fıdan, A.F., 2017. Efficacy of safranal to cisplatin-induced nephrotoxicity. Biochem. J. 474, 1195–1203.

Karimian, P., Kavoosi, G., Saharkhiz, M.J., 2012. Antioxidant, nitric oxide scavenging and malondialdehyde scavenging activities of essential oils from different chemotypes of Zataria multiflora. Nat. Prod. Res. 26, 2144–2147.

Kawabata, K., Tung, N.H., Shoyama, Y., Sugie, S., Mori, T., Tanaka, T., 2012. Dietary crocin inhibits colitis and colitis-associated colorectal carcinogenesis in male ICR mice. Evid Based Complement. Alternat. Med. 2012.

Kianbakht, S., Ghazavi, A., 2011. Immunomodulatory effects of saffron: a randomized double-blind placebo-controlled clinical trial. Phyther. Res. 25, 1801–1805.

Kianbakht, S., Mozaffari, K., 2009. Effects of saffron and its active constituents, crocin and safranal, on prevention of indomethacin induced gastric ulcers in diabetic and nondiabetic rats. J. Med. Plants 1, 30–38.

Kim, I.-S., Yang, M., Goo, T.-H., Jo, C., Ahn, D.-U., Park, J.-H., Lee, O.-H., Kang, S.-N., 2012. Radical scavenging-linked antioxidant activities of commonly used herbs and spices in Korea. Int. J. Food Sci. Nutr. 63, 603–609.

Koul, A., Abraham, S.K., 2017. Intake of saffron reduces γ-radiation-induced genotoxicity and oxidative stress in mice. Toxicol. Mech. Methods 27, 428–434.

Lari, P., Abnous, K., Imenshahidi, M., Rashedinia, M., Razavi, M., Hosseinzadeh, H., 2015. Evaluation of diazinon-induced hepatotoxicity and protective effects of crocin. Toxicol. Ind. Health 31, 367–376.

Lei, M., Guo, C., Hua, L., Xue, S., Yu, D., Zhang, C., Wang, D., 2017. Crocin attenuates joint pain and muscle dysfunction in osteoarthritis rat. Inflammation 40, 2086–2093.

Linardaki, Z.I., Lamari, F.N., Margarity, M., 2017. Saffron (Crocus sativus L.) tea intake prevents learning/memory defects and neurobiochemical alterations induced by aflatoxin B 1 exposure in adult mice. Neurochem. Res. 42, 2743–2754.

Li, K., Li, Y.A., Ma, Z., Zhao, J., 2015. Crocin exerts anti-inflammatory and anti-catabolic effects on rat intervertebral discs by suppressing the activation of JNK. Int J Mol Med 36, 1291−1299.

Liu, W., Sun, Y., Cheng, Z., Guo, Y., Liu, P., Wen, Y., 2018. Crocin exerts anti-inflammatory and anti-arthritic effects on type II collagen-induced arthritis in rats. Pharm. Biol. 56, 209−216.

Mahmoudabady, M., Neamati, A., Vosooghi, S., Aghababa, H., 2013. Hydroalcoholic extract of *Crocus sativus* effects on bronchial inflammatory cells in ovalbumin sensitized rats. Avicenna J. Phytomed. 3, 356.

Mahmoudzadeh, L., Najafi, H., Ashtiyani, S.C., Yarijani, Z.M., 2017. Anti-inflammatory and protective effects of saffron extract in ischaemia/reperfusion-induced acute kidney injury. Nephrology 22, 748−754.

Mashmoul, M., Azlan, A., Khaza'ai, H., Yusof, B., Noor, S., 2013. Saffron: a natural potent antioxidant as a promising anti-obesity drug. Antioxidants 2, 293−308.

Mehri, S., Abnous, K., Khooei, A., Mousavi, S.H., Shariaty, V.M., Hosseinzadeh, H., 2015. Crocin reduced acrylamide-induced neurotoxicity in Wistar rat through inhibition of oxidative stress. Iran. J. Basic Med. Sci. 18, 902.

Mohammadzadeh, L., Hosseinzadeh, H., Abnous, K., Razavi, B.M., 2018. Neuroprotective potential of crocin against malathion-induced motor deficit and neurochemical alterations in rats. Environ. Sci. Pollut. Res. 25, 4904−4914.

Mollazadeh, H., Emami, S.A., Hosseinzadeh, H., 2015. Razi's Al-Hawi and saffron (*Crocus sativus*): a review. Iran. J. Basic Med. Sci. 18, 1153.

Nader, M., Chahine, N., Salem, C., Chahine, R., 2016. Saffron (*Crocus sativus*) pretreatment confers cardioprotection against ischemia-reperfusion injuries in isolated rabbit heart. J. Physiol. Biochem. 72, 711−719.

Naghizadeh, B., Mansouri, S.M.T., Mashhadian, N.V., 2010. Crocin attenuates cisplatin-induced renal oxidative stress in rats. Food Chem. Toxicol. 48, 2650−2655.

Nam, K.N., Park, Y.-M., Jung, H.-J., Lee, J.Y., Min, B.D., Park, S.-U., Jung, W.-S., Cho, K.-H., Park, J.-H., Kang, I., 2010. Anti-inflammatory effects of crocin and crocetin in rat brain microglial cells. Eur. J. Pharmacol. 648, 110−116.

Ohba, T., Ishisaka, M., Tsujii, S., Tsuruma, K., Shimazawa, M., Kubo, K., Umigai, N., Iwawaki, T., Hara, H., 2016. Crocetin protects ultraviolet A-induced oxidative stress and cell death in skin in vitro and in vivo. Eur. J. Pharmacol. 789, 244−253.

Oruc, S., Gönül, Y., Tunay, K., Oruc, O.A., Bozkurt, M.F., Karavelioğlu, E., Bağcıoğlu, E., Coşkun, K.S., Celik, S., 2016. The antioxidant and antiapoptotic effects of crocin pretreatment on global cerebral ischemia reperfusion injury induced by four vessels occlusion in rats. Life Sci. 154, 79−86.

Pan, T., Wu, T., Wang, P., Leu, Y., Sintupisut, N., Huang, C., Chang, F., Wu, Y., 2013. Functional proteomics reveals the protective effects of saffron ethanolic extract on hepatic ischemia-reperfusion injury. Proteomics 13, 2297−2311.

Premkumar, K., Thirunavukkarasu, C., Abraham, S.K., Santhiya, S.T., Ramesh, A., 2006. Protective effect of saffron (*Crocus sativus* L.) aqueous extract against genetic damage induced by anti-tumor agents in mice. Hum. Exp. Toxicol. 25, 79−84.

Rahiman, N., Akaberi, M., Sahebkar, A., Emami, S.A., Tayarani-Najaran, Z., 2018. Protective effects of saffron and its active components against oxidative stress and apoptosis in endothelial cells. Microvasc. Res. 118, 82−89.

Rahmani, A.H., Khan, A.A., Aldebasi, Y.H., 2017. Saffron (*Crocus sativus*) and its active ingredients: role in the prevention and treatment of disease. Pharmacogn. J. 9.

Rajaei, Z., Hosseini, M., Alaei, H., 2016. Effects of crocin on brain oxidative damage and aversive memory in a 6-OHDA model of Parkinson's disease. Arq. Neuropsiquiatr. 74, 723−729.

Rashedinia, M., Lari, P., Abnous, K., Hosseinzadeh, H., 2015. Protective effect of crocin on acrolein-induced tau phosphorylation in the rat brain. Acta Neurobiol. Exp. 75, 208−219.

Razavi, B.M., Hosseinzadeh, H., 2015. Saffron as an antidote or a protective agent against natural or chemical toxicities. DARU J. Pharm. Sci. 23, 31.

Razavi, M., Hosseinzadeh, H., Abnous, K., Motamedshariaty, V.S., Imenshahidi, M., 2013. Crocin restores hypotensive effect of subchronic administration of diazinon in rats. Iran. J. Basic Med. Sci. 16, 64.

Rezaee, R., Hosseinzadeh, H., 2013. Safranal: from an aromatic natural product to a rewarding pharmacological agent. Iran. J. Basic Med. Sci. 16, 12.

Riahi-Zanjani, B., Balali-Mood, M., Mohammadi, E., Badie-Bostan, H., Memar, B., Karimi, G., 2015. Safranal as a safe compound to mice immune system. Avicenna J. phytomedicine 5, 441.

Rios, J.L., Recio, M.C., Giner, R.M., Manez, S., 1996. An update review of saffron and its active constituents. Phyther. Res. 10, 189−193.

Sadeghnia, H.R., Shaterzadeh, H., Forouzanfar, F., Hosseinzadeh, H., 2017. Neuroprotective effect of safranal, an active ingredient of *Crocus sativus*, in a rat model of transient cerebral ischemia. Folia Neuropathol. 55, 206−213.

Salem, I.B., Boussabbeh, M., Helali, S., Abid-Essefi, S., Bacha, H., 2015. Protective effect of Crocin against zearalenone-induced oxidative stress in liver and kidney of Balb/c mice. Environ. Sci. Pollut. Res. 22, 19069−19076.

Salem, I.B., Boussabbeh, M., Neffati, F., Najjar, M.F., Abid-Essefi, S., Bacha, H., 2016. Zearalenone-induced changes in biochemical parameters, oxidative stress and apoptosis in cardiac tissue: protective role of crocin. Hum. Exp. Toxicol. 35, 623−634.

Samarghandian, S., Asadi-Samani, M., Farkhondeh, T., Bahmani, M., 2016a. Assessment the effect of saffron ethanolic extract (*Crocus sativus* L.) on oxidative damages in aged male rat liver. Der Pharm. Lett. 8, 283−290.

Samarghandian, S., Azimi-Nezhad, M., Borji, A., Farkhondeh, T., 2016b. *Crocus sativus* L.(saffron) extract reduces the extent of oxidative stress and proinflammatory state in aged rat kidney. Prog. Nutr. 18, 299−310.

Samarghandian, S., Azimi-Nezhad, M., Farkhondeh, T., 2017a. Immunomodulatory and antioxidant effects of saffron aqueous extract (*Crocus sativus* L.) on streptozotocin-induced diabetes in rats. Indian Heart J. 69, 151−159.

Samarghandian, S., Azimi-Nezhad, M., Samini, F., 2014. Ameliorative effect of saffron aqueous extract on hyperglycemia, hyperlipidemia, and oxidative stress on diabetic encephalopathy in streptozotocin induced experimental diabetes mellitus. BioMed Res. Int. 2014.

Samarghandian, S., Azimi-Nezhad, M., Samini, F., 2015. Preventive effect of safranal against oxidative damage in aged male rat brain. Exp. Anim. 64, 65−71.

Samarghandian, S., Azimi-Nezhad, M., Samini, F., Farkhondeh, T., 2017b. The role of saffron in attenuating age-related oxidative damage in rat hippocampus. Recent Pat. Food Nut.r Agric. 8, 183−189.

Samarghandian, S., Samini, F., Azimi-Nezhad, M., Farkhondeh, T., 2017c. Anti-oxidative effects of safranal on immobilization-induced oxidative damage in rat brain. Neurosci. lett. 659, 26−32.

Sapanidou, V., Taitzoglou, I., Tsakmakidis, I., Kourtzelis, I., Fletouris, D., Theodoridis, A., Lavrentiadou, S., Tsantarliotou, M., 2016. Protective effect of crocetin on bovine spermatozoa against oxidative stress during in vitro fertilization. Andrology 4, 1138−1149.

Santhosh, S.M., Hemshekhar, M., Thushara, R.M., Devaraja, S., Kemparaju, K., Girish, K.S., 2013. Vipera russelli venom-induced oxidative stress and hematological alterations: Amelioration by crocin a dietary colorant. Cell Biochem. Funct. 31, 41−50.

Soeda, S., Ochiai, T., Paopong, L., Tanaka, H., Shoyama, Y., Shimeno, H., 2001. Crocin suppresses tumor necrosis factor-α-induced cell death of neuronally differentiated PC-12 cells. Life Sci. 69, 2887−2898.

Sun, Y., Yang, J., Wang, L.Z., Sun, L.R., Dong, Q., 2014. Crocin attenuates cisplatin-induced liver injury in the mice. Hum. Exp. Toxicol. 33, 855−862.

Tamaddonfard, E., Farshid, A.A., Maroufi, S., Kazemi-Shojaei, S., Erfanparast, A., Asri-Rezaei, S., Taati, M., Dabbaghi, M., Escort, M., 2014. Effects of safranal, a constituent of saffron, and vitamin E on nerve functions and histopathology following crush injury of sciatic nerve in rats. Phytomedicine 21, 717−723.

Tsantarliotou, M.P., Poutahidis, T., Markala, D., Kazakos, G., Sapanidou, V., Lavrentiadou, S., Zervos, I., Taitzoglou, I., Sinakos, Z., 2013. Crocetin administration ameliorates endotoxin-induced disseminated intravascular coagulation in rabbits. Blood Coagul. Fibrinolysis 24, 305−310.

Tseng, T.-H., Chu, C.-Y., Huang, J.-M., Shiow, S.-J., Wang, C.-J., 1995. Crocetin protects against oxidative damage in rat primary hepatocytes. Cancer Lett. 97, 61−67.

Vakili, S., Savardashtaki, A., Moghaddam, M.A.M., Nowrouzi, P., Shirazi, M.K., Ebrahimi, G., 2017. The effects of saffron consumption on lipid profile, liver enzymes, and oxidative stress in male hamsters with high fat diet. Trends Pharm. Sci. 3, 201−208.

Vijayabhargava, K., Asad, M., 2011. Effect of stigmas of Crocus sativus L.(saffron) on cell mediated and humoral immunity. Nat. Prod. J. 1, 151−155.

Vosooghi, S., Mahmoudabady, M., Neamati, A., Aghababa, H., 2013. Preventive effects of hydroalcoholic extract of saffron on hematological parameters of experimental asthmatic rats. Avicenna J. Phytomed. 3, 279.

Wang, X., Zhang, G., Qiao, Y., Feng, C., Zhao, X., 2017. Crocetin attenuates spared nerve injury-induced neuropathic pain in mice. J. Pharmacol. Sci. 135, 141−147.

Wang, Y., Sun, J., Liu, C., Fang, C., 2014. Protective effects of crocetin pretreatment on myocardial injury in an ischemia/reperfusion rat model. Eur. J. Pharmacol. 741, 290−296.

Wang, Y., Wang, Q., Yu, W., Du, H., 2018. Crocin attenuates oxidative stress and myocardial infarction injury in rats. Int. Heart J. 17−114.

Xiong, Y., Wang, J., Yu, H., Zhang, X., Miao, C., 2015. Anti-asthma potential of crocin and its effect on MAPK signaling pathway in a murine model of allergic airway disease. Immunopharmacol. Immunotoxicol. 37, 236−243.

Xu, G., Yu, S., Gong, Z., Zhang, S., 2005. [Study of the effect of crocin on rat experimental hyperlipemia and the underlying mechanisms]. Zhongguo Zhongyao Zazhi 30, 369−372.

Yang, L., Dong, X., 2017. Crocin attenuates hemorrhagic shock-induced oxidative stress and organ injuries in rats. Environ. Toxicol. Pharmacol. 52, 177−182.

Yang, L., Qian, Z., Yang, Y., Sheng, L., Ji, H., Zhou, C., Kazi, H.A., 2008. Involvement of Ca^{2+} in the inhibition by crocetin of platelet activity and thrombosis formation. J. Agric. Food Chem. 56, 9429−9433.

Yang, R., Tan, X., Thomas, A.M., Shen, J., Qureshi, N., Morrison, D.C., Van Way III, C.W., 2006. Crocetin inhibits mRNA expression for tumor necrosis factor-α, interleukin-1β, and inducible nitric oxide synthase in hemorrhagic shock. J. Parenter. Enter. Nutr. 30, 297−301.

Yang, R., Yang, L., Shen, X., Cheng, W., Zhao, B., Ali, K.H., Qian, Z., Ji, H., 2012. Suppression of NF-κB pathway by crocetin contributes to attenuation of lipopolysaccharide-induced acute lung injury in mice. Eur. J. Pharmacol. 674, 391−396.

Yang, X., Huo, F., Liu, B., Liu, J., Chen, T., Li, J., Zhu, Z., Lv, B., 2017. Crocin inhibits oxidative stress and Pro-inflammatory response of microglial cells associated with diabetic retinopathy through the activation of PI3K/Akt signaling pathway. J. Mol. Neurosci. 6, 581−589.

Yaribeygi, H., Mohammadi, M.T., Sahebkar, A., 2018. Crocin potentiates antioxidant defense system and improves oxidative damage in liver tissue in diabetic rats. Biomed. Pharmacother. 98, 333−337.

Yosri, H., Elkashef, W.F., Said, E., Gameil, N.M., 2017. Crocin modulates IL-4/IL-13 signaling and ameliorates experimentally induced allergic airway asthma in a murine model. Int. Immunopharmacol. 50, 305−312.

Yousefi, E., Eskandari, A., Javad Gharavi, M., Khademvatan, S., 2014. In vitro activity and cytotoxicity of Crocus sativus extract against Leihmania major (MRHO/IR/75/ER). Infect. Disord. Drug Targets 14, 56−60.

Yousefsani, B.S., Mehri, S., Pourahmad, J., Hosseinzadeh, H., 2018a. Crocin prevents sub-cellular organelle damage, proteolysis and apoptosis in rat hepatocytes: a justification for its hepatoprotection. Iran. J. Pharm. Res. IJPR 17, 553.

Yousefsani, B.S., Pourahmad, J., Hosseinzadeh, H., 2018b. The mechanism of protective effect of crocin against liver mitochondrial toxicity caused by arsenic III. Toxicol. Mech. Methods 28, 105−114.

Zeinali, M., Zirak, M.R., Rezaee, S.A., Karimi, G., Hosseinzadeh, H., 2019. Immunoregulatory and anti-inflammatory properties of *Crocus sativus* (Saffron) and its main active constituents: a review. Iran. J. Basic Med. Sci.

Zhang, C., Ma, J., Fan, L., Zou, Y., Dang, X., Wang, K., Song, J., 2015. Neuroprotective effects of safranal in a rat model of traumatic injury to the spinal cord by anti-apoptotic, anti-inflammatory and edema-attenuating. Tissue Cell 47, 291−300.

Zhang, R., Zhi-Yu, Q., Xiao-Yuan, H.A.N., Zhen, C., Jun-Ling, Y.A.N., Hamid, A., 2009. Comparison of the effects of crocetin and crocin on myocardial injury in rats. Chin. J. Nat. Med. 7, 223−227.

Zhang, W., Li, Y., Ge, Z., 2017. Cardiaprotective effect of crocetin by attenuating apoptosis in isoproterenol induced myocardial infarction rat model. Biomed. Pharmacother. 93, 376−382.

Zhou, C., Bai, W., Chen, Q., Xu, Z., Zhu, X., Wen, A., Yang, X., 2015. Protective effect of crocetin against burn-induced intestinal injury. J. Surg. Res. 198, 99−107.

Zhu, K.-J., Yang, J.-S., 2014. Anti-allodynia effect of safranal on neuropathic pain induced by spinal nerve transection in rat. Int. J. Clin. Exp. Med. 7, 4990.

CHAPTER 17

Crocus sativus L. (Saffron) and Its Components Relaxant Effect on Smooth Muscles and Clinical Applications of This Effect

MOHAMMAD HOSSEIN BOSKABADY • AMIN MOKHTARI-ZAER • MOHAMMAD REZA KHAZDAIR • ARGHAVAN MEMARZIA • ZAHRA GHOLAMNEZHAD

INTRODUCTION

Crocus sativus L. (*C. sativus*) or saffron belongs to the family of Iridaceae, from the Liliaceae, is growing up to 8- to 30-cm high. The leaves are right and high with a ciliate margin and keel. This plant grows in dry climate especially in Iran as well as another region of the world such as Spain, Italia, France, Turkey, Greece, India, Egypt, Switzerland, United Arab Emirate, Morocco, Azerbaijan, Pakistan, Chania, New Zealand, and Japan (Fernández, 2004). Saffron is used as an herbal medicine in addition to its usage as a food additive in cooking because of its remarkable color and odor (Nilakshi et al., 2011).

The major components of *C. sativus* are picrocrocin, crocetin, and safranal. All saffron properties such as color, taste, odor, and aroma are dependent on these components. In addition, the plant contained volatile aroma and nonvolatile active fractions including lycopene, zeaxanthin, alpha- and beta-carotenes, as well as carotenoids (Srivastava et al., 2010). Chemical studies also showed the presence of glycoside components such as kaempferol and quercetin in the petals of *C. sativus* (Hosseinzadeh and Younesi, 2002).

This plant has been used in herbal medicine for the treatment of different diseases. The therapeutic effects of saffron have been demonstrated by pharmacological and clinical studies. The findings have shown that the plant is effective for neurodegenerative disorders such as multiple sclerosis (MS) (Hosseinzadeh and Younesi, 2002),

coronary artery disorders (Xu et al., 2005), respiratory disease (Boskabady and Aslani, 2006), and gastrointestinal (GI) disease (Rios et al., 1996). Several studies also showed various pharmacological effects for saffron including antiinflammatory, antiantigenotoxic, antiatherosclerotic (Premkumar et al., 2001), antioxidant (Hosseinzadeh et al., 2009), anticancer (Abdullaev, 2002; Aung et al., 2007; Mousavi et al., 2011), memory improvement (Abe and Saito, 2000; Ghadrdoost et al., 2011), antidepressant (Hosseinzadeh and Noraei, 2009), genoprotective (Hosseinzadeh and Sadeghnia, 2007), and antitussive effects (Hosseinzadeh and Ghenaati, 2006).

The lowering blood pressure properties of the plant and its components, crocin and safranal, were also demonstrated in previous research (Fatehi et al., 2003). Crocin also showed an improving effect on cardiac arrhythmia (Jahanbakhsh et al., 2012), and it can reduce contractility and heart rate (Boskabady et al., 2008).

The therapeutic effects of the *C. sativus* extract and its constituent, safranal, on an animal model of asthma (sensitized guinea pig) including their effects on pathological changes, tracheal responsiveness, inflammatory cells, and mediators and Th1/Th2 balance were shown in previous studies (Bayrami and Boskabady, 2012; Byrami et al., 2013; Gholamnezhad et al., 2013). The effects of the saffron extract and safranal on Th1/Th2 balance in PHA-stimulated human peripheral

Saffron. https://doi.org/10.1016/B978-0-12-818462-2.00017-6

219

mononuclear cells were also demonstrated (Boskabady et al., 2011b; Feyzi et al., 2016). Antiinflammatory, immunomodulatory, and antioxidant properties of *C sativus* and its components were also reviewed previously (Boskabady and Farkhondeh, 2016). The purpose of this chapter is reviewing the saffron and its component relaxant effect on smooth muscles and clinical application of this effect.

METHOD

Various databases including Medline/PubMed, Science Direct, ISI Web of Knowledge, Scopus, Embase, Google Scholar, Chemical Abstracts, and Biological Abstracts were searched to find available articles on the relaxant effect of saffron and its constituent on various types of smooth muscles until the end of December 2018. Keywords such as saffron, *Crocus sativus*, crocin, safranal, crocetin, relaxant effect, cardiovascular, GI, respiratory, and urogenital were used for this purpose.

SAFFRON AND ITS COMPONENTS RELAXANT EFFECT ON SMOOTH MUSCLES
Saffron and Its Components Relaxant Effect on Tracheal Smooth Muscle

Saffron aqueous ethanolic extract relaxant effect comparable to the effect of theophylline was reported. The plant extracts (0.15, 0.3, 0.45, and 0.60 g %) and theophylline (0.15, 0.30, 0.45, and 0.60 mM) exhibited relaxant action on guinea-pig tracheal smooth muscle (TSM) precontracted by 10-μM methacholine compared to saline. Also, there was a positive correlation between increasing concentrations of the extract and its relaxant effects (Boskabady and Aslani, 2006). Furthermore, administration of safranal (0.15, 0.30, 0.45, and 0.60 mL of 0.2 mg/mL solution) also showed a relaxant effect in a dose-dependent manner on TSM. The results also showed lower relaxant effect for safranal than the extract and theophylline effect (Boskabady and Aslani, 2006).

Decreased responsiveness of TSM to methacholine and ovalbumin (OVA) was also reported due to long-term oral administration of *C. sativus* extracts and safranal in sensitized guinea pigs (Byrami et al., 2013). Quercetin (20 mg/kg) showed significant bronchodilatory effects in both in vivo and in vitro studies (Joskova et al., 2011). These effects could be produced from the relaxant effect of the plant extract on TSM.

The antitussive effect of the saffron ethanolic extract (100–800 mg/kg, intraperitoneally [i.p.]) and safranal (0.25–0.75 mL/kg, i.p.) in guinea pigs was also

reported that it may be attributed to their relaxant action on TSM (Hosseinzadeh and Ghenaati, 2006).

Saffron and Its Components Relaxant Effect on Vascular Smooth Muscle

Intravenous administration of aqueous extract of *C. sativus* (2.5, 5, and 10 mg/kg), safranal (0.25, 0.5, and 1 mg/kg), and crocin (50, 100, and 200 mg/kg) in normotensive and hypertensive animals reduced the mean arterial blood pressure and heart rate in a dose-dependent manner. Administration of 10 mg/kg of saffron, 200 mg/kg of crocin, and 1 mg/kg of safranal lowered mean systolic blood pressure (MSBP) by 60 ± 8.7, 51 ± 3.8, and 50 ± 5.2 mmHg, respectively. These results suggested that *C. sativus* extract and its two active components showed hypotensive properties in the rats. Moreover, the lowering blood pressure effect of safranal was more potent than crocin (Imenshahidi et al., 2010).

Ethanolic and aqueous extracts of *C. sativus* petals dose-dependently reduced blood pressure in the rats. In this work, aqueous extract (50 mg/g) lowered blood pressure by 17 mmHg compared with the control group. It has been suggested that *C. sativus* petal extracts induced this effect by relaxation of vascular smooth muscle or affecting the heart or both. Nonetheless, the more probable mechanism of the hypotensive effect of extract may contribute to a reduction in peripheral vascular resistance due to the relaxation of vascular smooth muscle (Fatehi et al., 2003).

Reduction of deoxycorticosterone acetate–induced hypertension or increase in MSBP due to treatment with aqueous extract of saffron (10, 20, and 40 mg/kg/day) was also shown in a dose-dependent manner, but this effect on blood pressure was absent in normotensive rats. Furthermore, evidence showed that saffron generates the antihypertensive effects for relatively a short period of time. Therefore, it was suggested that saffron induced short-term blood pressure regulation (Imenshahidi et al., 2013). Likewise, admiration of saffron aqueous ethanolic extract (0.1, 0.5, 1.0, and 5.0 mg%) produced a negative inotropic and chronotropic effect, which was comparable to the effects of diltiazem. It was suggested that the muscle relaxant properties of the extract could be responsible for the heart contractility of the extract (Boskabady et al., 2008).

In the isoproterenol-induced myocardial injury model in rats, the effects of *C. sativus* were evaluated. In this model, isoproterenol enhanced the level of troponin in the serum and reduced the activity of glutathione peroxidase in the heart muscle compared with control group. In addition, isoproterenol-induced heart muscle damages by more than 70%. Saffron remarkably decreased excessive destruction of the tissue and significantly decreased serum levels of heart troponin I (Joukar et al., 2010). On heart ischemia-reperfusion—induced lethal cardiac arrhythmias model, *C. sativus* (100 mg/kg/day) administration significantly decreased ventricular tachycardia (VT)/ventricular fibrillation (VF) numbers, durations, and also the severity of arrhythmia compared with the untreated group. The PR and QTcn intervals of electrocardiogram were significantly longer in the *C. sativus* (200 mg/kg/day) group (Joukar et al., 2013).

Responses to the endothelium-dependent relaxant effect of acetylcholine (ACh) were improved by treatment with crocetin (15, 30 mg/kg) in a dose-dependent manner in aorta isolated from high cholesterol diet—fed rabbits. Oral admiration of crocetin restored the maximal relaxation compared with the control group dose-dependently. Crocetin increased the of serum nitric oxide (NO) concentration, increased vessel cyclic GMP (cGMP) content as well as unregulated mRNA expression of endothelial NO synthase (eNOS) compared with control group (Tang et al., 2006).

Increased systolic blood pressure (SBP) and heart rate after administration of diazinon (DZN) normalized by the crocin (50 mg/kg) which might be due to relation response of vascular smooth muscle (Razavi et al., 2013).

The effects of kaempferol on endothelium-dependent (bradykinin) and independent (sodium nitroprusside) relaxation of porcine coronary arteries were indicated. Kaempferol (3×10^{-6} M) increased relaxations created by bradykinin and sodium nitroprusside (Xu et al., 2015). It was demonstrated that crocin (1 μM) has preventive effects on the cell apoptosis induced by H_2O_2, in cardiovascular diseases (Xu et al., 2006).

Quercetin, 10^{-6} and 10^{-4} M, inhibited the contractions induced by noradrenaline, high KCl, and Ca^{2+} in a concentration-dependent manner. This effect was observed when the quercetin was added before or after the induction of contractions. Quercetin also increased the aortic cyclic AMP content (Duarte et al., 1993a).

The contractions elicited by KCl, noradrenaline, or phorbol 12-myristate,13-acetate were also relaxed by kaempferol and quercetin (Duarte et al., 1993a,b).

Saffron and Its Components Relaxant Effect on GI and Urogenital Smooth Muscle

Saffron petals extract relaxant effect was examined on isolated ileum of guinea pig. Findings revealed that administration of *C. sativus* aqueous and ethanol extracts decreased contractile responses to electrical field stimulation (EFS) of guinea pig ileum. Furthermore, the aqueous extract (560 mg/mL) reduced the contractile responses to epinephrine (1 μM) in guinea pig ileum (Fatehi et al., 2003).

Kaempferol (3—60 μM) and quercetin (1—100 μM) reversed contractions induced by KCl (60 μM) in rat uterus in a concentration-dependent way. However, the inhibitory effect of cAMP-dependent protein kinases (TPCK, 3 μM) antagonized the effect of quercetin and kaempferol. To sum up, cAMP contributes to the relaxant effects of quercetin and kaempferol on KCl (60 mM)-induced tonic contraction (Revuelta et al., 1997). Table 17.1 presents the saffron and its components' relaxant effect on different types of smooth muscles.

MECHANISMS RESPONSIBLE FOR THE RELAXANT EFFECT OF SAFFRON AND ITS COMPONENTS ON SMOOTH MUSCLES

The saffron and its components' relaxant effect could be due to different mechanisms such as stimulatory effect on β2-adrenoreceptors, inhibitory effect on muscarinic receptor, inhibitory effect on histaminic (H_1) receptors, inhibitory effect on calcium channel, endothelium-dependent relaxation (EDR) effect, and the effect of saffron and its constituent on intracellular cAMP as well as their effect on intracellular cAMP.

β2-Adrenoreceptors Stimulatory Effect of Saffron and Its Components

The β-adrenoceptors have been divided into at least three groups, β1, β2, and β3, which are commonly expressed in cardiac muscle, airway smooth muscle, and adipose tissue, respectively (Somlyo and Somlyo, 1994). Inhalation of selective β2-agonists is commonly used as the most effective bronchodilatory drug and therefore, for the management of obstructive airway diseases. Selective β2-agonists drugs bind to the β2-adrenoceptor and trigger the activation of certain G-proteins followed by the production of cyclic adenosine monophosphate (cAMP) in airway smooth muscle leading to bronchodilation (Cazzola et al., 2013). Cyclic AMP induces its effect through activating several effector molecules such as cAMP-dependent protein kinase (PKA). Probably, PKA decreases the cytosolic Ca^{2+} level via preventing the influx of Ca^{2+} by the cell membrane K^+ channels activation and via stimulation of the sarcoplasmic reticulum (SR) Ca^{2+} uptake, which results in decreased Ca^{2+}-dependent myosin light-chain kinase (MLCK) activity. In addition, stimulation of PKA directly increased the activity of myosin light-chain phosphatase (MLCP). Subsequently, diminished MLCK activity and increased MLCP activity results in reduced phosphorylation of MLC and vasodilatation (Morgado et al., 2012).

TABLE 17.1
Saffron and Its Components' Relaxant Effect on Smooth Muscles.

Smooth Muscle (SM) Type	Solution	Effect	Reference
Trachea smooth muscle	AE and EE of stigma	Relaxant effects on TSM precontracted by methacholine	Boskabady and Aslani (2006)
	Safranal	TSM relaxant effect	Boskabady and Aslani (2006)
	AE of stigma	Reduced tracheal responsiveness to methacholine	Byrami et al. (2013)
	Safranal	Reduced tracheal responsiveness to methacholine in sensitized animals by OVA	Byrami et al. (2013)
	AE of stigma and safranal	Antitussive effect	Hosseinzadeh and Ghenaati (2006)
	Quercetin	In vivo and in vitro bronchodilatory effect	Joskova et al. (2011)
Vascular smooth muscle	AE of stigma, safranal and crocin	Lowered MAP and heart rate	Imenshahidi et al. (2010)
	AE and EE of petals	Lowers BP dose-dependently in isolated rat vas deferens	Fatehi et al. (2003)
	AE of stigma	Decreased MSBP in hypertensive rats	Imenshahidi et al. (2013)
	AE and EE of stigma	Reduced cardiac contractile and heart rate	Boskabady et al. (2008)
	AE of stigma	Decreased intensity of tissue destruction	Joukar et al. (2010)
	AE of stigma	Decreased durations and also arrhythmia severity	Joukar et al. (2013)
	Crocetin	Improved EDR in response to acetylcholine	Tang et al. (2006)
	Crocin	Restored elevation of HR and reduction of SBP induced by diazinon	Razavi et al. (2013)
	Kaempferol	Enhanced relaxations produced by bradykinin and sodium nitroprusside	Xu et al. (2015)
	Crocin	Preventive effects on the cell apoptosis, in cardiovascular diseases	Razavi et al. (2013)
	Quercetin	Inhibitory effects on contractions produced by NA, high KCl and Ca^{2+} in a concentration-dependent manner	Duarte et al. (1993a)
	Quercetin and kaempferol	Relaxant effects on rat aortic strips contraction	Duarte et al. (1993a,b)
Gastrointestinal smooth muscle	AE and EE of petals	Decreased EFS of guinea-pig ileum	Fatehi et al. (2003)
	Kaempferol and quercetin	Relaxed the tonic contraction induced by KCl	Revuelta et al. (1997)

AE, aqueous extract; EE, ethanolic extract; TSM, tracheal smooth muscle; OVA, ovalbumin; SBP, systolic blood pressure; HR, heart rate; EFS, electrical field stimulation; MAP, mean arterial blood pressure; BP, blood pressure; MSBP, mean systolic blood pressure; EDR, endothelium-dependent relaxation; NA, noradrenaline.

The stimulatory effect on the β2-adrenergic receptor is one of the possible mechanisms for natural products such as saffron and its constituents inducing smooth muscles relaxation (Chaudhary et al., 2012). In fact, saffron and safranal β2-adrenergic stimulatory effect were demonstrated in isolated guinea pig TSM (Nemati et al., 2008). The safranal β2-adrenergic stimulatory effect was evaluated by conducting isoprenaline cumulative concentration-response curves (nonspecific β-adrenergic agonist) induced relaxation of precontracted TSM. The study was performed in the presence of two components of aqueous ethanolic extracts of saffron (0.1 and 0.2 g %), safranal (1.25 and 2.5 μg), propranolol (10 nM), and saline. Although the extract and safranal induced leftward shifts in isoprenaline curves when compared to saline, propranolol showed a rightward shift in the curve. Therefore, *C. sativus* extract and its components safranal showed a stimulatory effect of the on β2-adrenoreceptors (Nemati et al., 2008). Consequently, these findings suggested β2-agonistic activities of the *C. sativus* and its constituent, as a potential medicinal plant in the treatment of obstructive airways disorders.

Although stimulation of β2-adrenoreceptors might account for *C. sativus*–induced relaxation of TSM, the adrenergic receptors blocking the effect of the plant petal on vas deferens smooth muscle was also suggested (Fatehi et al., 2003). It was shown that the *C. sativus* petals' extract decreased contractile responses to EFS in isolated rat vas deferens (Fatehi et al., 2003). This study suggested that adrenergic receptors involved in the relaxation of vas deferens by *C. sativus* petals' extract.

Muscarinic Receptor Blocking Effects of Saffron and Its Components

Five subtypes including M 1 to 5 are located in various organs, such as vascular and airway smooth muscles (Harvey, 2012). It has been well known that muscarinic receptor agonists such as acetylcholine, methacholine, and carbachol cause contraction of airway smooth muscle in vivo and in vitro. In addition, anticholinergic drugs, for instance, the atropine, have been used to treat asthma and obstructive airway diseases for several years (Gosens et al., 2006). It was shown that the relaxant effect of *C. sativus* and safranal was mediated by the blocking of muscarinic receptors of TSM. Methacholine concentration-response curves were nonparallelly shifted to right due to saffron extract and safranal caused significant, but the maximum response to methacholine was not achieved in the presence of the extract and safranal. These results indicated a functional antagonism effect of the plant and its component on TSM (Neamati and Boskabady, 2010).

Histaminic Antagonistic Activity of Saffron and Its Components

Evidence revealed that histamine affects the smooth muscle of numerous tissues, including bronchioles, intestine, uterus, arterioles, and spleen. Administration of exogenous histamine to guinea pigs generates symptoms and signs of respiratory changes similar to those generated after challenge with the certain antigen (Togias, 2003). Three types of histamine receptors have currently been identified. H_1-receptors mediate bronchoconstriction and H_1-receptor activation, which seems to stimulate inositol trisphosphate (IP3) generation and transient Ca^{2+} release from intracellular stores, followed by continued generation of IP, IP_2, and IP_3, which is linked to prolonged Ca^{2+} influx in cultured human bronchial smooth muscle cells (Goldie et al., 1986).

In a number of studies, the histaminic (H_1) antagonistic effect of plants in smooth muscle cells have been reported (Boskabady et al., 2011a, 2006). Saffron inhibitory effect on histamine (H_1) receptors was evaluated by the effect of aqueous-ethanolic extracts of the plant on the histamine-induced contraction of guinea pig TSM. Three concentrations of the extracts (0.025 g%, 0.05 g %, and 0.1 g%) lead to a parallel rightward shift in histamine concentration-response curve, and the maximum response to histamine was obtained in the presence of the extract. Chlorpheniramine also showed a similar effect to that of saffron (Boskabady et al., 2010).

Therefore, saffron showed a competitive antagonistic (inhibitory) effect on histamine H_1 receptors that could be contributed to the plant relaxant effect on TSM. Similarly, the effect of safranal (0.63, 1.25, and 2.5 μg/mL) on histamine (H_1) receptors in guinea pig TSM were evaluated. The findings showed that safranal shifted histamine-response curves to the right, causing achievement of maximum response to histamine and increased EC50 (effective concentration of histamine causing 50% of maximum response). These results indicated competitive antagonistic effect of safranal at histamine H_1 receptors which may be considered as one possible mechanism for the relaxant action of safranal on TSM (Boskabady et al., 2011a).

Calcium Channel Antagonist Activity of Saffron and Its Components

Intracellular calcium and associated calcium channels play a significant role in the regulation of smooth muscle activity. Therefore, any change in intracellular/extracellular calcium concentration results in various disturbance such as intestinal spasm and bronchoconstriction. In this regard, calcium channel antagonists commonly used in different abnormalities such as cardiovascular disorders and hypertension. These drugs induce a common inhibition on the L-type calcium channels in smooth muscle cells and result in relaxation.

Several studies have demonstrated that medicinal plants induce a relaxant effect on smooth muscles via blocking of the calcium channels (Boskabady et al., 2005a, 2005b; Rakhshandah et al., 2010). For instance, crocin could inhibit the influx of extracellular Ca^{2+} and also release intracellular Ca^{2+} stores in the endoplasmic reticulum in cultured bovine aortic smooth muscle cells (He et al., 2004). Furthermore, the effect of saffron on Ca^{2+} influx in the aorta smooth muscle of rat was evaluated by radioactive tracer ^{45}Ca. Data showed that the Ca^{2+} influxes induced by norepinephrine (1.2 µmol/L and KCl of 100 mmol/L) were remarkably inhibited by saffron concentration-dependently. The finding indicated that the plant can block the influx of extracellular Ca^{2+} via potential-dependent Ca^{2+} channels and receptor-operated Ca^{2+} channels (Liu et al., 2005). Similarly, in another study, the chronic treatment with saffron had a hypotensive effect that was attributed to the smooth muscles inhibitory effect through calcium channel blocking or inhibition of sarcoplasmic reticulum Ca^{2+} release into the cytosol (Boskabady and Aslani, 2006).

In addition, crocin could inhibit the elevation of intracellular Ca^{2+} in the smooth muscle cells in an atherosclerosis model. When the cells were treated with Ox-LDL in the presence of extracellular Ca^{2+}, maximum intracellular Ca^{2+} have generated. However, preincubation of cells with crocin for 4 h, concentration-dependently, inhibited the Ox-LDL-induced intracellular Ca^{2+} elevation. In the lack of extracellular Ca^{2+}, Ox LDL-treated smooth muscle cell revealed maximum intracellular Ca^{2+}, and preincubation with crocin for 4 h significantly blocked the maximum response (He et al., 2005).

Flavonoid compounds, which are widely found as secondary metabolites in various plants including saffron, have an important function such as vasodilation. It has been suggested that the vasodilatory effect of these plants attributed to inhibition of PKC (protein kinase C) or reduction of Ca^{2+} uptake (Duarte et al., 1993a,b). It was proposed that crocetin attenuated the PKC activity in the fraction of membrane, which leads to a reduction of blood pressure by an inhibitory effect on proliferation in vascular smooth muscle cells (Zhou et al., 2010).

EDR Effect of Saffron and Its Components

Nitric oxide (NO) predominantly regulates the vascular tone. NO exerted vasodilatation largely through the activation of soluble guanylyl cyclase (sGC), resulting in cGMP production (Gao, 2010). The endothelium-dependent vasodilatation of crocetin has also been documented by upregulation of the mRNA expressions of eNOS in both in vitro and in vivo studies by its action on eNOS activity and NO production. These results suggest increased NO synthesized in response to crocetin by endothelial cells, which is the major endothelium-derived relaxing factor in the rat aortas (Tang et al., 2006).

Kaempferol may also have relaxation effects by endothelium-derived and exogenous NO as well as endothelium-dependent hyperpolarization through large-conductance calcium-activated potassium channel ($K_{Ca}1.1$ channels) (Xu et al., 2015).

Intracellular cAMP Effects of Saffron and Its Components

Substantial evidence indicates that kaempferol exerts significant relaxation in KCl-induced tonic contraction in isolated rat uterus, which largely mediated through the cAMP and antagonized by Rp-cAMPS, an antagonist of cAMP. In fact, the cAMP, transcription, and protein synthesis are involved in the kaempferol-induced relaxation in rat uterus (Revuelta et al., 2000). However, this mechanism also should be evaluated for saffron and its components in further studies. Table 17.2 presents the possible mechanisms of the saffron and its components relaxant effect.

CLINICAL APPLICATIONS OF SAFFRON AND ITS COMPONENTS RELAXANT EFFECT ON SMOOTH MUSCLES

There are evidence regarding the clinical applications of saffron and its active ingredients in various disorders (Pourmasoumi et al., 2018; Razak et al., 2017). For instance, the effect of saffron and its constituents was studied in patients with depression (Tabeshpour et al., 2017), premenstrual syndrome (Agha-Hosseini et al., 2008), erectile dysfunction (Mohammadzadeh-Moghadam et al., 2015), Alzheimer's disease (Farokhnia et al., 2014), and Metabolic syndrome (Kermani et al., 2017a,b). With regard to the plant relaxant effect on various types of smooth muscle, saffron may also have therapeutic values in the disorders including cardiovascular, respiratory, GI, and urogenital tracts disorders (summarized in Table 17.3).

Cardiovascular System

In most cardiovascular disorders such as heart failure, coronary artery disease, stroke, and peripheral vascular disease, hypertension is the major risk factor worldwide (Ogihara et al., 2005). Several adverse effects have been reported for the available antihypertension drugs for

TABLE 17.2
The Possible Mechanisms of Saffron and Its Components' Relaxation Effect on Smooth Muscles.

Smooth Muscle (SM) Type	Possible Mechanisms	Extract/Constituent and Studied Dose/Concentration	Reference
Trachea	β2-adrenoceptor stimulatory effects	Saffron AE extract (0.1 and 0.2 g%) and safranal (1.25 and 2.5 µg)	Nemati et al. (2008)
Trachea	Muscarinic and cholinergic receptor blocking effects	Saffron AE extract and safranal	Neamati and Boskabady (2010)
Trachea	Histaminic antagonistic activity	Saffron AE extract (0.02, 0.05 and 0.1 g%) Safranal (0.63, 1.25, and 2.5 µg/mL)	Boskabady et al. (2010) Boskabady et al. (2011a,b)
Vascular	Calcium channel antagonist activity	Crocin (1×10^{-8}, 1×10^{-7}, 1×10^{-6} mol/L)	He et al. (2004)
Vascular	Inhibitory effect on PKC or Ca^{2+} uptake	Kaempferol	(Duarte et al. 1993b)
Vascular	Inhibitory effect on PKC activity	Crocetin	Zhou et al. (2010)
Vascular	Increased endothelial NOS activity and production of NO	Crocetin	Tang et al. (2006)
Vascular	Activation of K_{Ca} 1.1 channels	Kaempferol (3×10^{-6} M)	Xu et al. (2015)
Uterus	Increased intracellular cAMP and PKA	Kaempferol (3–60 mM)	Revuelta et al. (2000)

PKC, protein kinase C; PKA, protein kinase A.

these drugs. It was suggested that saffron and its components produced hypotensive and cardiovascular protective effects (Mancini et al., 2014; Razavi et al., 2018). Intravenous administration of saffron aqueous extract (2.5, 5, and 10 mg/kg), safranal (0.25, 0.5, and 1 mg/kg), and crocin (50, 100, and 200 mg/kg) lowered the mean arterial blood pressure in normotensive and hypertensive rats induced by desoxycorticosterone acetate dose-dependently (Imenshahidi et al., 2010). Furthermore, administration of crocin (50, 100, and 200 mg/dL) for 5 weeks in hypertensive animals also showed that crocin reduced mean arterial blood pressure dose-dependently (Imenshahidi et al., 2014).

In the study conducted in healthy volunteers by Modaghegh and colleagues, saffron with a higher dose (400 mg) significantly decreased systolic blood pressure and mean arterial pressures (Modaghegh et al., 2008). However, in a double-blind, randomized clinical trial which was conducted on metabolic syndrome patients, no significant change in BP after the administration of 100 mg of crocin for 6 weeks was observed (Kermani et al., 2017a). In addition, a meta-analysis of 11 published studies did not exhibit any significant change in systolic blood pressure

after saffron consumption (Pourmasoumi et al., 2018). Based on contradictory results, further experiments are required to fully evaluate effects of saffron and its constituents on cardiovascular disorders.

Respiratory System

In vitro or in vivo animal studies indicated the bronchodilator effect of saffron in asthma and COPD through several mechanisms including antihistamine, anticholinergic, and β2-adrenoreceptors stimulation (Mokhtari-Zaer et al., 2015). Unfortunately, there have not yet been any controlled clinical studies investigating the bronchodilatory effect of the plant and its components on respiratory disorders such as asthma, COPD, or other obstructive pulmonary diseases. To confirm the bronchodilatory effects of saffron and its active compound, clinical studies should be performed. However, saffron and its components showed a potent relaxant effect on TSM as well as their stimulatory effect on β2-adrenoreceptors, inhibitory effect on muscarinic and histamine (H_1) receptors, as well as the effect on calcium channels, strongly suggest the bronchodilatory effect of saffron and its component.

TABLE 17.3

Possible Clinical Applications of Saffron and Its Components' Relaxant Effect on Smooth Muscles.

System	Disease	Effects	Possible Mechanism	Extract/ Constituents	Reference
Respiratory	Asthma COPD Other obstructive diseases	Relaxant effects on guinea pig tracheal chains	—	Safranal, AE, and EE of stigma	Boskabady and Aslani (2006)
		Reduction of TR		AE of stigma	Byrami et al. (2013)
		Antitussive effect		AE of stigma and safranal	Hosseinzadeh and Ghenaati (2006)
		In vivo and in vitro bronchodilation		Quercetin	Joskova et al. (2011)
		Bronchodilatory	β2— adrenoreceptors stimulatory	Aq, Eth Ext of stigma, safranal	Nemati et al. (2008)
		Bronchodilatory	Anticholinergic and antimuscarinic	Aq, Eth Ext of stigma, safranal	Neamati and Boskabady (2010)
		Bronchodilatory	Histaminic (H$_1$) receptor antagonism		Boskabady et al. (2011a)
Cardiovascular	Hypertension	Reduction of blood pressure	—	Aq. Ext., safranal, crocin	Imenshahidi et al. (2010)
		Reduction of blood pressure	—	Aq. and Eth. Ext of petals	Fatehi et al. (2003)
		Reduction of blood pressure	—	Aq. Ext of stigma	Imenshahidi et al. (2013)
		Decreased SBP and heart rate induced	Vascular SM relaxation	Crocetin	Razavi et al. (2013)
		Endothelium-dependent relaxation of aorta	Increased expression of eNOS, and cGMP	Crocetin	Tang et al. (2006)
		Relaxation of porcine coronary arteries	Preventive effects on the cell apoptosis	Kaempferol	Xu et al. (2006)
		Relaxation of rat aortic strips	Increased the aortic cAMP	Quercetin and kaempferol	Duarte et al. (1993a,b)
		Reduced heart rate and contractility	Vascular SM relaxation	Aq-Eth. Ext of stigma	Boskabady et al. (2008)
Gastrointestinal	constipation	Decreased EFS of guinea-pig ileum	—	AE and EE of petals	Fatehi et al. (2003)
Urogenital	Sexual dysfunctions	Improved erectile dysfunction	—	saffron gel	Mohammadzadeh-Moghadam et al. (2015)
	Premenstrual syndrome	Relieving premenstrual syndrome symptoms	—	capsule saffron 30 mg	Agha-Hosseini et al. (2008)
		Relaxed tonic contraction	Muscarinic stimulation	Kaempferol and quercetin	Revuelta et al. (1997)

Ext, extract; Aq., aqueous; Eth, ethanolic; TR, tracheal responsiveness; SM, smooth muscle; SBP, systolic blood pressure.

GI Tract

Rezaee Khorasany and his colleagues have published a review detailing the therapeutic effects of saffron in GI disorder including hepatotoxicity, liver cancer, fatty liver, colon cancer, stomach cancer, pancreas cancer, hyperlipidemia, peptic ulcer, ulcerative colitis, and ileum contractions (Khorasany and Hosseinzadeh, 2016). However, most of the studies have been carried out on isolated tissues or murine models of GI disorders. For instance, It has been reported that the petal extracts of *C. sativus* diminished the evoked contractions in isolated guinea-pig ileum (Fatehi et al., 2003). In fact, the saffron extract exhibited a spasmolytic effect in tissues precontracted by EFS. In fact, it was shown that electrical stimulation resulted in ACh released from activated synapses (Bornstein et al., 2004). It is suggested that ACh binds to M3 postsynaptic smooth muscle receptors and cause contraction of ileum smooth muscles. Nonetheless, the efficacy of saffron in GI tract disorders remains an open empirical question. Controlled clinical studies of saffron have yet to be conducted to determine the efficacy of this plant for people who have suffered from GI disorders.

Urogenital Tracts

Several experimental and clinical studies have shown a therapeutic effect of saffron and its component on sexual disfunction (Hosseinzadeh et al., 2008; Shamsa et al., 2009). In a study on male rats, crocin (100, 200, and 400 mg/kg) and the extract of the plant (160 and 320 mg/kg) enhanced mounting frequency, erection frequency, and intromission frequency. However, they reduced mounting latency, ejaculation latency, and intromission latency, while safranal did not have any effect on the mentioned parameters (Hosseinzadeh et al., 2008).

Although the previous studies conducted to determine the relaxant effect of saffron on smooth muscle, some studies have revealed the spasmodic action on smooth muscle-like uterine (Sadraei et al., 2003). In fact, *C. sativus* is regarded as an abortifacient agent, as it increases uterine muscle contraction (Hosseinzadeh

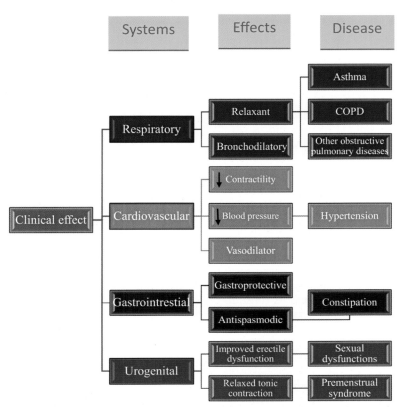

FIG. 17.1 Possible clinical applications of the relaxant effect of saffron and its constituents.

and Nassiri-Asl, 2013). In an *in vitro* experiment, saffron extract (200−1600 lg/mL) increased the spontaneous rhythmic contraction in isolated rat uterine (Sadraei et al., 2003). Furthermore, it has been reported that saffron consumption, particularly in the last trimester of gestation, can generate preterm delivery due to increased uterine contractions in female mice (Zeinali et al., 2009). It should be noted that *C. sativus* contained various components so each component could have different actions on muscular tissue. Interestingly, kaempferol, as a flavonol from saffron petal, showed a potent relaxant effect on KCl-precontracted rat uterus (Revuelta et al., 2000). In addition, in Chinese medicine, saffron usage is recommended for difficult labor, menorrhagia, and postpartum hemorrhage (Gruenwald, 1998).

However, little research has been performed to investigate the potential therapeutic effects of saffron in the urogenital tract disorders. Thus, based on such preclinical evidence, saffron could be extensively evaluated in clinical trials for urogenital tract diseases, and future studies should fill this knowledge gap. Possible clinical effect of saffron and its constituents are presented in Table 17.2 and Fig. 17.1.

CONCLUSION

The results of those evaluated in vivo and in vitro animal studies demonstrated relaxant effects of saffron extract, safranal, and quercetin, which approved the bronchodilatory and antitussive properties of the plant. In different hypertensive animal models and in vitro isolated vascular and heart preparations, the relaxant and hypotensive effects of *C. sativus* extract and its constituents (safranal, crocetin, crocin, quercetin, and kaempferol) have been shown. Several pathways, including protecting effect against heart toxic agent, antiarrhythmia property, improving endothelium-dependent relaxation response to acetylcholine, increasing serum level of nitric oxide (NO), upregulating vessel activity and mRNA expression of endothelial NO synthase (eNOS), as well as vessel cyclic GMP (cGMP) content, have been suggested for cardioprotective and vasodilatory effects of plant and its constituents. In addition, saffron petal extracts and its flavonoids kaempferol and quercetin showed relaxant effects on GI (ileum) and urogenital (uterus) smooth muscle preparations.

The saffron and its components' relaxant effect on smooth muscles of various organs, including blood vessels, trachea, GI, and urogenital, have been shown to be mediated via different mechanisms such as stimulatory effect on β2-adrenoreceptors, inhibitory effect on

muscarinic receptor, inhibitory effect on histaminic (H$_1$ receptor) receptors, inhibitory effect on calcium channel, EDR effect, and effect of saffron and its constituent on intracellular cAMP and effect of saffron and its constituent on intracellular cAMP.

The result of the reviewed studies suggested the therapeutic effect of saffron and its constituents on cardiovascular, GI, respiratory, and urogenital disorders. However, few clinical studies investigated those beneficial effects on related systems. Therefore, more clinical trials should be designated for demonstration of preventive and therapeutic effects of saffron and its constituents due to their smooth muscle relaxant effect.

REFERENCES

Abdullaev, F.I., 2002. Cancer chemopreventive and tumoricidal properties of saffron (*Crocus sativus* L.). Exp. Biol. Med. 227, 20−25.

Abe, K., Saito, H., 2000. Effects of saffron extract and its constituent crocin on learning behaviour and long-term potentiation. Phytother. Res. 14, 149−152.

Agha-Hosseini, M., Kashani, L., Aleyaseen, a, Ghoreishi, a, Rahmanpour, H., Zarrinara, a R., Akhondzadeh, S., 2008. *Crocus sativus* L. (saffron) in the treatment of premenstrual syndrome: a double-blind, randomised and placebo-controlled trial. BJOG 115, 515−519.

Aung, H.H., Wang, C.Z., Ni, M., Fishbein, A., Mehendale, S.R., Xie, J.T., Shoyama, A.Y., Yuan, C.S., 2007. Crocin from *Crocus sativus* possesses significant anti-proliferation effects on human colorectal cancer cells. Exp. Oncol. 29, 175.

Bayrami, G., Boskabady, M.H., 2012. The potential effect of the extract of *Crocus sativus* and safranal on the total and differential white blood cells of ovalbumin-sensitized Guinea pigs. Res. Pharm. Sci. 7, 249−255.

Bornstein, J.C., Costa, M., Grider, J.R., 2004. Enteric motor and interneuronal circuits controlling motility. Neurogastroenterol. Motil. 16 (Suppl. 1), 34−38.

Boskabady, M.H., Aslani, M.R., 2006. Relaxant effect of *Crocus sativus* (saffron) on Guinea-pig tracheal chains and its possible mechanisms. J. Pharm. Pharmacol. 58, 1385−1390.

Boskabady, M.H., Farkhondeh, T., 2016. Antiinflammatory, antioxidant, and immunomodulatory effects of *Crocus sativus* L. And its main constituents. Phytother. Res. 30, 1072−1094.

Boskabady, M.H., Kiani, S., Azizi, H., 2005a. Relaxant effect of *Cuminum cyminum* on Guinea pig tracheal chains and its possible mechanism (s). Indian J. Pharmacol. 37, 111.

Boskabady, M.H., Kiani, S., Haghiri, B., 2005b. Relaxant effects of *Ocimum basilicum* on Guinea pig tracheal chains and its possible mechanism (s). DARU J. Pharm. Sci. 13, 28−33.

Boskabady, M.H., Kiani, S., Rakhshandah, H., 2006. Relaxant effects of *Rosa damascena* on Guinea pig tracheal chains and its possible mechanism (s). J. Ethnopharmacol. 106, 377−382.

Boskabady, M.H., Rahbardar, M.G., Jafari, Z., 2011a. The effect of safranal on histamine (H1) receptors of Guinea pig tracheal chains. Fitoterapia 82, 162–167.

Boskabady, M.H., Rahbardar, M.G., Nemati, H., Esmaeilzadeh, M., 2010. Inhibitory effect of *Crocus sativus* (saffron) on histamine (H1) receptors of Guinea pig tracheal chains. Pharmazie 65, 300–305.

Boskabady, M.H., Seyedhosseini Tamijani, S.M., Rafatpanah, H., Rezaei, A., Alavinejad, A., 2011b. The effect of *Crocus sativus* extract on human lymphocytes' cytokines and T helper 2/T helper 1 balance. J. Med. Food 14, 1538–1545.

Boskabady, M.H., Shafei, M.N., Shakiba, A., Sefidi, H.S., 2008. Effect of aqueous-ethanol extract from *Crocus sativus* (saffron) on Guinea-pig isolated heart. Phytother. Res. 22, 330–334.

Byrami, G., Boskabady, M.H., Jalali, S., Farkhondeh, T., 2013. The effect of the extract of *Crocus sativus* on tracheal responsiveness and plasma levels of IL-4, IFN-gamma, total NO and nitrite in ovalbumin sensitized Guinea-pigs. J. Ethnopharmacol. 147, 530–535.

Cazzola, M., Page, C.P., Rogliani, P., Matera, M.G., 2013. β2-agonist therapy in lung disease. Am. J. Respir. Crit. Care Med. 187, 690–696.

Chaudhary, M.A., Imran, I., Bashir, S., Mehmood, M.H., Rehman, N., Gilani, A.-H., 2012. Evaluation of gut modulatory and bronchodilator activities of Amaranthus spinosus Linn. BMC Complement Altern. Med. 12, 166.

Duarte, J., Perez-Vizcaino, F., Zarzuelo, A., Jimenez, J., Tamargo, J., 1993a. Vasodilator effects of quercetin in isolated rat vascular smooth muscle. Eur. J. Pharmacol. 239, 1–7.

Duarte, J., Pérez, F.V., Utrilla, P., Jiménez, J., Tamargo, J., Zarzuelo, A., 1993b. Vasodilatory effects of flavonoids in rat aortic smooth muscle. Structure-activity relationships. Gen. Pharmacol. 24, 857–862.

Farokhnia, M., Shafiee Sabet, M., Iranpour, N., Gougol, A., Yekehtaz, H., Alimardani, R., Farsad, F., Kamalipour, M., Akhondzadeh, S., 2014. Comparing the efficacy and safety of *Crocus sativus* L. with memantine in patients with moderate to severe Alzheimer's disease: a double-blind randomized clinical trial. Hum. Psychopharmacol. 29, 351–359.

Fatehi, M., Rashidabady, T., Fatehi-hassanabad, Z., 2003. Effects of *Crocus sativus* petals' extract on rat blood pressure and on responses induced by electrical field stimulation in the rat isolated vas deferens and Guinea-pig ileum. J. Ethnopharmacol. 84, 199–203.

Fernández, J.-A., 2004. Biology, biotechnology and biomedicine of saffron. Recent Res. Dev. Plant Sci. 2, 127–159.

Feyzi, R., Boskabady, M.H., Seyedhosseini Tamijani, S.M., Rafatpanah, H., Rezaei, S.A., 2016. The effect of safranal on Th1/Th2 cytokine balance. Iran. J. Immunol. 13, 263–273.

Gao, Y., 2010. The multiple actions of NO. Pflügers Arch. J. Physiol. 459, 829–839.

Ghadrdoost, B., Vafaei, A.A., Rashidy-Pour, A., Hajisoltani, R., Bandegi, A.R., Motamedi, F., Haghighi, S., Sameni, H.R., Pahlvan, S., 2011. Protective effects of saffron extract and its active constituent crocin against oxidative stress and spatial learning and memory deficits induced by chronic stress in rats. Eur. J. Pharmacol. 667, 222–229.

Gholamnezhad, Z., Koushyar, H., Byrami, G., Boskabady, M.H., 2013. The extract of Crocus sativus and its constituent safranal, affect serum levels of endothelin and total protein in sensitized Guinea pigs. Iran. J. Basic Med. Sci. 16, 1022–1026.

Goldie, R.G., Spina, D., Henry, P.J., Lulich, K.M., Paterson, J.W., 1986. In vitro responsiveness of human asthmatic bronchus to carbachol, histamine, beta-adrenoceptor agonists and theophylline. Br. J. Clin. Pharmacol. 22, 669–676.

Gosens, R., Zaagsma, J., Meurs, H., Halayko, A.J., 2006. Muscarinic receptor signaling in the pathophysiology of asthma and COPD. Respir. Res. 7, 73.

Gruenwald, J., 1998. PDR for Herbal Medicines. Medical Economics Company.

Harvey, R.D., 2012. Muscarinic receptor agonists and antagonists: effects on cardiovascular function. In: Muscarinic Receptors. Springer, pp. 299–316.

He, S.-Y., Qian, Z.-Y., Tang, F.-T., 2004. Effect of crocin on intracellular calcium concentration in cultured bovine aortic smooth muscle cells. Acta Pharm. Sin. 39, 778–781.

He, S.-Y., Qian, Z.-Y., Tang, F.-T., Wen, N., Xu, G.-L., Sheng, L., 2005. Effect of crocin on experimental atherosclerosis in quails and its mechanisms. Life Sci. 77, 907–921.

Hosseinzadeh, H., Ghenaati, J., 2006. Evaluation of the antitussive effect of stigma and petals of saffron (*Crocus sativus*) and its components, safranal and crocin in Guinea pigs. Fitoterapia 77, 446–448.

Hosseinzadeh, H., Nassiri-Asl, M., 2013. Avicenna's (Ibn sina) the canon of medicine and saffron (*Crocus sativus*): a review. Phytother. Res. 27, 475–483.

Hosseinzadeh, H., Noraei, N.B., 2009. Anxiolytic and hypnotic effect of *Crocus sativus* aqueous extract and its constituents, crocin and safranal, in mice. Phytother. Res. 23, 768–774.

Hosseinzadeh, H., Sadeghnia, H.R., 2007. Effect of safranal, a constituent of *Crocus sativus* (saffron), on methyl methanesulfonate (MMS)-induced DNA damage in mouse organs: an alkaline single-cell gel electrophoresis (comet) assay. DNA Cell Biol. 26, 841–846.

Hosseinzadeh, H., Shamsaie, F., Mehri, S., others, 2009. Antioxidant activity of aqueous and ethanolic extracts of *Crocus sativus* L. stigma and its bioactive constituents, crocin and safranal. Pharmacogn. Mag. 5, 419.

Hosseinzadeh, H., Younesi, H.M., 2002. Antinociceptive and anti-inflammatory effects of *Crocus sativus* L. stigma and petal extracts in mice. BMC Pharmacol. 2, 7.

Hosseinzadeh, H., Ziaee, T., Sadeghi, a, 2008. The effect of saffron, *Crocus sativus* stigma, extract and its constituents, safranal and crocin on sexual behaviors in normal male rats. Phytomedicine 15, 491–495.

Imenshahidi, M., Hosseinzadeh, H., Javadpour, Y., 2010. Hypotensive effect of aqueous saffron extract (*Crocus sativus* L.) and its constituents, safranal and crocin, in normotensive and hypertensive rats. Phytother. Res. 24, 990–994.

Imenshahidi, M., Razavi, B.M., Faal, A., Gholampoor, A., Mousavi, S.M., Hosseinzadeh, H., 2013. The effect of chronic administration of saffron (*Crocus sativus*) stigma aqueous extract on systolic blood pressure in rats. Jundishapur J. Nat. Pharm. Prod. 8, 175.

Imenshahidi, M., Razavi, B.M., Faal, A., Gholampoor, A., Mousavi, S.M., Hosseinzadeh, H., 2014. Effects of chronic crocin treatment on desoxycorticosterone acetate (doca)-salt hypertensive rats. Iran. J. Basic Med. Sci. 17, 9.

Jahanbakhsh, Z., Rasoulian, B., Jafari, M., Shekarforoush, S., Esmailidehaj, M., Mohammadi, M.T., Aghai, H., Salehi, M., Khoshbaten, A., 2012. Protective effect of crocin against reperfusion-induced cardiac arrhythmias in anaesthetized rats. EXCLI J 11, 20–29.

Joskova, M., Franova, S., Sadlonova, V., 2011. Acute bronchodilator effect of quercetin in experimental allergic asthma. Bratisl. Lek. Listy 112, 9–12.

Joukar, S., Ghasemipour-Afshar, E., Sheibani, M., Naghsh, N., Bashiri, A., 2013. Protective effects of saffron (Crocus sativus) against lethal ventricular arrhythmias induced by heart reperfusion in rat: a potential anti-arrhythmic agent. Pharm. Biol. 51, 836–843.

Joukar, S., Najafipour, H., Khaksari, M., Sepehri, G., Shahrokhi, N., Dabiri, S., Gholamhoseinian, A., Hasanzadeh, S., 2010. The effect of saffron consumption on biochemical and histopathological heart indices of rats with myocardial infarction. Cardiovasc. Toxicol. 10, 66–71.

Kermani, T., Kazemi, T., Molki, S., Ilkhani, K., Sharifzadeh, G., Rajabi, O., 2017a. The efficacy of crocin of saffron (*Crocus sativus* L.) on the components of metabolic syndrome: a randomized controlled clinical trial. J. Res. Pharm. Pract. 6, 228.

Kermani, T., Zebarjadi, M., Mehrad-Majd, H., Mirhafez, S.-R., Shemshian, M., Ghasemi, F., Mohammadzadeh, E., Mousavi, S.H., Norouzy, A., Moghiman, T., Sadeghi, A., Ferns, G., Avan, A., Mahdipour, E., Ghayour-Mobarhan, M., 2017b. Anti-inflammatory effect of Crocus sativus on serum cytokine levels in subjects with metabolic syndrome: a randomized, double-blind, placebo-controlled trial. Curr. Clin. Pharmacol. 12, 122–126.

Khorasany, A.R., Hosseinzadeh, H., 2016. Therapeutic effects of saffron (*Crocus sativus* L.) in digestive disorders: a review. Iran. J. Basic Med. Sci. 19, 455.

Liu, N., Yang, Y., Mo, S., Liao, J., Jin, J., 2005. Calcium antagonistic effects of Chinese crude drugs: preliminary investigation and evaluation by 45Ca. Appl. Radiat. Isot. 63, 151–155.

Mancini, A., Serrano-Diaz, J., Nava, E., D'Alessandro, A.M., Alonso, G.L., Carmona, M., Llorens, S., 2014. Crocetin, a carotenoid derived from saffron (Crocus sativus L.), improves acetylcholine-induced vascular relaxation in hypertension. J. Vasc. Res. 51, 393–404.

Modaghegh, M.-H., Shahabian, M., Esmaeili, H.-A., Rajbai, O., Hosseinzadeh, H., 2008. Safety evaluation of saffron (*Crocus sativus*) tablets in healthy volunteers. Phytomedicine 15, 1032–1037.

Mohammadzadeh-Moghadam, H., Nazari, S.M., Shamsa, A., Kamalinejad, M., Esmaeeli, H., Asadpour, A.A., Khajavi, A., 2015. Effects of a topical saffron (*Crocus sativus* L) gel on erectile dysfunction in diabetics: a randomized, parallel-group, double-blind, placebo-controlled trial. J. Evid. Based Complement. Altern. Med. 20, 283–286.

Mokhtari-Zaer, A., Khazdair, M.R., Boskabady, M.H., 2015. Smooth muscle relaxant activity of Crocus sativus (saffron) and its constituents: possible mechanisms. Avicenna J. Phytomed. 5, 365.

Morgado, M., Cairrao, E., Santos-Silva, A.J., Verde, I., 2012. Cyclic nucleotide-dependent relaxation pathways in vascular smooth muscle. Cell. Mol. Life Sci. 69, 247–266.

Mousavi, S.H., Moallem, S.A., Mehri, S., Shahsavand, S., Nassirli, H., Malaekeh-Nikouei, B., 2011. Improvement of cytotoxic and apoptogenic properties of crocin in cancer cell lines by its nanoliposomal form. Pharm. Biol. 49, 1039–1045.

Neamati, N., Boskabady, M.H., 2010. Effect of Crocus sativus (saffron) on muscarinic receptors of Guinea pig tracheal chains. Funct. Plant Sci. Biotechnol. 4, 128–131.

Nemati, H., Boskabady, M.H., Ahmadzadef Vostakolaei, H., 2008. Stimulatory effect of *Crocus sativus* (saffron) on β 2-adrenoceptors of Guinea pig tracheal chains. Phytomedicine 15, 1038–1045.

Nilakshi, N., Gadiya, R.V., Abhyankar, M., Champalal, K.D., 2011. Detailed profile of Crocus sativus. Int. J. Pharma Bio Sci. 2, 530–540.

Ogihara, T., Matsuzaki, M., Matsuoka, H., Shimamoto, K., Shimada, K., Rakugi, H., Umemoto, S., Kamiya, A., Suzuki, N., Kumagai, H., 2005. The combination therapy of hypertension to prevent cardiovascular events (COPE) trial: rationale and design. Hypertens. Res. 28, 331.

Pourmasoumi, M., Hadi, A., Najafgholizadeh, A., Kafeshani, M., Sahebkar, A., 2018. Clinical evidence on the effects of saffron (Crocus sativus L.) on cardiovascular risk factors: a systematic review meta-analysis. Pharmacol. Res. 139, 348–359.

Premkumar, K., Abraham, S.K., Santhiya, S.T., Gopinath, P.M., Ramesh, A., 2001. Inhibition of genotoxicity by saffron (Crocus sativus L.) in mice. Drug Chem. Toxicol. 24, 421–428.

Rakhshandah, H., Boskabady, M.H., Mossavi, Z., Gholami, M., Saberi, Z., 2010. The Differences in the relaxant effects of different fractions of Rosa damascena on Guinea pig tracheal smooth muscle. Iran. J. Basic Med. Sci. 13, 126–132.

Razak, S.I.A., Anwar Hamzah, M.S., Yee, F.C., Kadir, M.R.A., Nayan, N.H.M., 2017. A review on medicinal properties of saffron toward major diseases. J. Herbs, Spices, Med. Plants 23, 98–116.

Razavi, B.M., Alyasin, A., Hosseinzadeh, H., Imenshahidi, M., 2018. Saffron induced relaxation in isolated rat aorta via endothelium dependent and independent mechanisms. Iran. J. Pharm. Res. 17, 1018–1025.

Razavi, M., Hosseinzadeh, H., Abnous, K., Motamedshariaty, V.S., Imenshahidi, M., 2013. Crocin restores hypotensive effect of subchronic administration of diazinon in rats. Iran. J. Basic Med. Sci. 16, 64.

Revuelta, M.P., Cantabrana, B., Hidalgo, A., 1997. Depolarization-dependent effect of flavonoids in rat uterine smooth muscle contraction elicited by $CaCl_2$. Gen. Pharmacol. 29, 847–857.

Revuelta, M.P., Cantabrana, B., Hidalgo, A., 2000. Mechanisms involved in kaempferol-induced relaxation in rat uterine smooth muscle. Life Sci. 67, 251−259.

Rios, J.L., Recio, M.C., Giner, R.M., Manez, S., 1996. An update review of saffron and its active constituents. Phytother. Res. 10, 189−193.

Sadraei, H., Ghannadi, A., Takei-bavani, M., 2003. Effects of Zataria multiflora and Carum carvi essential oils and hydroalcoholic extracts of Passiflora incarnata, Berberis integerrima and Crocus sativus on rat isolated uterus contractions. Int. J. Aromather. 13, 121−127.

Shamsa, A., Hosseinzadeh, H., Molaei, M., 2009. Evaluation of *Crocus sativus* L . (saffron) on male erectile dysfunction : a pilot study. Phytomedicine 16, 690−693.

Somlyo, A.P., Somlyo, A.V., 1994. Signal transduction and regulation in smooth muscle. Nature 372, 231.

Srivastava, R., Ahmed, H., Dixit, R.K., others, 2010. Crocus sativus L.: a comprehensive review. Pharmacogn. Rev. 4, 200.

Tabeshpour, J., Sobhani, F., Sadjadi, S.A., Hosseinzadeh, H., Mohajeri, S.A., Rajabi, O., Taherzadeh, Z., Eslami, S., 2017. A double-blind, randomized, placebo-controlled trial of saffron stigma (*Crocus sativus* L.) in mothers suffering from mild-to-moderate postpartum depression. Phytomedicine 36, 145−152.

Tang, F.T., Qian, Z.Y., Liu, P.Q., Zheng, S.G., He, S.Y., Bao, L.P., Huang, H.Q., 2006. Crocetin improves endothelium-dependent relaxation of thoracic aorta in hypercholesterolemic rabbit by increasing eNOS activity. Biochem. Pharmacol. 72, 558−565.

Togias, A., 2003. H1-receptors: localization and role in airway physiology and in immune functions. J. Allergy Clin. Immunol. 112, S60−S68.

Xu, G.-L., Qian, Z.-Y., Yu, S.-Q., Gong, Z.-N., Shen, X.-C., 2006. Evidence of crocin against endothelial injury induced by hydrogen peroxide in vitro. J. Asian Nat. Prod. Res. 8, 79−85.

Xu, G., Yu, S., Gong, Z., Zhang, S., 2005. [Study of the effect of crocin on rat experimental hyperlipemia and the underlying mechanisms]. Zhongguo Zhongyao Zazhi 30, 369−372.

Xu, Y.C., Leung, S.W.S., Leung, G.P.H., Man, R.Y.K., 2015. Kaempferol enhances endothelium-dependent relaxation in the porcine coronary artery through activation of large-conductance Ca(2+) -activated K(+) channels. Br. J. Pharmacol. 172, 3003−3014.

Zeinali, F., Anvari, M., Dashti, R.M.H., Hosseini, S.M., 2009. The effects of different concentrations of saffron (Crocus sativus) decoction on preterm delivery in mice. Planta Med. 75, PI29.

Zhou, C., Xiang, M., He, S., Qian, Z., 2010. Protein kinase C pathway is involved in the inhibition by crocetin of vascular smooth muscle cells proliferation. Phytother. Res. 24, 1680−1686.

CHAPTER 18

Medicinal Properties of Saffron With Special Reference to Cancer—A Review of Preclinical Studies

HIFZUR R. SIDDIQUE • HOMA FATMA • MOHAMMAD AFSAR KHAN

INTRODUCTION

Saffron (*Crocus sativus*) is a perennial herb, popularly called as a golden condiment, used mainly for spice derived from the dried stigmas of the flower. Saffron is one of the most expensive spices in the world due to its medicinal values, taste, and complications that take place in its cultivation, harvesting, and handling. The herb is cultivated in Iran, Greece, Spain, Italy, and India. The saffron plants are divided by means of bulbs (or corms) and the flowers. A flower has three mauve-colored stigmas and three yellow-colored stamens. The stigmas are discarded, and only the mauve-colored stigmas that are almost 25−30 mm long are essential as the source of saffron. Phenotypic variation can be noted in the saffron sample from different regions, but very little genetic diversity is noted among saffron plants. These reduced genetic variations are due to the absence of sexual reproduction among saffron as they propagate through asexual/vegetative for reproduction. The variation in saffron quality depends upon how the stigmas are processed, sowing time, and environmental attributes (Namayandeha et al., 2013; Cenci-Goga et al., 2018). The dried stigmas are used as spices, coloring agents, food colorant, cosmetics, and other uses (Wani et al., 2011; Bhargava et al., 2011).

Plants are the source of different medicines due to the presence of different phytochemicals/active ingredients. Phytochemicals are the nonnutritive secondary metabolites produced in the different parts of the plants based on the physiology of the plant. Saffron also contains almost 150 phytochemicals that are known to have different medicinal properties. The important phytochemicals are mainly crocin, crocetin, picrocrocin, safranal, terpenes alcohol, terpenes, and their esters (Fig. 18.1). Other important phytochemicals found in saffron are kaempferol, taxifolin, naringenin, zeaxanthin, lycopene, and vitamins especially thymine, etc. These compounds are accountable for color, aroma, taste, and odor of saffron, respectively (Samarghandian and Borji, 2014). It is a well-known fact that different plant-derived active ingredients/phytochemicals interfere with different cellular functions at the molecular level and similar interferences are also observed with the phytochemicals found in saffron (Rios et al., 1996; Schmidt et al., 2007; Siddique and Saleem, 2011; Siddique et al., 2011, 2012a,b; Samarghandian and Borji, 2014; Cenci-Goga et al., 2018).

Saffron is considered as a natural medicine since ancient times. Saffron has been reported to act as anticatarrhal, antispasmodic, antitumor, analgesic, antigenotoxic, neuroprotective, antidepressive, nerve-sedative, diaphoretic, antiinflammatory, anticonvulsant, antianxiety, antihypersensitive, and antihyperlipidemic (Fig. 18.2) (Rios et al., 1996; Schmidt et al., 2007; Bathaie et al., 2010). Saffron is also reported to have effects on cardiovascular disease and diabetes. Thus, saffron exhibits a broad spectrum of pharmacological activities. Saffron is gaining popularity as an alternative medicine option and has been reported to show effective disease prevention and treatment effects. In this chapter, we discuss the different pharmacological effects of saffron with particular emphasis on cancer.

Saffron. https://doi.org/10.1016/B978-0-12-818462-2.00018-8

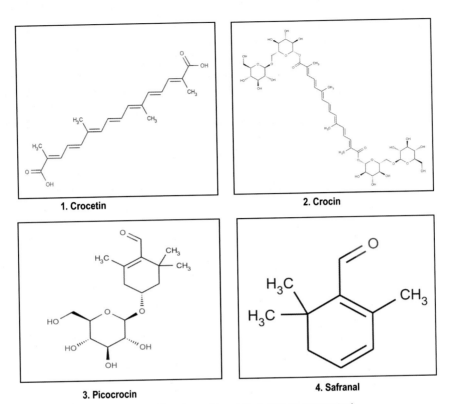

1. Crocetin

2. Crocin

3. Picocrocin

4. Safranal

FIG. 18.1 Structure of important saffron component.

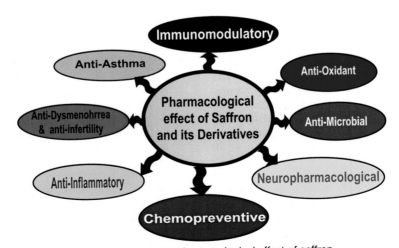

FIG. 18.2 Important pharmacological effect of saffron.

SAFFRON AND METABOLIC SYNDROME

High blood glucose level and triglycerides, reduced level of high-density lipoprotein (HDL), hypertension, and ectopic fat accumulation resulting in the expanded waistline are the specific components for the metabolic syndrome and risk factors for cardiovascular disease and diabetes mellitus (Han et al., 2016; Razavi et al., 2016). Saffron and its ingredients are reported to have a beneficial role against different risk factors of metabolic syndrome (Fig. 18.3). Saffron is said to be cardioprotective and hypotensive in rats. Nasiri et al. (2015) reported that saffron inhibits the platelet aggregation and atherosclerosis both in humans and rabbits, respectively. In a different study, Mueller and Beck (2011) reported a significant decrease in serum triglyceride, total cholesterol, low-density lipoprotein, and very low-density lipoprotein in diet-induced hyperlipidemic rats when treated with saffron. The hypolipidemic effect of saffron is found to be exerted by interfering with the pancreatic lipase that further hinders with the absorption of fat and cholesterol (Sheng et al., 2006). Saffron is also reported to stimulate low-to-moderate peroxisome proliferator-activated receptor α (PPARα) with the transactivation efficacy of almost 40.4%. The hypolipidemic activity of saffron may be through the transactivation of PPARα (Mueller and Beck. 2011). Similarly, Hemmati et al. (2015) reported that oral treatment of saffron in streptozotocin-induced diabetic rats, lead to the significant increase in the serum adiponectin levels that has an inverse relation with metabolic syndrome risk factors and direct relationship with HDL. Level of adiponectin was found to increase in all the saffron-treated groups, thus indicating the beneficial role of saffron in metabolic syndrome (Hemmati et al., 2015).

Saffron is reported to affect DOCA-salt-induced hypertensive rats. Safranal and crocin are the two main constituents found in saffron, and these compounds are reported to reduce systolic blood pressure although, no effect was observed on the blood pressure of normotensive rats (Nasiri et al., 2015). A significant decrease in the aortic area, media thickness, and elastic lamellae number were also observed in the saffron-treated rats. The aortic area, media thickness, and elastic lamellae were found to be increased in hypertension patients. Thus, this study established that saffron is beneficial for hypertension and its related complications (Nasiri et al., 2015). Shemshian et al. (2014) reported that saffron treatment reduced the production of heat shock proteins (HSPs) that are known to be the risk factors in cardiovascular diseases. Interestingly, when studying the effect of saffron on the antibody titers to HSPs, a significant decrease in the anti-HSP27, anti-HSP70 was found in the patients with metabolic syndrome that were treated with saffron.

Obesity is a medical condition in which the total amount of adipose tissue increases. With the increase in fat content of the body, a significant increase in body weight is observed in the obese patient. Studies have contemplated the antiobesity effect of saffron. Saffron exhibited weight reducing properties in slightly overweight women (Gout et al., 2010). One of the marks of obesity is hyperleptinemia. Saffron was found to affect the blood leptin level (Mashmoul et al., 2013). Blood leptin level can act as a parameter for measuring body fat mass and insulin sensitivity. A significant decrease in the blood leptin level was observed in the saffron-treated rats. The antiobesity properties are majorly due to the anorectic effect (Kianbhakt and Hasheem, 2015). Antiinflammatory, antioxidant

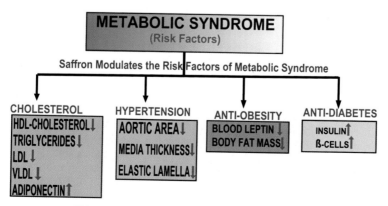

FIG. 18.3 Role of saffron in metabolic syndrome.

action, and increased metabolism of lipid and glucose are also the possible mechanisms of the antiobesity properties (Mashmoul et al., 2013; Kianbhakt and Hasheem, 2015).

SAFFRON AND ANTIDIABETIC AGENT

Diabetes is characterized by a high blood sugar level and is one of the most prevalent diseases in the world. Diabetes seldom visits alone and is always surrounded by various complications that may turn out to be life threatening (Zareba et al., 2005). Saffron extracts are reported to have antihyperglycemic activity in the alloxan-induced diabetic rats. Nondiabetic rats were seen to have a hypoglycemic effect when provided with saffron extracts (Arasteh et al., 2010). Saffron is found to be the cause of regeneration of the β-cells in alloxan-induced diabetic rats and subsequently, increase in the level of insulin (Kianbhakt and Hajiahghee, 2011). Saffron-treated L6 myoblast cells showed a significant increase in glucose uptake, in a dose-dependent manner, under both hyperglycemic and normoglycemic condition. Furthermore, saffron consumption along with resistance exercise can cause a reduction in the fasting glucose level in rats (Dehgan et al., 2016). Significant reduction in the glycated hemoglobin has also been observed in various studies. Furthermore, GLUT-4 and AMPkα have been found to be upregulated both in vitro and in vivo studies (Dehgan et al., 2016). A summary of the targeted molecules that are known to be significant risk factors in metabolic syndrome by saffron and its derivatives (Fig: 18.3).

SAFFRON AND ANTIOXIDANT PROPERTY

Antioxidant properties of saffron are mainly due to crocin, one of the carotenoid components of the saffron (Mashmoul et al., 2013; Dehgan et al., 2016). Studies have shown that chronic treatment with saffron has resulted in a reduced level of glutathione, superoxide dismutase (SOD), and catalase (CAT) (Dehgan et al., 2016). Increased activity of SOD and glutathione peroxidase (GPx) can be related to the administration of crocin. Furthermore, the reduced level of malondialdehyde content in the ischemic cortex of rat has been reported when treated with crocin (Vakili et al., 2013). Saffron is reported to scavenge the cellular reactive oxygen species (ROS) (Samarghandian et al., 2014b). Linardaki et al. (2013) reported that saffron extracts reverse the monoamine oxidase activity and lipid peroxidation level when coadministered with aluminum (Linardaki et al., 2013).

SAFFRON AND NEUROPHARMACOLOGY EFFECT

Saffron and its active components such as crocin, crocetin, and safranal are supposed to have neuropharmacological effects in the peripheral and central nervous systems (Nassiri-Asl and Hosseinzadeh, 2015). Clinical trials have shown the beneficial role of saffron extracts in many of the neurodegenerative diseases and also in reducing opioid withdrawal syndrome (Nassiri-Asl., 2015). Furthermore, saffron is reported to protect neurons against different toxic insults. Crocin significantly inhibited the acrylamide-induced neurotoxicity through inhibition of oxidative stress and improved the behavioral and histopathological parameter (Mehri et al., 2015).

Cognitive Deficits

Cognition can be defined as the high processing of information, and cognitive deficit is an inclusive term that can be used to describe any variable that may hinder the cognition process (Trivedi et al., 2006). Continuous supplement of saffron is reported to have ameliorative effects on cognitive deficits. Saffron is also implicated in the prevention of learning and memory impairment. Moreover, saffron is said to have an enhancing effect on the memory (Pitsikas et al., 2007; Samarghandian et al., 2014b).

Anticonvulsant Effects

The anticonvulsant effect of saffron extract is studied where ethanolic and aqueous extracts of saffron were reported to be interfering with the pentylenetetrazole seizure and maximal electroshock seizure tests (Hosseinzadeh et al., 2002). Alcoholic extracts of saffron possess sleep-inducing effect, and this sedative potential of saffron aids in the anticonvulsant property of the saffron (Zhang et al., 1994). When safranal and crocin were studied for their probable effect on anticonvulsant effect; safranal was associated with the delayed onset of convulsions, decrease in the duration of seizure, and decrease in the mortality rate due to convulsion. On the other hand, crocin seems to have no anticonvulsant properties (Hosseinzadeh et al., 2005).

Antidepressant

Saffron is proved to be an important soldier in the battle against depression and anxiety—two of the most common mental health problems in the world. cAMP response element binding protein (CREB) is a transcription factor and is activated by phosphorylation at a specific serine residue. Furthermore, CREB regulates the neurotrophic factor brain-derived neurotrophic factor (BDNF)—one of the important molecules that is targeted in antidepressant treatment. BDNF is known to decrease in depressive condition. The protein level of phosphorylated CREB was observed to increase in the mice treated with saffron (Hassani et al., 2014; Asrari et al., 2018). Phosphorylated CREB then increases the level of BDNF. Saffron extracts are also found to decrease the Hamilton depression rating scale to about 10%—14% (Burke et al., 1995).

Learning Memory Effect

Alzheimer is a chronic ongoing condition with varied cognitive damage in different patients. Formation of neuritic plaques made up of amyloid peptides is associated with the pathophysiology of Alzheimer's disease (Goldsworthy and Vallence, 2013). Studies have shown that crocin and safranal exhibit a protective effect against Alzheimer's disease by inhibiting the amyloid protein aggregation and plaque formation (Howes and Perry, 2011). Thus, safranal is beneficial in the prevention of dementia. Ahmad et al. (2005) reported the beneficial effect of crocetin against Parkinson's disease. They observed that saffron improved the health of the neurons by reducing the utilization of dopamine in a rat model. A similar observation was made by Purushothuman et al. (2013) in an induced Parkinson mouse model where saffron protects substantia nigra pars compacta dopaminergic cells.

SAFFRON AND ANTIMICROBIAL EFFECT

Different parts of the saffron plant are reported to have antimicrobial properties. Ethyl acetate extract of stigma, stamen, leaves, and Corolla are reported to have antimicrobial efficacy against some fungi and bacteria (Vahidi et al., 2002). Methanol extracts, safranal, and crocin are demonstrated to inhibit the growth of *Helicobacter pylori* (Nakhaei et al., 2008). Aqueous and alcoholic extracts of saffron have been reported to have a significant bacteriostatic effect on the *Streptococcus mutans, Lactobacillus*, and antifungal effects on *Candida albicans*. Although alcoholic extracts seem to be more efficient bacteriostat and antifungal as compared to the aqueous extract (Karabasaki et al., 2016). Saffron can be utilized as an antimicrobial agent in food products as natural additives although, it has some limitations such as strong flavor and decrease in antimicrobial activity, which can be overcome by the use of other preservatives (Cenci-Goga et al., 2018).

SAFFRON AND IMMUNOMODULATORY EFFECT

Saffron has found to have a beneficial role in improving the immune system. An increase in the IgG level and a decrease in the IgM level have been reported in saffron-treated groups (Kianbakht and Ghazavi, 2011b). Saffron has found to regulate immune reactivity by inhibiting the histamine (H1) and muscarine receptors (Bani et al., 2011).

SAFFRON AND RESPIRATORY DISORDER

Saffron extracts were reported to have a significant effect on the respiratory system. Saffron and its bioactive compound have a relaxant effect on the smooth muscles of the trachea. The relaxant effect on smooth muscles leads to a bronchodilatory effect, which has a relieving effect in asthma effect (Bayrami et al., 2012).

SAFFRON AND ANTICANCER PROPERTIES

Anticancer properties of saffron have been established in different preclinical models both in vitro and in vivo. All the major constituents of saffron such as crocin, crocetin, and safranal were found to have significant anticancer activity in various tumors including prostate cancer (CaP), leukemia, lung cancer, etc. (Samargandhian and Shabestari, 2013, Samarghandian et al., 2013; Samarghandian and Borji, 2014; Samarghandhian et al., 2014a; Makhlouf et al., 2016). As saffron is composed of different phytochemicals and a number of phytochemicals inhibit tumor cells proliferation, it is believed that the additive and synergistic effect of various phytochemicals could enhance the efficacy against tumorigenesis (Festuccia et al., 2014; Milajerdi et al., 2016). Interestingly, saffron is found to be more effective when given orally, although its chemopreventive efficiency might be increased with liposome encapsulation (Zhang et al., 2013). Hoshyar and Mollaei (2017) observed that crocin, a major constituent of the saffron, inhibits the growth of cancerous cells but spare the normal/or noncancerous cells. In this direction, numerous studies reported that saffron extracts and its derivatives significantly inhibited the invasion, migration, and adhesion activity of cancer cell (Zhang et al., 2013; Hoshyar and Mollaei, 2017; Arzi et al., 2018). Saffron extracts were reported to possess antiinflammatory properties due to its strong antioxidant activity. The antiinflammatory effect of saffron is mainly due to crocin and crocetins (Poma et al., 2012). The extracts of saffron were found to be effective in decreasing the proinflammatory cytokines such as NO, TNF-α, and Il-β level in cultured microglia cells that were stimulated by lipopolysaccharide, a strong proinflammatory agent (Nam et al., 2010).

The antimetastatic properties of saffron were also documented in the triple negative breast cancer cells (4T1) (Arzi et al., 2018). The antimetastatic properties by crocin are suggested to be due to the interference with Wnt/β-catenin, downregulation of *NEDD9* and *VEGF-α* genes, and upregulation of *E-CAD* gene (Arzi et al., 2018). Crocin and crocetin show comparable inhibition of cancer cells invasion in 4T1 cells (Arzi et al., 2018). In another study, Al-Snafi. (2016) reported that cell viability of malignant carcinomic human alveolar basal epithelial cells was significantly decreased in a concentration and time-dependent manner when treated with ethanolic extract of saffron suggesting the antiproliferative effect of saffron. Similarly, saffron reduces the number and incidence of hepatic dyschromatic nodules in rats and delimits cell proliferation (Amin et al., 2011). Interestingly, Amin et al. (2011) also observed that saffron treatment significantly increased the cell cycle arrest in the liver cancer cells, HepG2, and altered the preneoplastic foci of hepatocytes. The same group in another study reported that crocin treatment prevents the preneoplastic events leading to Hepatocellular carcinoma (HCC) in an in vivo condition (Amin et al., 2015).

Saffron aqueous extract has been found to inhibit 1-methyl-3-nitro-1-nitrosoguanidine-induced gastric adenocarcinoma (Bathaie et al., 2013). Hoshyar et al. (2013) reported that saffron exhibited concentration and time-dependent cytotoxicity against a gastric adenocarcinoma cell line. In addition to its anticancer effect against gastric adenocarcinoma, saffron extract treatment on the colorectal cell lines (HCT-116, SW-480, and HT-29) showed a significant reduction in the survival and proliferation of cancer cells (Aung et al., 2007). Saffron derivatives were also reported to intervene with the proliferation of prostate cancer (CaP) cells (D'Alessandro and Mancini, 2013; Festuccia et al., 2014). Saffron derivatives, crocin, and crocetin treatment were reported to be associated with increased apoptosis and reduction in blood vessels, although crocetin seemed to have higher anticarcinogenic potential than crocin (Festuccia et al., 2014). D'Alessandro and Mancini. (2013) reported when malignant CaP cell lines were treated with saffron extracts and pure crocin, a significant dose- and time-dependent decrease in cell proliferation. Moradzadeh et al. (2019) observed that saffron derivatives were found to be effective against leukemia cells by inducing antiproliferative and

proapoptotic activity in the cells. When human T-cell leukemia cell line, MOLT-4 was evaluated for the chemopreventive effect of crocin, it exhibited a cytotoxic effect on leukemia cell line through DNA fragmentation (Rezaee et al., 2013). Crocin was also observed to downregulate antiapoptotic, proliferative, invasive, and angiogenic protein and upregulate proapoptotic protein in liver cancer cells (Kim and Park, 2018).

There are many probable mechanisms proposed on how saffron extracts exhibit chemopreventive activity (Fig. 18.4). Inhibition of synthesis of RNA and DNA is one of the proposed mechanisms by which crocin exerts its anticarcinogenic activity. Abdulaev and Frenkel (1992) had noted that when HeLa cells were treated with saffron, RNA and DNA synthesis was inhibited along with interference in the colony formation. In a study done by Sun et al. (2011), it was observed that 0.4 mM of crocin could downregulate the cellular RNA and DNA content of the tongue squamous carcinoma cell line Tca8113. In this study, they also observed that crocin capable of inducing both early and late apoptosis of the cell line. Saffron tends to show dose-dependent inhibitory effect on colony formation capability of tumor cells whereas normal cells remain unaffected (Zhang et al., 2013). Crocetin also shows chemopreventive activity in neoplastic cells by inhibiting RNA, DNA, and protein synthesis, RNA polymerase II. It also inhibits the histone H1 and H1-DNA structure interaction (Milajerdi et al., 2016). Epithelial-mesenchymal transition (EMT) is one of the characteristics of cancer cells and is marked by the E-cadherin, and cytokeratin repression failed cell-to-cell adhesion and increased cell migration. Saffron and its ingredient were found to reverse the EMT responses by increasing the E-cadherin expression and reducing the expression of N-cadherin and β-catenin (Festucci et al., 2014).

Oxidative stress is the apparent disturbance in the oxidant and antioxidant balance in scavenging reactive species production in the biological system (Siddique et al., 2007). Excess free radicals cause damages to all types of macromolecules and play a significant role in different stages of cancer. There are multiple reports available where researchers reported that saffron significantly reduces oxidative stress. Thus, the anticancer effect of saffron might be correlated to its ability to reduce oxidative stress by preventing the formation of free radicals. Antioxidant defense system plays an important role in defending the body against the damage instilled by the intermediate reactive species. Various signaling pathways that are involved in carcinogenesis are modulated by ROS (Saha et al., 2017). Oral treatment of

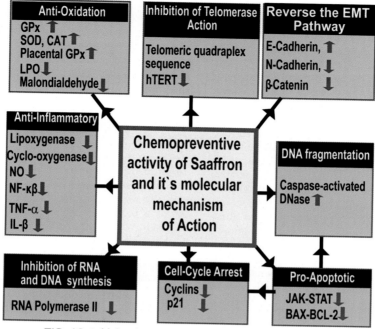

FIG. 18.4 Molecular targets of saffron and its components.

saffron on 7,12 dimethylbenz[a]anthracene-treated mice had revealed the beneficial role of saffron (Das et al., 2010). Saffron treatment slowdowns the 7,12-Dimethylbenz[a]anthracene (DMBA)-induced skin carcinoma with the help of antioxidant defense systems. Saffron helps in elevating the serum level of antioxidant enzymes such as SOD, CAT, GPx, and GST (Das et al., 2010). In another study, Nair et al. (1995), suggested that saffron exerted its chemopreventive effect by regulating lipid peroxidation and antioxidant activity. Nair et al. (1995) treated the animals simultaneously with saffron and cyclophosphamide and observed that saffron significantly decreases the bladder toxicity without affecting its antitumor activity.

Magesh et al. (2006) reported that crocetin could reverse the carcinogen effect on induced lung cancer model. Crocetin treatment was observed to restore normal levels of Lipid Peroxidation (LPO) and other enzyme markers in benzo(a) pyrene-induced lung cancer-bearing mice. (Magesh et al., 2006). Saffron is also reported to increase the antioxidant capability in 1-methyl-3-nitro-1-nitrosoguanidine-induced cancer groups. Saffron was found to improve the level of antioxidants in a dose-dependent manner in rats (Bathaie et al., 2013). Placental glutathione S-transferase (GST) belongs to the antioxidant family of GST enzymes and

serves as a marker of liver preneoplastic lesions in rats (Suzuku et al., 2004). When diethyl nitrosamine (DEN)-treated rats were treated with saffron, a significant decrease in the number of placental GST positive foci was observed in the liver. Saffron was also observed to reverse the DEN-induced oxidative stress in rat's liver (Amin et al., 2011). Restoration of the activity of major antioxidant enzymes such as SOD, CAT, and GPx was noticed, and decreased activity of myeloperoxidase decreased the level of malondialdehyde and protein carbonyl was observed in the liver (Amin et al., 2011).

Telomeres are G-rich nucleotides repeats that are present at the chromosome terminus and replicate with the help of telomerase. In normal cells, telomere shortens continuously with every cell division and activates the senescence. However, in cancer cell lines, telomeres continue to divide withholding the senescent period and acquiring immortality (Artendi and DePinho, 2010). It was reported that crocin-treated HepG2 cell line shows decreased telomerase activity as compared to untreated cancer cell lines. This is due to the interaction of crocin with telomeric quadruplex sequences and downregulation hTERT gene (Noureini and Wink, 2012).

Saffron is observed to have a proapoptotic effect in cancerous cells. Mousavi et al. (2009) has reported that saffron extract decreases cell viability in the MCF-7 breast cancer cell line. Saffron induces apoptosis in the MCF-7 cell line through caspase-dependent pathway. Moreover, activation of caspase was found to be responsible for the activation of caspase-activated DNase (CAD). CAD participates in the chromatin cleavage at internucleosomal sites and DNA fragmentation (Mousavi et al., 2009). Crocin was found to be regulating growth and apoptosis of the cancer cell by regulating the IL-6/STAT3 pathway. Crocin also reported to inhibit STAT3 in Hep3B and HepG2 cells by inactivating Janus Kinases (JAK1, JAK2) and Src Kinase. Crocin was reported to demonstrate the antiproliferative and antitumorigenicity effect on human HL-60 cells through apoptosis and cell cycle arrest (Sun et al., 2013). In another study, N-nitroso-N-methyl urea-induced breast tumors were reported to be suppressed by crocin treatment. A significant decrease in the expression of Cyclin D1, p21 in p53 dependent manner has been observed indicating that crocin treatment induced apoptosis and cell cycle arrest in the tumor cells (Ashrafi et al., 2015).

In a study done by Zhong et al. (2011), it has been observed that crocetin can induce apoptosis in HeLa, A549, and SKOV3 cells, in a time and concentration-dependent manner with highest cell death accounted at 72 h before treatment. The viability of various cancer cells was found to be significantly decreased when they were incubated with saffron in a time and concentration-dependent manner. High Bax/Bcl-2 ratio was found in the sample that suggests that saffron induces apoptosis in the cancer cell (Behdani et al., 2016). Saffron was reported to exhibit apoptosis in alveolar human lung cancer cells through the activation of caspase-dependent pathways (Samargandhian and Shabestari, 2013). Safranal exhibited a potential chemopreventive effect on prostate cancer cells by activating apoptosis in the cells (Makhlouf et al., 2016).

Serum level of many inflammatory cytokines has been reported to be upregulated in many cancers. Crocin eliminated chronic inflammation in HCC-induced rats by restoring the level of proinflammatory cytokines such as NO, TNF-α, and NF-$\kappa\beta$. Furthermore, a significant decrease in the number of TNF-R1 positive cells has been observed (Amin et al., 2015). Chen et al. (2015) reported that crocetin could reduce the interleukin-1β and tumor necrosis factor-α in methylcholanthrene-induced cervical cancer in mice. Saffron extracts were also reported to inhibit the enzymes that are involved in inflammation in cancer pathologies. Studies have shown that phenolic compounds of saffron inhibit 5-lipoxygenase and cyclooxygenase (Behdani et al., 2016).

There are several other hypotheses that have been discussed and put forward; however, the exact mechanism by which saffron exerts the anticarcinogenic and chemopreventive effect is warranted for further investigations.

OTHER APPLICATIONS

Saffron has been reported to have aphrodisiac properties in both animal and human. Simultaneous administration of saffron and selective serotonin reuptake inhibitors has a beneficial role in sexual functions and also seem to improve the libido, lubrication, and act as a pain reliever in sexual dysfunction patients (Hosseinzadeh et al., 2008; Modabberina et al., 2012; Kashani et al., 2013).

PERSPECTIVE ON CLINICAL TRIAL

Data obtained from all the preclinical and clinical trials have shown that the saffron might help in the treatment of many diseases but need thorough investigation. Promising results have been seen from a few clinical studies, but solid conclusions are yet to be drawn from them. Various useful effects have already been documented about this phytomedicine, and many effects are ready to be sent to clinical trials.

CONCLUSION

Saffron has started its journey as a spice and traditional herb since centuries and has gained its significance in the pharmaceutical and clinical field. Saffron contains some bioactive phytochemical compounds that have been found useful against several diseases such as metabolic disorder, neurological, and cancer. Cancer is one of the deadliest diseases around the world, and the limited therapeutic action requires more rigorous effect. Although not much is known about its mechanism of action, the ongoing research suggested that saffron could be a potential therapeutic agent against cancer. However, further evidence and extensive research are needed to guarantee the use of saffron as a chemopreventive agent in clinical trials.

ACKNOWLEDGMENTS

The authors are thankful to the chairman, Department of Zoology, AMU, Aligarh for timely help. HF and MAK express their sincere gratitude to UGC and CSIR, India for fellowships, respectively. HRS is thankful to the UGC [Grant no. F.30-377/2017(BSR)] and DST-SERB (Grant No. EMR/20l7/001758), New Delhi, for providing financial help.

Conflict of interest: All the authors declare that there is no conflict of interest.

REFERENCES

Abdullaev, F.I., Frenkel, G.D., 1992. Effect of saffron on cell colony formation and cellular nucleic acid and protein synthesis. Biofactors 3, 201–204.

Ahmad, A.S., Ansari, M.A., Ahmad, M., Saleem, S., Yousuf, S., Hoda, M.N., Islam, F., 2005. Neuroprotection by crocetin in a hemi-Parkinsonian rat model. Pharmacol. Biochem. Behav. 81 (4), 805–813.

Al-Sanafi, A.E., 2016. Medicinal plants with anticancer effects (part 2)- Plant based review. SAJP 5 (5), 175–193.

Amin, A., Hamza, A.A., Bajbouj, K., Ashraf, S.S., Saffron, S.D., 2011. A potential candidate for a novel anticancer drug against hepatocellular carcinoma. Hepatology 54 (3), 857–867.

Amin, A., Hamza, A.A., Daoud, S., Khazanehdari, K., Hrout, A.A., Baig, B., Chaiboonchoe, A., Adrian, T.E., Salehi-Ashtiani, Zaki, N., 2015. Saffron-based crocin prevents early lesions of liver cancer: in vivo, in vitro and network analyses. Recent Pat. Anticancer Drug Discov. 10 (999), 1–13.

Arasteh, A., Aliyev, A., Khamnei, S., Delazar, A., Mesgari, M., Mehmannavaz, Y., 2010. Effects of hydromethanolic extract of saffron (Crocus sativus) on serum glucose, insulin and cholesterol levels in healthy male rats. J. Med. Plants Res. 4, 397–402.

Artandi, S.E., DePinho, R.A., 2010. Telomeres and telomerase in cancer. Carcinogenesis 31 (1), 9–18.

Arzi, L., Riazi, G., Sadeghizadeh, M., Hoshyar, R., Jafarzadeh, N., 2018. A comparative study on anti-invasion, antimigration, and antiadhesion effects of the bioactive carotenoids of saffron on 4T1 breast cancer cells through their effects on Wnt/β-catenin pathway genes. DNA Cell Biol. 37 (8), 697–707.

Ashrafi, M., Bathaie, S.Z., Abroun, S., Azizian, M., 2015. Effect of crocin on cell cycle regulators in N-nitroso-N-Methylurea-induced breast cancer in rats. DNA Cell Biol. 34 (11), 684–691.

Asrari, N., Yazdian-Robati, R., Abnous, K., Razavi, B.M., Rashednia, M., Hasani, F.V., Hosseinzadeh, H., 2018. Antidepressant effects of aqueous extract of saffron and its effects on CREB, P-CREB, BDNF, and VGF proteins in rat cerebellum. J. Pharmacopuncture 21 (1), 35–40 (2018).

Aung, H.H., Wang, C.Z., Ni, M., Fishbein, A., Mehendale, S.R., Xie, J.T., Shoyama, C.Y., Yuan, C.S., 2007. Crocin from Crocus sativus possesses significant anti-proliferation effects on human colorectal cancer cells. Exp. Oncol. (3), 175–180.

Bani, S., Pandey, A., Agnihotri, V.K., Pathania, V., Singh, B., 2011. Selective Th2 Upregulation by Crocus Sativus: A Neutraceutical Spice. Hindawi Publishing Corporation, pp. 1–9. Evid Based Complement Alternat Med (2011).

Bathaie, S.Z., Mousavi, Z., 2010. New applications and mechanisms of action of saffron and its important ingredients. Crit. Rev. Food Sci. Nutr. 50, 761–786.

Bathaie, S.Z., Miri, H., Mohagheghi, M.A., Mokhtari-Dizaji, M., Shahbazfar, A.A., Hasanzadeh, H., 2013. Saffron aqueous extract inhibits the chemically-induced gastric cancer progression in the Wistar albino rat. Iran J Basic Med Sci 16 (1), 27–38.

Bayrami, G., Boskabadi, M.H., 2012. The potential effect of the extract of Crocus sativus and safranal on the toral and different white blood cells of ovalbumine-sensitized Guinea pigs. RPS 7, 249–255.

Behdani, M.A., Hoshyar, R., 2016. Phytochemical properties of Iranian organic saffron stigma: antioxidant, anticancer and apoptotic approaches. Cell. Mol. Biol. 62 (14), 69–73.

Bhargava, V., 2011. Medicinal uses and pharmacological properties of Crocus sativus LINN (saffron). Int. J. Pharm. Pharm. Sci. 3 (3), 22–26 (2011).

Burke, M.J., Preskorn, S.H., 1995. Standard antidepressant pharmacotherapy for the acute treatment of mood disorders. In: Bloom, E.F., Kupfer, D.J. (Eds.), Psychopharmacology – 4th Generation of Progress. Raven Press, New York.

Cenci-Goga, B.T., Torricelli, R., Gonabad, Y.H., Ferradini, N., Venanzoni, R., Sechi, P., Iulietto, M.F., Albertini, E., 2018. In vitro bactericidal activities of various extracts of saffron (Crocus sativus L.) stigmas from Torbat-e Heydarieh, Gonabad and Khorasan, Iran. Microbiol. Res. 9, 7583.

Chen, B., Hou, Z.H., Dong, Z., Li, C.D., 2015. Crocetin down-regulates the proinflammatory cytokines in methylcholanthrene-induced rodent tumor model and inhibits COX-2 expression in cervical cancer cells. BioMed Res. Int. 829513.

D'Alessandro, A.M., Mancini, A., Lizzi, A.R., 2013. Crocus sativus stigma extract and its major constituent crocin possess significant antiproliferative properties against human prostate cancer. Nutr. Cancer 65 (6), 930–942.

Das, I., Das, S., Saha, T., 2010. Saffron suppresses oxidative stress in DMBA-induced skin carcinoma: a histopathological study. Acta Histochem. 112 (4), 317–327.

Dehghan, F., Hajiaghaalipour, F., Yusof, A., Muniandy, S., Hosseini, S.A., Heydari, S., Salim, L.Z., Azarbayjani, M.A., 2016. Saffron with resistance exercise improves diabetic parameters through the GLUT4/AMPK pathway in-vitro and in-vivo. Sci. Rep. 28 (6), 25139.

Festuccia, C., Mancini, A., Gravina, G.L., Scarsella, L., Llorens, S., Alonso, G.L., Tatone, C., Di Cesare, E., Jannini, E.A., Lenzi, A., D'Alessandro, A.M., Carmona, M., 2014. Antitumor Effects of Saffron-Derived Carotenoids in Prostate Cancer Cell Models, p. 135048.

Goldsworthy, M.R., Vallence, A.M., 2013. The role of β-amyloid in alzheimer's disease-related neurodegeneration. J. Neurosci. 33 (32), 12910–12911.

Gout, B., Bourges, C., Paineau-Dubreuil, S., 2010. Satiereal, a Crocus sativus L extract, reduces snacking and increases satiety in a randomized placebo-controlled study of mildly overweight, healthy women. Nutr. Res. 30, 305–313.

Han, T.S., Lean, M.E.J., 2016. A clinical perspective of obesity, metabolic syndrome and cardiovascular disease. JRSM Cardiovascular Dis. 5, 2048004016633371.

Hassani, F.V., Naseri, V., Razavi, B.M., Mehri, S., Abnous, K., Hosseinzadeh, H., 2014. Antidepressant effects of crocin and its effects on transcript and protein levels of CREB, BDNF, and VGF in rat hippocampus. Daru 22 (1), 16.

Hemmati, M., Zohoori, E., Mehrpour, O., Karamian, M., Asghari, S., Zarban, A., Nasouti, R., 2015. Anti-atherogenic potential of Jujube, saffron and barberry: anti-diabetic and antioxidant actions. Excli. J. 14, 908–915.

Hoshyar, R., Mollaei, H., 2017. A comprehensive review on anticancer mechanisms of the main carotenoid of saffron, crocin. J. Pharm. Pharmacol. 69 (11), 1419–1427.

Hoshyar, R., Bathaie, S.Z., Sadeghizadeh, M., 2013. Crocin triggers the apoptosis through increasing the Bax/Bcl-2 ratio anFd caspase activation in human gastric adenocarcinoma, AGS, cells. DNA Cell Biol. 32 (2), 50–57.

Hosseinzadeh, H., Khosravan, V., 2002. Anticonvulsant effects of aqueous and ethanolic extracts of Crocus sativus L. Stigmas in mice. Arch. Irn. Med. 5 (1), 44–47.

Hosseinzadeh, H., Talebzadeh, F., 2005. Anticonvulsant evaluation of safranal and crocinfrom Crocus sativus in mice. Fitoterapia 76 (7–8), 722–724.

Hosseinzadeh, H., Ziaee, T., Sadeghi, A., 2008. The effect of saffron, Crocus sativus stigma, extract and its constituents, safranal and crocin on sexual behaviors in normal male rats. Phytomedicine 15 (6–7), 491–495.

Howes, M.L., Perry, E., 2011. The role of phytochemicals in the treatment and prevention of dementia. Drugs Aging. 2, 439–468 (2011).

Karbasaki, B.F., Hosseinzadeh, H., Sedigheh, F.B.B., Hoda, V., Kiarash, G., Molok, A.B., 2016. Evaluation of antimicrobial effects of aqueous and alcoholic extracts of saffron on oral pathogenic microbes (Streptococcus mutans, Lactobacillus, Candida albicans). J. Mash. Dent. Sch. 40 (3), 203–212.

Kashani, L., Raisi, F., Saroukhani, S., Sohrabi, H., Moddaberina, A., Nasehi, A.A., Jamshedi, A., Ashrafi, M., Mansouri, P., Ghaeli, P., Akhondzadeh, S., 2013. Saffron for treatment of fluoxetine-induced sexual dysfunction in women: randomized double-blind placebo-controlled study. Hum. Psychopharmacol. Clin. Exp. 28 (1), 54–56.

Kianbakht, S., Ghazavi, A., 2011. Immunomodulatory effects of saffron: a randomized double-blind placebo-controlled clinical trial. Phytother Res. 25 (12), 1801–1805.

Kianbakht, S., Hajiahghee, R., 2011. Anti-hyperglycemic effects of saffron and its active constituents, crocin and safranal, in alloxan-induced diabetic rats. J. Med. Plant 10 (39), 82–89.

Kianbakht, S., Hasheem, D.F., 2015. Anti-obesity and anorectic effects of saffron and its constituent crocin in obese Wistar rat. J. Med. Plant 14 (53), 25–33.

Kim, B., Park, B., 2018. Saffron carotenoids inhibit STAT3 activation and promote apoptotic progression in IL-6-stimulated liver cancer cells. Oncol Rep. 39 (4), 1883–1891.

Linardaki, Z.I., Orkoula, M.G., Kokkosis, A.G., Lamari, F.N., Margarity, M., 2013. Investigation of the neuroprotective action of saffron (Crocus sativus L.) in aluminum exposed adult mice through behavioral and neurobiochemical assessment. Food Chem. Toxicol. 52, 163–170.

Magesh, V., Singh, J.P., Selvendiran, K., Ekambaram, G., Sakthisekaran, D., 2006. Antitumour activity of crocetin in accordance to tumor incidence, antioxidant status, drug metabolizing enzymes and histopathological studies. Mol. Cell. Biochem. 287 (1–2), 127–135.

Makhlouf, H., Diab, M., Alghabsha, M., Tannoury, M., Chahine, R., Saab, A., Saab, M.T.A., 2016. In vitro antiproliferative activity of saffron extracts against human acute lymphoblastic T-cell human leukemia. Indian J. Tradit. Knowl. 15 (1), 16–21.

Mashmoul, M., Azlan, A., Khaza'ai, H., Nisak, B., Yusof, M., Saffron, S.M.N., 2013. A natural potent antioxidant as a promising anti-obesity. Drug. Antioxidants. 2, 293–308.

Mehri, S., Abnous, K., Khooei, A., Mousavi, S.H., Shariaty, V.M., Hosseinzadeh, H., 2015. Crocin reduced acrylamide-induced neurotoxicity in Wistar rat through inhibition of oxidative stress. Iran J Basic Med Sci 18 (9), 902–908 (2015).

Milajerdi, A., Djafarian, K., Hosseini, B., 2016. The toxicity of saffron (Crocus sativus L.) and its constituents against normal and cancer cells. Nutr. Intermed. Metab. 3, 23–32.

Modabbernia, A., Sohrabi, H., Nasehi, A.A., Raisi, F., Saroukhani, S., Jamshidi, A., Tabrizi, M., Ashrafi, M., Akhondzadeh, S., 2012. Effect of saffron on fluoxetine-induced sexual impairment in men: randomized double-blind placebo-controlled trial. Psychopharmacology (Berl) 223 (4), 381–388.

Moradzadeh, M., Kalani, R.M., Avan, A., 2019. The antileukemic effects of saffron (Crocus sativus L.) and its related molecular targets: a mini review. J. Cell. Biochem. 120 (4), 4732–47388.

Mousavi, S.H., Tavakkol-Afshari, J., Brook, A., Jafari-Anarkooli, I., 2009. Role of caspases and Bax protein in saffron-induced apoptosis in MCF-7 cells. Food Chem. Toxicol. 47, 1909–1913 (2009).

Mueller, M., Beck, V., Jungbauer, A., 2011. PPARα activation by culinary herbs and spices. Planta Med. 77, 497–504.

Nair, S.C., Kurumboor, S.K., Hasegawa, J.H., 1995. Saffron chemoprevention in biology and medicine: a review. Cancer Biother. 10 (4), 257–264.

Nakhaei, M., Khaje-Karamoddin, M., Ramezani, M., 2008. Inhibition of Helicobacter pylori growth in vitro by saffron (Crocus sativus L.). Iranian J. Basic Med. Sci. 11, 91–96.

Nam, K.N., Park, Y.M., Jung, H.J., Lee, J.Y., Min, B.D., Park, S.U., Jung, W.S., Cho, K.H., H Park, J., Kang, I., Hong, J.W., Lee, E.H., 2010. Anti-inflammatory effects of crocin and crocetin in rat brain microglial cells. Eur. J. Pharmacol. 648 (1–3), 110–116.

Namayendeha, A., Nemati, Z., Kamelmanesch, M., 2013. Genetic relationships among species of Iranian crocus (Crocus spp.). Crop Breed J 3 (1), 61–67.

Nasiri, Z., Sameni, H.R., Vakili, A., Jarrahi, M., Khorasani, M.Z., 2015. Dietary saffron reduced the blood pressure and prevented remodeling of the aorta in L-NAME-induced hypertensive rats. Iranian J. Basic Med. Sci. 18, 1143–1146.

Nassiri-Asl, M., Hosseinzadeh, H., 2015. Neuropharmacology effects of saffron (Crocus sativus) and its active constituents. In: Bioactive Nutraceuticals and Dietary Supplements in Neurological and Brain Disease, 1, pp. 29–39.

Noureini, S.K., Wink, M., 2012. Antiproliferative effects of crocin in HepG2 cells by telomerase inhibition and hTERT down-regulation. Asian Pac. J. Cancer Prev. 13 (5), 2305–2309.

Pitsikas, N., Zisopoulou, S., Tarantilis, P.A., Kanakis, C.D., Polissiou, M.G., Sakellaridis, N., 2007. Effects of the active constituents of Crocus sativus L., crocins on recognition and spatial rats' memory. Behav. Brain Res. 183 (2), 141–146, 2007.

Poma, A., Fontecchio, G., Carlucci, G., Chichiriccò, G., 2012. Anti-inflammatory properties of drugs from saffron crocus. Antiinflamm Antiallergy Agents Med Chem 11 (1), 37–51.

Purushothuman, S., Nandasena, C., Peoples, C.L., El-Massri, N., Johnstone, D.M., Mitrofanis, J., Stone, J., 2013. Saffron pre-treatment offers neuroprotection to Nigral and retinal dopaminergic cells of MPTP-Treated mice. J. Parkinson's Dis. 3, 77–83.

Razavi, B.M., Saffron, H.H., 2016. A promising natural medicine in the treatment of metabolic syndrome. J. Sci. Food Agric. 97 (6), 1679–1685.

Rezaee, R., Mahmoudi, M., Abnous, K., Zamini, S.R.T., Hashemzaei, M., Karimi, G., 2013. Cytotoxic effects of crocin on MOLT-4 human leukemia cells. J. Complement. Integr. Med. 10 (1) jcim.2013.

Rios, J., Recio, M., Giner, R., Manez, S., 1996. An update review of saffron and its active constituents. Phytother Res. 10, 189–193.

Saha, S.K., Lee, S.B., Won, J., Choi, H.Y., Kim, K., Yang, G.M., Dayem, A.A., Cho, S.G., 2017. Correlation between oxidative stress, nutrition and cancer initiation. Int. J. Mol. Sci. 18 (7), 1544.

Samargandhian, S., Shabestari, M.M., 2013. DNA Freagmentation and apoptosis induced by safranal in human Prostate cancer cell line. Indian J. Urol. 29 (3), 177–183.

Samarghandhian, S., Shoshtari, M.E., Sargolzaei, J., Hossinimoghadam, H., Farahzad, J.A., 2014a. Antitumor activity of saffranal against neuroblastoma cells. Pharmacogn. Mag. 10 (2), 419–424.

Samarghandian, S., Borji, A., 2014. Anticarcinogenic effect of saffron (Crocus sativus L.) and its ingredients. Pharmacogn. Res. 6 (2), 99–107.

Samarghandian, S., Borji, A., Farahmand, S.K., Afshari, R., Davoodi, S., 2013. Crocus sativus L. (Saffron) stigma aqueous extract induces apoptosis in alveolar human lung cancer cells through caspase-dependent pathways activation. BioMed Res. Int. 2013, 1–12.

Samarghandian, S., Azimi-Nezhad, M., Samini, F., 2014. Ameliorative effect of saffron aqueous extract on hyperglycemia, hyperlipidemia, and oxidative stress on diabetic encephalopathy in streptozotocin induced experimental diabetes mellitus. BioMed Res. Int. 920857.

Schmidt, M., Betti, G., Hensel, A., 2007. Saffron in phytotherapy: pharmacology and clinical uses. Wien. Med. Wochenschr. 157, 315–319.

Shemshian, M., Mousavi, S.H., Norouzy, A., Kermani, T., Moghiman, T., Sadeghi, A., Ghayour-Mobarhan, M., Ferns, G.A., 2014. Saffron in metabolic syndrome: its effects on antibody titers to heat-shock proteins 27, 60, 65 and 70. J. Complement. Integr. Med. 11 (1), 43–49.

Sheng, L., Qian, Z., Zheng, S., Xi, L., 2006. Mechanism of hypolipidemic effect of crocin in rats: crocin inhibits pancreatic lipase. Eur. J. Pharmacol. 543 (1–3), 116–122.

Siddique, H.R., Saleem, M., 2011. Beneficial health effects of lupeol triterpene: a review of preclinical studies. Life Sci. 88 (7–8), 285–293.

Siddique, H.R., Gupta, S.C., Mitra, K., C Murthy, R., Saxena, D.K., Chowdhari, D.K., 2007. Induction of biochemical stress markers and apoptosis in transgenic Drosophila melanogaster against complex chemical mixtures: role of reactive oxygen species. Chem. Biol. Interact. 169 (3), 171–188.

Siddique, H.R., Mishra, S.K., Karnes, R.J., Lupeol, M.S., 2011. A novel androgen receptor inhibitor: implications in prostate cancer therapy. Clin. Cancer Res. 17 (16), 5379–5391.

Siddique, H.R., Liao, D.J., Mishra, S.K., Schuster, T., Wang, L., Matter, B., Campbell, P.M., Villalta, P., Nanda, S., Deng, Y., Saleem, M., 2012a. Epicatechin-rich cocoa polyphenol inhibits Kras-activated pancreatic ductal carcinoma cell growth in vitro and in a mouse model. Int. J. Cancer 131 (7), 1720–1731.

Siddique, H.R., Schuster, T., Lupeol, M.S., 2012b. A novel inhibitor of Wnt/β-catenin signaling: implications in colon cancer therapy. Cancer Res. 72 (8), pp. 3847–3847.

Sun, J., Xu, X.M., Ni, C.Z., Zhang, H., Li, X.Y., Zhang, C.L., Liu, Y.R., Li, S.F., Zhou, Q.Z., Zhou, H.M., 2011. Crocin inhibits proliferation and nucleic acid synthesis and induces apoptosis in the human tongue squamous cell carcinoma cell line Tca8113. Asian Pac. J. Cancer Prev. 12 (10), 2679–2683.

Sun, Y., Hu, H.J., Zhao, Y.X., Wang, L.Z., Sun, L.R., Wang, Z., Sun, X.F., 2013. Crocin exhibits antitumor effects on human leukemia HL-60 cells in vitro and in vivo. Evid. Based Complementary Alter. Med. E690164.

Suzuku, S., Asamoto, M., Tsujimura, K., Shirai, T., 2004. Specific differences in gene expression profile revealed by cDNA microarray analysis of glutathione S-transferase placental form (GST-P) immunohistochemically positive rat liver foci and surrounding tissue. Carcinogenesis 25 (3), 439–443 (2004).

Trivedi, J.K., 2006. Cognitive deficits in psychiatric disorders: current status. Indian J. Psychiatr. 48 (1), 10–20.

Vahidi, H., Kamalinejad, M., Sedaghati, N., 2002. Antimicrobial properties of Crocus sativus L. Int. J. Pharmacol. Res. 1, 33–35.

Vakili, A., Einali, M.R., Bandegi, A.R., 2013. Protective effect of crocin against cerebral ischemia in a dose- dependent manner in a rat model of ischemic stroke. J. Stroke Cerebrovasc. Dis. 23 (1), 106–113.

Wani, B.A., Hamza, A.K.R., Mohiddin, F.A., 2011. Saffron: A repository of medicinal properties. J. Med. Plants Res. 5 (11), 2131–2135.

Zareba, G., Serradell, R., Castaner, R., Davies, S.L., Prous, J., Mealy, N., 2005. Phytotherapies for diabetes. Drugs Future 30, 1253–1282.

Zhang, Y., Shoyama, Y., Sugiura, M., Saito, H., 1994. Effect of *Crocus sativus* L. on the ethanol-induced impairment of passive avoidance performances in mice. Biol. Pharm. Bull. 17, 217–221.

Zhang, Z., Wang, C.Z., Wen, X.D., Shoyama, Y., Yuan, C.S., 2013. Role of saffron and its constituents on cancer chemoprevention. Pharm. Biol. 51 (7), 920–924.

CHAPTER 19

The Remarkable Pharmacological Efficacy of Saffron Spice via Antioxidant, Immunomodulatory, and Antitumor Activities

HAMID A. BAKSHI • HAKKIM L. FARUCK • SANGILIMUTHU ALAGAR YADAV • MURTAZA M. TAMBUWALA

INTRODUCTION

Cancer is considered as the uncontrolled unnatural proliferation of cells in the human tissue system, which may end in fatality. Cells having abnormality with cancer are also called malignant; these cells naturally attack to kill the good cells. The birth of these cells is due to disequilibrium in the body, which can be handled by removing the disequilibrium, which would cure the cancer. Multimillion dollars are being spent yearly on cancer research, but still, the cause of cancer is far from our reach (Jemal et al., 2005). Several million people are new victims of this disease yearly and go on the verge of death. About 2%–3% deaths worldwide are due to cancer as per report published in 2006 by American Cancer Society. Owing to cancer, around 3500 million people are killed yearly in the world. Many chemical agents are used to cure the diseases, but the treatment leads to severe adverse effects, prohibiting the administration of these chemical agents (Kathiresan et al., 2006).

Cancer is considered as the world's second major cause of death. The main reasons for occurrence of the diseases are chewing of tobacco, smoking, imbalances in diet and hormones, and chronic inflammation (Ames et al., 1995). Worldwide breast cancer is considered to be widespread among women (Koduru et al., 2007). Among South-African women, about 3% of women are affected by breast cancer (Koduru et al., 2007). Further in line is the spread of colon cancer in the United States. Among US men, carcinoma of the prostate is widespread and identified with an estimate of around 0.2 million new cases and 37K deaths expected yearly, as per 1999 report of American Cancer Society. With increased longevity in India, the cancer disease is going to be a threat, as most common cancer in elderly is digestive tract cancer.

About 6% men and women are detected with gastrointestinal cancer at certain stage in their life in the United States. Many people are seeking alternative or complimentary line of treatment because of threat of death by cancer and severe side effects associated with chemotherapy and radiation therapy. The significant line of treatment for cancers include lifestyle changes such as dietary changes, avoiding of tobacco products, treating inflammation efficiently with intake of nutritional supplements to enhance immune response. Contemporary study is seeking solutions to find effective drugs for chemotherapy without any side effect having new horizons in understanding cell biology.

In current standard treatment system, chemotherapy is the most prominent option for advanced stages of cancer which leads to metastasis. However, cause serious side effects to normal tissues(Somkumar 2003; Pandey and Madhuri, 2006).

Traditional medicines from plants are being used since thousands of years all over the world for various ailments in human and animals. They cure ailments including cancer with no toxicity and not affecting the health and vitality of the patient. Around half of the contemporary drugs are from plant origin, and most of them have the capability to control spread of cancer cells (Rosangkima and Prasad, 2004). As per the World Health Organisation about four-fifth of the people in developing world opt for natural drugs of plant origin for their main source for cure. A contemporary study indicated more than 60% people rely on vitamins or herbs for their cancer cure (Madhuri and Pandey, 2008; Sivlokanathum et al., 2005).

Since a decade, natural drugs are being accepted world over and have made a difference in health as well as international trade of these herbal medicines.

This also made possible the world's large population to use these medicines and improve the health (Akerele, 1988). India is a major user of herbal medicines. The United States has also been using the plants and phytomedicines on large scale since last 2 decades. The United States has established a National Center for Complementary and Integrative Health (NCCIH). The natural herbal medicines are being used as diet supplements along with essential vitamins, amino acids, and minerals (Rao et al., 2004). Consuming natural herbal products is considered a routine for any ailment in the South-African cultural life. As per an estimate, about 27 million South Africans normally consume herbs from more than 1000 varieties of plants (Koduru et al., 2007; Meyer et al., 1996). Number of herbal products, world over, including India, are used from ancient times for cancer prevention and therapy. Select medicinal plants have been of interest to scientists for study of the natural products and for cure of carcinoma or tumor.

CHEMOPREVENTION

By avoiding the exposure to known carcinogens, cancer risk can be reduced, but many of the unknown carcinogens do exist, and it is difficult to avoid their exposure unless proper identifications are done. Moreover, the prevention of exposure to some of these compounds being used in daily life requires major lifestyle changes, which are difficult to achieve. Lifestyle modification alone can help prevent almost 66% cancer cases according to researchers. Doll and Petro (1981) indicated that about 10%–70% (mean 35%) cancers are associated to diet, based on the study of diseases in humans and statistical data, significantly covering the food items that enhance the risk. Although the exact number is ambiguous, there are numerous evidences from clinical, epidemiological, and laboratory research that confirm cancer risk to be associated to the dietary factors.

The contemporary study uses modified diets and nutritional supplements to prevent cancer. It is envisaged that people may need to consume exclusive pills or two, prepared from herbal products, to prevent or delay the outbreak of cancer (Greenwald, 1996). However, an appropriate study of the mechanisms and the constituents of fruit and vegetables help fight cancer is mandatory prior to recommendation for their inclusion in supplementary diet or prior to the clinical study.

Biologically active compounds known as phytochemicals are low-energy compounds in traditional natural diet that have significant anticarcinogenic and antimutagenic properties. Having known the large structural variations of phytochemicals, it is difficult to define structure–activity correlation to infer their basic molecular mechanisms. An improved technique would be to study their impact on cancer-related signal transduction pathways.

It has been indicated by studies that the risk of developing cancer in South East Asian population is far lower than those in North America and is attributed to the routine use of ingredients such as cruciferous vegetables, turmeric, cayenne, soy, garlic, and ginger in their diet, which work as chemoprevention.

Several studies have mentioned plant-based chemopreventive ingredients or compounds and their capabilities for prevention and control of cancer. Since these chemopreventive compounds are obtained from natural food products, they are considered safe pharmacologically. The content of these dietary ingredients are wide range of different compounds such as polyphenols from green tea, curcumin from turmeric, and organosulfur compounds from garlic (Sporn, 1976).

Cancer prevention, control, and management by these phytochemical compounds is recognized as accessible, acceptable, inexpensive, and readily applicable. Promoting the awareness to consume these natural phytochemicals for prevention and control of cancer would be appreciated, specially with rising cost of health care for people at large. Many natural components such as carbohydrates, fats, and proteins, as well as vitamins, minerals, and fibers from plants are under study for their use as cancer-preventive drugs. In spite of important advances in mechanism of understanding cancer spread, very little is known about cancer preventive agent's mechanism of action. The action of natural phytochemical drugs is likely to have a combination of many distinct chemopreventive mechanisms. Disturbance or irregularity of intracellular-signaling cascades leads to growth of cancer cell from healthy cells; hence, it is significant to understand chemical signaling mechanism and the network, which get affected by individual chemopreventive natural product to get improved idea of their basic mechanisms.

FREE RADICALS AND ANTIOXIDANTS

Toxic byproducts of oxygen metabolism are recognized as free radicals and are highly sensitive species. Ordinary function of cells such as ovulation or fertilization, mitochondrial respiratory chain, phagocytosis, and arachidonic acid metabolism may give rise to extremely reactive oxygen species (ROS). Increase in the formation of ROS has been seen in several pathophysiological state. When cerebral tissue encounters noxious stimuli, they produce oxygen free radicals during recovery phase (Beal, 2000). Oxygen can immediately take unpaired electrons from organic species and convert them to partly reactive species, together they are called ROS, including oxide ($O2$), alkoxy (RO), peroxyl (ROO), hydrogen peroxide (H_2O_2), hydroxyl (HO), and (NO) nitric oxide till converted to water. Halliwell and Gtteridge (1999) reported that the majority of the free reactive species are developed in the mitochondrial as well as microsomal electron transport chain.

In mitochondrial respiratory chain, moderately ROS are retained by cytochrome oxidase. However, ubiquinone directly transfers electron to oxygen compared with retained moderately reduced species. Autooxidation of semiquinones may generate super oxide anion in the internal mitochondrial membrane. Mitochondrial electron transport chains are enzymatically dismutated to H_2O_2 for majority of superoxide radicals. The alkoxy and hydroxyl free radicals quickly attack the macromolecules inside cells being highly reactive (Hemnani and Parihar, 1998).

Lipids, enzymes, proteins, carbohydrates, and DNA in cells and tissues are damaged by free radicals, the ROS. ROS leads to protein modification and DNA damage, which leads to cell fatality because of DNA fragmentation, lipid peroxidation, and membrane damage. The damage due to oxidation by ROS includes the toxicity of xenobiotics as well as the pathophysiological leading to skin aging, cognitive dysfunction, atherosclerosis, diabetic retinopathy, abnormal growth of cells—neoplasm (benign or malignant), cataract, adult acute respiratory attack, organ failure, vital illness such as sepsis, shock, long lasting inflammation of the gastrointestinal tract, condition in which blood clots form throughout the body, disseminated intravascular coagulation (DIC), tissue injuries, deterioration of the immune system and its phagocytic cells, nitric oxide production by the endothelium, ischemia reperfusion injury leading to vascular damage and liberate copper and iron ions from metalloprotein (Boveris et al., 1972).

Deficiency of iron content leads to different neurodegeneration diseases such as amyotrophic lateral sclerosis, spastic paraplegia, gliosis and multiple sclerosi (Heinonen et al., 1998).

Antioxidant Activity

A significant role such as health protection is played by antioxidant compounds. The hazard for chronic ailments including cancer and cardiac disease is reduced by antioxidants as per scientific evidence. Fruits, vegetables, and whole grains are some of the main supplies of natural antioxidants. Substances which protect from oxidation, like phytate and phytoestrogens, phenolic acids, vitamin E, vitamin C, and carotenes, present in plant-sourced food are recognized to have the capability to reduce the cancer disease risk. Almost all antioxidant compounds derived from plant sources in a typical diet have different properties as well as physical and chemical characteristics.

The ability to nullify the free electron species is the main characteristic of antioxidants. Biological systems have harsh free radicals and oxygen species from several sources. The oxidation of proteins, nucleic acids, lipids or DNA by free radicals may initiate degeneration. Free radicals such as peroxide, hydroperoxide, and lipid peroxyl are scavenged by antioxidant compounds such as polyphenols, phenolic acids, and flavonoids for prevention of oxidation of cell components leading to degeneration. The antioxidants in fruits, red wine, tea, and vegetables have the efficacy of natural foods for reduction of the degenerative chronic diseases including cardiac ailments and cancers, according to a number of clinical studies. The literature mentions several studies about the free radical reduction properties of antioxidants in foods (Miller et al., 2000).

IMMUNOMODULATION ACTIVITY

The principal function of immunomodulator is to balance the immune system components by either regulation and suppression or stimulation and normalization. If pathogens or infectious chemicals attack and disturb balance of immune system and shift it into disease state, immune system activates and provides primary protection against such attacks. The starting point in immunomodulation is to hunt for natural chemicals that can cure residual cancer (Yamamoto, 1996). The adjuvant biological therapy results in the discovery of Bacillus Calmette Guerin (BCG) as an antituberculosis vaccination (Petard et al., 1998) and systematic utilization of levamisol (Kurman, 1993) proved to be quite promising. Most important advancement in immunomodulation is the discovery of cyclosporine (Walsh et al., 1992). For the prevention of graft rejection, it is used as a powerful immunosuppressant and is found to be a blessing for many. For the treatment of several autoimmune diseases, the cyclosporine is being used.

To increase the efficacy of vaccine, immunoadjuvants are used, because a specific adjuvant is used with particular vaccines, hence this could be considered as specialized immunostimulants. The major impediment in development of antimalarial vaccine was lack of a proper biological adjuvant (Allison, 1997).

Nonspecific immunostimulants were used to enhance the body immunity against disease. Immunostimulants can work with innate immune reaction and with adaptive immune action. For a normal individual, the immunostimulants are intended to serve as preventive or promoting immune reaction, i.e., immune potentiators, by enhancing the primary stage of immune reaction and for the individual having a poor immune reaction as immunotherapeutic drugs. For conditions such as autoimmune diseases, graft rejection, and quick immune response or delayed type of hypersensitivity, immunosuppressants might be used for their management.

There are many applications of immunomodulation as conformed by contemporary scientists.

In modern treatment, the aspect of immunomodulation viz. immunopotentiation is significant, when the host safeguarding systems are to be enhanced with a condition of poor immune reaction.

Indian Traditional Medicine called *Rasaynas* that deals with medicine from plants has gained attention of many researchers. Majority of the studies have been conducted irrespective of a significant interdisciplinary technique. References of several plants that have the immunomodulatory effect were found, and several of them are being studied by contemporary scientific methodologies and have these characteristics. These plants include *Aloe vera* (Gharila kumari), *Allium sativum* (Lasun), *Asparagus racemose* (Satawar), *Curcuma longa* (Haldi), *Ocimum sanctum* (Tulsi), *Tinospora cordifolia* (Giloe), and *Withania somnifera* (Ashvaganda).

ANTITUMOR ACTIVITY

The basic curative techniques for cancer are surgery and radiation, but these are most successful if the tumor is detected at an initial stage. For later stage of tumors, chemotherapy is chosen, and though these medicines are efficient, they have major adverse effects and drug resistance (Kelloff et al., 2000), hence new therapeutic alternatives are required. In the realm of alternate cancer medicines with very minor toxicity and low adverse effects, herbal Indian drugs are considered a good choice.

In the hunt for alternate antitumor agents, researchers put in efforts to find the suitable natural drugs for their efficacy in controlling cancer risks, delaying carcinogenesis, or preventing tumor development. Many plants such as *Taxus brevifolia* (Taxceae) which is a source of taxanes (paclitaxel and docetaxel), Pacific yew, *Digitalis purpurea* (Plantaginaceae), which are sources of digitalins, and purple foxglove have attracted researchers for their medicinal properties (Rocha et al., 2001; Lindholm et al., 2002; Ruskin et al., 2002). Contemporary studies indicate the efficacy of many

edible herbs, spices, fruits, and vegetables in decreasing the cancer incidence, due to the content of natural compounds present in them (Aruna and Sivarama krishnan, 1990; Unni and Kuttan, 1990; Dragsted et al., 1993).

SIGNIFICANCE OF SAFFRON (CROCUS SATIVUS L.) SPICE

C. sativus L. (*Iiridaceae*), generally called saffron, is the most expensive species of the world and is composed of orange-red color pungent stigmas; they are used in a dried form for flavoring and coloring foods as dye (Bakshi et al., 2007). Saffron is a perennial herb grown in Algeria, Azerbaijan, Australia, China, Egypt, France, Greece, Iran, India, Israel, Italy, Mexico, Morocco, New Zealand, Spain, Switzerland, Turkey, and United Arab Emirates. Folk's herbal medicines have included saffron as a remedy for several ailments because of its pain-relieving and sedative properties (Basker et al., 1983; Locock, 1995; Robinson, 1995) (Fig. 19.1). Owing to high demand, saffron is produced *in vitro*, and faster regeneration protocols have been developed for mass propagation (Bakshi et al., 2008). Saffron's biochemical characteristics have generated the interest of researchers during the last few years (Abdullaev et al., 1993, 2002; Souret and Weathers, 1999). Hartwell (1982) mentioned that in ancient era, saffron was made use of as an anticancer remedy as well as for preparations containing saffron extracts against different kinds of tumors and cancers. The stomach, spleen, liver, kidney, and uterus tumors have been treated with pharmaceutical preparations of saffron. In the early 1990s, some authors proved that natural saffron extracts presented antitumor, anticarcinogenic, antimutagenic effects, and cytotoxic properties (Nair et.al., 1995).

PHYTOCHEMISTRY OF SAFFRON (C. SATIVUS L.)

The approximate chemical assay of commonly available saffron (*C. sativus* L.,) had been done by several authors (Basker and Negbi, 1985; Skrubis, 1990; International Standards Organization, 1980a; Melchior and Kastner, 1974; Sampathu et al. 1984; Triebold and Aurand, 1963; Stecher, 1968; Nicholls, 1945; Sastry et al., 1955; Indian Standard, 1969). The main purpose of *C. sativus* analysis is for the estimation of retrievable color intensity on macroscale or microscale amounts. The guarantee of correct botanical identification and mixing of low-quality materials such as floral waste were major difficulties faced for chemical analysis of saffron. It is practically unavoidable in supply to find the parts of the yellow-to-uncolored stigma, anthers, and some petals or even

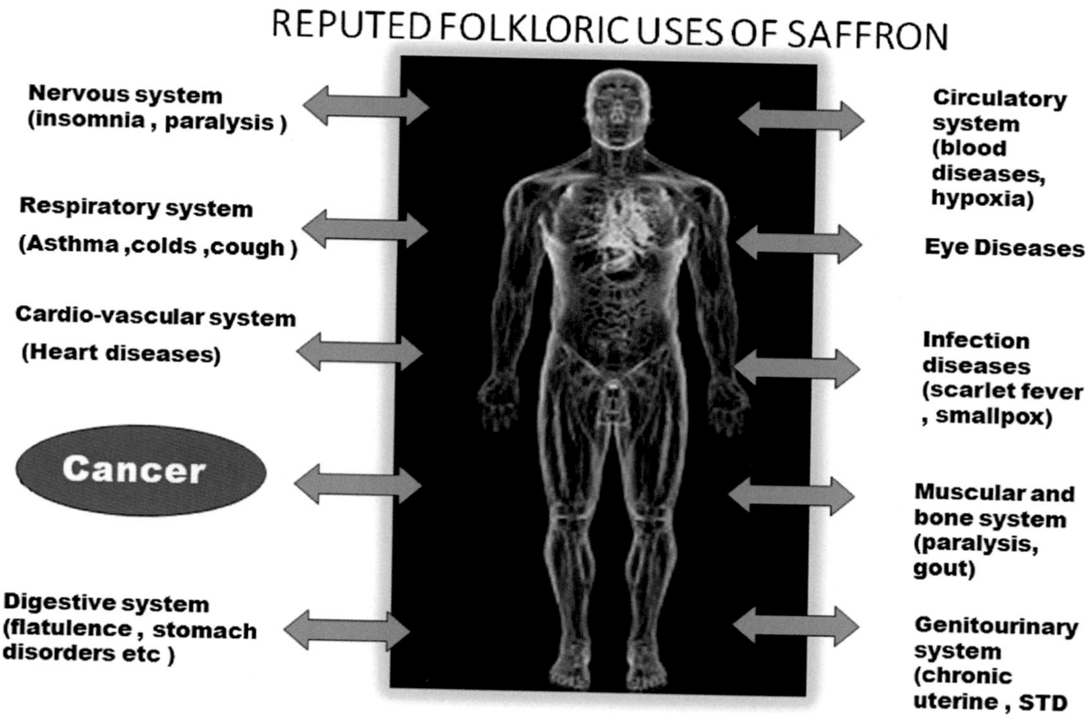

REPUTED FOLKLORIC USES OF SAFFRON

Nervous system
(insomnia , paralysis)

Respiratory system
(Asthma ,colds ,cough)

Cardio-vascular system
(Heart diseases)

Cancer

Digestive system
(flatulence , stomach
disorders etc)

Circulatory
system
(blood
diseases,
hypoxia)

Eye Diseases

Infection
diseases
(scarlet fever
, smallpox)

Muscular and
bone system
(paralysis,
gout)

Genitourinary
system
(chronic
uterine , STD

FIG. 19.1 Folkloric uses of saffron (Bakshi et al., 2008).

leaves (International Standard organization 1980a, 1980b; Hanson, 1973; Basker and Negbi, 1985).

Zechmeister (1962) reported that saffron is red-orange fundamentally because of a water-soluble carotenoid, a-crocin, a diester made from the disaccharide gentiobiose and dicarboxylic corrosive crocetin. The substance bond skeleton of alpha-crocin is made of shorter carbon chains of crocetin, which has nine conjugated twofold bonds; alpha crocin is additionally a glycoside, a concoction with a sugar displayed at the two finishes of carotenoid atom which makes it water solvent. Furthermore, water-soluble and water-insoluble carotenoid structures are available with a minor dimensional variation as detailed by different examiners (Pander and Witter 1975; Dhingra et al., 1975).

Complete constituent analyses have indicated that saffron contains approximately 10% moisture, 12% protein, and 5% each of minerals, fat, and crude fiber, and the rest is sugars, starch, dextrins, pectin, pentosans, and gums, including reducing sugars (% w/w).

Saffron at a trace level also contains vitamins such as riboflavin and thiamine (Rios et al., 1996). Biochemical research has been accomplished for portrayal of many biochemically dynamic medications found in saffron.

The significant mixes in saffron found with bioactivity are crocetin (a characteristic carotenoid dicarboxylic corrosive forerunner of crocin), crocin (monoglycosyl or diglycosyl polyene esters), picrocrocin (monoterpene glycoside antecedent of safranal and result of zeaxanthin debasement), and safranal (Fig. 19.2), all these ingredients have the capacity to add to the shade, taste, and smell to enhance the quality (Rios et al., 1996).

There is a huge effect of atmosphere and genotype on compositional constituents of saffron, number of blooms, and disgrace yield, which were significantly changed by condition of the plant. The constituents of crocetin esters, namely (1) transcrocetin di-(b-Dgentibiosyl)ester, (2) transcrocetin (b-D-gentibiosyl) ester, (3) transcrocetin (b-D-glucosyl) (b-D-gentibiosyl) ester, (4) picrocrocin, and (5) trans-crocetin (b-D-glucosyl) ester were assessed by the spectrophotometric ISO standard technique, which positioned the examples into three subjectively diminishing classes (I—III); arrangement was assessed principally through the use of HPLC outfitted with a bright noticeable diode exhibit locator and electro-shower mass spectrometer identifiers (HPLC—UV—vis-DAD—ESI-MS), which made it conceivable to assess the metabolic qualities of disgrace

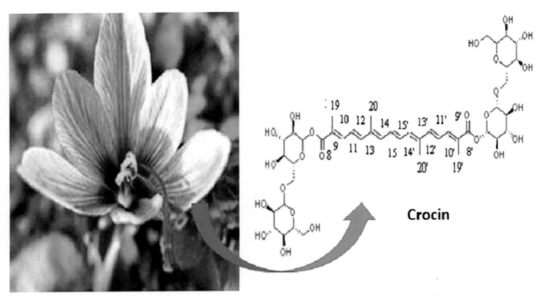

FIG. 19.2 Chemical structure of Crocin from saffron (Bakshi et al., 2008).

tests as far as picrocrocin and crocetin esters content. The mix of biochemical examination information with the natural conditions and genotype demonstrated that crocetin esters 1 and 2 make up the real parts of all-out crocetin ester sum, which likewise appears with a high positive connection (0.971 and 0.833, separately). In addition, the concentration of crocetin esters 2 (0.794) and 3 (0.818) and absolute crocetin esters (0.678) are closely related to the concentration of picrocrocin. In long term, a Pearson connection was performed so as to assess any conceivable connection between yield attributes (bloom number, complete yield, and unitary shame weight) and the subjective parameters of saffron (Siracusa et al., 2010).

The complete phenolics content in *C. sativus L.* corms in the torpid state and dynamic state was evaluated by the Folin-Ciocalteu strategy. The trial was performed on gas chromatography-mass spectrometry (GC-MS) after silylation by N-methyl-N-trimethylsilyl trifluroacetamide + %1 trimethyl iodosilane. A few synthetics were found, and 11 mixes were assessed. The most elevated phenolics content in dynamic corms was watched for genetic corrosive (5.693 ± 0.057 μg/g) and the least for gallic corrosive (0.416 ± 0.006 μg/g). These two phenolic mixes are the most noteworthy (0.929 ± 0.015 μg/g) and least (0.017 ± 0.001 μg/g) phenolics in torpid corms, individually (Esmaeiliet .al 2011). The outcomes from quantization and GC-MS investigation demonstrated a high centralization of phenolic mixes in dynamic corms than the idle state.

What's more, the extreme purifying exercises of saffron corms were inspected by 1,1-diphenyl-2-pycrylhydrazyl test, and EC (50) values were resolved around 2055 and 8274 ppm for dynamic and torpid corms separately (Esmaeiliet.al 2011).

Carotenoids as Anti-Oxidative Damage Modifier

All carotenoids are oxidized by opening of C=C bonds to get oxygen molecules and, in this way, lessening the trademark shading. This procedure is improved by light. The conjugative sort security gives moderate assurance from oxidation; however, the oxidation response on these carotenoids shields the living cells from serious oxidation harm.

Mathews et al., (1982) reported the effect of gardenia crocetin on experimental skin tumors in nude mice and encountered a minor inhibitory activity on the progress of skin tumors induced by the application of croton oil and 9, 10-dimethyl-1, 2-benzanthracene. In rats, Gardenia crocin triggered major inhibitory activity against hepatocarcinogenic chemicals such as aflatoxin B1 and dimethyl nitrosamine as well as mildly reducing chronic hepatic damage in rats. This work was in agreement with that of Lin and Wang, 1986.

Tseng et al. (1995) reported that carotenoid plays essential functions in plant tissues protecting against oxidative damage. Consistent with this function in plants, gardenia crocetin decreased lipid peroxidation induced by reactive oxygen species in rat primary hepatocytes. A similar work was also conducted on Gardenia crocin, and the water-soluble form also shows antioxidant properties at concentrations up to 40 ppm. At 20 ppm, the antioxidant activity of crocin is comparable to that of butylated hydroxyanisole (BHA).

Pham et al. (2001) reported that extracts from saffron and other carotenoid-containing spices showed significant hydrogen peroxide scavenging activity as measured by using peroxidase-based assay systems.

Martı́nez et al. (2001) revealed that carotenoids are soluble in lipids and might go about as a layer of connected free-radical controllers; the cancer prevention agent properties of these mixes could counteract DNA harm prompted by free radicals and free extreme chain responses.

Maggi et al. (2009) detailed that the drying is critical for saving the state of saffron, as it is required for discharging of safranal from picrocrocin by means of enzymatic procedure, the activity of releasing D-glucose and safranal, the unstable oil in saffron. There are six fundamental natural synthetic compounds found in saffron, and all are unstable; these include safranal, isophorone 2, 2, 6trimethyl-1, 4-cyclohexanedione, 4-ketoisophorone, 2-hydroxy-4, 4, 6-trimethyl-2, 5-cyclohexadien-1-one, just as 2, 6, 6-trimethyl-1,4-cyclohexadiene-1-carboxaldehyde.

PHARMACOLOGICAL AND BIOLOGICAL ACTIVITIES OF SAFFRON (*C. SATIVUS L.*)

From old occasions saffron reaped from dried, dull red marks of shame of *C. sativus L.* harvested in different occasions and their blossoms used as a medication to treat different human wellbeing conditions including hack, tooting, stomach issue, colic, a sleeping disorder, perpetual uterine hemorrhages, amenorrhea, dysmenorrheal, gynecological scatters (counting guideline of monthly cycle, reducing awkward period or absence of feminine cycle), red fever, smallpox, colds, asthma, and cardiovascular issue. Saffron (*C. sativus*) is a bulbous perpetual of the iris family (Iridaceae) cherished for its brilliant shaded, impactful marks of disgrace, which are dried and used to flavor and shade sustenances. Saffron is a zest known distinctly in development and mainly developed in Spain and Iran; in addition, they are grown on a lower scale in Greece, Turkey, India, Azerbaijan, France, Italy, India, China, Morocco, Turkey, Israel, Egypt, United Arab Emirates, Mexico, Switzerland, Algeria, Australia, and New Zealand (Abdullaev, 1993, 2002; Bakshi et al., 2007, 2008).

Gainer et al. (1976) reported that gardenia crocetin postponed the beginning and diminished the quantity of skin papillomas and Rous sarcoma tumors. The effect of gardenia crocetin on experimental skin tumors in nude mice showed a small inhibitory effect on the development of skin tumors induced by the application of 9, 10-dimethyl-1, 2-benzanthracene and croton oil (Mathews et al., 1982). In rats, gardenia crocins revealed a great protective effect against hepatocarcinogenic compounds such as aflatoxin B1 and dimethylnitrosamine, partially reducing chronic hepatic damage (Lin and Wang, 1986).

The orally controlling saffron ethanolic concentrates upgraded the life expectancy of Swiss pale-skinned person mice intraperitoneally joined with sarcoma-180 (S-180) cells, Ehrlich ascites carcinoma (EAC) or Dalton's lymphoma ascites (DLA) tumors. At this point, the creators did not distinguish the precise kind of the dynamic compound from saffron; however, they reported that this atom demonstrated the nearness of glycosidic security (Nair et al., 1991). Encapsulation of saffron can be done by liposome to efficiently increase its antitumor activity against S-180 and EAC solid tumors and potentiating it sufficiently to inhibit the growth of the tumors. Also, saffron stimulated nonspecific proliferation of lymphocytes in vitro because of the existence of the T-cell mitogen phytohemagglutinin. The antitumor activity might be immunologically mediated (Nair et al., 1992).

Abdullaev and Frenkel (1992) detailed for the first time that saffron reduce restrained development of harmful cells in vivo and in vitro. During the most recent decade, various examinations in a creature model framework exhibited the antitumor impact of saffron and its constituents on various dangerous cells. The carotenoid plays fundamental roles in plant tissues ensuring protection against oxidative harm. Reliably, with this capacity in plants, gardenia crocetin diminished lipid peroxidation actuated by receptive oxygen species in rodent essential hepatocytes (Tseng et al., 1995). The inhibitory action on the in vitro development of HeLa cells delivered by saffron extricates (ID50 ¼ 2.3 mg/mL) was mostly due to crocin (ID50 of 3 mM), although picrocrocin and safranal, with an ID50 of and 0.8 mM, individually, assumed a minor job in the cytotoxicity of saffron removes. These outcomes proposed that sugars may assume a job in saffron's cytotoxic impact as crocetin (the deglycosylated carotenoid) did not cause cell development restraint even at high dosages (Escribano et al., 1996). The treatment of creatures with cysteine (20 mg/kg body weight) alongside saffron extracts (50 mg/kg body wt) considerably decreased the dangerous harm done by cisplatin, similar to changes in chemical movement and nephrotoxicity (Daly, 1998).

Verma and Bordia (1998) announced that 50 milligrams of saffron in 100 mL of milk was given two times per day to human subjects, as revealed in an Indian investigation in 1998. The noteworthy reduction in lipoprotein oxidation powerlessness in patients with coronary artery disease (CAD) demonstrates the capability of saffron as a cell reinforcement.

It was demonstrated that crocin analogs secluded from saffron essentially expanded the blood stream in the retina and choroids just as encouraged retinal capacity recuperation. It was proposed that crocin analogs could be used to treat ischemic retinopathy as well as age-related macular degeneration (Xuan et al., 1999; Escribano et al., 1999a,b) detailed that the initiation of macrophages by the bioactive part separated from saffron corms at noncytotoxic focuses, estimated by the arrival of nitric oxide (NO). Treatment with 50 mg/mL multiplied the arrival of nitrate and nitrite by these cells. Higher fixations (up to 500 mg/mL) brought about a diminished NO creation in parallel with a checked fall in cell practicality. On the other hand, Garcı́a-Olmo et al. (1999) reported the effects of long-term treatment with saffron crocin (the glyosidic form of crocetin) on tumor growth and lifespan of rats bearing syngeneic colorectal tumors, induced by rat adenocarcinoma DHD/K12-PROb cells injected subcutaneously. Crocin treatment of those animals increased significantly their life span and reduced tumor-enlarging rate, faster in female mice. The selective action of crocin in female rats as compared with male rats suggests that the effects of crocin in animals might be partially dependent on hormonal factors.

An investigation on saffron, ginsenoside, and cannabinoid subordinates to decide potential film-related antitumor impacts of these substances. Saffron subordinates were ineffectual on the inversion of multidrug opposition of lymphoma cells (the inversion of multidrug obstruction is the after effect of the restraint of the efflux siphon work in the tumor cells). Crocetin esters were less intense than crocin itself in the restraint of early antigen articulation. In any case, diglucosylcrocetin and crocin averted early tumor antigen articulation of adenovirus-tainted cells, triglucosylcrocetin being less compelling. Crocin did not demonstrate any antiviral impacts on tainted Vero cells (Molnar et al., 2000). Gardenia crocin, the water-solvent structure, has likewise appeared at fixations up to 40 ppm. At 20 ppm, the cancer-prevention agent movement of crocin is tantamount to that of BHA. Concentrates from saffron and other carotenoid-containing flavors demonstrated huge hydrogen peroxide rummaging movement as estimated by using peroxidase-based test frameworks (Pham et al., 2001).

Premkumar et al. (2001) reported that the impacts of watery concentrates of saffron (created principally via carotenoids) in Swiss pale skinned person mice and recommended that pretreatment with saffron can essentially repress the dangerous impact on genetic materials of cells by cisplatin, cyclophosphamide, mitomycin, and urethane. Saffron extricate crocetin likewise diminishes bladder poisonous quality of the anticancer specialist cyclophosphamide without influencing its antitumor property (Nair et al., 1993). The most lipid-dissolvable carotenoids go about as layer-related free-radical foragers, and the cancer prevention agent properties of these mixes could avoid DNA harm initiated by free radicals and free extreme chain responses (Martı́nez et al., 2001)

The crocin detached from saffron shows antiapoptotic activity in PC-12 cells treated with daunorubicin. These discoveries propose that crocin hinders neuronal demise initiated by both inward and an outer apoptotic upgrade in exceedingly separated cells (neurons). This particular conduct proposes significant helpful ramifications, identified with the way that customized cell demise is diminished in malignancy and expanded in neurodegenerative illness (Soeda et al., 2001). Ozaki et al. (2002) announced no mutagenic action due to crocetin, while genipin, shaped by geniposide hydrolysis, caused DNA harm and initiated tetraploidy.

In Iranian conventional medication, the saffron had been used as an anticonvulsant cure. As of late, in investigations with mice using maximal electroshock seizure (MES) and pentylenetetrazole (PTZ) tests, it was exhibited that the fluid and ethanolic concentrates of saffron have anticonvulsant movement. It was recommended that saffron concentrates may be valuable in both nonattendance and tonic clonic seizures (Hosseinzadeh and Khosravan, 2002).

Since antiquated occasions, saffron collected from the dried, dim red marks of shame of C. sativus L. blossoms has been used as a medication to treat different human wellbeing conditions including hack, fart, stomach issue, colic, sleep deprivation, gynecological issue (counting guideline of feminine cycle, easing awkward period or absence of monthly cycle), red fever, little pox, colds, asthma, and cardiovascular issue (Abdullaev, 2003).

Fatehi et al. (2003) revealed the impacts of saffron petal on pulse in anesthetized rodents and on reactions of the segregated rodent vas deferens and guinea pig ileum incited by electrical field incitement (EFS). It was demonstrated that water and ethyl liquor concentrates of saffron decreased the circulatory strain in a portion subordinate way. EFS of the separated rodent vas deferens likewise were diminished by these saffron extracts.

The crocin family biosynthesis process was performed by using high pressure liquid chromatography (HPLC) to choose the glucosyltransferase activity and to make procedure for consolidating remedy from saffron cells. It was discovered that two glucosyltransferases are locked in with the advancement of crocetin glucosyl and gentiobiosyl-esters. GTase1 formed an ester bond between crocetin carboxyl social events and glucose moieties, while GTase2 catalyzed the course of action of glucosidic bonds with glucosyl ester packs at the two terminations of the molecule. Synthetic compounds can catalyze the improvement of crocetin glucosides in vitro. GTase1 activity is higher during introductory 4 days of crocin glucosides biosynthesis yet decreases in the following 4 days. The content of crocin increases in C. sativus cell cultures for the first six days and declined in subsequent experimental days (Yang et al., 2005). The flawlessness standards of crocin were surveyed in Indian saffron by clear, fast, and a preservationist crocin test system, and it was assumed that Indian saffron is rich in crocin, and excellence of blends exhibited relative results that stood out from sigma crocin (Chatterjee et al., 2005). The vital foe of secretory and antiulcer activities incited by the liquid suspension of saffron were evaluated against pylorus ligation (shay rodents), indomethacin, and distinctive narcotizing administrators in rodents. Histopathological assessment of rat stomach did not show any malicious ramifications for extreme and interminable toxic quality (Mofleh et al., 2006).

Saffron is promising alternative approach to achieve cure; the technique for saffron's anticancer activity is generally unknown, and several experts have proposed the part of development of the medicine Saffron. Scientists reported that saffron may unequivocally attack DNA courses of action and change quality verbalization. Bathaie demonstrated that carotenoids (crocin, crocetin, and dimethylcrocetin) of saffron clearly bind to DNA minor scores and produce conformational changes of express DNA (Bathaie et al., 2007).

The little yield of saffron and related more noteworthy cost actuated determined workers tragically to pollute as far back as a couple of hundreds of years. In the fourteenth century, Nuremberg, Germany, was the point of convergence of the European saffron business with saffron created in Austria, Sicily, France, Crete, Greece, and Spain, encountering its dealers. In any case, an incredible piece of the saffron was sullied in a guile and dumbfounded way, tragically. The Safranschou Code was familiar and maintained all together with a guarantee of the validity of saffron, the code containing unequivocal saffron measures and disciplines for defilement. The coercion disciplines were not kidding in light of the fact that experts were endorsed by the code to keep or execute people found at risk of defiling saffron. Trading of saffron is very attractive due to its market price and its increasing demand is an extensive beguiling (Hagh-Nazari and Keifi, 2007).

In the twofold outwardly weakened randomized and counterfeit treatment controlled primer, 30 mg/day of saffron compartment supplementation (15 mg twice step by step: morning and night) was convincing in treating premenstrual cycle issue (PMS) in women developed 20−45 with standard menstrual cycles and PMS system experience for at any rate a half year (Agha-Hosseini et al., 2008). The anxiolytic properties of crocin were considered in animals, and it was seen that 50 mg/kg bt wt segment of crocin extended motor development when stood out from diazepam. It was also shown that lower measurements of crocin did not modify animals lead (Pitsikas et al., 2008).

C. sativus liquid concentrate's sexual enhancement activities were evaluated in male rodents in addition to its constituents safranal and crocin. Mounting repeat (MF), intromission repeat (IF), erection repeat (EF), mount inertness (ML), intromission torpidity (IL), and release idleness (EL) were the factors evaluated during the sexual lead consider. Crocin, at all doses, and the concentrate, especially at bits 160 and 320 mg/kg body wt., extended MF, IF, and EF rehearses and reduced EL, IL, and ML parameters. Safranal did not show a sexual enhancement property however the crocin major constituent of saffron derived from its aqueous extract demonstrated for sexual enhancement (Hossinzadeh et al., 2008).

The counter ulcer capability of saffron is observed in mice, which also affirms its customary use against gastric disorders. The study was intended to examine the viability of three unique medications (ethanol saffron extricate, business saffron remove, and crocin) and to exhibit that every one of the three segments showed antiulcer action, such as omeprazole, the proton siphon inhibitor being utilized to treat peptic ulcer. Saffron, crocin, and safranal showed cancer prevention agent properties that repressed ulcer arrangement by stifling indomethacin-caused gastric mucosa harm by raising glutathione levels and hampering lipid oxidation (Kianbakht and Mozaffari, 2009; Xu et al., 2009). Nabavizadeh et al. (2009) revealed that 100 mg/kg of fluid saffron separate caused elevated yields of gastric corrosive and pepsin in Wister rodents and demonstrated process improvement of saffron.

Mousavi et al. (2009) detailed that saffron concentrate of 200−2000 μg/mL inhibited portion subordinate multiplication of MCF-7 cells, IC50 = 400 ± 18.5 μg/mL after 48 h. Similarly detailed were the entrancing, anxiolytic loco engine, and engine coordination movement of saffron, saffronal and crocin in mice using a pentorbital rest time test, an assessed maze test, an open field test, and a rotarod test (Hossinzadeh and Noraci, 2009).

The job of caspases and Bax protein in MCF-7 cells in saffron-actuated apoptosis is in the arrangement of cell culture for bosom malignancy in in vitro investigations. Saffron-delivered apoptosis can be avoided by master caspase inhibitors, proposing caspase-subordinate pathway was initiated by saffron in MCF-7 cells. Bax protein articulation was likewise expanded in saffron-treated cells. Along these lines, saffron has genius apoptotic impacts on a bosom malignancy inferred cell line and could be considered as a potential chemotherapeutic operator in bosom disease (Mousavi et al., 2009).

Shamsa et al. (2009) detailed the impact of C. sativus (saffron) contemplated on male erectile dysfunction (ED). Twenty male patients with ED were pursued for 10 days in which every morning they took a table containing 200 mg of saffron. Patients underwent the nighttime penile bloat (NPT) test and the worldwide record of erectile capacity poll (IIEF15) toward the beginning of the treatment and toward the end of the 10 days of trial. After the 10 days of taking saffron, there was a factually huge improvement in tip unbending nature and tip distension just as base inflexibility and base tumescence. ILEF-15 aggregates' centers were essentially higher in patients after saffron treatment (before treatment 22.15$\pm$71.44; after treatment 39.20$\pm$71.90, p<0.001). Saffron demonstrated a constructive outcome on sexual capacity with an expanded number and span of erectile occasions found in patients with ED even simply subsequent to taking it for 10 days.

The free radical rummaging and lipid peroxidation avoidance of crocin from C. sativus is discussed. The preclinical examination exhibits that crocin is compelling in restraining free extreme development and furthermore to assault the free radicals (Bakshi et al., 2009). The toxicological impacts and in vitro cancer-prevention agent property of the ethanolic concentrates of C. sativus and Propolis were inspected. These concentrates did not cause any mortalities or indications of poisonous quality in mice when regulated orally at dosages of up to 5 g/kg b.wt. In the subendless investigation, the tried concentrates did not cause any critical change in liver and kidney elements of rodents, after oral administration for eight progressive weeks at dosages of 500 mg/kg b.wt. of each. Propolis indicated noteworthy in vitro cancer prevention agent action at concentrations of 40–100 mg/mL. Conversely, the ethanolic extract of C. sativus indicated frail cell reinforcement movement in convergences

of 1–10 mg/mL while at 20–100 mg/mL concentration it failed to show any cancer-prevention agent action. Oral administration of C. sativus every day, propolis ethanolic separates alone or in blend, for eight progressive weeks to rodents was found to be safe and did not cause any poisonous changes in the liver and kidney. Cell reinforcement study demonstrated that propolis ethanolic concentrate was a more powerful cancer-prevention agent than C. sativus (Ramadan et al., 2010). In our examination to analyze the impact of crocin, the vital compound in saffron, against in vitro and in vivo xenograft counteractive action of Dalton's lymphoma, we uncovered huge increment in life expectancy of Dalton's lymphoma–bearing creatures with 95.6% reduction of strong tumor in crocin-treated creatures on the 31st day of tumor vaccination. This examination urged us to further proceed with our exploration on crocin (Bakshi et al., 2009).

To completely and distinctively comprehend, regardless of whether crocin or crocetin stifles, microglial enactment was considered. Crocin and crocetin were demonstrated to be successful in restraining LPS-initiated nitric oxide (NO) discharge from refined rodent cerebrum microglial cells. These mixes decreased the LPS-animated preparations of tumor rot factor-α, interleukin-1β, and intracellular responsive oxygen species. The mixes additionally successfully diminished LPS-evoked NF-κB enactment. What's more, crocin diminished NO discharge from microglia animated with interferon-γ and amyloid-β. In organotypic hippocampal cut societies, both crocin and crocetin hindered the impact of LPS on hippocampal cell passing. These outcomes recommend that crocin and crocetin give neuroprotection by reducing the creation of different neurotoxic atoms from initiated microglia (Nam et al., 2010).

Crocetin is a pharmacologically dynamic carotenoid compound of Gardenia jasminoides Ellis which is used as a customary home-grown prescription and regular colorant. The pilot analysis was intended to comprehend the impact of crocetin on rest. The clinical study involved a twofold, visually impaired, fake treatment controlled, hybrid preliminary of 21 sound grown-up men with a gentle rest objection. It included two mediation times of about 14 days each, isolated by a 2-week washout period. The target rest quality was estimated by using an actigraph and evaluated the emotional side effects utilizing St. Mary's Hospital Sleep Questionnaire. Actigraph information demonstrated that after administration of crocetin, the quantity of arousing scenes decreased in contrast with that of the fake treatment (P = .025). Emotional information from St. Mary's Hospital Sleep Questionnaire demonstrated that crocetin would, in general, improve the nature of rest contrasted with rest before its admission. Furthermore, no reactions from crocetin admission were watched. The outcomes recommend that crocetin may add to improving the nature of sleep (Kuratsune et al., 2010; Kuratsune et al., 2010).

The protective effects of crocin against cisplatin-induced renal oxidative stress in rats were studied. Blood chemistry and biochemical and histopathological examination were done, and it was concluded that crocin significantly protects against cisplatin-induced renal toxicity (Naghizadeh et al., 2010). To study antidepressant properties of stigmas and corms of C. sativus L., the aqueous ethanol extract of C. sativus corms was fractionated on the basis of polarity. Among the different fractions, the petroleum ether fraction and dichloromethane fraction at doses of 150, 300, and 600 mg/kg showed significant antidepressant-like activities in dose-dependent manners, by means of behavioral models of depression (Yang et al., 2010). All these results suggest that the low polarity parts of C. sativus corms should be considered as a new plant material for curing depression, which merit further studies regarding antidepressive-like activities of chemical compounds isolated from the two fractions and mechanism of action (Yang et al., 2010).

The impacts of three convergences of macerated concentrate of saffron (C. sativus L.), dexamethasone, and saline on cell practicality and generation of cytokines, including interleukin (IL)-4, IL-10, and interferon-γ (IFN-γ), were assessed. In cells animated with PHA, various groupings of the concentrate essentially hindered cell feasibility of lymphocytes. High groupings of the concentrate (500 μg/mL) additionally restrained emission of IFN-γ in invigorated cells and IL-10 discharge in both animated and nonstimulated cells. The impacts of high and low convergences of the concentrate (500 and 50 μg/mL, individually) on IL-4 emission were lower than those of dexamethasone. The concentrate demonstrated a stimulatory impact on IFN-γ and IL-4 emission in no invigorated cells. The proportions of IFN-γ to IL-4 within the sight of all groupings of saffron on animated cells were essentially higher than those for the control gathering results showed that the concentrate of saffron has the potential to intervene provocative markers (Boskabadyet.al 2011).

Potential of Dietary Crocin the Marker Compound in Saffron (C. sativus L.) Against Different Malignancies

Previous studies have shown a variety of pharmacological effects of dietary crocin (Aung et al., 2007; Bakshi et al., 2009); however, the mechanism underlying antitumor

activity of crocin remains unclear. Different hypotheses had been propounded to explain its anticarcinogenic and antitumor action. The crocin induced apoptosis in HeLa and K562 cells (Escribano et al., 1996), while other studies have indicated the role of free radicals chain reaction in its antitumor action (Premkumar et al., 2001). The induction of apoptosis by saffron in human cancer cell lines was also shown in our previous study (Bakshi et al., 2008). In-vivo experiments on athymic bare mice had reasoned that crocetin, a carotenoid compound got from saffron, could actuate apoptosis in pancreatic tumors in athymic naked mice (Dhar et al., 2009). In 2011, Sun et al., through their examinations, had inferred that the preventive impact of crocin was on DNA and RNA amalgamation yet not on protein union, and in any case, it is hypothesized that it could be the conceivable component of crocin-actuated apoptosis (Sun et al., 2011).

Various speculations for the methods against cancer-causing and antitumor activities of saffron and its constituents have been recommended. One of the instruments for the antitumor or cancer-causing activity of saffron and its parts is the preventive impact on cell DNA and RNA union and not on protein combination (Sun et al., 2011; Nair et.al., 1995; Abdullaev et al., 1995/1996). The second component for the antitumor activity of saffron and its constituents is the preventive impact on free extreme chain responses, as carotenoids are lipid soluble and might go about as film bound high-effectiveness free extreme destroyer, which is associated with their cell reinforcement properties (Molnar et al., 2000; Verma et al., 1998; Tseng et al., 1995). The third proposed system by which the saffron concentrate demonstrates its antitumor activity is the metabolic change of carotenoids to retinoids (Tarantilis et al.,1994; Dufresne et al., 1997), yet, as of late, it was accounted for that transformation of carotenoids to nutrient. Anti cancer activity of C. sativus derived active principles is unquestionable (Smith, 1998). The fourth estimated instrument is that the cytotoxic impact of saffron is associated with cooperation of carotenoids with topoisomerase II, a chemical related with cell DNA-protein communication (Smith, 1998; Molnar et al., 2000). Notwithstanding, these examinations give signs to the examinations of the biochemical and subatomic instruments of antitumor impacts of crocin. With this scenery, in this venture, I am proposing to explore the activity of dietary crocin in different human disease cell lines and concentrate the adjustment in the outflow of apoptosis qualities in connection to its cytotoxic dimensions.

Past specialists have strived to clarify against disease and chemopreventive impact of crocin through their investigations; however, no agreement can be reached upon its method of activity. An ongoing report had demonstrated that crocin hinders telomerase action by downdirecting interpretation of hTERT quality in HepG2 cell line (Noureini and Wink, 2012). The abatement of telomerase movement in HepG2 cell treated with crocin concurs with an ongoing report demonstrating that crocin displays hostile to proliferative impacts in human colorectal malignant growth cell lines while not influencing typical cells (Aung et al., 2007). The perception of decrease in telomerase action additionally acclimates with aftereffects of another report that presumed that crocin subordinates were increasingly dynamic in tumor cell settlement arrangement in an in vitro examine ponder than different carotenoids (Bakshi et al., 2010; Sun et al., 2011), in this manner diminishing clearness on its method of action. In option, crocin and crocetin were appeared to restrain bosom malignant growth cell expansion (Chryssanthi et al., 2007). The in vitro and in vivo investigations have effectively affirmed a fixation and time subordinate development restraint by crocin in xenograft mouse models (Bakshi et al., 2009). Another examination had demonstrated the improvement of cytotoxic and apoptogenic properties of crocin in malignant growth cell lines, HeLa and MCF-7, utilizing its nanoliposomal structure, which make it increasingly productive at impressively lower IC50 values (Mousavi et al., 2011). Apoptosis enlistment by saffron and its constituents has appeared in few investigations without clarifying the component of activity. Saffron concentrate prompted apoptosis in human malignancy cell line (Bakshi et al., 2008). The crocetin, a carotenoid compound got from saffron, could actuate apoptosis in pancreatic cells just as athymic naked mice tumor (Dhar et al., 2009). The restraint of caspases could square saffron-initiated apoptosis in MCF-7 cells in this manner, demonstrating caspase-subordinate pathways were incited by saffron in MCF-7 cells and a few factors other than caspases, for example, apoptosis actuating factor (AIF) may not be especially included. Bax articulation was discovered expanded, proposing a mitochondrial pathway including apoptosis (Mousavi et al., 2009). However, the precise atomic mechanism(s) of crocin incited cell demise in disease is as yet not clear.

In later past, a portion of our work on dietary crocin has showed free radical searching and lipid peroxidation hindrance (Bakshi et al., 2009), apoptosis and cell cycle capture in pancreatic malignancy cell lines (Bakshi et al., 2010), cytotoxic and apoptogenic impact of "CS" on various Human disease cell lines (Bakshi et al., 2008), in vitro and in vivo xenograft restraint of Daltons lymphoma (Bakshi et al., 2009), breast disease cell (MCF-7) passing by enacting caspase flagging (Bakshi et al., 2016a), and low centralization of crocin can execute the cervical malignant growth (Hep-2) cell by saving ordinary vero cells (Bakshi et al., 2016b). Moreover pervious examination demonstrated that saffron concentrate is protected in in vivo model (Bakshi et al., 2016a) and that dietary crocin hinders dangerous melanoma in in vivo model (Bakshi et al., 2017a) and turns around melanoma metastasis (Bakshi et al., 2017b). This demonstrated crocin can possibly convert into centers. However, progressively future unthinking exploration is expected to completely comprehend job of crocin in malignant growth counteractive action.

HINDERING IMPACTS OF SAFFRON

The absence of saffron wellbeing data has prompted research focusing on this significant issue. The few investigations that have been directed have delivered conflicting results. In few cases, infusions of 1.2–2 g/per normal saffron body weight may cause sickness, spewing, loose bowels, and dying, while in different cases, no unfriendly impacts have been related with ingestion of 4 g of saffron for every day for a few days, incorporating into pregnant ladies. Anyway it is not evident whether these German investigations utilized C. sativus or if the investigations were completed utilizing knoll saffron (Colchicum autumnale), which is rich in Germany (Schmidt et al., 2007). As per another examination, portions of in excess 10 g of saffron may initiate premature birth with announced symptoms including diminished hunger, drowsiness, queasiness, regurgitating, uterine dying, hematuria, the gastrointestinal mucosal dying, vertigo, and dazedness (Schmidt et al., 2007). Safran concentrate causes unfavorably susceptible responses in extremely uncommon cases (Lucas et al., 2001). Saffron has a high LD50 = 20 g/kg that clarifies why toxicology specialists think of it as safe for human utilization right now (Bisset and Wichtl, 1994). The real measure of saffron utilized in nourishment regularly is much lower than the portion that causes any of the announced symptoms. The portion required in this survey for positive medical advantages is reliable within the measure of saffron utilized in various kitchens. In vivo examinations in creatures demonstrate an extremely low or even nonexistent danger of both saffron and its concentrates in contrast to many human investigations (Karimi et al., 2001; Nair et al., 1991, 1995). It ought to be noticed that the utilization of in vitro or in vivo creature studies has demonstrated huge number of the beneficial outcomes of saffron;

however, it stays hazy whether these constructive outcomes are indistinguishable in people. Further clinical research is justified so as to explain the potential advantages or destructive impacts in people.

CONCLUSION

The overall population acknowledges the utilization of saffron for nourishment, shading, and seasoning all through the world and by numerous social groups. Scientists around the globe are anyway more pulled in to the capability of saffron for natural or pharmacological capacity, which is because of the huge number of phytochemicals found in saffron. In numerous in vitro and in vivo examinations, safranal, crocetin, crocins, and picrocrocin are considered among these phytochemicals to be the most restoratively bioactive and the most analyzed. These tests unmistakably demonstrate that saffron utilization is emphatically related with lower sickness hazard, including metabolic issue (gastric turmoil), premenstrual disorder, despondency, a sleeping disorder and uneasiness, cardiovascular illness, and numerous malignancies. Notwithstanding, the best perceptions were seen in creature models, bringing up numerous issues: How do these potential advantages convert into human models? Is there any distinction between saffron creature resistance and human resilience? How sheltered is man's saffron. It must be viewed as that different impacts could be conceivable because of saffron rough concentrates (which contain all phytochemicals) and their bioactive mixes (filtered phytochemicals). Further preliminaries are required so as to understand the refinement in wellbeing points of interest attributable to unrefined concentrates and cleaned types. Regarding medicinal use, further large-scale epidemiological examinations, clinical investigations, and research facility study are required to explain the procedures and effects of saffron on human wellbeing.

REFERENCES

Abdullaev, F.I., 1993. Biological effects of saffron. Biofactors 4 (2), 83−86.

Abdullaev, F.I., Gonzalez, de, Mejia, E., 1995-1996. Inhibition of colony formation of HeLa cells by naturally occurring and synthetic agents. Biofactors 5 (3), 133−138.

Abdullaev, F.I., 2002. Cancer chemopreventive and tumouricidal properties of saffron (Crocus sativus L.). Exp. Biol. Med. 227 (1), 20−25.

Abdullaev, F.I., 2003. Saffron (Crocus sativus L.) and its possible role in the prevention of cancer. In: Majumdar, D.K., Govil, J.N., Sing, V.K. (Eds.), Recent Progress in Medicinal Plants, vol. 8. SCI Tech Publishing LLC, Houston, TX, USA, pp. 53−67.

Abdullaev, F.I., Frenkel, G.D., 1992. Effect of saffron on cell colony formation and cellular nucleic acid and protein synthesis. Biofactors 3, 201−204.

Agha-Hosseini, M., Kashani, L., Aleyaseen, A., Ghoreishi, A., Rahmanpour, H., Zarrinara, A.R., et al., 2008. Crocus sativus L. (saffron) in the treatment of premenstrual syndrome: a double-blind, randomised and placebo-controlled trial. BJOG 115 (4), 515−519.

Akerele, O., 1988. Medicinal plants and primary health care: an agenda for action. Fitoterapia 59, 355−363.

Allison, A.C., 1997. Immunological adjuvant and their mode of actions. Arch .Immunol. Ther. Exp. 45, 1410−1447.

Ames, B.N., Gold, L.S., Willett, W.C., 1995. The causes and prevention of cancer. Proc. Natl. Acad. Sci. USA 92, 5258−5265.

Aruna, K., Sivarama krishnan, V.M., 1990. Plant products as protective agents against cancer. Ind. J. Exp. Biol. 28, 1008−1011.

Aung, H.H., Wang, C.Z., Ni, M., et al., 2007. Crocin from Crocus sativus possesses significant anti-proliferation effects on human colorectal cancer cells. Exp. Oncol. 29, 175−180.

Bakshi, H., Sultan, P., Kusha, B., Shawal, A.S., 2007. Invitro studies of saffron (Crocus sativus). Ind. J. Appl. Life Sci. 2 (1−2), 82−84.

Bakshi, H., Smitha, S., Jitender, M., Binamin, B., 2008. The faster Regeneration protocol for saffron (Crocus sativus). Ind. J. Bot. Res. 4 (1), 13−22.

Bakshi, H., Smitha, S., Anna, F., Zeinab, R., Shah, G.A., Manik, S., 2009a. Crocin from Kashmiri saffron induces invitro and in vivo xenograft growth inhibition of Dalton's lymphoma in mice. Asian Pac. J. Cancer Prev. (10), 887−890.

Bakshi, H., Smitha, S., Tajamul, I., Pryeim, S., Manik, S., 2009b. The free radical and the lipid peroxidation inhibition of crocin isolatedfrom Kashmiri saffron (Crocus sativus) occurring in northern part of India. Int. J. Pharmatech. Res. 1 (4), 1317−1321.

Bakshi, H., Smitha, S., Roya, R., Phalisteen, S., et al., 2010. DNA fragmentation and Cell cycle arrest: a hallmark of apoptosis induced by crocin from kashmirir saffron against pancreatic cancer cell Line (BX-PC-3). Asia Pac. J. Cancer Prev. (11), 1−6.

Bakshi Hamid, A., Sam, S., Rozati, R., et al., 2010. DNA fragmentation and cell cycle arrest, A Hallmark of apoptosis induced by crocin from Kashmiri saffron in a human pancreatic cancer cell line. Asian Pac. J. Cancer Prev. 11, 675−679.

Bakshi Hamid, A., Faruck, L.H., Sam., S., 2016a. Molecular mechanism of saffron induced caspases mediated MCF-7 cell death and in vivo toxicity profiling and ex vivo macrophage activation in normal Swiss albino mice. Asian Pac. J. Cancer Prev. 17, 1499−1506.

Bakshi Hamid, A., Faruck, L.H., Sam, S., Al-Buloshi, M., 2016b. Assessment of in vitro cytotoxicity of saffron (Crocus sativus L.) on cervical cancer cells (HEp-2) and their in vivo preclinical toxicity in normal Swiss albino mice. Int. J. Herb. Med. 4 (5), 80−83.

Bakshi Hamid, A., Faruck, L.H., Sam., S., Javid, F., 2017. Role of dietary crocin in invivo melanoma remission. Asian Pac. J. Cancer Prev. 18, 841−846.

Basker, D., Negbi, M., 1983. Uses of saffron. Econ. Bot. 3, 228−235.

Basker, D., Negbi, M., 1985. Crocetin equivalent of saffron extracts: comparison of three extraction methods. J. Assoc. Public Anal. 23, 65–69.

Bathaie, S.Z., Bolhasani, A., Hoshyar, R., Ranjbar, B., Sabouni, F., Moosavi-Movahedi, A., 2007. Interaction of saffron carotenoids as anticancer compounds with ctDNA, Oligo (dG.dC) 15, and Oligo (dA.dT)15. DNA Cell Biol. 26 (8), 533–540.

Beal, M.F., 2000. Energetic in the pathogenesis of neurodegenerative disease. Trends Neurosci. 23, 298–303.

Bisset, N.G., Wichtl, M., 1994. Herbal Drugs and Phytopharmaceuticals, third ed. Medpharm GmbH Scientific Publishers, Stuttgart.

Boskabady, M.H., Hosseini, S., Tamijani, S.M., Rafatpanah, H., Rezaei, A., Alavinejad, A., 2011. The effect of crocus sativus extract on human lymphocytes' cytokines and T helper 2/T helper 1 balance. J. Med. Food 14, 1538–1545.

Boveris, A., Oshino, N., Chance, B., 1972. The cellular production of hydrogen peroxide. Biochem. J. 128, 617–630.

Chatterjee, S., Balakrishna Poduval, T., Tilak, J.C., Devasagayam, T.P.A., 2005. A modified, economic, sensitive method for measuring total antioxidant capacities of human plasma and natural compounds using Indian saffron (Crocus sativus). Clin. Chim. Acta 352, 155–163.

Chryssanthi, D.G., Lamari, F.N., Iatrou, G., et al., 2007. Inhibition of breast cancer cell proliferation by style constituents of different Crocus species. Anticancer Res. 27, 357–362.

Daly, E.S., 1998. Protective effect of cysteine and vitamine E, Crocus sativus and Nigella sativa extracts on cisplatin-induced toxicity in rats. J. Pharm. 53, 87–93.

Dhar, A., Mehta, S., Dhar, G., 2009. Crocetin inhibits pancreatic cancer cell proliferation and tumor progression in a xenograft mouse model. Mol. Cancer Ther. 8, 315–323.

Dhingra, V.K., Seshadri, T.R., Mukerjee, S.K., 1975. Minor carotenoid glycosides from saffron (Crocus sativus). Indian J. Chem. 3, 339–341.

Doll, R., Petro, R., 1981. The causes of cancer:quantitative estimate of aviodiable risk of cancer in the United States today. J. Natl. Cancer Inst. 66 (6), 1191–1308.

Dragsted, L.O., Strube, M., Larsen, J.C., 1993. Cancer-protective factors in fruits and vegetables: biochemical and biological background. Pharmacol. Toxicol. 72 (Suppl. 1), 116–135.

Dufresne, C., Cormier, F., Dorion, S., 1997. In vitro formation of crocetin glucosyl esters by Crocus sativus callus extract. Planta Med. 63 (2), 150–153.

Escribano, J., Alonso, G.L., Coca-Prados, M., et al., 1996. Crocin, safranal and picrocrocin from saffron (Crocus sativus L.) inhibit the growth of human cancer cells in vitro. Cancer Lett. 100, 22–30.

Escribano, J., Piqueras, A., Medina, J., Rubio, A., Alvarez-Ortí, M., Fernández, J.A., 1999a. Production of a cytotoxic proteoglycan uses callus culture of saffron corms (Crocus sativus L.). J. Biotechnol. 73, 53–59.

Escribano, J., Díaz-Guerra, M.J.M., Riese, H.H., Ontañ, n J., García-Olmo, D., García-Olmo, D.C., Rubio, A., Fernández, J.A., 1999b. In vitro activation of macrophages by a novel proteoglycan isolated from corms of Crocus sativus L. Cancer Lett. 144, 107–114.

Esmaeili, N., Ebrahimzadeh, H., Abdi, K., Safariani, S., 2011. Determination of some phenolic compounds in Crocus sativus L. corms and its antioxidant activities study. Pharmacogn. Mag. 7 (25), 74–80.

Fatehi, M., Rashidabady, T., Fatehi-Hassanabad, Z., 2003. Effects of Crocus sativus L. petals extract on rat blood pressure and on responses induced by electrical field stimulation in the rat isolated vasdeferens and Guinea-pigileum. J. Ethanopharmacol. 84, 199–203.

Gainer, J.L., Wallis, D.A., Jones, J.R., 1976. The effect of crocetin on skin papillomas and Rous sarcoma. Oncol. Times 33, 222–224.

García-Olmo, D.C., Riese, H.H., Escribano, J., Ontañ ó, n J., Ferná ndez, J.A., Atiénzar, M., García- Olmo, D., 1999. Effects of long-term treatment of colon adenocarcinoma with crocin, a carotenoid from saffron (Crocus sativus L.): an experimental study in the rat. Nutr. Cancer 35, 120–126.

Greenwald, P., 1996. Cancer risk factors for selecting cohorts for large scale chemoprevention trials. J. Cell. Biochem. Suppl. 25, 29–36.

Hagh-N, S., Keifi, N., 2007. Saffron and various fraud manners in its production and trades. Acta Hortic. 739, 411–416.

Halliwell, B., Gutteridge, J.M.C., 1999. Free Radicals in Biology and Medicine. Oxford University Press, Oxford.

Hanson, N.W. (Ed.), 1973. Official, Standardised and Recommended Methods of Analysis, second ed. Society for Analytical Chemistry, London, p. 674.

Hartwell, J.L., 1982. Plants Used against Cancer. A Survey. Quaterman Publications, Lawrence, pp. 284–289.

Heinonen, I.M., Meyer, A.S., Frankel, E.N., 1998. Antioxidant activity of berry phenolics on human low density lipoprotein and liposome oxidation. J. Agric. Food Chem. 46 (10), 41074112.

Hemnani, T., Parihar, M.S., 1998. Reactive oxygen species and oxidative DNA damage. Ind J Physiol Pharmacol 42 (4), 44–52.

Hosseinzadeh, H., Khosravan, V., 2002. Anticonvulsant effects of aqueous and ethanolic extracts of Crocus sativus L. Stigmas in mice. Arch. Iran. Med. 5, 44–47.

Hosseinzadeh, H., Noraei, N.B., 2009 Jun. Anxiolytic and hypnotic effect of Crocus sativus aqueous extract and its constituents, crocin and safranal, in mice. Phytother Res 23 (6), 768–774.

Indian Standard, 1969. Specification for Saffron. Indian Standards Institution IS, 5453.

International Standards Organization, 1980a. Saffron: Specification. ISO 3632. Geneva.

International Standards Organization, 1980b. Spices and Condiments—Determination of Cold Water Extract.ISO 941. Geneva.

Jemal, A., Murray, T., Ward, E., et al., 2005. Cancer statistics, 2005. Ca - Cancer J. Clin. 55, 10–30.

Karimi, G., Hosseinzadeh, H., Khaleghpanah, P., 2001. Study of antidepressant effect of aqueous and ethanolic extracts of Crocus sativus in mice. Iran. J. Basic Med. Sci. 4 (3–11), 11–15w.

Kathiresan, K., Boopathy, N.S., Kavitha, S., 2006. Coastal vegetation—an underexplored source of anticancer drugs. Nat. Product. Radiance 5, 115—119.

Kelloff, G.J., Crowell, J.A., Steele, V.E., Lubert, R.A., Malone, W.A., Boone, C.W., Kopelovich, L., Hawk, E.T., Lieberman, R., Lawrence, J.A., Ali, I., Viner, J.L., Sigman, C.C., 2000. Progress in cancer chemoprevention: development of diet-derived chemopreventive agents. J. Nutr. 130 (2S), 467—471.

Kianbakht, S., Mozaffari, K., 2009. Effects of saffron and its active constituents,crocin and safranal on prevention of indomethacin induced gastric ulcers in diabetic and non diabetic rats. J. Med. Plants 8 (5), 30—38.

Koduru, S., Grierson, D.S., Afolayan, A.J., 2007. Ethnobotanical information of medicinal plants used for treatment of cancer in the Eastern Cape Province, South Africa. Curr. Sci. 92, 906—908.

Kurman, M.R., 1993. Recent clinical trials with levamisole. Ann. NY Acad. Sci. 685, 269—277.

Lin, J.K., Wang, C.J., 1986. Protection of crocin dyes on the acute hepatic damage induced by aflatoxin B1 and dimethylnitrosamine in rats. Carcinogenesis 7, 595—599.

Lindholm, P., Gullbo, J., Claeson, P., Goransson, U., Johansson, S., Backlund, A., Larsson, R., Bohlin, L., 2002. Selective cytotoxicity evaluation in anticancer drug screening of fractionated plant extracts. J. Biomol. Screen 7, 333—340.

Locock, R.A., 1995. Alternatives saffron. Can. Pharmaceut. J. 127, 45—46.

Lucas, C.D., Hallagan, J.B., Taylor, S.L., 2001. The role of natural color additives in food allergy. Adv. Food Nutr. Res. 43, 195—216.

Madhuri, S., Pandey, G., 2008. Some dietary agricultural plants with anticancer properties. Plant Arch. 8, 13—16.

Maggi, L., Carmona, M., del Campo, C.P., Kanakis, C.D., Anastasaki, E., Tarantilis, P.A., et al., 2009. Worldwide market screening of saffron volatile composition. J. Sci. Food Agric. 89 (11), 1950—1954.

Martínez-Tomé, M., Jiménez, A.M., Ruggieri, S., Frega, N., Strabbioli, R., Murcia, M.A., 2001. Antioxidant properties of Mediterranean spices compared with common food additives. J. Food Prot. 64, 1412—1419.

Mathews-Roth, M.M., 1982. Effects of crocetin on experimental skin tumours in hairless mice. Oncology 39, 362—364.

Melchior, H., Kastner, H., 1974. Gewurze. Verlag Paul Parey, Berlin, pp. 147—150.

Meyer, J.J.M., Afolayan, A.J., Taylor, M.B., Engelbrecht, L., 1996. Inhibition of herpes simlex virus type I by aqueous extracts from shoots of Helichrysum aureonitens. J. Ethnopharmacol. 52, 41—43.

Miller, H.E., Rigelhof, F., Marquart, L., Prakash, A., Kanter, M., 2000a. Whole-grain products and antioxidants. Cereal Foods World 45 (2), 59—63.

Miller, H.E., Rigelhof, F., Marquart, L., Prakash, A., Kanter, M., 2000b. Antioxidant content of whole grain breakfast cereals, fruits and vegetables. J. Am. Coll. Nutr. 19 (3), 312S—319S.

Al-Mofleh, I.A., AlHaider, A.A., Mossa, J.S., Al-Sohaibani, M.O., Qureshi, S., Rafatuallh, S., 2006. Antigastric Ulcer studies on saffron (Crocus sativus) in rats. Pak. J. Biol. Sci. 9 (6), 1009—1013.

Molnar, J., Szabo, D., Pusztai, R., Mucsi, I., Berek, L., Ocsovski, I., KawataE, Shoyama, Y., 2000. Membrane associated antitumor effects of crocine-,ginseniside and cannabinoid derivates. Anticancer Res. 20 (2a), 861—867.

Mousavi, S.H., Tavakkol-Afshari, J., Brook, A., Jafari-Anarkooli, I., 2009. Role of caspases and Bax protein in saffron-induced apoptosis in MCF-7 cells. Food Chem. Toxicol. 47 (8), 1909—1913.

Mousavi, S.H., Moallem, S.A., Mehri, S., et al., 2011. Improvement of cytotoxic and apoptogenic properties of crocin in cancer cell lines by its nanoliposomal form. Pharm. Biol. 49, 1039—1045.

Nabavizadeh, F., Salimi, E., Sadroleslami, Z., Karimian, S.M., Vahedian, J., 2009. Saffron (Crocus sativus) increases gastric acid and pepsin secretions in rats: role of nitric oxide (NO). Afr.J Pharm.Pharmacol. 3 (5), 181—184.

Naghizadeh, B., Mansouri, S.M., Mashhadian, N.V., 2010. Crocin attenuates cisplatin-induced renal oxidative stress in rats. Food Chem. Toxicol. 48, 2650—2655.

Nair, S.C., Pannikar, B., Panikkar, K.R., 1991. Antitumour activity of saffron (Crocus sativus). Cancer Lett. 57 (2), 109—114.

Nair, S.C., Salomi, M.J., Varghese, C.D., Panikkar, B., Panikkar, K.R., 1992. Effect of saffron on thymocyte proliferation, intracellular glutathione levels and its antitumour activity. Biofactors 4, 51—54.

Nair, S.C., Panikkar, K.R., Parathod, R.K., 1993. Protective effects of crocetin on bladder cytotoxicity induced by cyclophosphamide. Cancer Biother. 8, 339—343.

Nair, S.C., Kurumboor, S.K., Hasegawa, J.H., 1995. Saffron chemoprevention in biology and medicine, a review. Cancer Biother. 10, 257—264.

Nam, K.N., Young, -M.P., Hoon-, J.J., Jung, Y.L., Byung, D.M., Seong-U, P., 2010. Anti- inflammatory effects of crocin and crocetin in rat brain microglial cells. Eur. J. Pharmacol. 648, 110—116.

Nicholls, J.R., 1945. Aid to the Analysis of Food and Drugs, sixth ed. Bailliere, Tindall and Cox, London, p. 195.

Noureini, S.K., Wink, M., 2012. Antiproliferative effects ofcrocin in HepG2 cells by telomerase inhibition and hTERTdown-regulation. Asian Pac. J. Cancer Prev 13 (5), 2305—2309.

Ozaki, A., Kitano, M., Furusawa, N., Yamaguchi, H., Kuroda, K., Endo, G., 2002. Genotoxicity of gardenia yellow and its components. Food Chem. Toxicol. 40, 1603—1610.

Pandey, G., Madhuri, S., 2006. Medicinal plants: better remedy for neoplasm. Indian Drugs 43, 869—874.

Petard, J.J., Guille, J., Lobel, B., Abbou, C.C., Cheopin, D., 1998. Current state of knowledge concerning the mechanism of action of BCG. Prog. Urol. 8, 415—421.

Pfander, H., Witter, F., 1975. Carotenoid glycosides. 2. Carotenoid content of safran. Helv. Chim. Acta. 58, 1608—1620.

Pham, T.Q., Cormier, F., Farnworth, E., Tong, V.H., Van Calsteren, M.R., 2001. Antioxidant properties of crocin from Gardenia jasminoides Ellis and study of the reactions of crocin with linoleic acid and crocin with oxygen. J. Agric. Food Chem. 48, 1455–1461.

Pitsikas, N., Boultadakis, A., Georgiadou, G., Tarantilis, P.A., Sakellaridis, N., 2008. Effects of the active constituents of Crocus sativus L., crocins, in an animal model of anxiety. Phytomedicine 15, 1135–1139.

Premkumar, K., Abraham, S.K., Santhiya, S.T., et al., 2001. Inhibition of genotoxicity by saffron (Crocus sativus L.) in mice. Drug Chem. Toxicol. 24, 421–428.

Ramadan, A., Soliman, G., Mahmoud, S.S., Nofal, S.M., Abdel-Rahman, R.F., 2010. Evaluation of the safety and antioxidant activities of Crocu sativus and Propolis ethanolic extracts. J. Saudi Chem. Soc. (in press).

Rao, K.V.K., Schwartz, S.A., Nair, H.K., Aalinkeel, R., Mahajan, S., Chawda, R., Nair, M.P.N., 2004. Plant derived products as a source of cellular growth inhibitory phytochemicals on PC-3M, DU-145 and LNCaP prostate cancer cell lines. Curr. Sci. 87, 1585–1588.

Rios, J.L., Recio, M.C., Giner, R.M., Manez, S., 1996. A update review of saffron and its active constituents. Phytother Res. 10, 189–193.

Robinson, A., 1995. Notes on the saffron plant (Crocus sativus L.). Pharm. Hist. 25, 2–3.

Rocha, A.B., Lopes, R.M., Schwartsmann, G., 2001. Natural products in anticancer therapy. Curr. Opin. Pharmacol. 1, 364–369.

Rosangkima, G., Prasad, S.B., 2004. Antitumour activity of some plants fromMeghalaya and Mizoram against murine ascites Dolton's lymphoma. Indian J. Exp. Biol. 42, 981–988.

Ruskin, A., Ribnicky, D.M., Komarnytsky, S., Ilic, N., Poulev, A., Borisjuk, N., Brinker, A., Moreno, D.A., Ripoll, C., Yakoby, N., O'Neal, J.M., Cornwell, T., Pastor, I., Fridlender, B., 2002. Plants and human health in the twenty-first century. Trends Biotechnol. 20, 522–531.

Sampathu, S.R., Shivashankar, S., Lewis, Y.S., 1984. Saffron (Crocus sativus Linn.)— cultivation, processing, chemistry and standardization. CRC Crit. Rev. Food Sci. Nutr. 20, 123–157.

Sastry, L.V.L., Srinivasan, M., Subrahmanyan, V., 1955. Saffron (Crocus sativus linn.). Sci. Ind. Res. (14-A), 178–184. India.

Schmidt, M., Betti, G., Hensel, A., 2007. Saffron in phytotherapy: pharmacology and clinical uses. Wien. Med. Wochenschr. 157 (13–14), 315–319.

Siracusa, L., Gresta, F., Avola, G., Lombardo, G.M., Ruberto, G., 2010. Influence of corm provenance and environmental condition on yield and apocarotenoid profiles in saffron (Crocus sativus L.). J. Food Compos. Anal. 23, 394–400.

Sivalokanathan, S., Ilayaraja, M., Balasubramanium, M.P., 2005. Efficacy of Terminalia arjuna (Roxb.) on N-nitrosodiethylamine induced hepatocellular carcinoma in rats. Indian J. Exp. Biol. 43, 264–267.

Skrubis, B., 1990. The cultivation in Greece of Crocus sativus L. In: Tammaro, F., Marra, L. (Eds.), Lo Zafferano. Proc. Internat. Conf. On Saffron, L'Aquila, Italy. Università Della Studi L'Aquila e Accademia Italiana delli Cucina, L'Aquila, pp. 171–182.

Smith, T.A.D., 1998. Carotenoids and cancer: prevention and potential therapy. Br. J. Biomed. Sci. 55 (4), 268–275.

Soeda, S., Ochiai, T., Paopong, L., Tanaka, H., Shoyama, Y., Shimeno, H., 2001. Crocin suppresses tumour necrosis factor-alpha-induced cell death of neuronally differentiated PC12 cells. Life Sci. 69, 2887–2898.

Somkumar, A.P., 2003. Studies on Anticancer Effects of Ocimum sanctum and Withania somnifera on Experimentally Induced Cancer in Mice (Ph.D. thesis), J. N. K. V. V., Jabalpur.

Souret, F.F., Weathers, P.J., 1999. Cultivation, in vitro culture, secondary metabolite production, and phytopharmacognosy of saffron (Crocus sativus L.). J. Herbs, Spices, Med. Plants 6, 99–116.

Sporn, M.B., 1976. Approaches to prevention of epithelial cancer during thepreneoplastic period. Cancer Res. 36, 2699–2702.

Stecher, P.G. (Ed.), 1968. The Merck Index, eighth ed. Merck & Co., Inc., Rahway, NJ. 928, 831.

Sun, J., Xu, X., Ni, C., et al., 2011. Crocin inhibits proliferation and nucleic acid synthesis and induces apoptosis in the human tongue squamous cell carcinoma cell line Tca8113. Asian Pac. J. Cancer Prev 12, 2679–2683.

Tarantilis, P.A., Morjani, H., Polissiou, M., Manfait, M., 1994a. Inhibition of growth and induction of differentiation promyelocytic leukemia (HL- 60) by carotenoids from Crocus sativus L. Anticancer Res. 14 (5A), 1913–1918.

Tarantilis, P.A., Polissiou, M., Manfait, M., 1994b. Separation of picrocrocin, cistranscrocins and safranal of saffron using high-performance liquid chromatography with photodiode-array detection. J. Chromatogr. A 664 (1), 55–61.

Triebold, H.O., Aurand, L.W., 1963. Food Composition and Analysis. Van Nostrand Company, Inc., Princeton, NJ, p. 463.

Tseng, T.H., Chu, C.Y., Huang, J.M., Shiow, S.J., Wang, C.J., 1995. Crocetin protects against oxidative damage in rat primary hepatocytes. Cancer Lett. 97 (1), 61–67.

Unni, K.M.C., Kuttan, R., 1990. Tumour reducing and anticarcinogenic activity of selected spices. Cancer Lett. 51, 85–89.

Verma, S.K., Bordia, A., 1998. Antioxidant property of saffron in man. Indian J. Med. Sci. 52 (5), 205–207.

Walsh, C.T., Zydowasky, L.D., MC-keom, 1992. Cyclosporine A , the cyclopin class of peptidylpropyl isomerase, the blockade of the Tcell induction. J. Biol. Chem. 267, 1315–1318.

Xu, G.L., Li, G., Ma, H.P., Zhong, H., Liu, F., Ao, G.Z., 2009. Preventive effect of crocin in inflamed animals and in LPS-challenged RAW 264.7 cells. J. Agric. Food Chem. 57 (18), 8325–8330.

Xuan, L., Tanaka, H., Xu, Y., Shoyama, Y., 1999. Preparation of monoclonal ;antibody with linoleic acid and crocin with oxygen. J. Agric. Food Chem. 48, 1455–1461.

Yamamoto, K., 1996. Elimination of minimal residual leukemic cells by biological response modifiers. Rinsho Ketsueki 37, 666–670.

Yang, B., Guo, Z., Lui, P., 2005. Crocin synthesis mechanism in crocus sativus. Tsinghua Sci. Technol. 8 (20), 567–572.

Yang, W., Ting, H., Yu, Z., Chang, J.Z., Qian, L.M., Khalid, R., Luping, Q., 2010. Antidepressant properties of bioactive fraction from the extract of Crocus sativus. J. Nat. Med. 64, 24–30.

Zechmeister, L., 1962. Cis-trans Isomeric Carotenoids Vitamins A and Arylpolyenes, vol. 3. Springer-Verlag, Vienna, pp. 102–114.

FURTHER READING

Abdullaev, F.I., 1994. Inhibitory effect of crocetin on intracellular nucleic acid and protein synthesis in malignant cells. Toxicol. Lett. 70, 243–251.

Abdullaev, F.I., 2001. Plant-derived agents against cancer. In: Gupta, S.K. (Ed.), Pharmacology and Therapeutics in the New Millennium. Narosa Publishing House, New Delhi, India, pp. 345–354.

Abdullaev, F.I., Gonzalez de Mejia, E., 1995/1996. Inhibition of colony formation of Hela cells by naturally occurring and synthetic agents. Biofactors 5 (3), 133–138.

Aggarwal, B.B., Takada, Y., Oommen, O.V., 2004. From chemoprevention tochemotherapy: common targets and common goals. Expert Opin. Investig. Drugs 13, 1327–1338.

American Cancer Society, 1999. Facts and Figures. National Cancer Institute.

American Cancer Society, 2006. A Biotechnology Company Dedicated to Cancer Treatment, Viewed on 25 January.

Bagchi, D., Preuss, H., 2005. Phytopharmaceuticals in Cancer Chemoprevention. CRC Press, Boca Raton.

Bajaj, S., Ahmad, I., Fatima, M., Raisuddin, S., Vohora, S.B., 1999. Immunomodulatory activity of a Unani gold preparation used in Indian system of medicine. Immunopharmacol. Immunotoxicol. 21, 151–161.

Bakshi Hamid, A., Trak, T., Fassal, G., Naseer, A., 2012. Crocus sativus L. Prevents progression of cell growth and enhances cell toxicity in human breast cancer and Lung cancer cell lines. Int. J. Inst. Pharm. Life Sci. 2 (2), 120–124.

Bakshi Hamid, A., Faruck, L.H., Sam, S., Javid, F., 2018. Dietary crocin reverses melanoma metastasis. J. Biomed. Res. 32 (1), 39–50.

Brandt, H.D., Osuch, E., Mathibe, L., Tsipa, P., 1995. Plants associated with accidental poisoned patients presenting at Ga-Rankuwa Hospital, Pretoria. S. Afr. J. Sci. 91, 57–59.

Cheesbrough, M., 1988. District Laboratory Practice in Tropical Countries, Part 1. Cambridge University press; ICSH: International Committee for Standardization in Haematology. Haematological Tests, Cambridge, UK, pp. 282–298.

Chen, C., Kong, A.N., 2005. Dietary cancer-chemopreventive compounds: from signaling and gene expression to pharmacological effects. Trends Pharmacol. Sci. 26, 318–326.

Chen, C.C., Hsu, J.D., Wang, S.F., Chiang, H.C., Yang, M.Y., Kao, E.S., Ho, Y.C., Wang, C.J., 2003. Hibiscus sabdariffa extract inhibits the development of atherosclerosis in cholesterolfed rabbits. J. Agric. Food Chem. 51 (18), 5472–5477.

Conney, A.H., 2003. Enzyme induction and dietary chemicals as approaches to cancer chemoprevention: the seventh DeWitt S. Goodman lecture. Cancer Res. 63, 7005–7031.

Dorai, T., Aggarwal, B.B., 2004. Role of chemopreventive agents in cancer therapy. Cancer Lett. 215, 129–140.

Feizzdeh, B., Tavakkol Afshari, J., Rakhshandeh, H., Rahimi, A., Brook, A., Doosti, H., 2008. Cytotoxic effect of Saffron stigma aqueous extract on human transitional cell carcinoma and mouse fibroblast. Urol. J. 5, 161–167.

Freshney, R.I., 1987. Culture of Animal Cells: A Manual of Basic Techniques. Wiley-Liss.

Friebolin, H., 1998. Basic -One and Two-Dimensional NMR Spectroscopy, third ed. (New York).

Gerster, H., 1993. Anticarcinogenic effect of common carotenoids. Int. Nutr. Res. 63, 92–121.

Giaccio, M., 2004. Crocetin from saffron: an active component of an ancient spice. Crit. Rev. Food Sci. Nutr. 44 (3), 155–172.

Guzman, M., 2003. Cannabinoids: potential anticancer agents. Nat. Rev. Cancer 3, 745–755.

Harborne, J.B., 1984. Phytochemical Methods: A Guide to Modern Techniques of Plant Analysis. Chapman and Hall, London, UK.

Hariri, A.T., Moallem, S.A., Mahmoudi, M., Hosseinzadeh, H., 2011. The effect of crocin and safranal, constituents of saffron, against subacute effect of diazinon on hematological and genotoxicity indices in rats. Phytomedicine 18 (6), 499–504.

Hosseinzadeh, H., Noraei, N.B., 2009. Anxiolytic and hypnotic effect of Crocus Sativus aqueous extract and its constituents, crocin and safranal, in mice. Phytother Res. 23 (6), 768–774.

Hosseinzadeh, H., Ziaee, T., Sadeghi, A., 2008. The effect of saffron, Crocus Sativus stigma, extract and its constituents, safranal and crocin on sexual behaviors innormal male rats. Phytomedicine 15, 491–495.

International Standards Organization, 1970. Saffron, 3rd Draft proposal.ISO/TC 34/SC 7, 215E. Geneva.

Kanakis, C.D., Tarantilis, P.A., Pappas, C., Bariyanga, J., Tajmir-Riahi, H.A., Polissiou, M.G., 2009. An overview of structural features of DNA and RNA complexes with saffron compounds: Models and antioxidant activity. J. Photochem. Photobiol. B 95, 204–212.

Kasatsune, H., Umigai, N., Takeno, R., Kajimoto, Y., Nakono, T., 2010. Effect of crocetin from gardenia jasminoides Ellis on sleep : a pilot study. Phytomedicine 17, 840–843.

Lee, B.M., Park, K.K., 2003. Beneficial and adverse effects of chemopreventive agents. Mutat. Res. 523 (524), 265–78.

Lippmann, S.M., Lotan, R., 2000. Advances in the development of retinoids as chemopreventive agents. J. Nutr. 130 (2S), 479–482.

Magesh, V., Vijeya Singh, J.P., Selvendiran, K., Ekambaram, G., Sakthisekaran, D., 2006. Antitumour activity of crocetin inaccordance to tumor incidence, antioxidant status, drug metabolizing enzymes and histopathological studies. Mol. Cell. Biochem. 287 (1–2), 127–135.

Morini, P., Betta, C.E., 1991. The response of rat liver lipid peroxidation, antioxidant enzyme activities and glutathione concentration to the thyroid hormone. Int. J. Biochem. 23, 1025–1030.

Mosmann, T., 1983. Rapid colorimetric assay for cellular growth and survival: application to proliferation and cytotoxicity assays. J. Immunol. Methods 65, 55–63.

Nair, S.C., Varghese, C.D., Pannikar, K.R., Kurumboor, S.K., Parathod, R.K., 1994. Effects of saffron in vitamin A levels and its antitumour activity on the growth of solid timors in mice. Int. J. Pharmacogn. 32, 105–114.

Pfander, H., Wittwer, F., 1975. Untersuchungen zur Carotinoid Zusammensetzung im Saffran II. Helv. Chim. Acta 58, 1608–1620.

Rock, C.L., 1997. Carotenoids: biology and treatment. Pharmacol. Ther. 75, 185–197.

Sanchez-Moreno, C., Larrauri, J.A., Saura-Calixto, F., 1998. A procedure to measure the antiradical efficiency of polyphenols. J. Sci. Food Agric. 76, 270–276.

Shmsa, A., Hossein, H., Mahmood, M., Mohamed, T.S., Omid, R., 2009. Evauation of *Crocus sativus* (Saffron) on male erectile dysfunction: a Pilot study. Phytomedicine 16, 690–693.

Skeham, P., Storeng, D., Scudiero, D., Monks, A., McMahon, D., et al., 1990. The new colorimetric cytotoxicity assay for anticancer-drug screening. J. Natl. Cancer Inst. 82, 11071112.

Thornberry, N.A., Lazebnik, Y., 1998. Caspases: enemies within. Science 281, 1312–1316.

Velasco, M., Díaz-Guerra, M.J.M., Díaz-Achirica, P., Andreu, D., Rivas, L., Bosca, L., 1997. Macrophagetriggering with cecropin A and melittin-derived peptides induces type II nitricoxide synthase expression. J. Immunol. 158, 4437–4443.

Vrinda, B., 2002. Preclinical Studies on the Radio & Chemoprotective Potential of the Ocimum Flavonoids. A thesis supplemented to the Manipal Academy of Higher Education.. 29-35 & 76-84.

Winterhalter, P., Straubinger, M., 2000. Saffron-renewed interest in an ancient spice. Food Rev. Int. 16, 39–59.

CHAPTER 20

Role of *Crocus sativus* L. in the Modern Green Anticancer Approach

RUQAYA JABEEN • MIR AJAZ AKRAM • MUZAFAR AHMAD SHEIKH

INTRODUCTION

Cancer has emerged as an alarming causal agent of deaths around the world. There have been reports of around 8 million people being diagnosed with cancer every year. Since time immemorial, herbal plants have been in use almost in all cultures worldwide as a traditional medicine (Shultes, 1978; Abdullaev and Espinosa-Aguirre, 2004). Currently, chemoprevention strategies have earned a huge reputation as a prospective approach to cancer control (Abdullaev and Espinosa-Aguirre, 2004). Saffron (*Crocus sativus* L.) belongs to the Iridaceae family and is cultivated in Europe, Central Asia, Iran, Algeria, Turkey, India, and China (Javadi et al., 2013) (Table 20.1).

The most important constituents of saffron are crocin, crocetin, picrocrocin, and safranal, as well as many nonvolatile constituents, mainly consisting of carotenoids (Ferna'ndez, 2006). In addition to taste enhancement, saffron exhibits many health benefits such as antioxidant, antiinflammatory, antimutagen, antigenotoxic, chemopreventive, and tumoricidal activity (Abdullaev and Espinosa-Aguirre, 2004).

The aim of this review is to investigate and report the anticancer activity of saffron (*C. sativus* L.) and its principal ingredients.

CHEMICAL COMPOSITION OF SAFFRON

Since ancient times, Saffron has been extensively served as a herbal drug, spice, as well as for coloring and flavoring purposes (Jawadi et al., 2013). More than 150 components have been discovered in the chemical analysis of saffron stigmas, crocin, crocetin, and safranal being the most significant of them all. Research done on animals as well as on cultured human cancer cell lines has shown promising antitumor as well as cancer preventive properties in saffron and its main constituents (Samarghandian et al., 2014). Saffron comprises

around 10% moisture, 12% protein, 5% fat, 5% minerals, 5% crude fiber, and 63% sugars (% w/w) in addition to the trace amounts of riboflavin and thiamine vitamins (Rios et al., 1996). Crocin is 8,8-diapocarotene-8,8-dioic acid, and is the most effective anticancerous constituent among the three main chemical constituents of saffron stigma (Hoshyar et al., 2016). Crocin, can effectively stall the spread of cancer cells, and its extended use can destroy the cancer cells (Bolhassani et al., 2014). García-Olmo et al. (1999), in his research, found that crocin is effective in prolonging the longevity of female mice inflicted with colon adenocarcinoma as well as stop the growth of tumor. Gutheil et al. (2012) claimed that crocetin has exhibited a promising potential as an anticancerous agent in animals as well as the cell culture systems that the authors attributed to the inhibition of nucleic acid synthesis, enhancement in antioxidative system and induction of apoptosis as well as hindrance in growth factor signaling pathways. Safranal is an organic compound isolated from saffron, which is mainly accountable for the aroma in saffron. Samarghandian et al. (2014) found that safranal exerts activity against proliferation of N2A cells by arresting cells in the G1 phase of cell cycle and causing apoptosis.

CHEMOPREVENTION

Cancer chemoprevention involves using various chemicals to interfere in the early stages of the disease facilitating the reversal or suppression of tumor formation (Das et al., 2010). Cancer in the past few decades has been impacting the quality and expectancy of human life. The various substances found in herbs, vegetables, and some spices could prove to be an alternative approach in the cancer prevention or its treatment. *Crocus sativus* has been widely used in traditional medicine for treatment of various diseases since

Saffron. https://doi.org/10.1016/B978-0-12-818462-2.00020-6

TABLE 20.1
Anticancerous Studies of Saffron Components on Various Types of Cancers.

Type of Cancer	Study	Results
Gastric cancer	Bathaie et al. (2013a); Bathaie et al., (2013b); Zhou et al. (2019)	SAE treatment restrained the spread of gastric cancer. An MTT assay demonstrated significant dose- and time-dependent restraint of AGS cell proliferation. Crocin inhibits the EMT, migration, and invasion of gastric cancer cells.
Hepatic cancer	Parizadeh et al. (2011); Amin et al. (2011); Amin et al. (2016)	Gradual decrease in hepatic cancerous cells with the increase in saffron concentration. Notably reduced the increased frequency and the occurrence of hepatic dyschromatic nodules. Crocin decreases the amount as well as the spread of placental glutathione-S-transferase-positive foci in the liver of rats.
Breast cancer	Chryssanthi et al. (2007); Modaghegh et al., (2008); (Jemal et al., 2003)	The crocetin from *Crocus sativus* prevents the propagation of MDA-MB-231 and MCF-7 breast cancer cells. The *Crocus sativus* style extract prevented the multiplication cancer cells of the breast. *trans*-Crocin-4 significantly prevented the proliferation of the breast cancer cells at concentrations greater than 200 mg.
Ovarian cancer	Neyshaburinezhad et al. (2018)	Crocin might have a role in the suppression of drug resistance in the human ovarian cancer-resistant cell line through the downregulation of MRP transporters.
Skin cancer	Konoshima et al. (1998); Wang et al. (2018)	Crocin and crocetin derivatives suppress the spread of skin cancer in mice. Saffron can suppress the propagation of skin cancer cells, A431 and SCL-1
Lung cancer	Samarghandian et al. (2010); Liu et al. (2014); Magesh et al. (2006); Chen et al. (2015)	Ethanolic extract of saffron imparts proapoptotic effects in a lung cancer-derived cell line, thereby showing a promise as a possible chemotherapeutic agent against lung cancer. There was a decrease in xenograft tumor size using the saffron extracts at the concentration of 100 mg/kg/d at a stretch for 28 days. Crocetin intensely brought a reversal to the pathological changes shown by cancerous animals. Crocin caused a significant decrease in the propagation of human lung cancer cells.

ages in addition to its tremendous cancer chemoprevention potential. In different examinations, researchers have found that saffron possesses a remarkable capacity to slow down the cancer growth (Dhar et al., 2009). Saffron's anticancerous properties incorporate restraining the tumor advancement as well as avoiding synthetic changes to DNA that can actuate cancer genes or prompt fresh cancerous mutations (Aung et al., 2007 and Gutheil et al., 2012).

GASTRIC CANCER

Gastric cancer (GC) occupies the fourth position in the list of most widespread malignancies and is the second principal cause of cancer-linked death worldwide especially in the East Asian countries (Matysiak-Bundnik et al., 2006; Macdonald et al., 2006; Jemal et al., 2011). Gastric cancers are most often discovered in advanced stages, as respectable GC prognosis is poor and it is often diagnosed in advanced or metastatic stages; therefore, its treatment remains a great challenge. The conventional remedial approaches for stomach cancer treatment include surgical procedure, radiotherapy, and chemotherapy. In spite of the developing treatment methods for cancer patients, their worth is time constrained and noncurative. Subsequently, to conquer these disadvantages, an unremitting screening for superior and more secure drugs has been continuous for various decades, bringing about the discovery of anticancer potential of a few phytochemicals. Chemoprevention utilizing promptly accessible primal substances from vegetables, spices, fruits, as well as herbs is one of the vital approaches for cancer remedial action in the current era. Saffron, a spice as well as food coloring agent found in the stigmas of saffron, is utilized as home medication to cure various diseases that includes cancer by primeval Arabian, Indian, as well as Chinese civilizations. Various in vivo and in vitro studies have been carried out to validate the therapeutic potential of saffron, especially for treatment of gastric cancer. Bathaie et al. (2013a) explored the protective potential of saffron aqueous extract (SAE) on 1-methyl-3-nitro-1-nitrosoguanidine-induced gastric cancer in albino rats. Their study revealed that SAE administration restrained the progression in the gastric cancer as supported by the pathologic examination; 20% of the rats with cancer supplemented with elevated doses of SAE (175 mg/kg) were absolutely normal by the end of the experimentation, and no rat was found with the adenoma among the SAE-supplemented groups. Additionally, the domino effect of the flow cytometry and propidium iodide staining demonstrated that the ratio of the apoptosis and proliferation was augmented because of the SAE treatment in the cancerous rats. Furthermore, no evidence of metastasis and invasion was observed during necropsy. Thus, the researchers recommended saffron as a potent anticancer herb.

In the research done by Bathaie et al. (2013b), the restorative impact of crocetin on the gastric adenocarcinoma cells and 1-methyl-3-nitro-1-nitrosoguanidine-prompted stomach cancer in rats was explored. The MTT assay demonstrated a considerable restraint of AGS cell propagation owing to crocetin treatment. The flow cytometry and the assay of activity of caspases affirm that the apoptosis had got provoked in particular cells; Western blot as well as RT-PCR examination

uncovered the repression of the Bcl-2 as well as the increase in the Bax expression in the AGS cells supplemented with crocetin. Such types of alterations were not noticed in the normal human fibroblast (HFSF-PI3) cells. The pathological examination done on the tumorous tissue in MNNG (N-methyl-N'-nitro-N-nitrosoguanidine)-prompted stomach cancer in rats demonstrated an inhibition in the tumor progression. Besides this, crocetin showed restorative potential and prevented changes in the biochemical parameters like the antioxidant activity of the serum and the lactate dehydrogenase activity in rats. This investigation exhibits cell reinforcement, hostile to proliferative, and apoptotic exercises of crocetin against gastric cancer that may profit human stomach cancer treatment. This study clearly demonstrated the antioxidant and apoptotic potential of crocetin in treating the stomach cancer. Zhou et al. (2019) in his study found that crocin inhibits the EMT, migration, and invasion of gastric cancer cells.

HEPATIC CANCER

Hepatic cancer is one of the major cancers on the earth. Disappointingly, liver cancer is the third most cause of cancer-related deaths globally. Epidemiological studies have highlighted the reality of an inverse association between the consumption of herbs, vegetables, fruits, spices, and cancer risk. A number of in vivo and in vitro experiments discussed later clearly revealed that saffron and its main constituents encompass the potential to prevent and cure liver cancer. In the study undertaken by Parizadeh et al. (2011), the result of crocus aqueous extract on the production of nitric oxide (NO) by the hepatic cancer cell line (HepG-2) as well as the laryngeal cancer cell line (Hep-2) was explored. Both cell lines were treated with aqueous saffron extract; cell viability and measurable variations in the production of nitric oxide were assessed by the Griess test. The MTT assay clearly demonstrated a gradual decrease in cancerous cells with the increase in the crocus dose while in the Griess test, the elevation in the levels of saffron extract resulted in the gradual decrease in the amount of nitric oxide generated in the cancer cells. This clearly validates the cytotoxic effect of saffron on HepG2 and Hep-2 cell lines. Furthermore, the cytotoxic effect of saffron was doubtlessly credited to its potential ability to reduce NO concentration.

Amin et al. (2011) evaluated the efficacy of the crocus extract on the diethylnitrosamine-caused hepatic cancer in rats. Ethanolic extract of *Crocus sativus* notably reduced the increased count as well as the occurrence of liver dyschromatic nodules. In addition, saffron decreased the number and the outreach of glutathione-S-transferase (GST-p) in liver of diethylnitrosamine-treated rats. Furthermore, saffron neutralized diethylnitrosamine-caused oxidative stress in experimental animals through the restoration of the altered levels of endogenous antioxidants such as superoxide dismutase, catalase, and glutathione-S-transferase, and diminished the activity of myeloperoxidase, malondialdehyde, and protein carbonyl formation in liver tissue. This study provides exclusive confirmation about the chemopreventive potential of saffron against liver cancer through inhibition of cell proliferation, modulating oxidative damage, suppressing inflammatory response, and induction of apoptosis.

Crocin, a major constituent of *Crocus sativus* L., exerts a significant chemopreventive effect against diethylnitrosamine (DEN)-induced hepatic cancer through its antiproliferative, proapoptotic, and inflammatory properties. Crocin also decreases the amount and the outreach of the placental glutathione-S-transferase-positive foci in the livers of DEN-supplemented rats. In vitro studies done on (HepG2) hepatic cell line showed curative potential of crocin through the inhibition of cell proliferation, modulating oxidative damage, induction of apoptosis, and suppressing inflammatory responses by arresting the cell cycle at S and G2/M stages of cell cycle (Amin et al., 2016).

BREAST CANCER

Breast cancer accounts for around one-third of the cancerous occurring in women, worldwide. Epidemiological research has advocated that overindulgence in carotenoids might offer protection from the incidence of the breast cancer (Sato et al., 2002). The crocetin from *Crocus sativus* prevents the spread of breast cancer MDA-MB-231 as well as MCF-7 cells in the media having 10% serum. The efficacy was very prominent in the MCF-7 cells; whereas, the resultant effect was eloquent at the levels more than 200 μM in MDA-MB-231 cells (Chryssanthi et al., 2007).

The incubation of the breast cancer cells, MDA-MB-231 together with substantial treatment of crocetin (1 and 10 μM) in the serum-free situation, causes a vital decline in the propagation and presumptuousness of breast cancer cells. This disagreement of results may be justified by the phenomenon that with the presence of sera, the proliferation of the cells is aroused indicting that the preventive effect of crocetin is apparent at elevated concentrations. These results also advocated that crocetin is by no means cytotoxic when given in normal concentrations, which is endorsed by the fact that the consumption of saffron (200 and 400 mg) is considered secure for the consumption of humans (Modaghegh et al., 2008). The *Crocus sativus* style extract prevented the multiplication of cancer cells in the breast. It was observed that IC$_{50}$ values in Crocus *sativus* were 350 and 500 Ìg/mL, respectively, for MCF-7 and MDA-MB-231. In the aim of exploring the constituents responsible for the said action, the efficacy of *trans*-crocin-4, crocetin, and safranal was investigated on propagation of the breast cancer cells. The findings clearly showed that safranal at the concentration higher than 125 significantly declined the spread of the MDA-MB-231 as well as MCF-7 at levels higher than 500. Similarly, *trans*-crocin-4 prevented the propagation of MCF-7 and MDA-MB-231 at levels greater than 200 mg (Jemal et al., 2003).

OVARIAN CANCER

The cancer of the ovaries is regarded to be the main fatal gynecologic malignancy. Around under a half of the affected women stay alive for 5 years or more after the disease is diagnosed. The efforts are being made for early detection and new therapeutic approaches to lessen mortality but have been mostly ineffective because the pathogenesis of epithelial ovarian cancer is scantily understood. Ovarian cancer often remains hidden until it extends to the pelvis and abdomen. Ovarian cancers affect women of all age groups, and the diagnosis surfaces usually after the menopause. The greatest risk factors are the increasing age as well as the family history of the incidences of ovarian cancer.

Until now, 90% of the ovarian cancers are carcinomas with epithelial ovarian carcinoma being the common, followed by the malignant germ cell tumors (3%) such as yolk sac tumors, immature teratomas, dysgerminomas, and rare stromal cell tumors (1%–2%). In the last decade, much research has recommended new herbs with potential anticancerous effects that have generated an optimism of expansion to safer anticancerous treatments (Hemalswarya et al., 2006). Saffron compounds like crocin has been studied to have shown promising results against various types of tumors including leukemia, ovarian, and breast carcinoma, colon adenocarcinoma, liver, pancreas, and lung cancer (Gutheil et al., 2012). Neyshaburinezhad et al. (2018) studied the efficacy of crocetin on the Multiple drug resistance (MDR) phenotype in the human ovarian carcinoma cell lines (A2780 and A2780-RCIS) and proposed its usage together with traditional chemotherapeutic drugs in treating ovarian cancer. Mahdizadeh et al. (2016) in his study on ovarian cancer opined that crocin could suppress drug resistance via down regulation of MRP transporters in the human ovarian cancer-resistant cell line.

SKIN CANCER

Skin cancer includes any malignant epidermal growth. UV radiations (A and B) are the causal agents of skin cancer. Basal cell carcinoma is the most widespread type of skin cancer in addition to melanoma as well as the carcinoma of the squamous cells. Skin cancer is growing up to be one of the prominent malignancies around the world, and the deaths due to skin cancers are increasing year by year. Currently, there is not much prevention and treatment of skin cancers like squamous cell carcinoma and malignant melanoma. Das et al. (2010) opined that the saffron is effective in the inhibition of cell proliferation in addition to the dysplasia, hyperplasia, as well as papilloma growth. Konoshima et al. (1998) found that the crocin and crocetin derivatives inhibit skin tumor promotion in mice. Wang et al. (2018), in his study, opined that the crocus extract has the ability to curtail the growth of skin cancer cells (A431 and SCL-1). The flow cytometry results further revealed that the crocin can also stimulate the apoptosis of the skin cancer cells to a considerable degree in a dose-dependent manner. The authors attributed the probable cause of apoptosis to the inhibition of the Jak2/Stat3 pathway, downregulation of the anti-apoptotic protein, Bcl-2 expression, and enhancement in the levels of proapoptotic protein Bid and procaspase-3.

LUNG CANCER

Worldwide, lung cancer is the most common form of cancer. Saffron has been used in folk medicine for centuries. In addition to being one of the most difficult cancers to cure, lung cancer also tends to relapse easily besides having a high incidence of recurrence (Li et al., 2004; Molina et al., 2006). Lung cancers are divided into two major histological groups including nonsmall cell lung cancer (85%) and small cell lung cancer (15%) (Samarghandian et al., 2013). Carcinomic human alveolar basal epithelial cell (A549) is the most common and widely studied cell line in lung cancer (Brognard et al., 2001). Samarghandian et al. (2010) found that the ethanolic extract of saffron resulted in decrease of cell proliferation in cancerous cells in a concentration and time-dependent behavior. They further concluded that saffron extract imparts proapoptotic effect in lung cancer-derived cell line thereby showing a potent chemotherapeutic promise against lung cancer. Li et al. (2014) studied the anticancerous effect and the possible mechanism of Zhejiang saffron against A549 and H446 cell lines of lung cancer. They found that with the saffron concentration of 100 mg/kg/d for the duration of 28 days, there was a decline in the size of the xenograft tumor. Magesh et al. (2006) studied the effects of crocetin against lung cancer-bearing mice in preinitiation and postinitiation periods and found that crocetin intensely brought a reversal to the pathological changes shown by cancerous animals. Chen et al. (2015) found that the crocin significantly suppressed the proliferation of human lung adenocarcinoma cells.

BIOTECHNOLOGICAL APPROACH TO SAFFRON PRODUCTION

Given the high evidence of saffron and its constituents as anticancerous agents, its scarcity and the huge cost of acquiring large quantities of these compounds may hinder prevention and treatment of cancer using saffron. Low multiplication rates in addition to the fungal infestation of corms are the biggest hurdles for availability of sufficient quality planting material (Yasmin et al., 2013). It is therefore necessary to increase the productivity per unit area so as to enhance the net returns to farmers and encourage the saffron cultivation. Biotechnological approaches like micropropagation of saffron with direct or indirect shoot induction as well as plantlet regeneration via somatic embryogenesis followed by microcorm production can help in producing huge quantities of disease-free propagating material in less time (Ahmad et al., 2014). In vegetatively growing plants like saffron, in vitro mutagenesis of tissue explant, which is followed by clonal propagation, could serve as important tool to enhance genetic variation in the base population as well as quick multiplication of mutant clones (Kashtwari et al., 2018).

Use of molecular markers as a tool for identification of variability among different saffron clones is a significant part of improvement of saffron through breeding (Mir et al., 2015). For breeding new cultivars of saffron with economically superior traits, the selection of superior clones in existing plantations as well as creation of new valuable forms through induced mutations is an important approach (Ali et al., 2013).

CONCLUSIONS

Research in the last decade on saffron plant has suggested a great potential in saffron with cytotoxic, antitumoral, chemopreventive, antimutagenic, and immunostimulating properties. Among these phytochemicals, crocins, crocetin, and safranal have been recommended as the most pharmacologically effective because they have effective cell growth regulation besides modulating gene expression in cancer cells. Until now, the studies done on animals showed that saffron as well as the main constituents present in it has huge anticancerous potential. The proper clinical trials need to be undertaken on humans to establish the saffron efficacy against cancer. Moreover, extensive research needs to be taken up to understand the underlying mechanism(s) involved in the anticancerous properties in the saffron and its constituents.

REFERENCES

Abdullaev, F.I., Espinosa-Aguirre, J.J., 2004. Biomedical properties of saffron and its potential use in cancer therapy and chemoprevention trials. Cancer Detect. Prev. 28 (6), 426–432.

Ahmad, M., Zaffar, G., Habib, M., Arshid, A., Dar, N.A., Dar, Z.A., 2014. Saffron (Crocus sativus L.) in the light of biotechnological approaches: a review. Sci. Res. Essays 9 (2), 13–18.

Ali, G., Iqbal, A.M., Nehvi, F.A., Samad, S.S., Nagoo, S., Naseer, S., Dar, N.A., 2013. Prospects of clonal selection for enhancing productivity in Saffron (Crocus sativus L.). Afr. J. Agric. Res. 8 (5), 460–467.

Amin, A., Hamza, A.A., Bajbouj, K., Ashraf, S.S., Daoud, S., 2011. Saffron: a potential candidate for a novel anticancer drug against hepatocellular carcinoma. Hepatology 54 (3), 857–867.

Amin, A., Hamza, A.A., Daoud, S., Khazanehdari, K., Al Hrout, A., Baig, B., Chaiboonchoe, A., Adrian, T.E., Zaki, N., Salehi-Ashtiani, K., 2016. Saffron-based crocin prevents early lesions of liver cancer: in vivo, in vitro & network analyses. Recent Pat. Anti-Cancer Drug Discov. 11, 121–133.

Aung, H.H., Wang, C.Z., Ni, M., Fishbein, A., Mehendale, S.R., Xie, J.T., Yuan, C.S., 2007. Crocin from Crocus sativus possesses significant anti-proliferation effects on human colorectal cancer cells. Exp. Oncol. 29 (3), 175.

Bathaie, S.Z., Miri, H., Mohagheghi, M.A., Mokhtari-Dizaji, M., Shahbazfar, A.A., Hasanzadeh, H., 2013a. Saffron aqueous extract inhibits the chemically-induced gastric cancer progression in the Wistar albino rat. Iranian J. Basic Med. Sci. 16 (1), 27.

Bathaie, S.Z., Hoshyar, R., Miri, H., Sadeghizadeh, M., 2013b. Anticancer effects of crocetin in both human adenocarcinoma gastric cancer cells and rat model of gastric cancer. Biochem. Cell Biol. 91 (6), 397–403.

Bolhassani, A., Khavari, A., Bathaie, S.Z., 2014. Saffron and natural carotenoids: biochemical activities and antitumor effects. Biochim. Biophys. Acta Rev. Canc. 1845 (1), 20–30.

Brognard, J., Clark, A.S., Ni, Y., Dennis, P.A., 2001. Akt/protein kinase B is constitutively active in non-small cell lung cancer cells and promotes cellular survival and resistance to chemotherapy and radiation. Cancer Res. 61 (10), 3986–3997.

Chen, S., Zhao, S., Wang, X., Zhang, L., Jiang, E., Gu, Y., Shangguan, A.J., Zhao, H., Tangfeng, L.,V., Yu, Z., 2015. Crocin inhibits cell proliferation and enhances cisplatin and pemetrexed chemosensitivity in lung cancer cells. Transl. Lung Cancer Res. 4 (6), 775.

Chryssanthi, D.G., Lamari, F.N., Iatrou, G., Pylara, A., Karamanos, N.K., Cordopatis, P., 2007. Inhibition of breast cancer cell proliferation by style constituents of different Crocus species. Anticancer Res. 27 (1A), 357–362.

Das, I., Das, S., Saha, T., 2010. Saffron suppresses oxidative stress in DMBA-induced skin carcinoma: a histopathological study. Acta Histochemica 112 (4), 317–327.

Dhar, A., Mehta, S., Dhar, G., Dhar, K., Banerjee, S., Van Veldhuizen, P., Banerjee, S.K., 2009. Crocetin inhibits pancreatic cancer cell proliferation and tumor progression in a xenograft mouse model. Mol. Cancer Ther. 8 (2), 315–323.

Fernández, J.A., 2006. Anticancer properties of saffron, Crocus sativus Linn. Advances in phytomedicine 2, 313–330.

Gutheil, W.G., Reed, G., Ray, A., Anant, S., Dhar, A., 2012. Crocetin: an agent derived from saffron for prevention and therapy for cancer. Curr. Pharmaceut. Biotechnol. 13 (1), 173–179.

Garc-Olmo, D.C., Riese, H.H., Escribano, J., Ontañon, J., Fernandez, J.A., Atiénzar, M., Garcí-Olmo, D., 1999. Effects of long-term treatment of colon adenocarcinoma with crocin, a carotenoid from saffron (Crocus sativus L.): an experimental study in the rat. Nutr. Cancer 35 (2), 120–126.

Hemalswarya, S., Doble, M., 2006. Potential synergism of natural products in the treatment of cancer. Phytother Res. 20 (4), 239–249.

Hoshyar, R., Mostafavinia, S.E., Bathaie, S.Z., 2016. Anticancer effects of saffron stigma (Crocus Sativus): a review study. Razi J. Med. Sci. 22 (140), 69–78.

Javadi, B., Sahebkar, A., Emami, S.A., 2013. A survey on saffron in major islamic traditional medicine books. Iranian J. Basic Med. Sci. 16 (1), 1.

Jemal, A., Siegel, R., Ward, E., 2003. i wsp. Cancer statistics. CA A Cancer J. Clin. 53, 5–26.

Jemal, A., Bray, F., Center, M.M., Ferlay, J., Ward, E., Forman, D., 2011. Global cancer statistics. CA A Cancer J. Clin. 61 (2), 69–90.

Kashtwari, M., Wani, A.A., Dhar, M.K., Jan, S., Kamili, A.N., 2018. Development of an efficient in vitro mutagenesis protocol for genetic improvement of saffron (Crocus sativus L.). Physiol. Mol. Biol. Plants 24 (5), 951–962.

Konoshima, T., Takasaki, M., Tokuda, H., Morimoto, S., Tanaka, H., Kawata, K.,E., Xuan, L.,J., Saito, H., Sugiura, M., Molnar, J., Shoyama, Y., 1998. Crocin and crocetin derivatives inhibit skin tumour promotion in mice. Phytother Res. 12 (6), 400–404.

Li, Q., Wei, Y.Q., Wen, Y.J., Zhao, X., Tian, L., Yang, L., Deng, H.X., 2004. Induction of apoptosis and tumor regression by vesicular stomatitis virus in the presence of gemcitabine in lung cancer. Int. J. Cancer 112 (1), 143–149.

Liu, D.D., Ye, Y.L., Zhang, J., Xu, J.N., Qian, X.D., Zhang, Q., 2014. Distinct pro-apoptotic properties of Zhejiang saffron against human lung cancer via a caspase-8-9-3 cascade. Asian Pac. J. Cancer Prev. 15 (15), 6075–6080.

Macdonald, J.S., 2006. Gastric cancer-new therapeutic options. N. Engl. J. Med. 355 (1), 76–77.

Magesh, V., Singh, J.P.V., Selvendiran, K., Ekambaram, G., Sakthisekaran, D., 2006. Antitumour activity of crocetin in accordance to tumor incidence, antioxidant status, drug metabolizing enzymes and histopathological studies. Mol. Cell. Biochem. 287 (1–2), 127–135.

Mahdizadeh, S., Karimi, G., Behravan, J., Arabzadeh, S., Lage, H., Kalalinia, F., 2016. Crocin suppresses multidrug resistance in MRP overexpressing ovarian cancer cell line. Daru 24 (1), 17.

Matysiak-Bundnik, Megraud, T., Helicobacter, F., 2006. Pylori infectionand gastric cancer. Eur. J. Cancer 42, 708–716.

Mir, J.I., Ahmed, N., Singh, D.B., Khan, M.H., Zaffer, S., Shafi, W., 2015. Breeding and biotechnological opportunities in saffron crop improvement. Afr. J. Agric. Res. 10 (9), 970–974.

Modaghegh, M.H., Shahabian, M., Esmaeili, H.A., Rajbai, O., Hosseinzadeh, H., 2008. Safety evaluation of saffron (*Crocus sativus*) tablets in healthy volunteers. Phytomedicine 15 (12), 1032–1037.

Molina, J.R., Adjei, A.A., Jett, J.R., 2006. Advances in chemotherapy of non-small cell lung cancer. Chest 130 (4), 1211–1219.

Parizadeh, M.R., Ghafoori Gharib, F., Abbaspour, A.R., Tavakol Afshar, J., Ghayour-Mobarhan, M., 2011. Effects of aqueous saffron extract on nitric oxide production by two human carcinoma cell lines: hepatocellular carcinoma (HepG2) and laryngeal carcinoma (Hep2). Avicenna Journal of Phytomedicine 1 (1), 43–50.

Rios, J.L., Recio, M.C., Giner, R.M., Manez, S., 1996. An update review of saffron and its active constituents. Phytother Res. 10 (3), 189–193.

Samarghandian, S., Borji, A., 2014. Anticarcinogenic effect of saffron (*Crocus sativus* L.) and its ingredients. Pharmacogn. Res. 6 (2), 99.

Samarghandian, S., Boskabady, M.H., Davoodi, S., 2010. Use of in vitro assays to assess the potential antiproliferative and cytotoxic effects of saffron (*Crocus sativus* L.) in human lung cancer cell line. Pharmacogn. Mag. 6 (24), 309.

Samarghandian, S., Borji, A., Farahmand, S.K., Afshari, R., Davoodi, S., 2013. *Crocus sativus* L.(saffron) stigma aqueous extract induces apoptosis in alveolar human lung cancer cells through caspase-dependent pathways activation. BioMed Res. Int. 2013.

Sato, R., Helzlsouer, K.J., Alberg, A.J., Hoffman, S.C., Norkus, E.P., Comstock, G.W., 2002. Prospective study of carotenoids, tocopherols, and retinol concentrations and the risk of breast cancer. Cancer Epidemiology and Prevention Biomarkers 11 (5), 451–457.

Shultes, R.E., 1978. The kingdom of plants. In: Thomson, W.A.R. (Ed.), Medicines from the Earth. McGraw-Hill Book Co., New York, NY, p. 208.

Wang, G., Zhang, B., Wang, Y., Han, S., Wang, C., 2018. Crocin promotes apoptosis of human skin cancer cells by inhibiting the JAK/STAT pathway. Exp. Ther. Med. 16 (6), 5079–5084.

Yasmin, S., Nehvi, F.A., 2013. Saffron as a valuable spice: A comprehensive review. African Journal of Agricultural Research 8 (3), 234–242.

Zhou, Y., Xu, Q., Shang, J., Lu, L., &Chen, G., 2019. Crocin inhibits the migration, invasion, and epithelial-mesenchymal transition of gastric cancer cells via miR-320/KLF5/HIF-1α signaling. J. Cell. Physiol. https://doi.org/10.1002/jcp.28418.

FURTHER READING

Faridi, N., Heidarzadeh, H., Mohagheghi, M.A., Bathaie, S.Z., 2019. Breast cancer cell apoptosis induced by crocin, a saffron carotenoid. Basic Clin. Cancer Res. 11 (1), 241–250.

Festuccia, C., Mancini, A., Gravina, G.L., Scarsella, L., Llorens, S., Alonso, G.L., D'Alessandro, A.M., 2014. Antitumor effects of saffron-derived carotenoids in prostate cancer cell models. BioMed Res. Int. 2014, 1-12.

Giaccio, M., 2004. Crocetin from saffron: an active component of an ancient spice. Crit. Rev. Food Sci. Nutr. 44 (3), 155–172.

Gupta, S.K. (Ed.), 2001. Pharmacology and Therapeutics in the New Millennium. Springer Science & Business Media.

Melnyk, J.P., Wang, S., Marcone, M.F., 2010. Chemical and biological properties of the world's most expensive spice: Saffron. Food Res. Int. 43 (8), 1981–1989.

Premkumar, K., Thirunavukkarasu, C., Abraham, S.K., Santhiya, S.T., Ramesh, A., 2006. Protective effect of saffron (*Crocus sativus* L.) aqueous extract against genetic damage induced by anti-tumor agents in mice. Hum. Exp. Toxicol. 25 (2), 79–84.

Index

Note: Page numbers followed by "f" indicate figures and "t" indicate tables.

Printed in the United States
By Bookmasters